Asses
Long-Term
Health Effects of
Antimalarial Drugs
When Used for
Prophylaxis

David A. Savitz and Anne N. Styka, *Editors*

Committee to Review Long-Term Health Effects of Antimalarial Drugs

Board on Population Health and Public Health Practice

Health and Medicine Division

A Consensus Study Report of

The National Academies of
SCIENCES · ENGINEERING · MEDICINE

THE NATIONAL ACADEMIES PRESS
Washington, DC
www.nap.edu

THE NATIONAL ACADEMIES PRESS   500 Fifth Street, NW   Washington, DC 20001

This activity was supported by Contract Order No. VA 36C24E18C0067 between the National Academy of Sciences and the Department of Veterans Affairs. Any opinions, findings, conclusions, or recommendations expressed in this publication do not necessarily reflect the views of any organization or agency that provided support for the project.

International Standard Book Number-13:   978-0-309-67210-8
International Standard Book Number-10:   0-309-67210-4
Digital Object Identifier: https://doi.org/10.17226/25688

Additional copies of this publication are available for sale from the National Academies Press, 500 Fifth Street, NW, Keck 360, Washington, DC 20001; (800) 624-6242 or (202) 334-3313; http://www.nap.edu.

Suggested citation: National Academies of Sciences, Engineering, and Medicine. 2020. *Assessment of long-term health effects of antimalarial drugs when used for prophylaxis.* Washington, DC: The National Academies Press. https://doi.org/10.17226/25688.

The National Academies of
SCIENCES · ENGINEERING · MEDICINE

The **National Academy of Sciences** was established in 1863 by an Act of Congress, signed by President Lincoln, as a private, nongovernmental institution to advise the nation on issues related to science and technology. Members are elected by their peers for outstanding contributions to research. Dr. Marcia McNutt is president.

The **National Academy of Engineering** was established in 1964 under the charter of the National Academy of Sciences to bring the practices of engineering to advising the nation. Members are elected by their peers for extraordinary contributions to engineering. Dr. John L. Anderson is president.

The **National Academy of Medicine** (formerly the Institute of Medicine) was established in 1970 under the charter of the National Academy of Sciences to advise the nation on medical and health issues. Members are elected by their peers for distinguished contributions to medicine and health. Dr. Victor J. Dzau is president.

The three Academies work together as the **National Academies of Sciences, Engineering, and Medicine** to provide independent, objective analysis and advice to the nation and conduct other activities to solve complex problems and inform public policy decisions. The National Academies also encourage education and research, recognize outstanding contributions to knowledge, and increase public understanding in matters of science, engineering, and medicine.

Learn more about the National Academies of Sciences, Engineering, and Medicine at **www.nationalacademies.org**.

The National Academies of
SCIENCES · ENGINEERING · MEDICINE

Consensus Study Reports published by the National Academies of Sciences, Engineering, and Medicine document the evidence-based consensus on the study's statement of task by an authoring committee of experts. Reports typically include findings, conclusions, and recommendations based on information gathered by the committee and the committee's deliberations. Each report has been subjected to a rigorous and independent peer-review process and it represents the position of the National Academies on the statement of task.

Proceedings published by the National Academies of Sciences, Engineering, and Medicine chronicle the presentations and discussions at a workshop, symposium, or other event convened by the National Academies. The statements and opinions contained in proceedings are those of the participants and are not endorsed by other participants, the planning committee, or the National Academies.

For information about other products and activities of the National Academies, please visit www.nationalacademies.org/about/whatwedo.

v

Reviewers

This Consensus Study Report was reviewed in draft form by individuals chosen for their diverse perspectives and technical expertise. The purpose of this independent review is to provide candid and critical comments that will assist the National Academies of Sciences, Engineering, and Medicine in making each published report as sound as possible and to ensure that it meets the institutional standards for quality, objectivity, evidence, and responsiveness to the study charge. The review comments and draft manuscript remain confidential to protect the integrity of the deliberative process.

We thank the following individuals for their review of this report:

Paul Ahlquist, University of Wisconsin–Madison
Lesley H. Curtis, Duke University
Susan Ellenberg, University of Pennsylvania School of Medicine
Joshua J. Gagne, Brigham and Women's Hospital
Tobias Gerhard, Rutgers, The State University of New Jersey
K. Malcom Maclure, University of British Columbia
Ann Mckee, Boston University School of Medicine
William P. Nash, Veterans Affairs Greater Los Angeles Healthcare
  System
Laurence Slutsker, PATH Malaria and NTD Program
David Sullivan, Johns Hopkins Bloomberg School of Public Health
Carol S. Wood, Oak Ridge National Laboratory

Although the reviewers listed above provided many constructive comments and suggestions, they were not asked to endorse the conclusions or recommendations of this report nor did they see the final draft before its release. The review of this report was overseen by **Tracy Lieu,** Kaiser Permanente, Northern California, and **Brian L. Strom,** Rutgers, The State University of New Jersey. They were responsible for making certain that an independent examination of this report was carried out in accordance with the standards of the National Academies and that all review comments were carefully considered. Responsibility for the final content rests entirely with the authoring committee and the National Academies.

Preface

The men and women who serve in the U.S. Armed Forces and who are deployed to distant locations around the world encounter myriad health threats. In addition to those associated with the potential for combat, exposure to harmful agents, and disruption of their family life, they may face disease threats that are specific to the locations to which they are sent. Prominent among these is malaria, a parasitic disease that is endemic to several locations where U.S. forces have been posted over the years, including in parts of Afghanistan and Iraq. The threat of malaria—a debilitating and potentially deadly illness—can be significantly mitigated through the use of antimalarial drugs for prevention. Such drugs have known side effects, however, and concerns over whether adverse events related to taking the drugs persist after administration is stopped are well justified. This is a challenging issue, given the diversity of antimalarial drugs used, the wide range of potential adverse events, and the numerous other health concerns that service members encounter following deployment.

While there are many questions that could be asked regarding the use of anti-malarial drugs for deployed personnel, the committee's charge was very specific: assemble, examine, and assess the research that contributes to an understanding of whether the use of antimalarial drugs may cause persistent or latent health problems. The committee was not asked to review patient reports or to make recommendations regarding the use of such drugs (as the Food and Drug Administration does) nor to provide guidelines for those traveling to malaria-endemic areas (as the Centers for Disease Control and Prevention does). Instead, the committee was charged with evaluating the available scientific and medical information, and it did not speculate or conjecture beyond that body of knowledge. It is thus important to note that a determination that the evidence was not sufficient to draw a conclusion regarding a particular drug–outcome association should not be interpreted as a determination that the drug does not cause adverse health effects: the lack of evidence of adverse effects is not evidence of a lack of adverse effects. The committee looked carefully and exhaustively at the evidence and in this report describes the process by which the information it considered was gathered and presents its summary and assessment of what that research can tell us.

The committee hopes that its work will help the Department of Veterans Affairs, the Department of Defense, and other agencies, such as the Peace Corps and the Department of State, that send teams and workers to serve in malaria-endemic areas to provide guidance to its health care providers—in particular, regarding specific questions and symptoms in persons who have used the drugs of interest for prophylaxis and who may have concerns about their long-term health.

It is clear that some proportion of those who were deployed and prescribed antimalarial drugs became ill. The committee received accounts from a number of those who had experienced such illnesses, some quite severe, and there can be no doubt that their health problems are real and that they followed their use of antimalarial drugs. We very much appreciate the courage and commitment of those who took the time to educate the committee based on their personal experience.

The committee also wishes to acknowledge the Department of Veterans Affairs, Department of Defense, Food and Drug Administration, Peace Corps, Centers for Disease Control and Prevention, and Department of State who made presentations to the committee and responded to follow-up questions. We are extremely appreciative of the outstanding efforts of the staff of the National Academies of Sciences, Engineering, and Medicine's Health and Medicine Division; Anne Styka, who served as study director; Stephanie Hanson and Kristin White, who had a daunting task of identifying and culling the large and complex literature and more generally guiding and assisting the committee in its mission. We also are grateful to Rebecca Chevat who generously and capably provided logistical support to the committee. Finally, the committee would like to acknowledge a number of other individuals who helped make this work possible: Daniel Bearss, a senior research librarian who helped design and perform the initial literature searches and who sadly passed away during the course of this work; Jorge Mendoza, a senior research librarian who conducted the second set of literature searches; Audrey Thevenon, a program officer on the Board on Life Sciences, who provided expertise in malaria; Andy Koltun, a summer intern through Georgetown University School of Medicine's Population Health Scholars Track, who helped screen several thousand abstracts; Robert Pool for his editorial assistance; and Misrak Dabi, finance business partner who managed and led the financial and budgeting activities for the project.

David A. Savitz, *Chair*
Committee to Review Long-Term Health Effects of Antimalarial Drugs

Contents

Acronyms and Abbreviations

AFP	Australian Federal Police Association
AIDS	acquired immunodeficiency syndrome
A/P	atovaquone/proguanil
BMI	body mass index
CAS	Chemical Abstract Service
CDC	Centers for Disease Control and Prevention
CI	confidence interval
CNS	central nervous system
DEET	N,N-diethyl-3-metatoluamide
DNA	deoxyribonucleic acid
DoD	Department of Defense
DSM	*Diagnostic and Statistical Manual of Mental Disorders*
DSM-5	*Diagnostic and Statistical Manual of Mental Disorders, Fifth Edition*
ECG	electrocardiogram
FAERS	FDA Adverse Event Reporting System
FAF	fundus autofluorescence
FDA	Food and Drug Administration
FST	fluorescent spot test

G6PD	glucose-6-phosphate dehydrogenase
GFR	glomerular filtration rate
GPRD	General Practice Research Database
HIV	human immunodeficiency virus
HR	hazard ratio
IBD	irritable bowel disease
IBS	irritable bowel syndrome
ICD	*International Classification of Diseases*
ICD-9-CM	*International Classification of Diseases, Ninth Revision, Clinical Modification*
IPTp	intermittent preventive treatment in pregnancy
IR	incidence rate
IRR	incidence rate ratio
n	sample size
NewGen Study	National Health Study for a New Generation of U.S. Veterans
OEF	Operation Enduring Freedom
OIF	Operation Iraqi Freedom
OND	Operation New Dawn
OR	odds ratio
p	p value
PART	presumptive anti-relapse therapy
PCL-C	PTSD Checklist–Civilian version
PHQ	Patient Health Questionnaire
PICO	Participants, Inventions, Comparisons and Outcomes
PTSD	posttraumatic stress disorder
QTc	corrected QT interval (on an ECG)
RR	relative risk
SCID	Structured Clinical Interview for DSM-5
SD-OCT	spectral domain optical coherence tomography
SF-12	Medical Outcomes Study 12-item Short Form
SNP	single nucleotide polymorphism
UK	United Kingdom
UV-A	ultraviolet A
UV-B	ultraviolet B

VA   Department of Veterans Affairs

WHO   World Health Organization

Summary

Malaria is a constant threat for nearly half of the world's population, and people who travel to endemic areas for business, leisure, or military support operations are also at risk. In 2018 the World Health Organization estimated that there were 228 million cases of malaria, with 405,000 resulting in death (WHO, 2019). While preventive measures like mosquito repellents, window screens and bed nets, repellent-impregnated clothing, and large-scale use of insecticides are available to reduce the risk of infection, these measures are not as effective as prophylactic drugs. Several drugs are widely used for malaria prophylaxis, and as of 2019 six are approved by the Food and Drug Administration (FDA) and are available by prescription: chloroquine, primaquine, mefloquine, doxycycline, atovaquone/proguanil (A/P), and tafenoquine.

Malaria has affected nearly every U.S. military deployment since the Civil War, and it remains an ongoing threat to those engaged in current conflicts in Southwest Asia and peacekeeping missions to Africa and Southeast Asia. Department of Defense (DoD) policy requires that service members deployed to malaria-endemic areas be issued antimalarial drugs and adhere to the drug-taking regimens. Policies concerning which should be used as first-line and as second-line agents have evolved over time in response to malaria parasite resistance to antimalarials and new data about the drugs' adverse events and which precautions should be taken for specific underlying health conditions, areas of deployment, and other operational factors.

As is the case with any FDA-approved drug, each approved antimalarial drug has been tested for its safety and efficacy, so their risks of concurrent adverse events have been well characterized. However, the studies conducted to gain FDA approval are generally limited by small numbers of subjects and short follow-up periods, making it difficult to identify adverse events that are rare but potentially serious or that occur or develop over long periods of concurrent use or events that may persist post-cessation. The spectrum of potential adverse events may thus not be fully appreciated until the drug has been on the market for many years. Concern with the potential for long-term or persistent adverse events has been raised by veterans, service members, and other users. This is especially true for antimalarial drugs that have neurologic- or psychiatric-based effects, particularly mefloquine.

In response to these concerns, the Department of Veterans Affairs (VA) contracted with the National Academies of Sciences, Engineering, and Medicine (the National Academies) to convene an expert committee to assess the scientific evidence regarding the potential for long-term health effects resulting from the use of antimalarial drugs that have been approved by FDA and/or used by U.S. service members for malaria prophylaxis.

CHARGE TO THE COMMITTEE

At the committee's first meeting on January 28, 2019, a VA representative charged it to examine and "assess long-term health effects that might result from the use [by adults] of antimalarial drugs" that have been approved by FDA for use as prophylaxis in adults or used by DoD or that are of special interest to VA. Mefloquine and tafenoquine were specified as the two drugs of highest interest and importance to VA. Other antimalarial drugs that have been used by DoD in the past 25 years were also deemed to be important. Antimalarials that were used more than 25 years ago but are no longer in use were considered to be of lesser importance and were not assessed.

Although long-term health effects that might occur in any organ system were to be considered, VA specified that neurologic and psychiatric effects, including the potential development of posttraumatic stress disorder (PTSD), were particular areas of interest. VA stressed that long-term (which the committee interpreted to mean *persistent*, i.e., beginning during drug use and continuing after cessation, or *latent*, i.e., present only after cessation of drug use) health effects of antimalarial drugs should be the focus of the committee's work because short-term (or concurrent) adverse events are well recognized and indicated on a drug's FDA-mandated package insert. The committee defined a *health effect*—and preferentially uses the term "adverse event"—as any generally recognized symptom, condition, or diagnosis. As it was charged with addressing neurologic and psychiatric outcomes and because these outcomes were not assessed consistently across studies, the committee adopted a rubric for categorizing different outcomes; that rubric is explained in Chapter 3. The committee was asked to offer conclusions based on available evidence regarding associations of persistent or latent adverse events and to offer observations concerning the best use of available data as well as considerations for future research on the short-term and also the persistent or latent health effects of antimalarial drugs. In conducting its work, the committee operated independently of VA and other government agencies. It was not asked to make, and it did not make, judgments regarding specific cases in which individuals have claimed injury from the use of an antimalarial drug or such issues as the potential costs of compensation for veterans or policies regarding such compensation. The committee did not perform a cost–benefit analysis or a risk assessment regarding the use of these drugs. This report provides an evidence-based assessment of the scientific evidence regarding persistent and latent adverse events following the prophylactic use of the six antimalarial drugs of interest for the Secretary of Veterans Affairs to consider as VA exercises its responsibilities to veterans.

COMMITTEE'S APPROACH TO ADDRESSING ITS CHARGE

The committee's principal source of information on the potential persistent and latent health effects associated with the use of the antimalarials of interest was epidemiologic studies (observational studies and clinical trials) that were identified from comprehensive searches of the published peer-reviewed literature. In total, the committee considered more than 12,000 abstracts and examined more than 3,000 full-text articles and book chapters. Other supplemental sources of information included U.S. and foreign government documents and reports; information supplied by VA, DoD, and FDA; invited presentations on particular topics (such as neurotoxicology, antimalarials policy practiced by other government agencies, and adverse events monitoring through postmarketing surveillance), and comments offered by veterans and others, such as spouses and advocates, who are concerned about health issues that may be related to antimalarial drug use. The information provided by the public at the open meetings and over the course of the study was used to identify gaps in the literature regarding specific health outcomes of concern. The committee did not collect original data or perform any secondary data analyses.

A two-step process was used to screen the results of searches to identify potentially relevant literature for review. The first step entailed screening for relevance by title and abstract, and the second step was a full-text review to determine the final set of studies that the committee evaluated. For an epidemiologic analysis to be considered, it had to (1) have the drugs used in a prophylactic manner (not for treatment of active cases of malaria or for another disease or condition), (2) report on the presence or absence of adverse events or effects or other health outcome (such as blood counts), (3) have a comparison group, and (4) use adult populations (aged 16 years and older).[1] Additionally, the most important criterion was that there had to be empirical information about the adverse event (or indicate a lack of such an event) that began or persisted at least 28 days after the cessation (final dose) of the drug of interest. As long as a study met these criteria, it was included, even if it had severe methodologic limitations. Ultimately, 21 epidemiologic studies that met the committee's inclusion criteria were identified that addressed one or more of the six drugs of interest (Ackert et al., 2019; Andersen et al., 1998; DeSouza,

---

[1] If some of the subjects were less than 16 years old, the study was included.

1983; Eick-Cost et al., 2017; Green et al., 2014; Laothavorn et al., 1992; Leary et al., 2009; Lee et al., 2013; Lege-Oguntoye et al., 1990; Meier et al., 2004; Miller et al., 2013; Nasveld et al., 2010; Rueangweerayut et al., 2017; Schlagenhauf et al., 1996; Schneider et al., 2013, 2014; Schneiderman et al., 2018; Schwartz and Regev-Yochay, 1999; Tan et al., 2017; Walsh et al., 2004; Wells et al., 2006). These formed the basis for the committee's conclusions on the relationships between the use of antimalarial drugs and specific categories of persistent adverse health effects. Just over half of the identified studies (11) examined exposure to mefloquine; fewer examined the other drugs of interest: tafenoquine, 7; doxycycline, 7; A/P, 4; primaquine, 4; and chloroquine, 3.

Studies that did not follow their populations for at least 28 days after the final dose of a drug of interest was administered or that did not distinguish the timing of the adverse event (e.g., the follow-up time was more than 28 days after drug cessation, but the authors did not distinguish which adverse events occurred inside and outside the 28-day window) are briefly mentioned in this report but are not evaluated in depth. For example, several studies included only a brief mention that "no serious adverse events were reported" without further explanation of what adverse events were examined, how "serious" was defined, or the timing of those events; these were not considered informative for the committee's purposes. Likewise, studies that focused on derivatives of the drugs of interest (such as for drug discovery), drug-delivery systems (e.g., carriers, encapsulations), or the simultaneous administration of an antimalarial drug of interest in combination with any other antimalarial drug that is not an FDA-approved combination were considered to be outside of the committee's scope of work and were excluded from consideration.

The epidemiologic studies that met the inclusion criteria for primary evidence varied in their methods and quality. Each was assessed based on a common set of methodologic principles. The methods assessment included the selection of the study populations, study design, the length of follow-up, the sources of measurement for exposure and adverse events or health outcomes, the statistical analyses used, and control for confounding. A thorough evaluation was made of each study's strengths, limitations, and potential biases and their implications for the study results and for the precision of reported results, and this informed the evaluation of the study's contribution to the evidence base. If a study examined more than one drug or health outcome, it was considered separately for each drug and for each of those outcomes. It is important to note that a study could be well designed and well conducted but still have flaws, such as not distinguishing the timing of adverse events, that limited its information value to the committee.

EVIDENCE REVIEWED BY THE COMMITTEE

The committee reviewed epidemiologic studies that used different designs, populations, and analysis methods; examined disparate adverse events or outcomes; and used diverse methods to collect information. For assessment purposes, the committee categorized these studies by population, with studies of military and veterans presented first, followed by studies of other human populations (occupational groups, travelers, research volunteers, and residents of malaria-endemic areas). To supplement this information, other sources of adverse-event information, such as systematic reviews of concurrent adverse events, case reports, and studies of selected subpopulations, were also examined. The committee additionally drew on the knowledge of the biologic underpinnings of the adverse event or outcome of interest generated through experimental animal and cell culture studies in order to evaluate the degree to which the effect of a specific drug on a specific adverse event is grounded in knowledge of the pathways by which such an impact could occur.

Military and Veteran Populations

Because active-duty military and veterans are the population of interest, studies of these groups were accorded considerable weight in the committee's deliberations. The committee reviewed all identified studies of U.S. and foreign service members and veterans who used any of the antimalarials of interest. Few of these studies included objective measures of drug concentrations in the blood or tissue; more typically, the use of a particular antimalarial and its dosage was based on prescription data, self-report, or specified as part of the study design. Full adherence with the drug regimen was generally assumed when estimating and quantifying the risk of specific adverse events and health outcomes related to the use of a particular drug, although research has shown this is not always the case. As with other studies of health outcomes in military populations, where there is seldom any measure of exposure to a specific agent, comparisons between deployed and nondeployed veterans are considered the next most relevant comparison. Since sending service members to known malaria-endemic areas without prevention measures would be unethical, several studies of military populations compare the effects of two or more antimalarials. Because of the many other factors and stresses associated with deployed environments like combat, specific effects attributable to the use of an antimalarial drug may be difficult to tease out.

Studies of Non-Military and Non-Veteran Populations

Although U.S. service members and veterans constitute the primary population of interest, the committee also considered other populations that use antimalarial drugs (occupationally exposed persons, travelers, research volunteers, and people living in malaria-endemic areas) in which there was the potential for more precise quantification and evaluation of the risks of adverse events. These populations use antimalarial drugs but do not have some of the potentially confounding stressors, such as combat, typically found in military populations. Safety and tolerance studies performed in research volunteers from non-endemic areas who were followed for at least 28 days post-drug-cessation provide additional lines of evidence, as do the results of studies conducted using endemic populations. Finally, studies of adverse events associated with the prophylactic use of a drug in a population with a specific underlying condition (such as pregnancy or comorbid conditions) or demographic trait are described when appropriate.

Animal and Mechanistic Studies

The most commonly used experimental animal models for testing the potential toxicity of antimalarial drugs are mice, rats, dogs, and rhesus monkeys. The committee used studies of laboratory animal models to determine whether there is evidence of a pathophysiologic process or biologic mechanism that could provide evidence bearing on the relationship between exposure to an antimalarial drug in humans and a persistent or latent health effect. Several factors must be considered when extrapolating these results to human disease and disease progression, including the magnitude and duration of exposure, the timing of exposure during development or differentiation, the route of exposure, model-specific factors (such as sex, genetic background, and stress), and differences in pharmacokinetics and pharmacodynamics across species. Insights about biologic processes inform whether an observed pattern of statistical association might be interpreted as the product of more than error, bias, confounding, or chance. Discussions about biologic plausibility are presented after the evidence in humans is presented as part of the comprehensive synthesis of all the pertinent evidence.

WEIGHING THE EVIDENCE AND CONCLUSIONS

The quantitative and qualitative procedures underlying the committee's assessment of the evidence have been made as explicit and transparent as possible, as it focused its assessment on the potential for an *association* between the exposure to an antimalarial drug and health outcomes rather than a direct causal effect. A system of four categories of association for rating health outcomes based on the strength of the scientific evidence has gained wide acceptance by Congress, VA, researchers, and veterans groups, and has been used in the National Academies report series of assessments of veterans' health as well as in several other stand-alone reports including evaluations of safety and the adverse health outcomes of vaccines. The four categories are sufficient, limited or suggestive, inadequate or insufficient, and no association. The criteria for each category express a degree of confidence based on the quality of the evidence, specifically the timing and duration of the exposures, the nature of the specific adverse events or health outcomes, the populations exposed, and the quality, precision, and consistency of the studies examined. The conclusion does not take into account the benefit of the antimalarial to either population or individual health. Although both primary and supporting studies contributed to the committee's conclusion regarding the evidence of prophylactic use of an antimalarial to be associated with adverse events in a particular body system, primary studies were given more weight.

Conclusions were made independently of other reports or author conclusions. Several other groups have reviewed the available literature on a specific antimalarial drug, class, or a particular health outcome. However, they used different frameworks, inclusion criteria, or methods to judge association or causality, and therefore their conclusions may differ from those of the committee.

For each of the six drugs of interest, adverse events were categorized by neurologic, psychiatric, gastrointestinal, eye, cardiovascular, and other disorders. The committee assembled and discussed the evidence to reach a consensus on the level of the evidence for persistent or latent health effects for each drug of interest; these conclusions are presented in the Synthesis and Conclusion sections. In making its assessments, the committee was careful to note that a lack of informative data does not mean that there is no increased risk of a specific adverse event, only that the available evidence does not provide support for an increased risk. Each conclusion consists of two parts: the first sentence assigns the level of association, and the second sentence offers additional detail regarding whether further research in a particular area is merited based on a consideration of all the available evidence and any signals that may be present. For those health outcomes in which the committee concluded there is not a clear justification for additional research, the intention was to distinguish those issues for which there is presently an empirical basis for looking more closely and those for which such a basis is not present. As more research accumulates, the outcomes that warrant further research may change.

KEY FINDINGS AND GENERAL OBSERVATIONS

Nine of the 21 epidemiologic studies examined multiple drugs of interest, and they contribute to the evidence described in multiple chapters. In many cases, even when there were multiple studies of the same drug and same outcome, the characteristics of the study populations and methods were so divergent as to be of questionable relevance to one another. Almost no studies collected data prospectively for the purpose of assessing persistent or latent adverse events months to years after the cessation of antimalarial use.

The committee presents a total of 31 conclusions regarding the level of association between exposures to a drug of interest and persistent or latent adverse events (see Box S-1). For one association, there was determined to be a sufficient level of evidence to determine that an association exists. The committee concluded that there is sufficient evidence of an association between the use of tafenoquine and vortex keratopathy,[2] which although it was found to persist beyond 28 days post-cessation,

---

[2] Vortex keratopathy manifests as deposits in the inferior interpalpebal portion of the cornea. These deposits rarely result in reduction of visual acuity or ocular symptoms, and they typically resolve with discontinuation of the medication that caused them (AAO, 2019).

BOX S-1
Summary of Conclusions Regarding Categories of Association Between Exposure to Antimalarial Drugs and Persistent or Latent Adverse Events by System Outcome

Sufficient Evidence of an Association

Epidemiologic evidence is sufficient to conclude that there is a positive association between the prophylactic use of an antimalarial drug and the outcome in studies in which chance, bias, and confounding can be ruled out with reasonable confidence. For example, if several small studies without known bias and confounding show an association that is consistent in magnitude and direction, there could be sufficient evidence of an association. Experimental data supporting biologic plausibility strengthen the evidence of an association but are not a prerequisite and are not enough to establish an association without corresponding epidemiologic findings. There is sufficient evidence of an association between the following antimalarial drugs and health outcomes:

- Tafenoquine and vortex keratopathy

Limited or Suggestive Evidence of an Association

Epidemiologic evidence suggests an association between prophylactic use of an antimalarial drug of interest and the outcome in studies of humans, but the evidence can be limited by an inability to confidently rule out chance, bias, or confounding. For example, a high-quality study with strong findings of a positive association in conjunction with less compelling or inconsistent results from studies of populations with similar exposures could constitute such evidence. None of the associations between antimalarial drugs and health outcomes were determined to constitute limited or suggestive evidence.

Inadequate or Insufficient Evidence of an Association

The available epidemiologic studies are of insufficient quality, validity, consistency, or statistical power to support a conclusion regarding the presence or absence of an association. For example, such studies may have failed to control for confounding factors or had inadequate assessment of exposure or outcomes. Because the committee could not possibly address every rare condition or disease, it does not draw explicit conclusions about outcomes that are not discussed, and instead it makes conclusions by body system. It also notes whether the existing evidence, including nonepidemiologic information, merits additional research in a specific area. There is inadequate or insufficient evidence of an association between the following antimalarial drugs and health outcomes, grouped by whether the existing evidence supports additional research:

Basis for additional research
- Mefloquine and neurologic events
- Mefloquine and psychiatric events, including PTSD

- Mefloquine and eye disorders, including cataract
- Tafenoquine and psychiatric events
- Tafenoquine and eye disorders (other than vortex keratopathy)
- Atovaquone/Proguanil and eye disorders
- Doxycycline and gastrointestinal events

No basis for additional research

- Mefloquine and gastrointestinal events
- Mefloquine and cardiovascular events
- Tafenoquine and neurologic events
- Tafenoquine and gastrointestinal events
- Tafenoquine and cardiovascular events
- Atovaquone/Proguanil and neurologic events
- Atovaquone/Proguanil and psychiatric events
- Atovaquone/Proguanil and gastrointestinal events
- Atovaquone/Proguanil and cardiovascular events
- Doxycycline and neurologic events
- Doxycycline and psychiatric events
- Doxycycline and eye disorders
- Doxycycline and cardiovascular events
- Primaquine and neurologic events
- Primaquine and psychiatric events
- Primaquine and gastrointestinal events
- Primaquine and eye disorders
- Primaquine and cardiovascular events
- Chloroquine and neurologic events
- Chloroquine and psychiatric events
- Chloroquine and gastrointestinal events
- Chloroquine and eye disorders
- Chloroquine and cardiovascular events

Limited or Suggestive Evidence of No Association

Several adequate studies, which cover the full range of human exposure, are consistent in showing no association or reduced risk (not distinguished for the purposes of this evaluation, which was focused on the potential for adverse effects) with an exposure to an antimalarial of interest at any concentration and had relatively narrow confidence intervals. A conclusion of "no association" is inevitably limited to the conditions, exposures, and observation periods covered by the available studies, and the possibility of a small increase in risk related to the magnitude of exposure studied can never be excluded. However, a change in classification from inadequate or insufficient evidence of an association to limited or suggestive evidence of no association would require new studies that correct for the methodologic problems of previous studies and that have samples large enough to limit the possible study results attributable to chance. None of the associations between the antimalarial drugs and health outcomes were determined to constitute limited or suggestive evidence of no association.

was also found to resolve within 3 to 12 months and did not have a clinical implication, such as loss of vision.

For the other 30 conclusions across all drugs and outcome categories considered, the evidence between the drug of interest and persistent or latent adverse events was inadequate or insufficient. For all outcomes except for the potential of some eye disorders for A/P users, the occurrence of latent effects (those effects that did not manifest in individuals while taking the antimalarial and only emerged after drug cessation) was not supported. Based on information from the assessed epidemiologic studies and other studies of concurrent events, case reports, or biologic plausibility, the committee considers the existence of some persistent events for certain antimalarials to be highly plausible but not sufficiently studied. For this reason, in its conclusion for each outcome category the committee specifies whether the existing evidence warrants additional research in a specific area. The committee determined that there is a basis for further research for seven of the drug–outcome associations, and it views the most plausible persistent adverse events to be those that are the result of enduring concurrent events and thus gave additional weight to the evidence for concurrent events in determining whether there is a basis for further research.

The interpretation of studies that did not find increased risk associated with a particular drug took into account the extent to which they would have been capable of detecting associations had they been present. The informativeness of such studies depends in part on their statistical power, which is determined by factors that include the overall study size and frequency of the adverse events of interest. In a number of instances, studies that found no evidence of an association were of sufficient size and quality that it is unlikely that there are truly large increases in common adverse events, but this did not preclude smaller effects or effects on rarer outcomes. Even such modest increases in rare events may lead to substantial impairment for the individuals who are affected and result in a large absolute number of adverse events, given the number of people who use the antimalarial drugs.

Neurologic and Psychiatric Outcomes

As noted above, VA asked the committee to specifically address the evidence for persistent neurologic and psychiatric outcomes and the potential development of PTSD. Of the six drugs of interest, these concerns were greatest for mefloquine. Concurrent adverse neurologic events associated with the use of mefloquine are well recognized and include dizziness, vertigo, loss of balance, headache, memory impairment, confusion, encephalopathy, sensory or motor neuropathies, convulsions, and tinnitus. However, the post-cessation studies did not find these concurrent adverse events to be present at statistically different rates among users of mefloquine than with those who used other antimalarial drugs or who did not use any prophylaxis. Similarly, the evidence supporting concurrent adverse psychiatric effects (anxiety, depression, mood swings, panic attacks, abnormal dreams, insomnia, hallucinations, aggression, psychotic or paranoid reactions, and suicidal thoughts) with the use of mefloquine is compelling, but the epidemiologic studies that examined these outcomes at least 28 days post-drug-cessation do not indicate an increase of persistent psychiatric events relative to other antimalarial drugs or no use of antimalarial drugs.

Three high-quality studies—all conducted using active-duty U.S. military or veteran populations—reported PTSD diagnoses (based on *International Classification of Diseases, Ninth Revision, Clinical Modification* [ICD-9-CM] codes) or PTSD symptoms (based on validated instruments), taking into account deployment and combat exposure. In an analysis of active-duty service members, Eick-Cost et al. (2017) presented adjusted effect estimates of PTSD stratified by deployment status. Among the nondeployed, those who were prescribed mefloquine were found to have a statistically significant decrease in PTSD diagnoses relative to those prescribed doxycycline, but a statistically significantly increased risk relative to individuals who were prescribed A/P. There was no difference in PTSD diagnoses for deployed service members prescribed mefloquine versus those prescribed doxycycline or A/P. When service members were stratified by prior psychiatric history, no statistically significant differences between mefloquine and doxycycline for PTSD diagnoses were found. In their analysis of the hospitalizations of active-duty service members, Wells et al. (2006) reported no statistically significant differences for PTSD diagnoses for deployed service members who were prescribed mefloquine versus deployed service members who did not use an antimalarial drug or, separately, who were assigned to Europe or Japan. In their study of veterans who had responded to the 2009–2011 National Health Study for a New Generation of U.S. Veterans, Schneiderman et al. (2018), using a standardized instrument, also found no difference in PTSD symptoms between mefloquine users and nonusers of antimalarials after controlling for demographic characteristics and deployment. Therefore, based on the available evidence primarily from the epidemiologic studies, the committee concluded that there is insufficient or inadequate evidence of an association between the use of mefloquine for malaria prophylaxis and persistent or latent neurologic events or psychiatric events, including PTSD. However, given the concurrent adverse events, case reports, public submissions, and experimental animal studies, the committee concluded that there is a basis for further study of such associations.

Tafenoquine, like mefloquine, is contraindicated in persons with a history of psychotic disorders or current psychotic symptoms. None of the seven epidemiologic studies included data on psychiatric adverse events for which the timing post-tafenoquine-cessation was specified. In studies conducted pre-FDA approval, the most common concurrent psychiatric adverse reactions for tafenoquine were reported to be sleep disturbances, depression or depressed mood, and anxiety. Moreover, results from a combined set of studies submitted to FDA reported that psychiatric adverse events were similar between participants receiving tafenoquine and those receiving mefloquine and that the rates of adverse events for both groups were higher than those for participants receiving a placebo. Despite the issues with these studies—the timing of the events was not specified, the studies did not conduct systematic monitoring for the outcomes, and for several of the studies people with a history of psychiatric disorders were excluded—still these findings enhance the plausibility of psychiatric events being associated with use of tafenoquine. As such, although the committee concluded that there was insufficient or inadequate evidence of an association between the use of tafenoquine for malaria prophylaxis and persistent or latent psychiatric events, it also concluded that there was a basis for further study of persistent or latent psychiatric events.

Other Outcomes for Which There Is a Basis for Additional Research

The committee also identified several other indications of associations for specific outcomes in its review of post-cessation epidemiologic studies and supporting evidence (such as case reports of persistent adverse events, concurrent adverse events, or biologic plausibility) that would merit further study. For three of the drugs—mefloquine, tafenoquine, and atovaquone/proguanil—the committee believes there is a basis for additional research on persistent or latent eye disorders. For doxycycline there is a basis for additional research into persistent gastrointestinal events.

ADVANCING RESEARCH ON ANTIMALARIAL DRUGS

Given the seriousness of malaria and the billions of people at risk for it, there will be a continued need for antimalarial drugs. Studying the persistent and latent effects of exposures is challenging, and therefore it is important to recognize that a perfect or complete understanding is likely unrealistic. A key limitation of the existing literature is that very few studies were designed specifically to examine latent or persistent adverse events. To establish causal links between antimalarial exposure and persistent adverse events, it will be important to have a series of randomized trials and multiple well-designed observational studies of varying types that are designed to examine potential persistent outcomes and overcome the considerable weaknesses noted in past research. Ideally these studies would have explicit documentation of the timing of antimalarial drug use and symptom occurrence (with clear temporal ordering), an extended follow-up that includes assessments at multiple time points, and a validated collection of information regarding potential confounders, antimalarial exposure (dose and timing), and the outcomes of potential interest, including a careful collection of neurologic and psychiatric outcomes using validated instruments. Because some of the outcomes of concern are or may be rare, the samples will need to be of sufficient size to detect associations if they do exist. While it may not be realistic to carry out a large set of studies that have all of these components, there are strong designs that take advantage of existing data sets that would be feasible. In addition, a series of well-designed studies that each have a number of (but perhaps not all) these components could be quite informative, and they could be used to triangulate the evidence so as to develop an understanding of the potential mechanisms and persistent adverse events. Using standardized definitions and making exposure, outcome, and covariates as compatible as possible would better allow for a synthesis of the evidence across studies.

There has recently been more interest in assessing the potential persistent or latent adverse events of antimalarial drugs than there was when the first of the drugs were approved in the 1940s. For example, two required Phase IV trials are now being conducted to evaluate long-term tafenoquine safety. With regard to mefloquine specifically, several factors may influence whether additional studies of its use for malaria prophylaxis are conducted and how informative those results will be. Although mefloquine is still recommended for civilian use, the numbers of prescriptions for it have declined substantially, likely in part due to the 2013 FDA boxed warning regarding concurrent psychiatric symptoms (see Chapter 4), to media reports of adverse events, and to the availability of similarly efficacious drugs with comparatively fewer adverse events or different adverse event profiles. Since 2009, DoD policy has severely restricted the use of mefloquine for service members. Therefore, any prospective or retrospective studies conducted using service members since these policies went into effect will lack generalizability and will include people who have previously tolerated mefloquine, which may account for some of the findings of no difference in risk of most outcomes compared with other antimalarials.

Some of the most informative studies have used health care databases or other data sources that cover large populations. Therefore, a logical place to look for additional opportunities would be in other large databases that include a sufficiently large number of individuals who used antimalarial drugs and that provide documentation of their subsequent health experience; another option would be to link several large databases to obtain the data needed for both exposure and outcome assessment. Such data sources might include general VA and DoD health care databases, existing DoD and VA registries, cohorts of service members or veterans assembled previously, Medicare, FDA Sentinel, commercially available claims databases, and health care data from other countries with national health care systems. Other avenues of investigation that would likely be informative about persistent or latent adverse events are re-analyses of some of the existing studies to clarify the temporal course of drug use and health experience to enable inferences regarding concomitant versus persistent adverse events. It was clear to the committee that data on post-drug-cessation events had been collected for several epidemiologic studies, but the data were not reported in a manner that allowed the committee to distinguish the timing of the adverse events. A pooled data analysis effort using a standardized approach may also move this area of scientific inquiry forward.

Several other strategies and approaches were considered for advancing the evidence base on persistent adverse events associated with the use of antimalarial drugs. Conducting studies of adverse events up to 3–6 months post-cessation would be informative if focused and validated assessments of health status were performed over the subsequent weeks or months. This might involve extending clinical trials or systematically following returning travelers using clinical evaluations or even questionnaires that are sufficiently sensitive to discern even subclinical health status. To the extent that there are hypotheses regarding individuals with selected risk factors, smaller, more intensive evaluations could be used to target adverse events in these populations. Large case–control studies of specific adverse events could potentially generate additional evidence on associations of antimalarial drugs. Finally, well-conceived in vitro or in vivo studies could provide meaningful information to help in interpreting the evidence from human populations. Mechanistic links between antimalarial drugs and persistent or latent adverse outcomes have yet to be systematically and definitively explored through experimental studies, and the current literature in that area is relatively weak. Examples of research that would be required for suitable rigor include testing the impacts of prolonged exposure to biologically relevant antimalarial dosing across several behavioral tests with validity for persistent or latent psychiatric, neurologic, or other disorders and in vivo testing of lasting antimalarial-induced cell loss and toxicity using contemporary standards of assessment.

A number of approaches are unlikely to provide much additional insight regarding the persistent adverse events of antimalarial drugs. These include cross-sectional studies that do not allow for distinguishing between the use of a drug and correlates of symptoms or diagnoses; small clinical trials without sufficiently long post-cessation follow-up periods or sufficient numbers of participants to provide the needed statistical precision to address clinically significant outcomes; and studies of reports submitted to adverse event registries, such as that used by FDA.

FINAL OBSERVATIONS

There is a sharp contrast between the extensive evidence pertaining to concurrent adverse events that are experienced while a drug is being used or shortly following its cessation and the dearth of high-quality information pertaining to adverse experiences that are present after the use of that drug has ended. This remains true after combining the available studies across all the drugs of interest (some of which have been in use for more than 70 years) and types of possible adverse events. There appears to be a disconnect between the level of concern raised—millions of people have used the drugs, and there are recognized concurrent adverse events and case reports of adverse events—and the systematic research on persistent adverse events, particularly in areas such as the use of mefloquine and persistent neurologic or psychiatric outcomes. The available epidemiologic studies are highly variable in their methodologic quality and relevance and rarely can be considered replications, given the diversity of study populations and designs. Although conducting high-quality research on the persistent and latent effects of exposures is challenging, this should not prevent it from being done.

REFERENCES

AAO (American Academy of Ophthalmology). 2019. *Corneal verticillata.* https://www.aao.org/bcscsnippetdetail.aspx?id=27980840-6807-4c45-aaae-b8652b087987 (accessed October 30, 2019).

Ackert, J., K. Mohamed, J. S. Slakter, S. El-Harazi, A. Berni, H. Gevorkyan, E. Hardaker, A. Hussaini, S. W. Jones, G. C. K. W. Koh, J. Patel, S. Rasmussen, D. S. Kelly, D. E. Baranano, J. T. Thompson, K. A. Warren, R. C. Sergott, J. Tonkyn, A. Wolstenholme, H. Coleman, A. Yuan, S. Duparc, and J. A. Green. 2019. Randomized placebo-controlled trial evaluating the ophthalmic safety of single-dose tafenoquine in healthy volunteers. *Drug Saf* 42(9):1103-1114.

Andersen, S. L., A. J. Oloo, D. M. Gordon, O. B. Ragama, G. M. Aleman, J. D. Berman, D. B. Tang, M. W. Dunne, and G. D. Shanks. 1998. Successful double-blinded, randomized, placebo-controlled field trial of azithromycin and doxycycline as prophylaxis for malaria in western Kenya. *Clin Infect Dis* 26(1):146-150.

DeSouza, J. M. 1983. Phase I clinical trial of mefloquine in Brazilian male subjects. *Bull World Health Organ* 61(5):809-814.

Eick-Cost, A. A., Z. Hu, P. Rohrbeck, and L. L. Clark. 2017. Neuropsychiatric outcomes after mefloquine exposure among U.S. military service members. *Am J Trop Med Hyg* 96(1):159-166.

Green, J. A., A. K. Patel, B. R. Patel, A. Hussaini, E. J. Harrell, M. J. McDonald, N. Carter, K. Mohamed, S. Duparc, and A. K. Miller. 2014. Tafenoquine at therapeutic concentrations does not prolong Fridericia-corrected QT interval in healthy subjects. *J Clin Pharmacol* 54:995-1005.

Laothavorn, P., J. Karbwang, K. Na Bangchang, D. Bunnag, and T. Harinasuta. 1992. Effect of mefloquine on electrocardiographic changes in uncomplicated falciparum malaria patients. *Southeast Asian J Trop Med Public Health* 23(1):51-54.

Leary, K. J., M. A. Riel, M. J. Roy, L. R. Cantilena, D. Bi, D. C. Brater, C. van de Pol, K. Pruett, C. Kerr, J. M. Veazey, Jr., R. Beboso, and C. Ohrt. 2009. A randomized, double-blind, safety and tolerability study to assess the ophthalmic and renal effects of tafenoquine 200 mg weekly versus placebo for 6 months in healthy volunteers. *Am J Trop Med Hyg* 81:356-362.

Lee, T. W., L. Russell, M. Deng, and P. R. Gibson. 2013. Association of doxycycline use with the development of gastroenteritis, irritable bowel syndrome and inflammatory bowel disease in Australians deployed abroad. *Intern Med J* 43(8):919-926.

Lege-Oguntoye, L., G. C. Onyemelukwe, B. B. Maiha, E. O. Udezue, and S. Eckerbom. 1990. The effect of short-term malaria chemoprophylaxis on the immune response of semi-immune adult volunteers. *East Afr Med J* 67(11):770-778.

Meier, C. R., K. Wilcock, and S. S. Jick. 2004. The risk of severe depression, psychosis or panic attacks with prophylactic antimalarials. *Drug Saf* 27(3):203-213.

Miller, A. K., E. Harrell, L. Ye, S. Baptiste-Brown, J. P. Kleim, C. Ohrt, S. Duparc, J. J. Möhrle, A. Webster, S. Stinnett, A. Hughes, S. Griffith, and A. P. Beelen. 2013. Pharmacokinetic interactions and safety evaluations of coadministered tafenoquine and chloroquine in healthy subjects. *Br J Clin Pharmacol* 76:858-867.

Nasveld, P. E., M. D. Edstein, M. Reid, L. Brennan, I. E. Harris, S. J. Kitchener, P. A. Leggat, P. Pickford, C. Kerr, C. Ohrt, W. Prescott, and the Tafenoquine Study Team. 2010. Randomized, double-blind study of the safety, tolerability, and efficacy of tafenoquine versus mefloquine for malaria prophylaxis in nonimmune subjects. *Antimicrob Agents Chemother* 54:792-798.

Rueangweerayut, R., G. Bancone, E. J. Harrell, A. P. Beelen, S. Kongpatanakul, J. J. Möhrle, V. Rousell, K. Mohamed, A. Qureshi, S. Narayan, N. Yubon, A. Miller, F. H. Nosten, L. Luzzatto, S. Duparc, J.-P. Kleim, and J. A. Green. 2017. Hemolytic potential of tafenoquine in female volunteers heterozygous for glucose-6-phosphate dehydrogenase (G6PD) deficiency (G6PD *Mahidol* variant) versus G6PD normal volunteers. *Am J Trop Med Hyg* 97(3):702-711.

Schlagenhauf, P., R. Steffen, H. Lobel, R. Johnson, R. Letz, A. Tschopp, N. Vranjes, Y. Bergqvist, O. Ericsson, U. Hellgren, L. Rombo, S. Mannino, J. Handschin, and D. Sturchler. 1996. Mefloquine tolerability during chemoprophylaxis: Focus on adverse event assessments, stereochemistry and compliance. *Trop Med Int Health* 1(4):485-494.

Schneider, C., M. Adamcova, S. S. Jick, P. Schlagenhauf, M. K. Miller, H. G. Rhein, and C. R. Meier. 2013. Antimalarial chemoprophylaxis and the risk of neuropsychiatric disorders. *Travel Med Infect Dis* 11(2):71-80.

Schneider, C., M. Adamcova, S. S. Jick, P. Schlagenhauf, M. K. Miller, H. G. Rhein, and C. R. Meier. 2014. Use of anti-malarial drugs and the risk of developing eye disorders. *Travel Med Infect Dis* 12(1):40-47.

Schneiderman, A. I., Y. S. Cypel, E. K. Dursa, and R. Bossarte. 2018. Associations between use of antimalarial medications and health among U.S. veterans of the wars in Iraq and Afghanistan. *Am J Trop Med Hyg* 99(3):638-648.

Schwartz, E., and G. Regev-Yochay. 1999. Primaquine as prophylaxis for malaria for nonimmune travelers: A comparison with mefloquine and doxycycline. Clin Infect Dis 29(6):1502-1506.

Tan, K. R., S. J. Henderson, J. Williamson, R. W. Ferguson, T. M. Wilkinson, P. Jung, and P. M. Arguin. 2017. Long term health outcomes among returned Peace Corps volunteers after malaria prophylaxis, 1995–2014. *Travel Med Infect Dis* 17:50-55.

Walsh, D. S., C. Eamsila, T. Sasiprapha, S. Sangkharomya, P. Khaewsathien, P. Supakalin, D. B. Tang, P. Jarasrumgsichol, C. Cherdchu, M. D. Edstein, K. H. Rieckmann, and T. G. Brewer. 2004. Efficacy of monthly tafenoquine for prophylaxis of Plasmodium vivax and multidrug-resistant P. falciparum malaria. *J Infect Dis* 190(8):1456-1463.

Wells, T. S., T. C. Smith, B. Smith, L. Z. Wang, C. J. Hansen, R. J. Reed, W. E. Goldfinger, T. E. Corbeil, C. N. Spooner, and M. A. Ryan. 2006. Mefloquine use and hospitalizations among US service members, 2002-2004. *Am J Trop Med Hyg* 74(5):744-749.

WHO (World Health Organization). 2019. *World Malaria Report, 2019.* https://www.who.int/ publications-detail/world-malaria-report-2019 (accessed December 10, 2019).

1

Introduction

Despite the fact that malaria was eliminated in the United States in the 1950s, it continues to be a serious disease in many others countries around the world. The World Health Organization (WHO) estimated that in 2018 there were 228 million cases of malaria, and that an estimated 405,000 of these cases resulted in death (WHO, 2019). Malaria is a constant threat for nearly half of the world's population, while among the other half, there are many people who travel to areas where malaria is endemic for business, leisure travel, or to assist with military support operations, and they are also at risk of contracting malaria. The use of malaria prevention methods such as dermal mosquito repellents, chemical-repellent-impregnated clothing, and bed nets can help reduce the risk, but they are not as effective as prophylactic drugs.

A variety of malaria-preventing drugs have been discovered since quinine was first isolated from the bark of the cinchona tree in the early 1800s, and several are in widespread use today. As of 2019, six drugs have been approved by the Food and Drug Administration (FDA) that are currently available by prescription for malaria prophylaxis. They are, by order of the year of FDA approval, chloroquine, primaquine, mefloquine, doxycycline, atovaquone/proguanil, and tafenoquine. As is the case with any FDA-approved drug, each of these antimalarial drugs was tested in several studies to examine its safety and efficacy, so their risks of adverse drug events have been well characterized, at least for short-term effects. These adverse events, which include nausea, upset stomach, and drowsiness, are actually quite common but usually do no permanent harm to the user; in a small number of cases, however, they can have serious or persistent consequences. Studies conducted to gain FDA approval are generally limited by their small numbers of subjects, strict inclusion and exclusion criteria, and short follow-up periods, which makes it difficult during the approval process to identify adverse events that are rare but potentially serious or that occur or develop over long periods of time. As a result, some of the possible potential adverse events may be fully appreciated only after a drug has been on the market for many years.

Among the Americans most likely to be exposed to malaria are members of the military. Malaria has affected nearly every U.S. military deployment since the American Civil War and it remains an ongoing threat to service members involved in current conflicts in Southwest Asia and peacekeeping missions to Africa and Southeast Asia. Department of Defense (DoD) policy requires that service members deployed to malaria-endemic areas be issued antimalarial drugs and adhere to the drug-taking regimens. Policies concerning which should be used as first-line and as second-line agents have evolved over time in response to malaria parasite resistance to antimalarials and new data about the drugs' adverse events and which precautions should be taken for specific underlying health conditions, areas of deployment, and other operational factors.

Service members, veterans, and other users have raised concerns about the use of these antimalarial drugs, particularly mefloquine, resulting in long-term or persistent effects, especially those that are neurologic or psychiatric based. Furthermore, the number of veterans seeking disability compensation for conditions attributed to mefloquine use while in service is increasing. The Department of Veterans Affairs (VA) has responsibility for the health care of veterans and, therefore, has an interest in knowing which symptoms and health effects might persist in veterans long after service. Given its mission and in response to these concerns, VA contracted with the National Academies of Sciences, Engineering, and Medicine (the National Academies) to convene an expert ad hoc committee to conduct an assessment of the scientific evidence regarding the potential for long-term health effects resulting from the use of any of the currently available antimalarial drugs that were approved by FDA and/or used by U.S. service members for malaria prophylaxis.

IDENTIFICATION AND SELECTION OF PROPHYLACTIC ANTIMALARIAL DRUGS TO BE REVIEWED

To determine the antimalarial drugs that would be included in this report, a senior research librarian at the National Academies compiled a list of all antimalarial drugs that have been approved by FDA. This list contained 25 potential drugs of interest. Staff members of the National Academies' Health and Medicine Division then investigated each drug on the list to determine whether it was used for prophylaxis, treatment, or both prophylaxis and treatment of malaria. The drugs that are or have previously been used solely for the treatment of malaria were eliminated from further consideration; this included such agents as Artemisinins, Halofantrine, Fansidar, and Daraprim. The remaining drugs were cross-checked with policies from DoD on the use of antimalarial drugs for the prophylaxis of malaria with no time limits (Woodson, 2013) and also with the Centers for Disease Control and Prevention timeline summarizing the history of antimalarial drugs (Arguin and Magill, 2017). The resulting list of antimalarial drugs was then sent to DoD for verification of each drug's use as an antimalarial prophylactic in military populations. Representatives from DoD confirmed the drugs on the initial list and added two additional antimalarial agents, Dapsone (diaminodiphenyl sulfone) and combination chloroquine-primaquine (C-P pill) for the committee's consideration.

The initial list was also sent to VA for confirmation of the antimalarial drugs of interest to be assessed. When VA formally presented the Statement of Task to the committee, it added tafenoquine to the list of drugs for consideration. VA also stressed that those antimalarial prophylactic agents that are currently available or that have been used within the past 25 years were of highest interest. Based on the contract between VA and the National Academies and as specified in the committee's Statement of Task, this report includes the following antimalarial drugs that are used as prophylaxis, have been approved by FDA or used by U.S. military personnel, and are currently available or have been used in the recent past: mefloquine (Lariam®), tafenoquine (Arakoda™), atovaquone-proguanil (Malarone®), doxycycline (Acticlate®, Vibramycin®, Doryx®, Vibra-Tabs®, Doryx® MPC, doxycycline hyclate), chloroquine (Aralen®), and primaquine. Literature on other antimalarials, such as studies related to quinine's mechanisms of action, were also considered in order to inform the understanding of the mechanisms and the potential persistent or latent biologic effects of similar drugs. Although quinine, tetracycline, hydroxychloroquine, dapsone (diaminodiphenyl sulfone), and quinacrine (mepacrine, Atabrine) were used for prophylaxis of malaria by U.S. service members, these agents were all used more than 25 years ago and before the 1990–1991 Persian Gulf War and were not considered further.

CHARGE TO THE COMMITTEE

Box 1-1 shows the committee's Statement of Task. A VA representative delivered the charge to the committee during the open session of the committee's first meeting on January 28, 2019. As described above, the antimalarial drugs to be considered by the committee were approved by FDA for use as prophylaxis in adults or used by DoD or were of special interest to VA. Mefloquine (also sold under the trade name Lariam®) and tafenoquine (Arakoda™) were specified as the two drugs of highest interest and importance to VA, with other antimalarial drugs that are currently in use by DoD or that have been used by DoD in the past 25 years also to be considered important. Antimalarials that were used more than 25 years ago but that are no longer in use were considered to be of lesser importance. VA stressed that the focus of the committee's work should be the long-term health effects of antimalarial drugs that are used for prophylaxis because the short-term adverse events of the

---

BOX 1-1
Committee's Statement of Task

An ad hoc committee of the National Academies of Sciences, Engineering, and Medicine will conduct a study to assess the long-term health effects that might result from the use of antimalarial drugs by adults, in particular mefloquine, for the prophylaxis of malaria. The committee will examine the currently available medications, as approved by the Food and Drug Administration and/or used by the Department of Defense, and of interest to the Department of Veterans Affairs, and the long-term health effects that might occur in any organ system. These include latent effects that might be expected from their use by Service members during deployment to areas with endemic malaria, such as Afghanistan. Special attention will be given to possible long-term neurologic effects, long-term psychiatric effects and the potential development of Posttraumatic Stress Disorder (PTSD). Additionally, the committee will consider approaches for identifying short-term, long-term, and persistent adverse health effects of antimalarials. The committee will develop findings and conclusions based on its review of the evidence; the report will not include recommendations.

---

antimalarial drugs of interest are well recognized and are clearly indicated on the package inserts issued by FDA. Although the committee was asked to examine neurologic and psychiatric effects of the drugs—and the potential development of posttraumatic stress disorder (PTSD) in particular—the committee was to consider effects that might occur in any organ system. Instead of recommendations, the committee was asked to offer conclusions based on available evidence regarding the long-term effects and to provide observations on the best use of available data as well as considerations for future research in examining the persistent or latent health effects of antimalarial drugs.

Given the difficulty of conducting strict causality assessments, the committee chose instead to base its assessment on measures of association between exposure to an antimalarial drug and health outcomes. Assessing evidence for associations rather than causation means that the rigor of the evidence required to support a finding of statistical association is weaker than what is required to support causality, although some of the criteria that would contribute to determining causality may be met.

THE STUDY PROCESS AND INFORMATION GATHERING

The National Academies convened a 10-member interdisciplinary committee that included experts in epidemiology, biostatistics, pharmacology, drug safety, psychology, psychiatry, neurology, biochemistry, medicinal chemistry, toxicology, malaria, and military and veteran's health. The committee met in person for five 2-day meetings over 10 months. Between the in-person meetings, small groups of committee members held conference calls to review specific studies or to discuss the evidence base on a particular health outcome or topic.

In conducting its work, the committee operated independently of VA and any other government agency. It was not asked to make—and it did not make— judgments regarding specific cases in which individual people have claimed injury from the use of an antimalarial drug or regarding such broader issues as the potential costs of compensation for veterans or policies about such compensation. Several other groups have reviewed the available literature on specific antimalarial drugs, classes, or particular health outcomes. However, they used different frameworks, inclusion criteria, or methods to judge association or causality, and therefore the conclusions presented may differ from those of this committee. This report is intended to provide an evidence-based assessment of the scientific information available on long-term health effects following the prophylactic use of the antimalarial drugs which the Secretary of Veterans Affairs can consider as VA exercises its responsibilities to veterans. The committee did not perform a cost–benefit analysis or a risk assessment regarding the use of these drugs. This report, as with all National Academies' reports, is freely accessible online at the National Academies Press's website (www.nap.edu).

Several activities were undertaken to develop the scientific foundation for the report's findings and conclusions. The principal sources of information on potential long-term health effects associated with the use of the antimalarials of interest to the committee came from detailed searches of the published peer-reviewed literature which were not subject to time constraints. The committee did not collect original data, conduct original studies, or perform any secondary data analyses. In total the committee considered more than 12,000 abstracts of scientific and medical studies and read more than 3,000 full-text articles and book chapters. The literature search strategy and process for reviewing all results is discussed in detail in Chapter 3, Identification and Evaluation of the Evidence Base. This process was supplemented by examining other pertinent published literature, government documents and reports, and testimony and by consulting relevant National Academies reports.

As is the practice of nearly all National Academies consensus committees, the committee held two open sessions not only to gather additional information from people who have particular expertise on topics and subjects that arise during deliberations (such as experts in toxicology, agency representatives who are familiar with antimalarials policy and changes to it, and those who monitor reports of adverse events through postmarketing surveillance), but also especially to listen to individual veterans and others, such as spouses and advocates, who are concerned about aspects of health that may be related to use of these antimalarial drugs. Open sessions were held during the committee's first two meetings; the agendas and presentation topics are presented in Appendix A, and brief summaries of the presentations are found in Appendix B. The comments and information provided by the public at the open meetings and over the course of the study were used to identify information gaps in the literature regarding specific health outcomes of concern.

In addition to information provided by invited speakers and members of the public, the committee obtained information from VA and DoD via information requests that followed up on issues raised during presentations and on sources of data on policy. The committee also made two information requests to FDA to request the data or an explanation of the data that were used to support changes to the package insert or label associated with the adverse events of mefloquine. All presentations, responses to information requests, and written comments are available in the public access file for the project.[1]

ORGANIZATION OF THE REPORT

The remainder of this report is organized into nine chapters and four appendixes. Chapter 2 presents background information about the antimalarial drugs of interest as well as the military use of them and deployment factors that may exacerbate certain effects of some antimalarial drugs. Chapter 3 describes the considerations that guided the committee's identification, review, and evaluation of the scientific evidence.

The committee's evaluation of the epidemiologic literature and other supplemental information and its conclusions regarding the evidence are presented by drug in Chapters 4–9: Chapter 4, Mefloquine; Chapter 5, Tafenoquine; Chapter 6, Atovaquone/Proguanil; Chapter 7, Doxycycline; Chapter 8, Primaquine; and Chapter 9, Chloroquine. Because most of the attention concerning the adverse effects of antimalarials has been associated with the use of mefloquine, this drug is presented first. The other five drugs of interest are ordered by the FDA date of approval for use as a prophylactic for malaria, from most recent to earliest. Each drug-specific chapter begins with a brief history of the drug's development and use followed by a summary of the changes that have been made to the drug package insert or label since its approval as a prophylactic drug for malaria and then its pharmacokinetic properties. Known short-term adverse events associated with the use of the drug are then reported, followed by a summary and assessment of each of the identified epidemiologic studies that met the committee's inclusion criteria and were able to contribute some information on long-term health outcomes following cessation of the drug. Because neurologic and psychiatric outcomes, including PTSD, were specified in the committee's charge, results related to these outcomes are presented whenever they have been reported. Supplemental supporting evidence is then presented, including other identified studies of health

---

[1] Public access materials can be requested from paro@nas.edu.

outcomes in populations that used the drug of interest for prophylaxis but that did not meet the committee's inclusion criteria regarding the timing of follow-up; case reports of persistent adverse events; and information on adverse events of the drug when used in specific groups, such as women who are pregnant or those who have chronic health conditions. After the primary and supplemental evidence in humans is presented, supporting literature from experimental animal and in vitro studies is then summarized. Each chapter ends with a synthesis of all of the evidence presented and the inferences and conclusions that can be made from the available evidence, organized by body system category (neurologic disorders, psychiatric disorders, gastrointestinal disorders, eye disorders, cardiovascular disorders, and other disorders).

Chapter 10 contains a summary of the inferences from the available literature along with the methodologic challenges and limitations to investigating the persistent or latent effects of antimalarial drugs for prophylaxis. The committee discusses research considerations or approaches that can be implemented to improve the quality of data collected as well as the overall evidence base. Appendix A provides a list of open meeting agendas and invited presentation topics and Appendix B summarizes the invited presentations to the committee. A table that gives a high-level overview of each of the 21 epidemiologic studies that met the committee's inclusion criteria is presented in Appendix C. Committee and staff biographies can be found in Appendix D.

REFERENCES

Arguin, P. M., and A. J. Magill. 2017. For the record: A history of malaria chemoprophylaxis. https://wwwnc.cdc.gov/travel/yellowbook/2018/infectious-diseases-related-to-travel/emfor-the-record-a-history-of-malaria-chemoprophylaxisem (accessed December 18, 2018).

WHO (World Health Organization). 2019. *World Malaria Report, 2019.* https://www.who.int/publications-detail/world-malaria-report-2019 (accessed December 10, 2019).

Woodson, J. 2013. *Guidance on medications for prophylaxis of malaria.* Department of Defense Health Affairs. Memorandum prepared for Assistant Secretary of the Army (Manpower and Reserve Affairs), Assistant Secretary of the Navy (Manpower and Reserve Affairs), Assistant Secretary of the Air Force (Manpower and Reserve Affairs), Joint Staff Surgeon, Vice Commandant of the Coast Guard. https://health.mil/Reference-Center/Policies/2013/04/15/Guidance-on-Medications-for-Prophylaxis-of-Malaria (accessed November 5, 2019).

2

Background

This chapter provides background and information on several aspects of the committee's work. It begins with an overview of malaria as a disease and of the need for antimalarial drugs for prophylaxis. It then provides an overview of how the antimalarials under consideration interrupt the life cycle of the *Plasmodium* parasites and discusses the differences among causal prophylaxis, suppressive prophylaxis, presumptive anti-relapse therapy, and the treatment of malaria. An overview of differences among the classes of antimalarial drugs and their mechanisms of action is also provided. The next part of the chapter focuses on the use of prophylactic antimalarial drugs within military populations, including adherence and concurrent exposures that could occur during military service.

MALARIA IN HUMANS

The World Health Organization (WHO) has estimated that in 2018 there were 228 million cases of malaria (range, 206 million to 258 million) occurring in 87 countries and that 405,000 of these cases resulted in death. Nearly 50% of the world's population live in malaria-risk areas. WHO's Africa region carries the highest global burden of malaria, with 93% of the world's cases and almost 50% of its deaths occurring there. More than 60% of the malaria deaths in Africa are estimated to occur in children under 5 years of age. In 2018, just six countries in Africa accounted for more than half of all malaria cases worldwide: Nigeria (25%), the Democratic Republic of the Congo (12%), Uganda (5%), Côte d'Ivoire (4%), Mozambique (4%), and Niger (4%). By contrast, WHO's South-East Asia Region and Eastern Mediterranean Region accounted for 3.4% and 2.1% of cases, respectively (WHO, 2019). In 2016, 2,078 confirmed cases of (and 7 deaths from) malaria, nearly all imported, occurred in the United States, the majority of which (n = 1,729) originated in Africa (Mace et al., 2019). Increasing opportunities for international travel creates the risk of contracting malaria in populations that would otherwise not be exposed (Lalloo and Magill, 2019).

The vast majority of people residing in endemic areas experience malaria multiple times over their lifetimes, and very often the disease involves two or more species and stages of parasite. Consequently, as they age, these people often develop a partial immunity to each malaria species that they were infected with and subsequently experience less severe illness when infected with any of the species to which they have previously been exposed (Baird, 2012). WHO has made malaria case reduction a priority with the goal of reducing morbidity and mortality associated with malaria by 90% by the year 2030. Such an endeavor will require a multipronged approach to greatly reduce the transmission of malaria in endemic populations, primarily through the use of drugs for prophylaxis or treatment, vector control, and early diagnosis, and it will require improvements in access to and availability of antimalarial drugs for both prophylaxis and treatment, political leadership, increased resources, new tools (such as an efficacious vaccine), and education about antimalarial drugs and the need for increased drug adherence. Resistance to efficacious antimalarial drugs is a major concern, and this has been observed for several of the available drugs. Improvements in the availability of high-quality, correctly dosed drugs is particularly important, as antimalarial drugs of substandard quality or even falsified contents have been reported in endemic areas (Kaur et al., 2015; Newton et al., 2017). Low-quality drugs and falsified drugs contribute to drug resistance and higher levels of morbidity and mortality.

Disease

Infection with the *Plasmodium* parasite occurs after an infected female *Anopheles* mosquito takes a blood meal from a human host. Once the parasite infects a human, it migrates to the liver and enters into an incubation period during which the parasite establishes itself within the body and continues its life cycle. Depending on the *Plasmodium* species, the incubation period lasts from 7 to 30 days, and no symptoms of malaria are present during this time. For *P. falciparum*, typically about 10 to 15 days after the infective bite occurs, the first signs of disease will manifest. Most patients with uncomplicated malaria present with some combination of common symptoms including fever, chills, sweats, headaches, nausea, vomiting, body aches, or general malaise. Additional symptoms may include abdominal cramping, cough, muscle pains, and varying levels of mental disorientation. These symptoms are typically the result of the human immune response to massive hemolysis and malaria parasites being released into the bloodstream (Moss and Morrow, 2014).

If uncomplicated malaria is not treated in a timely manner, severe malaria can develop. Features of severe malaria generally appear 3 to 7 days after the onset of the symptoms associated with uncomplicated malaria. According to WHO, the case definition of severe malaria includes one or more of the following symptoms or clinical findings that occurs in the absence of an identified alternative cause and in the presence of *P. falciparum* asexual parasitemia: impaired consciousness, acidosis, hypoglycemia, severe malarial anemia, renal impairment or acute kidney injury, jaundice, pulmonary edema, significant bleeding, shock, or hyperparasitemia (WHO, 2014).

The current case definition of severe malaria by WHO no longer includes neurologic symptoms or abnormalities outside of those associated with a coma. Prior to the 2014 malaria case definition revision, cerebral malaria was defined as severe malaria in which patients who were not comatose also exhibited neurologic symptoms (e.g., headache, neck stiffness, drowsiness, agitation, delirium, febrile convulsions, focal neurologic signs, or behavioral disturbances). Neurologic symptoms were eliminated from the case definition because high fever alone, which is a common symptom of malaria, is known to produce mild impairment of consciousness (sometimes referred to as delirium, obtundation, obnubilation, confusion, and psychosis) (WHO, 2014). The removal of other neurologic symptoms or abnormalities from the case definition also allowed for comparability of clinical findings associated with severe malaria. Because it is difficult to differentiate between the symptoms caused by high fever and those caused by severe malaria, removing fever from the case definition allows for more precise diagnostic criteria in which fever is removed as a potential confounder.

Although WHO's case definition for severe malaria no longer includes neurologic symptoms not directly associated with coma, several studies have found that many survivors of severe malaria can develop long-term physiologic damage resulting in neurologic and cognitive deficits (Idro et al., 2006, 2010, 2016; John et al., 2008). Studies examining the relationship between uncomplicated malaria and long-term neurologic and psychiatric effects have been inconclusive (Dugbartey et al., 1998; Fernando et al., 2003).

In addition to neurologic and cognitive deficits that may be caused by clinical malaria, the Centers for Disease Control and Prevention (CDC) has reported that it has potential for other long-term health consequences as well. Serious long-term health effects can include severe anemia, rupture of the spleen, nephrotic syndrome, hyperreactive malarial splenomegaly, severe disease in a pregnant mother, premature birth or low-birth-weight infants, and recurrence of malaria infection. These symptoms can lead to severe disability and may even result in death if malaria infections remain untreated. Prompt and adequate treatment can prevent the development of these more serious health consequences (CDC, 2019a).

Infectious Agents

There are five species of the *Plasmodium* parasite that are known to cause disease in humans: *Plasmodium falciparum, Plasmodium vivax, Plasmodium ovale,*

Plasmodium malariae, and *Plasmodium knowlesi*. Figure 2-1 summarizes the life cycle of all *Plasmodium* parasites, although the specific details of the progression through the cycle vary among the five species. A result of this variation is that the timelines for symptom presentation and the targets of drug actions differ among the species (CDC, 2019a).

After the *Plasmodium* parasite enters the human body, it migrates to the liver and begins invading hepatocyctes; this is the exo-erythrocytic phase of the *Plasmodium* life cycle. Once in the hepatocytes, the incubation period varies, resulting in different timelines being observed between infection and the presentation of symptoms for different infective species. The *P. falciparium*, *P. malariae*, and *P. knowlesi* species enter the incubation period, and over the next several days replicate thousands of times inside the hepatocytes. The increasing parasitic load inside liver cells eventually causes the hepatocyte to swell and rupture, releasing thousands of parasites into the bloodstream. Once in the bloodstream, the parasite enters into the erythrocytic phase of its life cycle and continues replicating within the body (Moss and Morrow, 2014).

By contrast, *P. vivax* and *P. ovale* can, after invading the hepatocytes, either continue to progress through the life cycle (like *P. falciparum*, *P. malariae*, or *P. knowlesi*) or become hypnozoites and lie dormant within the hepatocyte for up to several years before reactivating and resuming their development, subsequently causing clinical symptoms of malaria. During this dormant period *P. vivax* and *P. ovale* hypnozoites remain undetectable by the human immune system or any current diagnostic techniques. These hypnozoites can differentiate at any time into the next stage of the life cycle, at which point they are released into the bloodstream (Moss and Morrow, 2014). Importantly, not all dormant parasites differentiate at the same time. This means some of the dormant parasites may differentiate and continue through the parasite life cycle, while others may remain dormant and undetectable. This complicates the prophylaxis and treatment needed for these two *Plasmodium* species; therefore, prophylactics that target the exo-erythrocytic stage of the *Plasmodium* life cycle are critical for preventing infection with *P. vivax* and *P. ovale*.

PROPHYLACTIC ANTIMALARIAL DRUGS

As described in Chapter 1, the antimalarial drugs covered by this report are those that are currently available and approved by the Food and Drug Administration (FDA) as of 2019 for malaria prophylaxis in adults and that are currently being used, or that have been used in the past 25 years by U.S. military personnel for malaria prophylaxis. Specifically, they are mefloquine, tafenoquine, atovaquone/proguanil (A/P), doxycycline, primaquine, and chloroquine.

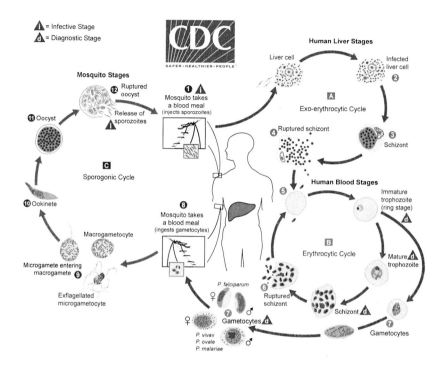

FIGURE 2-1 Life cycle of the *Plasmodium* parasite.
NOTES: "The malaria parasite life cycle involves two hosts. During a blood meal, a malaria-infected female *Anopheles* mosquito inoculates sporozoites into the human host ❶. Sporozoites infect liver cells ❷ and mature into schizonts ❸, which rupture and release merozoites ❹. (Of note, in *P. vivax* and *P. ovale* a dormant stage [hypnozoites] can persist in the liver [if untreated] and cause relapses by invading the bloodstream weeks, or even years later.) After this initial replication in the liver (exo-erythrocytic schizogony Ⓐ), the parasites undergo asexual multiplication in the erythrocytes (erythrocytic schizogony Ⓑ). Merozoites infect red blood cells ❺. The ring stage trophozoites mature into schizonts, which rupture releasing merozoites ❻. Some parasites differentiate into sexual erythrocytic stages (gametocytes) ❼. Blood stage parasites are responsible for the clinical manifestations of the disease. The gametocytes, male (microgametocytes) and female (macrogametocytes), are ingested by an *Anopheles* mosquito during a blood meal ❽. The parasites' multiplication in the mosquito is known as the sporogonic cycle Ⓒ. While in the mosquito's stomach, the microgametes penetrate the macrogametes generating zygotes ❾. The zygotes in turn become motile and elongated (ookinetes) ❿, which invade the midgut wall of the mosquito where they develop into oocysts ⓫. The oocysts grow, rupture, and release sporozoites ⓬, which make their way to the mosquito's salivary glands. Inoculation of the sporozoites ❶ into a new human host perpetuates the malaria life cycle" (CDC, 2017).
SOURCE: CDC, 2017.

Differences Between Causal Prophylaxis, Suppressive Prophylaxis, Presumptive Anti-Relapse Therapy, and Treatment of Malaria

There are two types of prophylaxis used to prevent the development of clinical malaria: causal and suppressive. Briefly, causal prophylaxis is begun in persons free of infection, and it prevents the formation of both tissue schizonts in the liver and hypnozoites of the malaria parasite. Suppressive prophylaxis refers to drugs that act only on parasites within the red blood cells (Schwartz, 2012). Neither type of prophylaxis prevents human infection with *Plasmodium* parasites; instead, the drugs inhibit the *Plasmodium* parasite's ability to further establish infection, replicate, and cause clinical disease; the drugs are also used to prevent recurrence of malaria. Two other categories of antimalarial drugs are approved for use by FDA: those for presumptive anti-relapse therapy (PART) and drugs for treatment of malaria. Precise definitions that clearly explain the differences between the different types of prophylaxis were not available from CDC, WHO, or FDA. As a result, the following definitions were compiled from other sources.

Richter et al. (2016) defines recurrence of malaria as a clinical malaria attack after it has been treated. Recurrence is further differentiated into recrudescence and relapse. Recrudescence is defined as "malaria recurrence originating from subclinical low-level circulating asexual erythrocytic stages, and the *Plasmodium* species associated with recrudescence are genetically identical to the ones of the first attack" (Richter et al., 2016, p. 2140). Relapse is defined as "malaria recurrence originating from the latent *Plasmodium* tissue stages (hypnozoites) associated with *P. vivax* and *P. ovale* species, and the *Plasmodium* species associated with relapse are heterologous and differ from those causing the first malaria episode" (Richter et al., 2016, p. 2140); however, relapses may be genetically identical, if the initial infection was monogenomic. Recrudescence is often linked to the failure or low efficacy of suppressive antimalarial prophylaxis, whereas relapse can be associated with the inappropriate use of suppressive prophylaxis for the prevention of hypnozoites from *P. vivax* or *P. ovale* infection or with the failure of causal prophylaxis.

Causal Prophylaxis

Of the six drugs included in this report, three exhibit causal prophylactic activity: A/P, primaquine, and tafenoquine. A/P exhibits causal prophylactic activity only against *P. falciparum*, and it is not effective against hypnozoites associated with *P. ovale* or *P. vivax*. Causal prophylaxis, also called exo-erythrocytic stage prophylaxis, kills the *Plasmodium* parasite before it can complete its development in the liver, thereby inhibiting the parasite's ability to replicate or cause clinical disease (60 Degrees Pharmaceuticals, 2018). The use of causal prophylaxis to prevent infection with *P. vivax* and *P. ovale* is critical; these species can remain dormant in the liver for long periods (up to several years) after an infection occurs and can result in relapse of disease. Causal prophylaxis should be taken for 7–14 days after returning from an area with endemic malaria because the parasites are killed early in their life cycle and they never enter the bloodstream. Figure 2-1 illustrates the way in which causal prophylaxis interferes with the exo-erythrocytic phase of the *Plasmodium* life cycle (A; steps 1–4). Because causal prophylaxis acts on the exo-erythrocytic stage of the life cycle, it can prevent human infection by all *Plasmodium* parasites. It is believed that causal prophylactic drugs work by interfering with some key cellular processes necessary for replication and cell survival, including deoxyribonucleic acid (DNA) replication and mitochondrial function (Schwartz, 2012).

Suppressive Prophylaxis

Whereas some of the drugs used for causal prophylaxis also demonstrate suppressive prophylactic activity (e.g., A/P, primaquine, and tafenoquine), mefloquine, chloroquine, and doxycycline are defined exclusively as suppressive antimalarial prophylactic drugs. Suppressive prophylaxis has no effect on *Plasmodium* parasites until the liver phase of the life cycle is complete and the parasite has invaded red blood cells. Suppressive prophylaxis is ineffective against hypnozoites of *P. vivax* or *P. ovale*, but it will kill *P. vivax* or *P. ovale* parasites that have entered the bloodstream (Schwartz, 2012). Figure 2-1 shows how suppressive prophylaxis interferes with the erythrocytic phase of the *Plasmodium* life cycle (B; steps 5–7). Taking suppressive prophylaxis as directed will suppress the symptoms of malaria in individuals who are infected with the malaria parasite. However, if suppressive prophylaxis is not taken as directed, symptoms of the disease will likely appear. Because these drugs act only on parasites in red blood cells, an individual must take them for 4 weeks after leaving an area with endemic malaria in order to eliminate parasites that may appear in the bloodstream during that time (Moss and Morrow, 2014).

The mechanisms of action for suppressive prophylactic drugs vary but are known to include blocking the production of hemozoin, which is a chemical that the parasite produces to protect itself from the toxic products produced as a result of its digestion of hemoglobin by turning them into a non-toxic compound; inhibiting vesicle functions that may interfere with phospholipid metabolism; binding to and altering the parasite's DNA; blocking transcription and translation of DNA into RNA and proteins; and impairing the expression of the apicoplast (a collection of structures present in *Plasmodium* parasites that allows for the invasion of host cells and the establishment of the parasite–host interaction) genes in the parasite, resulting in the inability of the parasite to replicate its DNA (Parhizgar and Tahghighi, 2017).

Presumptive Anti-Relapse Therapy

PART, also known as terminal prophylaxis, is the use of an antimalarial drug toward the end of the exposure period (or immediately thereafter) to prevent relapses or the delayed onset of clinical malaria caused by hypnozoites (dormant exo-erythrocytic stages) of *P. vivax* or *P. ovale*. PART is generally indicated for people who have had prolonged exposure in malaria-endemic areas (such as military personnel, Peace Corps volunteers, or missionaries) (CDC, 2019a). Two of the drugs included in this report, primaquine and tafenoquine, can be used both as primary prophylaxis and as PART. When used for PART, these drugs are often given in combination with chloroquine or another blood schizonticide. PART is an important factor in preventing relapse of malaria. Because PART agents act on both the exo-erythrocytic and erythrocytic stages, they affect the malaria life cycle at the same points as causal and suppressive prophylactic agents (see A and B in Figure 2-1).

Treatment

An inherent distinguishing factor between the prophylaxis and the treatment of malaria is how the antimalarial drugs are used: prophylaxis prevents disease, while the goal of treatment is to cure infection. Each of the drugs included in this report can be used for either prophylaxis or treatment; however, the dosage at which each drug is used for the treatment of malaria is significantly higher than when it is used for prophylaxis. For example, the treatment dose of A/P is four times higher than its prophylactic dose. As a result of the higher blood concentrations achieved with treatment regimens, adverse events may occur with treatment that are not observed when the drug is used for prophylaxis, or adverse events may be more severe in their presentation (Arguin and Magill, 2017; CDC, 2019b). Whereas the FDA package insert for A/P lists diarrhea, dreams, oral ulcers, and headache as common adverse events ($\geq 4\%$ of adults) when A/P is used as directed for prophylaxis, the common ($\geq 5\%$ of adults) adverse events when A/P is used for treatment include abdominal pain, nausea, vomiting, headache, diarrhea, asthenia, anorexia, and dizziness (FDA, 2019).

Distinguishing Between the Different Classes of Antimalarial Drugs

The antimalarial drugs under consideration in this report belong to several drug classes (based on chemical structure): 8-aminoquinolines (primaquine and tafenoquine), 4-aminoquinolines (chloroquine), tetracyclines (doxycycline), and quinoline methanols (mefloquine). A/P is a combination drug: atovaquone belongs to the class of naphthoquinones and proguanil is a synthetic arylbiguanide (antifolate). The adverse events of a given drug are often difficult to predict a priori, but sometimes the compounds of a certain drug class result in common adverse events. However, even though numerous non-antimalarial drugs contain quinoline (or quinolone) substructures, these structurally diverse drugs have adverse event profiles that are distinct from those of the antimalarial quinolines discussed in this report. The following text explains the different mechanisms of action that each drug class exhibits on the *Plasmodium* parasites; however, it is important to note that each drug class also exhibits unique pharmacokinetic and pharmaco-dynamic properties once inside the human body. The differences are not limited to the characteristics observed at a drug class level, but are also observed between individual drugs within the same drug class. Detailed information on the different pharmacokinetic and pharmacodynamic properties of each drug are presented in each drug-specific chapter.

8-Aminoquinolines

The 8-aminoquinoline class of antimalarials is unique in that it owes its ability to prevent the relapsing forms of malaria by acting against the malaria hypnozoites that lie dormant in the liver (Marcsisin et al., 2014). Primaquine, the prototype 8-aminoquinoline, was developed in 1945 and has prophylactic activity against the liver stage of all malaria parasites, against the asexual and sexual stages of *P. vivax*, *P. ovale*, *P. malariae*, and *P. knowlesi*, and the sexual stages of *P. falciparum* (it is only weakly active against the asexual blood stages of *P. falciparum*), and it has radical curative activity in *P. vivax* and *P. ovale* malaria. It is the most widely used 8-aminoquinoline for malaria prophylaxis, but its exact mechanism of action is still unknown. Primaquine localizes within the *Plasmodium* mitochondria and impairs the mitochondrial metabolism, which suggests drug-induced mitochondrial dysfunction as a potential mechanism of action (Schlagenhauf et al., 2019).

In general, 8-aminoquinolines are metabolized by the cytochrome P450 CYP2D family (particularly CYP2D6), which is required for both their anti-malarial activity and their toxicity. Several possible modes of action on the parasite have been proposed. One hypothesis is that active metabolites of 8-aminoquinolines may lead to mitochondrial dysfunction (Schlagenhauf et al., 2019) and the alteration of intracellular membrane structures in both erythrocytic and pre-erythrocytic stages of the parasite. Another hypothesis is that the highly reactive metabolites generate intracellular reactive species, which cause oxidative damage. The primaquine metabolite, 5-hydroxyprimaquine, and its downstream oxidation products such as the corresponding 5,6-orthoquinone (Fasinu et al., 2019) cause a substantial generation of reactive oxygen species, most notably hydrogen peroxide (Camarda et al., 2019). This leads to the killing of the malaria parasite (Camarda et al., 2019), methemoglobinemia (Liu et al., 2011), and oxida-tive damage to the erythrocyte cytoskeleton (Bowman et al., 2005).

Tafenoquine was first identified in 1978, but it was only recently approved (2018) for the prophylaxis and radical cure of malaria. Clinical trials of tafenoquine have not definitively determined whether it works via a causal or a suppressive prophylaxis mechanism (Baird, 2018). Tafenoquine is substantially more active against the erythrocytic stages of the *Plasmodium* life cycle than primaquine, and it is more slowly metabolized with a terminal elimination half-life of 14–17 days. Tafenoquine is active against all pre-erythrocytic and erythrocytic forms of human malaria as well as against the gametocytes of *P. falciparum* and *P. vivax* (FDA, 2018a).

Neither the precise mechanism of action of tafenoquine nor its molecular target have been determined. In vitro studies with the erythrocytic forms of *P. falciparum* suggest that tafenoquine may exert its effect by inhibiting hemozoin formation and inducing apoptotic-like death of the parasite (FDA, 2018b; Vennerstrom et al., 1999). This may explain why tafenoquine is active against the asexual blood stage of parasites, unlike primaquine, which does not inhibit hemozoin formation (Ebstie et al., 2016). Otherwise, the mechanism of action of tafenoquine is similar to that of primaquine (Ebstie et al., 2016) in which the spontaneous oxidation of metabolites generates hydrogen peroxide and hydroxyl radicals. The reactive oxygen species generated through *P. falciparum* ferredoxin-nicotinamide adenine dinucleotide phosphate ($NADP^+$) reductase and diflavin reductase enzymes are thought to result in parasite death, a theory that is supported by the upregulation of these enzymes in tafenoquine-sensitive stages of the parasite (Ebstie et al., 2016).

One limitation of antimalarial 8-aminoquinolines is that they are contra-indicated in people who have the X-linked glucose-6-phosphate dehydrogenase (G6PD) genetic defect. G6PD deficiency is the most common genetic human enzyme disorder, with 186 genetic variants that have been described. It is esti-mated to affect more than 400 million people worldwide, most of them in malaria-endemic areas and most commonly in males (Nkhoma et al., 2009). G6PD is the key enzyme in the oxidative pentose phosphate pathway. It converts $NADP^+$ into its reduced form, NADPH. NADPH is essential for protection against oxida-tive stress in erythrocytes. G6PD deficiency causes an increased susceptibility of erythrocytes to hydrogen peroxide and other reactive oxygen species which can lead to hemolysis (the rupture of red blood cells and release of their contents into the plasma) and hemolytic anemia (red blood cells being destroyed faster than they can be replaced), which in turn can lead to other serious complications, including arrhythmias, cardiomyopathy, heart failure, and death (NIH, n.d.; Peters and Van Noorden, 2009). The extent of hemolysis depends on the dose and dura-tion of drug exposure and the degree of G6PD deficiency. Persons with >80% of normal red-blood-cell G6PD activity are considered to be G6PD normal (WHO, 2016a). Males with <10% normal red-blood-cell G6PD activity are regarded as G6PD deficient; females with 30–80% of normal red-blood-cell G6PD activity are considered to be G6PD intermediate, and those with <30% are regarded as G6PD deficient. A study of more than 63,000 U.S. military personnel determined that 2.5% of men and 1.6% of women were G6PD deficient, with most of them having a moderate level of deficiency (Chinevere et al., 2006). The highest rates of deficiency were seen in African American men (12.2%) and women (4.1%) and Asian men (4.3%).

WHO recommends the use of ultraviolet spectrophotometry as the gold standard for measuring G6PD activity; however, this technique requires technol-ogy that is not suitable for field development or point-of-care testing. As a result, the most commonly used field test for G6PD deficiency is the fluorescent spot test (FST), a semi-quantitative assay that requires minimal laboratory supplies and does not require expertise for result interpretation. Several qualitative tests have been recently introduced that have better operational characteristics and similar detection capabilities as the FST. These tests can only distinguish G6PD homozygous females and hemizygous males with intermediate enzyme activities above 30% of normal from G6PD-normal individuals. Because G6PD deficiency is linked to the X chromosome, females can present with homozygous, heterozygous, or normal G6PD gene expression. The commonly used field tests are insufficient for detecting G6PD activity in heterozygous females with intermediate enzyme activities that fall outside of the 30% of normal threshold. As a result, heterozygous females may express G6PD-deficient characteristics that are not detected by the currently available field testing procedures (Ley et al., 2017); the presentation of these false-negative results may lead to inadvertent exposure to 8-aminoquinoline antimalarial drugs and their subsequent adverse events (Peters and Van Noorden, 2009). Recently, researchers have also begun exploring quantitative testing that can be administered in resource-limited settings; however, many of these tests are still in development or are undergoing evaluation (Pal et al., 2019).

Methemoglobinemia, usually mild and reversible, is a well-characterized feature in recipients of 8-aminoquinolines at therapeutic dosing (Baird, 2019). Methemoglobinemia occurs when the level of methemoglobin in red blood cells exceeds 1%, which can lead to decreased availability of oxygen to tissues (Denshaw-Burke et al., 2018). Severe methemoglobinemia can lead to complications, including abnormal cardiac rhythms, altered mental status, delirium, seizures, coma, and profound acidosis; if the level of methemoglobin in red blood cells exceeds 70%, death can result.

4-Aminoquinolines

As reviewed by Foley and Tilley (1998) and O'Neill et al. (2006), chloroquine, which was first discovered in 1934, is the prototype 4-aminoquinoline antimalarial drug. Both enantiomers of the racemic chloroquine have equivalent antimalarial activity. Chloroquine is active against the erythrocytic stages of all species of malaria, and it is also active against the gametocytes of *P. vivax*, *P. malariae*, and *P. ovale*. It is a diprotic weak base, and it works by concentrating in the parasite food vacuole and binding tightly to hematin as it is formed during the digestion of hemoglobin by the parasite. The binding of chloroquine to hematin interferes with the assembly of hematin into the non-toxic hemozoin, or malaria pigment, and this may increase the intrinsic toxicity of hematin to the parasite. As reviewed by Ecker et al. (2012), drug resistance to chloroquine in *P. falciparum* is mediated primarily by mutant forms of the chloroquine resistance transporter (PfCRT). These mutant forms of PfCRT effectively efflux chloroquine from the parasite digestive vacuole, the site of the drug's action. Mutations in PfCRT allow the parasite to persist at drug levels that kill chloroquine-sensitive parasites. Some researchers have suggested that chloroquine-sensitive *P. falciparum* is returning in parts of Africa due to the discontinuation of the widespread use of chloroquine in the early 1990s, which may have resulted in the parasite's reversal to a chloroquine-sensitive state (Schlagenhauf et al., 2019). Individuals who have G6PD deficiency should be closely monitored while receiving chloroquine because of the potential for hemolysis to occur; however, significant hemolysis is rare when the drug is given at prophylactic and therapeutic doses (Schlagenhauf et al., 2019).

Quinoline Methanols

Mefloquine is a synthetic structural analog of quinine (Hellgren et al., 1997). Mefloquine, as well as the other antimalarial quinolines such as chloroquine, primaquine, and tafenoquine, differs considerably from quinine with respect to both its mechanistic biology and the adverse events associated with its use. Furthermore, as numerous non-antimalarial drugs also contain quinoline substructures, overgeneralizations about adverse events of quinolines as a group are unwarranted (Dorwald, 2012). Mefloquine, a quinoline methanol, was first identified as a compound with antimalarial activity in animal models in the 1960s and was approved for prophylaxis and the treatment of malaria in humans in 1984. Mefloquine consists of a 50:50 racemic mixture of the erythro isomers available as tablets containing 250 mg of mefloquine salt. The formulation of mefloquine available in the United States contains 250 mg of mefloquine hydrochloride.

Mefloquine is a potent, long-acting blood schizonticide that is effective against all malarial species that infect humans (Schlagenhauf et al., 2010); however, it has no activity against the liver stages of parasite development (Palmer et al., 1993). Both the (+) and the (–) enantiomers are active against *P. falciparum,* but a higher activity for (+) mefloquine has been reported (Hellgren et al., 1997). One major reason for its importance in the malaria-prophylaxis armamentarium is its efficacy against chloroquine-sensitive and chloroquine-resistant *P. falciparum,* (Palmer et al., 1993), although resistance of *P. falciparum* to mefloquine is known to exist in parts of Cambodia, Laos, Myanmar, Thailand, and Vietnam (CDC, 2019a). The exact mechanism of action is unclear, but it is thought that inhibiting hemozoin formation in the *P. falciparum* food vacuole causes a toxic accumulation of the highly reactive hematin moiety, which in turn kills the parasite; oxidative damage is believed to play a role (Ridley et al., 1997; Sullivan et al., 1998). One study has found that in addition to inhibiting hemozoin, mefloquine can induce apoptosis in *Plasmodium* species by activating metacaspase and reactive oxygen species production (Gunjan et al., 2016). More recently, mefloquine was found to act by targeting the *P. falciparum* 80S ribosome to inhibit protein synthesis (Wong et al., 2017).

Antibiotics

Tetracyclines are a class of broad-spectrum antibiotic drugs that are used to treat a wide range of illnesses. Tetracyclines were first investigated for their antimalarial potential in the 1960s after the emergence of chloroquine-resistant *P. falciparum* parasites. The tetracycline drug doxycycline is a slow-acting schizonticidal agent. In addition to its activity against the erythrocytic stage of the parasite, doxycycline is thought to possess some pre-erythrocytic (causal) activity, but efficacy studies found unacceptably high failure rates for its use as a causal prophylactic. There is very limited evidence concerning doxycycline's effect on gametocytes of *Plasmodium* species, and it has been shown to have no effect on the hypnozoites. In one study that examined gametocytemia and doxycycline, *P. vivax* gametocytemia increased from 32% pre-treatment to 44% immediately post-treatment, and the median gametocyte clearance time was 62 hours. Gametocytemia has no clinical implications, but malaria may still be transmitted through mosquitoes if they bite an individual being treated for malaria with doxycycline (Tan et al., 2011).

Although doxycycline is known to be a blood schizontocide, the exact mechanism of its action is not well defined (Schlagenhauf et al., 2019). In *P. falciparum*, doxycycline impairs the expression of apicoplast genes, leading to nonfunctional apicoplasts in subsequent progeny, and it impedes the development of viable parasites. Doxycycline's antimalarial actions may be similar to its bacteriostatic actions of binding to ribosomal subunits and inhibiting protein synthesis, but this has only been observed in suprapharmacologic doses (Tan et al., 2011).

Combinations (Antifolates)

Atovaquone/proguanil (A/P) is a fixed drug combination made from atovaquone and proguanil for the prophylaxis of *P. falciparum* malaria. Atovaquone is a hydroxynaphthoquinone, and proguanil is a synthetic arylbiguanide (antifolate); the two drugs work synergistically against the erythrocytic stages of all the *Plasmodium* parasites and against the liver stage (causal prophylaxis) of *P. falciparum*. A/P is not active against hypnozoites in *P. vivax* or *P. ovale,* and it does not prevent relapse infections (Nixon et al., 2013).

Atovaquone acts by inhibiting the *Plasmodium* species' mitochondrial electron transport at the cytochrome bc_1 complex, which collapses mitochondrial membrane potential. The electron transport system of the *Plasmodium* species is 1,000 times more sensitive to atovaquone than this system in mammals, which is thought to explain the selective action and limited adverse events of the drug (Schlagenhauf et al., 2019). Inhibition of the *Plasmodium* bc_1 complex by atovaquone affects the concentrations of metabolites in the pyrimidine biosynthetic pathway and in the biosynthesis of purine, both of which are required for DNA replication in the *Plasmodium* parasite (Boggild et al., 2007). Proguanil is metabolized to cycloguanil, which inhibits dihydrofolate reductase, resulting in an impeding of the synthesis of folate cofactors required for parasite DNA synthesis.

When atovaquone and proguanil are given in combination, both in vitro and in vivo studies have found the mechanism of action to be synergistic between the two of them (Canfield et al., 1995; Looareesuwan et al., 1999). This leads to high cure rates of *P. falciparum* malaria, even in cases where the parasites have developed a resistance to cycloguanil conferred by DHFR mutations (Gay et al., 1997). The cause of the synergy between proguanil and atovaquone is thought to be found in the biguanide mode of action, not in the action of its metabolite(s) (Srivastava et al., 1999). Proguanil acts synergistically with atovaquone in individuals with proguanil-resistant parasites or in those who are unable to metabolize proguanil to cycloguanil because of CYP450 enzyme deficiencies (Helsby et al., 1990; Looareesuwan et al., 1999).

MILITARY USE OF ANTIMALARIALS

Malaria has affected almost all U.S. military deployments, actions, and overseas exercises since the American Civil War (see Table 2-1), and despite advances in antimalarial drugs and improvements in preventive equipment and supplies, it remains an ongoing threat (IOM, 2006). The number of malaria cases in U.S. service members varies each year and recently has ranged from a high of 124 cases in 2011 to a low of 30 cases in 2013 and 2015 (AFHSC, 2013, 2014, 2015, 2016; WHO, 2016b). A 65% increase in reported cases of malaria in military service members was reported between 2017 (35 cases) and 2018 (58 cases), and more than 25% of the cases in 2018 were due to *P. falciparum*, the most severe species of malaria (AFHSB, 2019). Successful control of malaria in the military demands effective prophylactic interventions, force-wide education about malaria and prevention, and prophylactic adherence by individual service members.

Keeping abreast of malaria medically and technologically has been a continuing effort for the U.S. military. During World War II the Japanese blockade of Javanese and Philippine quinine sources, Germany's monopoly on manufacturing available quinine and the antimalarial quinicrine (also known as mepacrine and under the trade name Atabrine), and intelligence that Germany was synthesizing new antimalarials all served to compel the United States to attempt to synthesize quinicrine based on a drug sample and to spur the United States and its allies to focus research into new synthetic antimalarials (IOM, 2006; Kitchen et al., 2006).

By 1942, the United States had successfully synthesized quinicrine, and U.S. service members were receiving it. The antimalarial research program, a collaboration among the military, scientific institutions, universities, and pharmaceutical firms, was established in 1941. Two of its early discoveries were chloroquine, which is effective against *P. falciparum* and which the U.S. military began using in 1945, and primaquine, which is effective against *P. vivax* and was first used on

TABLE 2-1 Major U.S. Military Actions, Deployments, or Overseas Exercises in Locations with a Malaria Threat, 1861–2003

Location	Year	Threat	Morbidity and Mortality
Civil War (Union)	1861–1865	*P. vivax,* *P. falciparum*	1.3 million cases, 10,000 deaths[a]
Panama Canal	1904–1914	*P. vivax,* *P. falciparum* *P. vivax*	1906 malaria rate 1,263/1,000/year 1913 malaria rate 76/1,000/year[b] Estimated 5,000 cases overseas
WWI	1914–1918	*P. falciparum*	1917: 7.5/1,000/year in United States[c]
WWII	1939–1945	*P. vivax*	600,000 cases mostly in Pacific theater. In some areas of South Pacific malaria rates were 4,000/1,000/year (4 cases per person per year) (Downs et al., 1947)
Korean War	1950–1953	*P. vivax*	Malaria rate 611/1,000/year 3,000 cases in troops returning to United States[d]
Vietnam War	1962–1975	*P. falciparum,* *P. vivax*	100,000 cases[e] 1.7/1,000 case fatality rate Hospital admissions 27/1,000/year 1965 malaria rate for U.S. Army forces: 98/1,000/year 1970: 2,222 cases (mostly *P. vivax*) Treated in United States
Panama	1988–1989	*P. falciparum*	Action primarily in Panama City
Persian Gulf	1991	*P. vivax*	Few cases in northern Iraq, Kurdish area
Somalia	1992–1994	*P. falciparum,* *P. vivax*	48 cases; 243 cases in forces on return home[f] (CDC, 1993)
Nigeria	2001	Chloroquine-resistant *P. falciparum*	Special forces 7 cases (2 deaths in 300 men)
Afghanistan	2003	*P. vivax,* chloroquine-resistant *P. falciparum*	8 cases in 725 Ranger task force members[g] (Kotwal et al., 2005)
Liberia	2003	*P. falciparum*	U.S. marines 80/290 (28% attack rate) with 40 Marines evacuated by air to Germany
Iraq War	2003–	*P. vivax*	Few cases

[a] Records for the Confederate forces were difficult to find (probably not kept). One example in South Carolina was 42,000 cases in 18 months in 1862–1863. (Malaria was endemic in the United States until the late 1940s.)

[b] 1913 malaria rate drop was due to control measures enforced by Colonel Gorgas.

[c] Malaria rate for troops training and/or garrisoned in southern states.

[d] In troops returning home there were at one point 629 cases/week.

[e] Some operational areas were intense: Ia Drang Valley (1966) malaria rate 600/1,000/year, equivalent of 2 maneuver battalions rendered inoperative.

[f] In Bardera in 1993 where malaria is hyperendemic: 53/490 cases in Marines.

[g] Attack rate (June–September 2002) 52.4/1,000/year.

SOURCE: IOM, 2006.

U.S. ships returning from Korea in 1951 (Brundage, 2003; IOM, 2006). By the early 1960s, *P. falciparum* resistance to chloroquine had been reported in South America, Southeast Asia, and Oceania (CDC, 2018; Kitchen et al., 2006). By 1962, the "C-P pill," a combination tablet of chloroquine and primaquine, had become the standard prophylactic regimen for soldiers in Vietnam. In 1963, however, the increasing toll of chloroquine-resistant *P. falciparum* in service members in Vietnam led to the launch of the U.S. Army Medical Research Program on Malaria at the Walter Reed Army Institute of Research (Brundage, 2003; IOM, 2006; Ockenhouse et al., 2005). Within 10 years, 27 new drugs or drug combinations had been developed, including dapsone, mefloquine, and halofantrine, which appeared to be the answers to chloroquine-resistant *P. falciparum* (Brundage, 2003; IOM, 2006). In 1966 dapsone was added to the C-P tablet given to troops at high risk of chloroquine-resistant *P. falciparum* (Brundage, 2003); hydroxychloroquine may also have also been used in Vietnam and during the Korean War, although records are unclear.[1]

In the late 1960s mefloquine was developed by F. Hoffmann-LaRoche in collaboration with the Walter Reed Army Institute and WHO (Kitchen et al., 2006). It was approved in 1989, was likely used by the military as early as 1990, and was used during Operation Restore Hope in Somalia (1992–1993) and Operation Iraqi Freedom (OIF; 2003–2011) (Kitchen et al., 2006, Sánchez et al., 1993).[2] Mefloquine was used as a first-line prophylactic agent only for deployments to certain high-malaria-risk areas in sub-Saharan Africa, such as for the Liberian Task Force in 2003, and it was used as a second-line agent in OIF and Operation Enduring Freedom (OEF) (Wiesen, 2019). The military began testing doxycycline for malaria prophylaxis in 1985, but it was not used routinely for prophylaxis until 1992 in Somalia (Sánchez et al., 1993; Wallace et al., 1996).[3] Doxycycline was used as the first-line agent in OIF (2003–2007) and OEF (2001–present), and it continues to be used in deployments to malaria-endemic regions (DoD, 2013).

A 2009 Department of Defense (DoD) memorandum advised that in chloroquine-resistant areas where doxycycline and mefloquine are equally efficacious, and when personnel have a history of neurobehavioral disorders, doxycycline should be the first-line agent and A/P the second-line agent, and in those who cannot take doxycycline or A/P, mefloquine should be used very cautiously and with clinical follow-up (DoD, 2009). The memo also stated, presumably regard-

---

[1] Personal communication to the committee, COL Andrew Wiesen, M.D., M.P.H., Director, Preventive Medicine, Health Readiness Policy and Oversight, Office of the Assistant Secretary of Defense (Health Affairs), April 16, 2019.

[2] Personal communication to the committee, COL Andrew Wiesen, M.D., M.P.H., Director, Preventive Medicine, Health Readiness Policy and Oversight, Office of the Assistant Secretary of Defense (Health Affairs), April 16, 2019.

[3] Personal communication to the committee, COL Andrew Wiesen, M.D., M.P.H., Director, Preventive Medicine, Health Readiness Policy and Oversight, Office of the Assistant Secretary of Defense (Health Affairs), April 16, 2019.

ing personnel with no history of neurobehavioral disorders, that mefloquine should only be used by those with contraindications to doxycycline and without contraindications to mefloquine. A 2013 DoD memo stated that doxycycline and A/P were to be considered first-line agents in chloroquine-resistant areas, with mefloquine reserved for use by those intolerant to or with contraindications to both doxycycline and A/P (DoD, 2013). A/P was approved in 2000, but its use in military service members was not significant until 2013, when it joined doxycycline as a first-line choice for chloroquine-resistant areas (DoD, 2013). The military medicine concept of force health protection is defined as "all measures taken by commanders, supervisors, individual service members, and the military health system to promote, protect, improve, conserve, and restore the mental and physical well-being of service members" (Raczniak et al., 2019). Force health protection policy positions in DoD are issued as directives and instructions and include the use of antimalarial drugs for prophylaxis. Although policy may be made at higher levels, the final decision to use malaria prophylaxis under force health protection is made by commanders in the field, guided by their medical staff (Raczniak et al., 2019). Final decisions regarding malaria prophylaxis policy can be directed by authorities at other levels as well.

When malaria prophylaxis is indicated, service members are required to receive it under proper medical supervision. If a drug is medically contraindicated, alternative agents may be used if they are available, and the unit medical officer is to document those who have not received standard preventive measures so that they may receive additional monitoring or treatment if they become ill. However, while ordinary travelers are encouraged to adhere to malaria prophylaxis, military personnel are required to do so. Moreover, military personnel often use malaria prophylaxis for longer periods than travelers (many deployments are for 1 year or more), and they do so under demanding, stressful, and dangerous circumstances (Fukuda et al., 2018).

Unlike the case with individual travelers, large military operations have operational constraints related to their forward planning. It is not easy to make rapid changes in policy concerning the widespread use of new medications, particularly when large numbers of personnel are deployed at short notice from a number of locations around the world. Moreover, many military missions to endemic areas are in places of conflict, where malaria control measures have been interrupted or impaired (Pergallo, 2001).

Current DoD policy requires that troops sent to endemic areas use personal protective measures, such as sleeping under mosquito nets, wearing insecticide-impregnated uniforms, using insect repellent (i.e., DEET [N,N-diethyl-3-metatoluamide]), and taking malaria prophylaxis drugs as prescribed. Although these requirements are particularly important for troops stationed in endemic areas for long periods of time, some individuals with certain military occupations, such as pilots and aircrews who transport goods and people and make short trips (generally less than 24 hours) to malaria-endemic areas, are subject to different requirements. For example, mefloquine is not approved for prophylactic use in pilots (DeJulio, 2016).

Adherence to Malaria Prophylaxis

One of the most important factors in choosing among the several drugs available for malaria prophylaxis is understanding the dosing regimen required to effectively prevent the development of clinical malaria. Efficacy rates are lower for individuals who incorrectly use antimalarial drugs than for those who use them correctly (Cunningham et al., 2014; Goodyer et al., 2011; Saunders et al., 2015). Although the terms *adherence* and *compliance* are often used interchangeably, the two terms are not synonymous. Medication adherence, as defined by WHO, is "the degree to which the person's behavior corresponds with the agreed recommendations from a health care provider." To assess adherence, investigators typically consider whether individuals actively fill or pick up newly prescribed medications from a pharmacy, or instead refill existing prescriptions on time (National Stroke Association, 2012). Compliance refers to the extent to which a person's behavior matches the prescriber's advice (Horne, 2006). Therefore, compliance refers to how much and how often an individual ingests a medication compared with the dosing regimen dictated on the medication's prescription label, packaging, or FDA package insert. It is important to distinguish between drug adherence and drug compliance because they may affect not only the efficacy of a drug but also the adverse events that may be associated with the drug's use. Despite this, many publications mix the terms. To avoid confusion, the committee preferentially uses the term "adherence" throughout the report when referring to behaviors regarding use of the antimalarial drugs of interest.

Adherence to prophylactic antimalarial drug regimens is often suboptimal. Studies specifically examining adherence in the case of drugs used for malaria prophylaxis have reported several reasons for the low rates of adherence, including forgetfulness, fear of adverse events, discomfort of swallowing or of swallowing too many pills, receiving inaccurate pre-travel advice from nonmedical or medical professionals, incorrect risk perception, failure to take any prophylaxis, and inaccurate understanding of malaria transmission (Adshead, 2014; Behrens et al., 1998; Cunningham et al., 2014; Goodyer et al., 2011; Hopperus Buma et al., 1996; Huzly et al., 1996; Landman et al., 2015; Laver et al., 2001; Ollivier et al., 2008; Phillips and Kass, 1996; Ropers et al., 2008; Saunders et al., 2015). In studies of people who are employed by or participate in organizations in which the use of antimalarial drugs for prophylaxis is required (e.g., military, Peace Corps, Department of State), reported adherence rates may be inflated. The dosing regimens vary for each antimalarial drug, so that adherence is more achievable for some drugs than others. For example, doxycycline and A/P must be taken every day, whereas mefloquine and tafenoquine only need to be taken once a week. One study of U.S. soldiers serving in Afghanistan in 2007 found that 60% were fully adherent with daily doxycycline and 80% reported full adherence with weekly mefloquine (Saunders et al., 2015). Similar rates of low adherence have been reported in other international military forces. In 2006 a study of French troops using daily doxycycline for prophylaxis found that 63.4% were nonadherent, based on measured plasma concentrations of doxycycline (Ollivier et al., 2008), while Dutch marine battalions stationed for 6 months in Cambodia reported 86.3% fully adhered with weekly mefloquine prophylaxis (Hopperus Buma et al., 1996). FDA and drug manufacturers note that even for individuals who adhere completely to drug dosing regimens, no drug is 100% efficacious, and it is still possible to develop clinical symptoms of malaria. Therefore, in addition to using antimalarial prophylaxis, the use of other preventative measures is recommended.

In malaria-endemic areas, DoD policy dictates that such personal protective measures as insect repellent (most commonly DEET), bed nets, and permethrin-impregnated uniforms be used in addition to a malaria prophylactic drug. Although DEET is known to be effective against mosquitos and other insects, during some deployments, such as Somalia, troops did not like that DEET caused dust to cake on the areas of exposed skin where it was used (Ledbetter et al., 1995). Similarly, the operational work and living environments of military personnel do not always lend themselves to the appropriate use of protective measures. For example, bed nets were reportedly not used in some combat environments for fear that the poles that bed nets were suspended on made the troops larger targets to the enemy (Ledbetter et al., 1995). One survey of U.S. soldiers who served in Afghanistan found that only 1% reported consistent use of bed nets, 4% reported consistent use of mosquito repellent, and 31% reported that all of their uniforms had been treated with permethrin; however, 44% and 20% of the survey respondents reported that bed nets and skin repellents, respectively, had not been issued during the deployment (Saunders et al., 2015).

While real or perceived side effects and adverse events of drugs used for malaria prophylaxis are common reasons given for the lack of adherence to them, other factors may contribute, especially during deployments. Forgetfulness, especially when troops have irregular schedules, have little or disrupted sleep, or go on leave, is common (Hopperus Buma et al., 1996; Ledbetter et al., 1995; Mayet et al., 2010; Saunders et al., 2015). Other reasons for a lack of adherence that have been reported in the published literature include not believing malaria is a serious threat or that the threat was "over," or accidently laundering pills (Hopperus Buma et al., 1996; Ledbetter et al., 1995; Saunders et al., 2015). Unit commanders may require that the taking of antimalarials is directly observed by unit medical personnel to improve adherence.

Concurrent Exposures of Military Service

This section focuses on the many natural and anthropogenic exposures that U.S. service members and veterans may have experienced that may confound associations between the use of antimalarial drugs and long-term health outcomes. As those antimalarial drugs that have been used in the past 25 years are of highest interest to the Department of Veterans Affairs (VA), this would include their use in service members who were deployed in support of OEF, OIF, and Operation New Dawn (OND) in Iraq and Afghanistan as well as surrounding areas included in the Southwest Asia Theater of Operations[4] and also peacekeeping, humanitarian, and engineering activities in Haiti, Liberia, Somalia, and other malaria-endemic areas around the world. Concurrent military exposures of the 1990–1991 Persian Gulf War (Operation Desert Storm and Operation Desert Eagle) are also considered because the antimalarials used for prophylaxis were chloroquine (DoD, 1993; VA, 1993) and doxycycline (Thornton et al., 2005) depending on the service branch and unit commander, with some reports of mefloquine use as well (see Kotwal et al., 2005), and these are antimalarial drugs that VA considers to be of high interest. Some of the potentially confounding exposures were unique to specific conflicts, such as the numerous oil-well fires and their smoke, the release of the nerve agents sarin and cyclosarin, and the use of pyridostigmine bromide as a prophylaxis for the nerve agents in the 1990–1991 Persian Gulf War. Other exposures, such as vaccinations against anthrax and botulinum, while uncommon, were used in the Persian Gulf War as well as the recent conflicts in Iraq and Afghanistan.

Understanding the adverse health effects of military service requires examining a combination of many complex issues, some of which may occur simultaneously for an individual. Some of these issues are explored below (and are based on information found in the National Academies *Gulf War and Health* report series as well as in several other reports that examined the health effects related to myriad exposures that service members received during their deployments). These issues include exposure to multiple biologic and chemical agents, combat and other psychologic stressors, the deployment environment, and individual variability factors.

Environmental and Chemical Exposures

During deployments, service members may have had a variety of environmental exposures related to their deployment including solvents, fumes from kerosene heaters in unvented tents, and exposure to petroleum-based combustion products including diesel fuel and leaded gasoline that were used in cooking stoves and portable generators and to suppress sand and dust in desert environments and aid in the burning of waste and trash in open air burn pits. Such combustion products may contain many hazardous agents such as polyaromatic hydrocarbons, dioxins, furans, and methane.

---

[4] VA defines the Southwest Asia Theater of operations to include the following locations: Iraq, Kuwait, Saudi Arabia, Bahrain, Gulf of Aden, Gulf of Oman, Oman, Qatar, and the United Arab Emirates; the waters of the Persian Gulf, Arabian Sea, and the Red Sea; and the airspace above these regions.

In areas of conflict, pesticide exposures are generally widespread among troops as their units attempt to resist the local insect and rodent populations. DEET and permethrin-impregnated uniforms are nearly ubiquitous in deployments to Southeast Asia, Southwest Asia, and Africa. Other pesticides that have been reportedly used, particularly in Iraq and Afghanistan, include methyl carbamates (e.g., proxpur, carbaryl), organophosphates (e.g., chlorpyrifos, diazinon, malathion), pyrethroids, lindane, and chlorinated hydrocarbons (DoD, 2001; RAND, 2000). However, objective information regarding individual levels of pesticide exposure is generally not available, and reports by individual veterans as to their use of and possible exposure to pesticides are subject to considerable recall bias.

Many environmental and chemical exposures could be related to particular activities related to a service member's or veteran's military occupational specialty. In the conflicts in Iraq and Afghanistan, the majority of occupational chemical exposures appear to have been related to repair and maintenance (chlorinated hydrocarbons), sandblasting (abrasive particles), vehicle repair (carbon monoxide and organic solvents), weapon repair (lead particles), and welding and cutting (chromates, nitrogen dioxide, and heated metal fumes). In addition, troops painted vehicles and other equipment used in the Persian Gulf region with a chemical-agent-resistant coating either before they were shipped to the Persian Gulf or while they were at ports in Saudi Arabia. Working conditions in the field were not ideal, and recommended occupational-hygiene standards might not have been followed at all times (NASEM, 2016).

In addition to the requirements for service members to be up to date on standard vaccines, certain military deployments require additional vaccines or prophylactic agents, such as for cholera, meningitis, and typhoid. Deployment to malaria-endemic locations, such as Southwest Asia, Southeast Asia, and Africa, require the issue of an approved antimalarial drug. In some combat theaters additional protective measures may be needed. For example, during the 1990–1991 Persian Gulf War, about 150,000 troops received anthrax vaccine and about 8,000 troops received botulinum toxoid vaccine, although medical records from this period are notably lacking information regarding who received these vaccines, how frequently the vaccines were administered, or the timing of vaccinations relative to other putative exposures (IOM, 2000).

Some environmental exposures resulted from the conflict itself, such as exposures to the depleted uranium used in munitions, excessive heat or humidity, additional vaccines administered, and smoke from open burn pits. Some of the exposures could be constant, such as dust, heat, and pesticides, while other exposures were intermittent or infrequent.

Combat Exposures

Although modern warfare has resulted in fewer deaths and casualties than earlier conflicts—those in Vietnam and Korea, World War I and World War II—

there are numerous opportunities for exposure to potentially harmful situations during deployment. Combat is widely acknowledged to be one of the most intense experiences that a person can have and may include many threatening situations such as killing or attempting to kill an enemy; being shot at by others; exposure to dead and wounded comrades, enemy combatants, and civilians; and being injured. For the 1990–1991 Gulf War and the OEF/OIF/OND conflicts, these situations included being in the vicinity of Scud missile explosions, contact with improvised explosive devices, contact with prisoners of war, direct combat duty, coming under small-arms fire, having artillery close by (Hoge et al., 2004; Kang et al., 2000; Unwin et al., 1999), and the fear of terrorist or chemical attacks. Many surveys have been conducted to assess veterans' combat experiences and exposures (e.g., Millennium Cohort Study, National Health Survey of Gulf War Era Veterans and Their Families, National Health Study for a New Generation of U.S. Veterans), and in nearly all of them, veterans have reported exposure to a wide variety of threatening or harmful situations during their deployments. In one study that conducted a survey of the combat experiences and mental health problems of Army or Marine Corps service members deployed to either OEF or OIF, researchers found that many of the respondents indicated having had several of these experiences. For example, among the marines deployed to Iraq (n = 815), 97% reported being shot at or receiving small arms fire, 95% reported being attacked or ambushed, 94% reported seeing dead bodies or human remains, and 92% reported receiving incoming artillery, rocket, or mortar fire. Although the percentages were slightly lower, soldiers deployed to Iraq (n = 894) also indicated having had similar combat experiences (Hoge et al., 2004).

Psychological Stressors

Deployment to a war zone in general, and combat exposure in particular, may result in psychiatric and physical sequelae among service members. In addition to the cramped and uncomfortable living conditions, the many potential environmental and chemical exposures, and the threat of combat, a variety of other stressors may also exert psychologic effects. Rapid mobilization may exert additional substantial pressure on those who are deployed, disrupting lives and separating families. Uncertainty about the duration of deployment was a continuing concern for U.S. troops during the Gulf War, OEF, and OIF, particularly during the early phases of the buildup. For the large numbers of reservists and National Guard members who were mobilized, there was added uncertainly about whether their jobs would be available when they returned to civilian life (VA, 2011). Although better mechanisms for and access to communication with family in the United States exist than was the case for earlier conflicts such as Vietnam, deployment can still add to the stress of maintaining family relationships, particularly for reserve and National Guard personnel who may not have deployed with a familiar or cohesive unit. Surveys of both active-duty and reserve and National Guard soldiers deployed to

Iraq in support of OIF found that the most important noncombat stressors were deployment length and family separation (MHAT, 2006a,b). Stressful working conditions, disrupted sleep patterns, and prolonged separation from families may exacerbate the psychological stressors (Adshead, 2014).

Although historically women who served in the military were not allowed to serve in direct combat specialties, they were deployed in combat support roles as administrators, air traffic controllers, logisticians, ammunition technicians, engineering equipment mechanics, ordnance specialists, communicators, radio operators, drivers, law enforcement specialists, aviators, and guards. Still others served on hospital, supply, oiler, and ammunition ships or served as public affairs officers and chaplains (DoD, 2004), and they experienced many of the same exposures and stressors as men when deployed. In addition, several studies of deployment experiences found that female military personnel were more likely to experience sexual harassment and assault than male personnel (Goldzweig et al., 2006; Kang et al., 2005; Vogt et al., 2005; Wolfe et al., 1998).

Following deployment, many veterans experience high levels of stress during the transition to civilian life (IOM, 2008, 2013; Mobbs and Bonanno, 2018). In particular, coming-home experiences may be challenging, with numerous stressors including relationships with spouses and family, and parenting roles (Mobbs and Bonanno, 2018; Steenkamp et al., 2017). Some of these coming-home stressors may be related to the military experience itself. Vietnam veterans, for example, frequently experienced social rejection and were stereotyped for being perceived as harming vulnerable Vietnamese populations, which placed them in a difficult position on top of other mental health issues they were experiencing (Marmar et al., 2015; Steenkamp et al., 2017). With a better understanding of those experiences by policy makers and professionals, Iraq and Afghanistan service members were treated more positively; however, a host of highly needed resources, such as access to mental health care, legal help, and vocational opportunities, has been limited (IOM, 2013). Whereas the lifetime prevalence of posttraumatic stress disorder (PTSD) in U.S. adults was estimated to be 6.8% according to the National Comorbidity Survey–Replication (Harvard Medical School, 2007), the prevalence of PTSD among post-9/11 veterans is much higher. Among post-9/11 veterans using VA health services, nearly one-quarter of them had a diagnosis of PTSD (IOM, 2014). Similarly, a meta-analysis of PTSD prevalence in post-9/11 veterans that included 33 studies published between 2007 and 2013 involving 4,945,897 OEF/OIF veterans estimated the overall prevalence of PTSD among these veterans to be 23% (Fulton et al., 2005). Despite some resources and programs available for returning veterans, the stresses of deployment and reintegration elevate their risk for a host of military-related psychiatric problems, including PTSD, depression, anxiety disorder, substance abuse, and suicidal ideation and attempts (Pietrzak et al., 2009; Thomas et al., 2017).

Living Conditions

Combat troops deployed to the conflicts in Southwest Asia were often crowded into warehouses and tents upon arrival in the Persian Gulf region and then often moved to isolated desert locations (NASEM, 2016). Most troops lived in tents and slept on cots lined up side by side, affording virtually no privacy or quiet. Sanitation was often primitive, with strains on latrines and communal washing facilities. Hot showers were infrequent, the interval between laundering uniforms was sometimes long, and desert flies were a constant nuisance, as were scorpions and snakes. Military personnel worked long hours and had narrowly restricted outlets for relaxation. Troops were ordered not to fraternize with local people, and alcoholic drinks were prohibited in deference to religious beliefs in the host countries. A mild traveler's type of diarrhea affected more than half of the troops in some units; one study of ground forces found that 57% of those surveyed had experienced at least one episode of diarrhea within the first 2 months of deployment and of those, 20% were unable to perform their military duties while affected (Hyams et al., 1991). Among British and Australian medical teams that were part of the coalition forces, 69% of British troops and 36% of Australian troops experienced diarrhea, with some episodes lasting for several days (Rudland et al., 1996). Fresh fruits and vegetables from neighboring countries were identified as the cause and were removed from the diet. Thereafter, the diet consisted mostly of packaged foods and bottled water.

Depending on the deployment location, weather may create additional stressors. During the summer months in Iraq, the air temperatures could reach as high as 115°F and the sand temperatures as high as 150°F. Except for coastal regions, the relative humidity was less than 40%. Troops had to drink large quantities of water to prevent dehydration. Although the summers were hot and dry, temperatures in winter in Iraq and Afghanistan were low, with wind chill temperatures at night dropping to well below freezing. Wind and blowing sand made the protection of skin and eyes imperative. Goggles and sunglasses helped somewhat, but visibility was often poor.

Interindividual Variability

Differences among people in their genetic, biologic, psychologic, and social vulnerabilities add to the complexity of determining health outcomes related to specific agents (NASEM, 2016). The likelihood of observing a particular health outcome may differ for people with increased sensitivity to an agent, such as G6PD deficiency as described earlier in the chapter. For example, a person who is a poor metabolizer of a particular substance, depending on his or her genetic makeup, might be at higher or lower risk for specific health effects if exposed to the substance.

All antimalarial drugs used for prophylaxis in adults are prescribed as fixed dose regimens in which the amount of drug (e.g., one tablet) and unit of time (e.g., once daily, weekly) is specified. For example, the recommended dosing for A/P is one tablet (250 mg atovaquone and 100 mg proguanil) per day beginning 1–2 days before entering and continuing throughout the stay, and for 7 days after leaving an endemic area. Consistent with FDA indications, the same fixed dose is prescribed to all adult individuals, regardless of sex, weight, or age. As such, certain anti-malarials may be more likely to be associated with side effects or adverse events in people with certain demographic characteristics. For example, among people who use mefloquine, more women report adverse events than men. Because in general women weigh less than men and have a smaller vascular volume, a fixed dose tablet of an antimalarial may result in higher plasma levels of the drug in people of lower weight (women) than in people of heavier weight (men). Some studies have shown that adverse events are related to the concentration of drug in the blood (Schwartz et al., 2001), not to the absolute dose of drug delivered. Therefore, if the target of drug delivery was for a specific plasma level across all adult users, then the drug would have to be dosed on a mg/kg basis. Since the goal of prophylaxis is protection against malaria, the fixed dose was determined based on the pharmacokinetic studies of a dose that offers the best combination of protection and tolerability and that was easy to mass produce.

REFERENCES

60 Degrees Pharmaceuticals. 2018. Arakoda™ (Tafenoquine Succinate) Tablets for the Prevention of Malaria in Adults. Washington, DC: 60 Degrees Pharmaceuticals.

Adshead, S. 2014. The Adverse Effects of Mefloquine in Deployed Military Personnel. *J R Nav Med Serv* 100(3):232-237.

AFHSB (Armed Forces Health Surveillance Branch). 2019. Update: Malaria, U.S. Armed Forces, 2018. *MSMR* 26(2):1-28.

AFHSC (Armed Forces Health Surveillance Center). 2013. Update: Malaria, U.S. Armed Forces, 2012. *MSMR* 20(1):2-5.

AFHSC. 2014. Update: Malaria, U.S. Armed Forces, 2013. *MSMR* 21(1):4-7.

AFHSC. 2015. Update: Malaria, U.S. Armed Forces, 2014. *MSMR* 22(1):2-6.

AFHSC. 2016. Update: Malaria, U.S. Armed Forces, 2015. *MSMR* 23(1):2-6.

Arguin, P. M., and A. J. Magill. 2017. For the record: A history of malaria chemoprophylaxis. https://wwwnc.cdc.gov/travel/yellowbook/2018/infectious-diseases-related-to-travel/emfor-the-record-a-history-of-malaria-chemoprophylaxisem (accessed December 18, 2018).

Baird, J. K. 2012. Elimination therapy for the endemic malarias. *Curr Infect Dis Rep* 14(3):227-237.

Baird, J. K. 2018. Tafenoquine for travelers' malaria: Evidence, rationale, and recommendations. *J Travel Med* 25(1):1-13.

Baird, J. K. 2019. 8-aminoquinoline therapy for latent malaria. *Clin Microbiol Rev* 32(4):e00011-19.

Behrens, R. H., R. B. Taylor, D. I. Pryce, and A. S. Low. 1998. Chemoprophylaxis compliance in travelers with malaria. *J Travel Med* 5(2):92-94.

Boggild, A., M. E. Parise, L. S. Lewis, and K. C. Kain. 2007. Atovaquone-proguanil: Report from the CDC Expert Meeting on Malaria Chemoprophylaxis (II). *Am J Trop Med Hyg* 76(2):208-223.

Bowman, Z. S., J. D. Morrow, D. J. Jollow, and D. C. McMillan. 2005. Primaquine-induced hemolytic anemia: Role of membrane lipid peroxidation and cytoskeletal protein alterations in the hemo-toxicity of 5-hydroxyprimaquine. *J Pharmacol Exp Ther* 314:833-845.

Brundage, J. 2003. Conserving the fighting strength: Milestones of operational military preventive medicine research. In *Military preventive medicine: Mobilization and deployment*. 1st ed. Vol. 1: Office of the Surgeon General, U.S. Army.

Camarda, G., P. Jirawatcharadech, R. S. Priestley, A. Saif, et al. 2019. Antimalarial activity of Primaquine operates via a two-step biochemical relay. *Nat Commun* 10(3226).

Canfield, C. J., M. Pudney, and W. E. Gutteridge. 1995. Interactions of atovaquone with other antimalarial drugs against *Plasmodium falciparum* in vitro. *Exp Parasitol* 80:373-381.

CDC (Centers for Disease Control and Prevention). 1993. Malaria among U.S. military personnel returning from Somalia, 1993. *MMWR* 42(27):523-526.

CDC. 2017. *DPDx—Laboratory identification of parasites of public health concern*. https://www.cdc.gov/dpdx/malaria/index.html (accessed March 13, 2019).

CDC. 2018. *Drug resistance in the malaria-endemic world*. https://www.cdc.gov/malaria/malaria_worldwide/reduction/drug_resistance.html (accessed November 12, 2019).

CDC. 2019a. Chapter 4: Travel related infectious diseases. In *CDC Yellowbook*. https://wwwnc.cdc.gov/travel/yellowbook/2020/travel-related-infectious-diseases/malaria (accessed March 14, 2019).

CDC. 2019b. *Treatment of malaria: guidelines for clinicians (United States)*. https://www.cdc.gov/malaria/resources/pdf/treatment_guidelines_101819.pdf (accessed December 27, 2019).

Chinevere, T. D., C. K. Murray, E. Grant, Jr., G. A. Johnson, F. Duelm, and D. R. Hospenthal. 2006. Prevalence of glucose-6-phosphate dehydrogenase deficiency in U.S. Army personnel. *Mil Med* 171(9):905-907.

Cunningham, J., J. Horsley, D. Patel, A. Tunbridge, and D. G. Lalloo. 2014. Compliance with long-term malaria prophylaxis in British expatriates. *Travel Med Infect Dis* 12:341-348.

DeJulio, P. A. 2016. You're the flight surgeon. *Aerosp Med Hum Perform* 87(4):429-432.

Denshaw-Burke, M., A. L. Curran, D. C. Savior, and M. Kumar. 2018. Methemoglobinemia. Medscape. https://webcache.googleusercontent.com/search?q=cache:MoqV2XjOJHIJ:https://emedicine.medscape.com/article/204178-overview+&cd=1&hl=en&ct=clnk&gl=us (accessed December 23, 2019).

DoD (Department of Defense). 1993. United States Army Reserve in Operation Desert Storm: Reservists of the Army Medical Department (monograph, J. R. Brinkerhoff, T. Silva, and J. Seitz, September 23, 1993). https://apps.dtic.mil/dtic/tr/fulltext/u2/a277591.pdf (accessed November 15, 2019).

DoD. 2001. *Environmental exposure report: Pesticides, final report*. Falls Church, VA: Department of Defense.

DoD. 2004. *Task force report on care for victims of sexual assault*. Washington, DC: Department of Defense. https://vawnet.org/material/task-force-report-care-victims-sexual-assault (accessed November 12, 2019).

DoD. 2009. Policy memorandum on the use of mefloquine (Lariam®) in malaria prophylaxis (September 4, 2009, #HA 09-017). Provided by COL Andrew Wiesen, M.D., M.P.H., Director, Preventive Medicine, Health Readiness Policy and Oversight, Office of the Assistant Secretary of Defense (Health Affairs), DoD, January 25, 2019.

DoD. 2013. Memorandum on guidance on medications for prophylaxis of malaria (April 15, 2013). Provided by COL Andrew Wiesen, M.D., M.P.H., Director, Preventive Medicine, Health Readiness Policy and Oversight, Office of the Assistant Secretary of Defense (Health Affairs), DoD, January 25, 2019.

Dorwald, F. Z. 2012. *Lead optimization for medicinal chemists: Pharmacokinetic properties of functional groups and organic compounds*. Mörlenbach, Germany: Wiley-VCH.

Downs, W. G., P. A. Harper, and E. T. Lisamsky. 1947. Malaria and other insect-borne diseases in the South Pacific Campaign, 1942-1945. II Epidemiology of insect-borne diseases in Army troops. *Am J Trop Med* 27:69-89.

Dugbartey, A. T., M. T. Dugbartey, and M. Y. Apedo. 1998. Delayed neuropsychiatric effects of malaria in Ghana. *J Nerv Ment Dis* 186(3):183-186.

Ebstie, Y. A., S. M. Abay, W. T. Tadesse, and D. A. Ejigu. 2016. Tafenoquine and its potential in the treatment and relapse prevention of *Plasmodium vivax* malaria: The evidence to date. *Drug Des Devel Ther* 10:2387-2399.

Ecker, A., A. M. Leane, J. Clain, and D. A. Fidock. 2012. PfCRT and its role in antimalarial drug resistance. *Trends Parasitol* 28(11):504-514.

Fasinu, P. S., N. P. Dhammika Nanayakkara, Y.-H. Wang, N. D. Chaurasiya, H. M. Bandara Herath, J. D. McChesney, B. Avula, I. Khan, B. L. Tekwani, and L. A. Walker. 2019. Formation primaquine-5, 6-orthoquinone, the putative active and toxic metabolite of primaquine via direct oxidation in human erythrocytes. *Malar J* 18(30).

FDA (Food and Drug Administration). 2018a. FDA briefing document. Tafenoquine tablet, 100 mg. Meeting of the Antimicrobial Drugs Advisory Committee (AMDAC). July 26, 2018. https://www.fda.gov/media/114753/download (accessed November 11, 2019).

FDA. 2018b. Package insert for Arakoda™ (tafenoquine) tablets. https://www.accessdata.fda.gov/scripts/cder/daf/index.cfm?event=overview.process&ApplNo=210607 (accessed October 29, 2019).

FDA. 2019. Package insert for Malarone (atovaquone and proguanil hydrochloride) tablets and Malarone (atovaquone and proguanil hydrochloride) pediatric tablets. https://www.accessdata.fda.gov/drugsatfda_docs/label/2019/021078s023lbl.pdf (accessed October 3, 2019).

Fernando, S. D., D. M. Gunawardena, M. R. Bandara, D. De Silva, R. Carter, K. N. Mendis, and A. R. Wickremasinghe. 2003. The impact of repeated malaria attacks on the school performance of children. *Am J Trop Med Hyg* 69(6):582-588.

Foley, M., and L. Tilley. 1998. Quinoline antimalarials: Mechanisms of action and resistance and prospects for new agents. *Pharmacol Ther* 79(1):55-87.

Fukuda, M., G. A. Raczniak, M. S. Riddle, M. Forgione, and A. J. Magill. 2018. Special considerations for U.S. military deployments. In *Yellow book*. Atlanta, GA: Centers for Disease Control and Prevention. https://relief.unboundmedicine.com/relief/view/cdc-yellowbook/204140/all/Special_Considerations_for_US_Military_Deployments (accessed November 12, 2019).

Fulton, J. J., P. S. Calhoun, H. R. Wagner, A. R. Schry, L. P. Hair, N. Feeling, E. Elbogen, and J. C. Beckham. 2005. The prevalence of posttraumatic stress disorder in Operation Enduring Freedom/Operation Iraqi Freedom (OEF/OIF) veterans: A meta-analysis. *J Anxiety Disord* 31:98-107.

Gay, F., D. Bustos, and B. Traore. 1997. In vitro response of *Plasmodium falciparum* to atovaquone and correlation with other antimalarials: Comparison between African and Asian strains. *Am J Trop Med* 56:315-317.

Goldzweig, C. L., T. M. Balekian, C. Rolon, E. M. Yano, and P. G. Shekelle. 2006. The state of women veterans' health research: Results of a systematic literature review. *J Gen Intern Med* 21(Suppl 3):S82-S92.

Goodyer, L., L. Rice, and A. Martin. 2011. Choice of and adherence to prophylactic antimalarials. *J Travel Med* 18(4):245-249.

Gunjan, S., S. K. Singh, T. Sharma, H. Dwivedi, B. S. Chauhan, M. Imran Siddiqi, and R. Tripathi. 2016. Mefloquine induces ROS mediated programmed cell death in malaria parasite: *Plasmodium. Apoptosis* 21(9):955-964.

Harvard Medical School. 2007. *Lifetime prevalence of DSM-IV/WMH-CIDI disorders by sex and cohort (n = 9,282)*. https://www.hcp.med.harvard.edu/ncs/ftpdir/NCS-R_Lifetime_Prevalence_Estimates.pdf (accessed September 25, 2019).

Hellgren, U., I. Berggren-Palme, Y. Bergvist, and M. Jerling. 1997. Enantioselective pharmacokinetics of mefloquine during long-term intake of the prophylactic dose. *Br J Clin Pharmacol* 44:119-124.

Helsby, N. A., S. A. Ward, R. E. Howell, and A. M. Breckenridge. 1990. The pharmacokinetics and activation of proguanil in man: Consequences of variability in drug metabolism. *Br J Clin Pharmacol* 30:287-291.

Hoge, C. W., C. A. Castro, S. C. Messer, D. McGurk, D. I. Cotting, and R. L. Koffman. 2004. Combat duty in Iraq and Afghanistan, mental health problems, and barriers to care. *NEJM* 351:13-22.

Hopperus Buma, A. P., P. P. van Thiel, H. O. Lobel, C. Ohrt, E. J. van Ameijden, R. L. Veltink, D. C. Tendeloo, T. van Gool, M. D. Green, G. D. Todd, D. E. Kyle, and P. A. Kager. 1996. Long-term malaria chemoprophylaxis with mefloquine in Dutch Marines in Cambodia. *J Infect Dis* 173:1506-1509.

Horne, R. 2006. Compliance, adherence, and concordance: Implications for asthma treatment. *Chest* 130(1):65S-72S.

Huzly, D., C. Schonfeld, W. Beuerle, and U. Bienzle. 1996. Malaria chemoprophylaxis in German tourists: A prospective study on compliance and adverse reactions. *J Travel Med* 3(3):148-155.

Hyams, K. C., A. L. Bourgeois, B. R. Merrell, P. Rozmajzl, J. Escamilla, S. A. Thornton, G. M. Wasserman, A. Burke, P. Echeverria, K. Y. Green, A. Z. Kapikian, and J. N. Woody. 1991. Diarrheal disease during Operation Desert Shield. *NEJM* 325(20):1423-1428.

Idro, R., J. A. Carter, G. Fegan, B. G. Neville, and C. R. Newton. 2006. Risk factors for persisting neurological and cognitive impairments following cerebral malaria. *Arch Dis Child* 91(2):142-148.

Idro, R., K. Marsh, C. C. John, and C. R. Newton. 2010. Cerebral malaria: Mechanisms of brain injury and strategies for improved neurocognitive outcome. *Pediatr Res* 68(4):267-274.

Idro, R., A. Kakooza-Mwesige, B. Asea, K. Sebyala, P. Bangirana, R. O. Opoka, S. K. Lubowa, M. Semrud-Clikeman, C. C. John, and J. Nalugya. 2016. Cerebral malaria is associated with long-term mental health disorders: A cross sectional survey of a long-term cohort. *Malar J* 15:184.

IOM (Institute of Medicine). 2000. *Gulf War and health, volume 1: Depleted uranium, pyridostigmine bromide, sarin, vaccines.* Washington, DC: National Academy Press.

IOM. 2006. *Battling malaria: Strengthening the U.S. military malaria vaccine program.* Washington, DC: The National Academies Press.

IOM. 2008. *Gulf War and health, volume 6: Psychologic, psychiatric, and psychosocial effects of deployment-related stress.* Washington, DC: The National Academies Press.

IOM. 2013. *Returning home from Iraq and Afghanistan: Assessment of readjustment needs of veterans, service members, and their families.* Washington, DC: The National Academies Press.

IOM. 2014. *Treatment for posttraumatic stress disorder in military and veteran populations: Final assessment.* Washington, DC: The National Academies Press.

John, C. C., A. Panoskaltsis-Mortari, R. O. Opoka, G. S. Park, P. J. Orchard, A. M. Jurek, R. Idro, J. Byarugaba, and M. J. Boivin. 2008. Cerebrospinal fluid cytokine levels and cognitive impairment in cerebral malaria. *Am J Trop Med Hyg* 78(2):198-205.

Kang, H. K., C. M. Mahan, K. Y. Lee, C. A. Magee, and F. M. Murphy. 2000. Illnesses among United States veterans of the Gulf War: A population-based survey of 30,000 veterans. *J Occup Environ Med* 42(5):491-501.

Kang, H., N. Dalager, C. Mahan, and E. Ishii. 2005. The role of sexual assault on the risk of PTSD among Gulf War veterans. *Ann Epidemiol* 15(3):191-195.

Kaur, H., E. L. Allan, I. Mamadu, Z. Hall, O. Ibe, M. El Sherbiny, A. van Wyk, S. Yeung, I. Swamidoss, M. D. Green, P. Dwivedi, M. J. Culzoni, S. Clarke, D. Schellenberg, F. M. Fernández, and O. Onwujekwe. 2015. Quality of artemisinin-based combination formulations for malaria treatment: Prevalence and risk factors for poor quality medicines in public facilities and private sector drug outlets in Enugu, Nigeria. *PLOS ONE* 10(5):e0125577.

Kitchen, L. W., D. W. Vaughn, and D. R. Skillman. 2006. Role of US military research programs in the cevelopment of US Food and Drug Administration-approved antimalarial drugs. *Clin Infect Dis* 43:67-71.

Kotwal, R. S., R. B. Wenzel, R. A. Sterling, W. D. Porter, N. N. Jordan, and B. P. Petruccelli. 2005. An outbreak of malaria in US Army Rangers returning from Afghanistan. *JAMA* 293(2):212-216.

Lalloo, D. G., and Magill. 2019. *Travel medicine: 14 - malaria: Epidemiology and risk to the traveler.* Edited by J. S. Keystone. 4th ed. Elsevier.

Landman, K. Z., K. R. Tan, and P. M. Arguin. 2015. Adherence to malaria prophylaxis among Peace Corps volunteers in the Africa region, 2013. *Travel Med Infect Dis* 12:61-68.

Laver, S. M., J. Wetzels, and R. H. Behrens. 2001. Knowledge of malaria, risk perception, and compliance with prophylaxis and personal and environmental preventive measures in travelers exiting Zimbabwe from Harare and Victoria Falls International Airport. *J Travel Med* 8:298-303.

Ledbetter, E., K. R. Hanson and M. R. Wallace. 1995. Malaria in Somalia: Lessons in prevention. *JAMA* 273(10):774-775.

Ley, B., G. Bancone, L. von Seidlein, K. Thriemer, J. S. Richards, G. J. Domingo, and R. N. Price. 2017. Methods for the field evaluation of quantitative G6PD diagnostics: A review. *Malar J* 16(1):361.

Liu, H., L. A. Walker, and R. J. Doerksen. 2011. DFT study on the radical anions formed by primaquine and its derivatives. *Chem Res Toxicol* 24(9):1476-1485.

Looareesuwan, S., J. D. Chulay, C. J. Canfield, and D. B. Hutchinson. 1999. Malarone (atovaquone and proguanil hydrochloride): A review of its clinical development for treatment of malaria. Malarone clinical trials study group. *Am J Trop Med Hyg* 60(4):533-541.

Mace, K. E., P. M. Arguin, N. W. Lucchi, and K. R. Tan. 2019. Malaria surveillance—United States, 2016. *MMWR Surveill Summ* 68(5):1-35.

Marcsisin, S. R., J. C. Sousa, G. A. Reichard, D. Caridha, Q. Zeng, N. Roncal, R. McNulty, J. Careagabarja, R. J. Sciotti, J. W. Bennett, V. E. Zottig, G. Deye, Q. Li, L. Read, M. Hickman, N. P. Dhammika Nanayakkara, L. A. Walker, B. Smith, V. Melendez, and B. S. Pybus. 2014. Tafenoquine and NPC-1161b require CYP 2D metabolism for anti-malarial activity: Implications for the 8-aminoquinoline class of anti-malarial compounds. *Malar J* 13(2):2.

Marmar, C. R., W. Schlenger, C. Henn-Haase, M. Qian, E. Purchia, M. Li, N. Corry, C. S. Williams, C. L. Ho, D. Horesh, K. I. Karstoft, A. Shalev, and R. A. Kulka. 2015. Course of posttraumatic stress disorder 40 years after the Vietnam War: Findings from the National Vietnam Veterans Longitudinal Study. *JAMA Psychiatry* 72(9):875-881.

Mayet, A., D. Lacassagne, N. Juzan, B. Chaudier, R. Haus-Cheymol, F. Berger, O. Romand, L. Ollivier, C. Verret, X. Deparis, and A. Spiegel. 2010. Malaria outbreak among French army troops returning from the Ivory Coast. *J Travel Med* 17(5):353-355.

MHAT (Mental Health Advisory Team). 2006a. *Mental Health Advisory Team (MHAT) III. Operation Iraqi Freedom 04-06: Final Report.* Washington, DC: Office of the Surgeon Multinational Force-Iraq and Office of the Surgeon General United States Army Medical Command. 29 May 2006. http://www.armymedicine.army.mil/news/mhat/mhat_iii/mhat-iii.cfm (accessed October 22, 2019).

MHAT. 2006b. *Mental Health Advisory Team (MHAT) IV Operation Iraqi Freedom 05-07: Final Report.* Washington, DC: Office of the Surgeon Multinational Force-Iraq and Office of the Surgeon General United States Army Medical Command. 17 November 2006. http://www.armymedicine.army.mil/news/mhat/mhat_iv/MHAT_IV_Report_17NOV06.pdf (accessed October 22, 2019).

Mobbs, M. C., and G. A. Bonanno. 2018. Beyond war and PTSD: The crucial role of transition stress in the lives of military veterans. *Clin Psychol Rev* 59:137-144.

Moss, W. J., and R. H. Morrow. 2014. The epidemiology and control of malaria. In K. E. Nelson and C. William, *Infectious disease epidemiology: Theory and practice.* Burlington, MA: Jones & Bartlett Learning.

NASEM (National Academies of Sciences, Engineering, and Medicine). 2016. *Gulf War and health, volume 10: Update of health effects of serving in the Gulf War.* Washington, DC: The National Academies Press.

National Stroke Association. 2012. Medication Adherence and Compliance. *National Stroke Association*: 1-9. https://oregon.providence.org/~/media/Files/Providence%20OR%20Migrated%20PDFs/Patients%20Toolkit/formsinstructions/nsa_med_adherencebooklet.pdf (accessed November 3, 2019).

Newton, P. N., K. Hanson, C. Goodman, and ACTwatch Group. 2017. Do anti-malarials in Africa meet quality standards? The market penetration of non-quality assured artemisinin combination therapy in eight African countries. *Malar J* 16:204.

NIH (National Institutes of Health). n.d. *Hemolytic anemia*. https://www.nhlbi.nih.gov/health-topics/hemolytic-anemia (accessed October 1, 2019).

Nixon, G. L., D. M. Moss, A. E. Shone, D. G. Lalloo, N. Fisher, P. M. O'Neill, S. A. Ward, and G. A. Biagini. 2013. Antimalarial pharmacology and therapeutics of atovaquone. *J Antimicrob Chemother* 68:977-985.

Nkhoma, E. T., C. Poole, V. Vannappagari, S. A. Hall, and E. Beutler. 2009. The global prevalence of glucose-6-phosphate dehydrogenase deficiency: A systematic review and meta-analysis. *Blood Cells Mol Dis* 42(3):267-278.

Ockenhouse, C. F., A. Magill, D. Smith, and W. Milhous. 2005. History of U.S. military contributions to the study of malaria. *Mil Med* 170(4):12-16.

Ollivier, L., R. Michel, M. P. Carlotti, P. Mahé, O. Romand, A. Todesco, R. Migliani, and J. P. Boutin. 2008. Chemoprophylaxis compliance in a French battalion after returning from malaria endemic area. *J Travel Med* 15:355-357.

O'Neill, P. M., S. A. Ward, N. G. Berry, J. P. Jeyadevan, G. A. Biagini, E. Asadollaly, B. K. Park, and P. G. Bray. 2006. A medicinal chemistry perspective on 4-aminoquinoline antimalarial drugs. *Curr Top Med Chem* 6(5):479-507.

Pal, S., P. Bansil, G. Bancone, S. Hrutkay, M. Kahn, G. Gornsawun, P. Penpitchaporn, C. S. Chu, F. Nosten, and G. J. Domingo. 2019. Evaluation of a novel quantitative test for glucose-6-phosphate dehydrogenase deficiency: Bringing quantitative testing for glucose-6-phosphate dehydrogenase deficiency closer to the patient. *Am J Trop Med Hyg* 100(1):213-221.

Palmer, K. J., S. M. Holliday, and R. N. Brogden. 1993. Mefloquine: A review of its antimalarial activity, pharmacokinetic properties and therapeutic efficacy. *Drugs* 45(3):430-475.

Parhizgar, A. R., and A. Tahghighi. 2017. Introducing new antimalarial analogues of chloroquine and amodiaquine: A narrative review. *Iran J Med Sci* 42(2):115-128.

Pergallo, M. S. 2001. The Italian Army standpoint on malaria chemoprophylaxis. *Med Trop* 61:59-62.

Peters, A. L., and C. J. Van Noorden. 2009. Glucose-6-phosphate dehydrogenase deficiency and malaria: Cytochemical detection of heterozygous G6PD deficiency in women. *J Histochem Cytochem* 57(11):1003-1011.

Phillips, M. A., and R. B. Kass. 1996. User acceptability patterns for mefloquine and doxycycline malaria chemoprophylaxis. *J Travel Med* 3:40-45.

Pietrzak, R. H., D. C. Johnson, M. B. Goldstein, J. C. Malley, and S. M. Southwick. 2009. Perceived stigma and barriers to mental health care utilization among OEF-OIF veterans. *Psychiatr Serv* 60(8):1118-1122.

Raczniak, G. A., M. S. Riddle, and M. Forgione. 2019. U.S. military deployments. In Chapter 9, Travel for work & other reasons, *Yellow book*. Atlanta, GA: Centers for Disease Control and Prevention. https://wwwnc.cdc.gov/travel/yellowbook/2020/travel-for-work-other-reasons/us-military-deployments (accessed November 12, 2019).

RAND Corporation. 2000. Review of the scientific literature as it pertains to Gulf War illnesses. Volume 8: Pesticides. Santa Monica, CA: RAND Corporation.

Richter, J., G. Franken, M. C. Holtfreter, S. Walter, A. Labisch, and H. Mehlhorn. 2016. Clinical implications of a gradual dormancy concept in malaria. *Parasitol Res* 115(6):2139-2148.

Ridley, R. G., A. Dorn, S. R. Vippagunta, and J. L. Vennerstrom. 1997. Haematin (haem) polymerization and its inhibition by quinoline antimalarials. *Ann Trop Med Parasitol* 91(5):559-566.

Ropers, G., M. Du Ry van Beest Holle, O. Wichmann, L. Kappelmayer, U. Stüben, C. Schönfeld, and K. Stark. 2008. Determinants of malaria prophylaxis among German travelers to Kenya, Senegal, and Thailand. *J Travel Med* 15(3):162-171.

Rudland, S., M. Little, P. Kemp, A. Miller, and J. Hodge. 1996. The enemy within: Diarrheal rates among British and Australian troops in Iraq. *Mil Med* 161(12):728-731.

Sánchez, J. L., R. F. DeFraites, T. W. Sharp, and R. K. Hanson. 1993. Mefloquine or doxycycline prophylaxis in U.S. troops in Somalia. *Lancet* 341(8851):1021-1022.

Saunders, D. L., E. Garges, J. E. Manning, K. Bennett, S. Schaffer, A. J. Kosmowski, and A. J. Magill. 2015. Safety, tolerability, and compliance with long-term antimalarial chemoprophylaxis in American soldiers in Afghanistan. *Am J Trop Med Hyg* 93(3):584-590.

Schlagenhauf, P., M. Adamcova, L. Regep, M. T. Schaerer, and H. G. Rhein. 2010. The position of mefloquine as a 21st century malaria chemoprophylaxis. *Malar J* 9(357).

Schlagenhauf, P., M. E. Wilson, E. Petersen, A. McCarthy, L. H. Chen, J. S. Keystone., P. E. Kozarsky, B. A. Connor, H. D. Nothdurft, M. Mendelson, and K. Leder. 2019. Malaria chemoprophylaxis. *Travel Med* (15):145-167.

Schwartz, E. 2012. Prophylaxis of malaria. *Mediterr J Hematol Infect Dis* 4(1):e2012045.

Schwartz, E., I. Potasman, M. Rotenberg, S. Almog, and S. Sadetzki. 2001. Serious adverse events of mefloquine in relation to blood level and gender. *Am J Trop Med Hyg* 65(3):189-192.

Srivastava, I. K., and A. B. Vaidya. 1999. A mechanism for the synergistic antimalarial action of atovaquone and proguanil. *Antimicrob Agents Chemother* 43(6):1334-1339.

Steenkamp, M. M., W. E. Schlenger, N. Corry, C. Henn-Haase, M. Qian, M. Li, D. Horesh, K. I. Karstoft, C. Williams, C. L. Ho, A. Shalev, R. Kulka, and C. Marmar. 2017. Predictors of PTSD 40 years after combat: Findings from the National Vietnam Veterans Longitudinal Study. *Depres Anxiety* 34(8):711-722.

Sullivan, D. J., Jr., H. Matile, R. G. Ridley, and D. E. Goldberg. 1998. A common mechanism for blockade of heme polymerization by antimalarial quinolines. *J Biol Chem* 273(47):31103-31107.

Tan, K. R., A. J. Magill, M. E. Parise, P. M. Arguin, and Centers for Disease Control and Prevention. 2011. Doxycycline for malaria chemoprophylaxis and treatment: Report from the CDC expert meeting on malaria chemoprophylaxis. *Am J Tropl Med Hyg* 84(4):517-531.

Thomas, M. M., I. Harpaz-Rotem, J. Tsai, S. M. Southwick, and R. H. Pietrzak. 2017. Mental and physical health conditions in U.S. combat veterans: Results from the National Health and Resilience in Veterans Study. *Prim Care Companion CNS Disord* 19(3).

Thornton, S. A., S. S. Sherman, T. Farkas, W. Zhong, P. Torres, and X. Jiang. 2005. Gastroenteritis in US Marines during Operation Iraqi Freedom. *Clin Infect Dis* 40(4):519-525.

Unwin, C., N. Blatchley, W. Coker, S. Ferry, M. Hotopf, L. Hull, K. Ismail, I. Palmer, A. David, and S. Wessely. 1999. Health of UK servicemen who served in Persian Gulf War. *Lancet* 353(9148):169-178.

VA (Department of Veterans Affairs). 1993. Unstructured information for: Post-operations Desert Shield/Desert Storm. https://gulflink.health.mil/va/va_refs/n46en031/osd.html (accessed November 5, 2019).

VA. 2011. *Caring for Gulf War 1 veterans*. Veterans Health Administration. http://www.publichealth. va.gov/docs/vhi/caring-for-gulf-war-veterans-vhi.pdf (accessed October 20, 2015).

Vennerstrom, J. L., E. O. Nuzum, R. E. Miller, A. Dorn, L. Gerena, P. A. Dande, W. Y. Ellis, R. G. Ridley, and W. K. Milhous.1999. 8-Aminoquinolines active against blood stage *Plasmodium falciparum* in vitro inhibit hematin polymerization. *Antimicrob Agents Chemother* 43(3):598-602.

Vogt, D. S., A. P. Pless, L. A. King, and D. W. King. 2005. Deployment stressors, gender, and mental health outcomes among Gulf War I veterans. *J Trauma Stress* 18(2):115-127.

Wallace, M. R., T. W. Sharp, B. Smoak, C. Iriye, P. Rozmajzl, S. A. Thornton, R. Batchelor, A. J. Magill, H. O. Lobel, C. F. Longer, and J. P. Burans. 1996. Malaria among United States troops in Somalia. *Am J Med* 100(1):49-55.

WHO (World Health Organization). 2014. Severe malaria. *Trop Med Int Health* 19(Suppl 1):7-131.

WHO. 2016a. *Testing for G6PD deficiency for safe use of primaquine in radical cure of* P. vivax *and* P. ovale. Policy brief, October 2016. https://www.who.int/malaria/publications/atoz/g6pd-testing-pq-radical-cure-vivax/en (accessed September 27, 2019).

WHO. 2016b. Fact sheet: World malaria 2016. https://www.who.int/malaria/media/world-malaria-report-2016/en (accessed January 12, 2019).

WHO. 2019. World Malaria Report, 2019. https://www.who.int/publications-detail/world-malaria-report-2019 (accessed December 10, 2019).

Wiesen, A. 2019. Overview of DoD antimalarial use policies. Presentation to the Committee to Review Long-Term Health Effects of Antimalarial Drugs on January 28, 2019.

Wolfe, J., E. J. Sharkansky, J. P. Read, R. Dawson, J. A. Martin, and P. C. Ouimette. 1998. Sexual harassment and assault as predictors of PTSD symptomatology among U.S. female Persian Gulf War military personnel. *J Interpers Violence* 13(1):40-57.

Wong, W., X. C. Bai, B. E. Sleebs, T. Triglia, A. Brown, J. K. Thompson, et al. 2017. The antimalarial mefloquine targets the *Plasmodium falciparum* 80S ribosome to inhibit protein synthesis. *Nat Microbiol* 2(17031).

3

Identification and Evaluation
of the Evidence Base

In this chapter the committee describes its two-phase approach for identifying and screening the literature and other existing evidence addressing potential long-term adverse health effects of the antimalarial drugs of interest. The process that the committee used to assess individual studies, including considerations concerning specific methodologic factors (such as study design, exposure assessment, outcomes assessment, and potential biases), is presented along with the types of studies identified and considered. How these methodologic considerations were applied to interpret the evidence is presented in the specific antimalarial drug chapters. The chapter concludes with a discussion on the process and classification system used to draw conclusions regarding the strength of evidence concerning the long-term health effects associated with the drugs of interest.

IDENTIFICATION OF THE EVIDENCE

The committee was tasked with comprehensively reviewing, evaluating, and summarizing the scientific literature related to long-term health effects that might be related to the use of currently available drugs for the prophylaxis of malaria in adults. Because some terms are used interchangeably in the literature, the committee endeavored to be as precise as possible in its terminology, and thus it adopted the definitions in Box 3-1 and uses them throughout the report. A conservative cutoff time of 28 days (which was considered equivalent to expressions of 4 weeks or 1 month) post-cessation of drug use was used to distinguish between events that are of short-term duration (and thus considered to be outside of the committee's scope) and those that are persistent or of long-term duration. The 28-day cutoff was chosen because it allowed for a sufficient washout period for the drugs of interest (the longest half-lives are approximately 14 days for both mefloquine and tafenoquine). *Long term* has been used in the literature with different interpretations. Given that prophylactic drugs for malaria should be used for the duration of a stay in a malaria-endemic area (as well as for multiple days or weeks after leaving the endemic area, depending on the antimalarial used), "long term" may refer to the timing of the drug use rather than to the timing of events that persist after drug use has been terminated. Therefore, the committee preferentially uses *persistent* to describe those adverse events that began during the period of drug use and that continued after drug cessation and beyond the period that the drug would still be present, which is defined as ≥28 days post-cessation. Adverse events that occur or change in their severity with prolonged use of an antimalarial drug are considered to be acute events because they occur while the drug is in use; if they do not persist once the use of the drug has ceased, they are outside the committee's charge of examining the evidence related to persistent health effects. Events that occur during drug use or that continue for a period extending from a few hours to less than 28 days after drug cessation have been referred to in the literature as acute or short-term events, but the committee uses the term *concurrent* events. The committee uses *concurrent* to identify events that begin with the use of a drug, not outcomes that may be present before use is begun (e.g., an individual starts a drug and then displays symptoms of hypertension rather than has hypertension and then starts a drug). *Latent* events refer to those adverse events that were not apparent during the period that the drug was in use but that were present at any time after the cessation of malaria prophylaxis. The focus of the assessment was on research that examined persistent or latent adverse events, both of which indicate the pres-

---

BOX 3-1
Common Terms Used Throughout the Report

Adverse event: Any unfavorable and unintended sign (e.g., an abnormal laboratory finding, symptom, or disease) associated with the use of a drug, without any judgment about causality or relationship to the drug.

Concurrent event: Incident adverse event that arises during antimalarial prophylaxis use or within 28 days of use.

Latent event: Incident adverse event that arises following the cessation of antimalarial prophylaxis use and that may become persistent.

Persistent event: Incident adverse event that arises during the antimalarial prophylaxis use and continues at least 28 days post-cessation.

ence of adverse health outcomes that extend beyond the period during which the user was taking the drug.

To begin, the committee oversaw extensive searches of the scientific and medical literature using a comprehensive strategy. Although antimalarial drugs used by the U.S. military currently or within the past 25 years were the primary focus, the committee's review also included studies of antimalarials used for prophylaxis in populations other than U.S. service members or veterans.

Literature Search Strategy

Under the direction of the committee, a National Academies of Sciences, Engineering, and Medicine staff research librarian conducted comprehensive electronic searches of the medical and scientific literature using three primary databases: TOXLINE, Index Medicus, and Embase. These three searchable databases index biologic, chemical, medical, and toxicologic publications. If any of the search terms were included in the title, abstract, or key words of the article (or the full text if available for search), the article was included in the results of the search. Search terms included full and abbreviated chemical names, common and manufacturer trade names, and the chemical abstracts service numbers for each of the antimalarial drugs of interest. A multi-purpose field code was included in the search parameters to ensure that all of the synonyms for the drugs of interest were retrieved in the searches. The search strategy was designed to ensure that all potentially relevant articles were captured, and it was not restricted by specific dates, publication types, populations, or species (experimental animal studies were included). The language was restricted to English.

For those drugs of interest that are indicated for uses other than malaria prophylaxis, additional terms and MeSH[1] descriptors were added. For example, doxycycline is approved for many uses, and more than 5,500 titles and abstracts were initially captured, so the search was revised to include additional terms related to "prophylaxis" and "malaria." As a result, the identified list was reduced to a more manageable 2,200 publications which were more likely to be relevant, while avoiding concerns about excluding any potentially relevant articles. Any adaptations made regarding the search strategy or screening criteria for a drug is discussed in the drug-specific chapters that follow.

Using the search terms in Box 3-2, the databases were searched twice. The first search of the literature included the earliest date of the database up to December 2018. A subsequent search was conducted in August 2019 to capture any relevant articles published or indexed after the initial search through July 31, 2019.

---

[1] MeSH descriptors are sets of terms naming descriptors in a hierarchical structure that permits searching at various levels of specificity. For example, MeSH terms for "malaria" include nine terms such as "falciparum," "vivax," and "Blackwater fever," without those terms having to be specified individually.

BOX 3-2
Generic and Trade Names of Antimalarial Drugs and CAS Numbers

Drug Name	Chemical Abstract Service Numbers
Atovaquone/Proguanil Malarone®	156879-69-5
Doxycycline Acticlate®, Vibramycin®, Doryx®, Vibra-Tabs®, Doryx® MPC, Doxycycline hyclate	564-25-0, 24390-14-5, 17086-28-1,10592-13-9, 94088-85-4
Chloroquine Aralen®, Chloroquine phosphate	54-05-7, 50-63-5, 3545-67-3
Mefloquine Lariam®, Mefloquine hydrochloride	53230-10-7, 51773-92-3
Primaquine Primaquine phosphate	90-34-6, 63-45-6
Tafenoquine succinate Arakoda™, Krintafel™	106635-81-8, 106635-80-7

TOXLINE (1840s–present) is a bibliographic database published by the National Library of Medicine which contains more than 4 million records, with new records added weekly. The database contains an assortment of citations from specialized journals and other sources including PubMed citations. It provides references covering the biochemical, pharmacologic, physiologic, and toxicologic effects of drugs and other chemicals. Most of TOXLINE's bibliographic citations contain abstracts or indexing terms and chemical abstract service registry numbers.

Index Medicus, a second database produced by the National Library of Medicine, covers citations indexed in PubMed and Medline. Citations in PubMed are fully indexed from 1966 to the present and selectively from 1809 to 1966, with a total of more than 25 million records. Index Medicus covers scientific literature in the areas of medical, biomedical, and life sciences and provides automatic mapping of search terms with MeSH terms. The focus of citations found in PubMed includes "in process" or "before print" citations as well as some citations from non-medical journals (particularly in public health, social science, psychology, and sociology) and ebooks (including several reports from the National Academies of Sciences, Engineering, and Medicine [the National Academies]). Medline

(1946–present) contains more than 22 million records on medical and biomedical sciences from approximately 5,600 journals (most of which are published in the United States).

Embase is an Elsevier database that contains more than 30 million records from more than 8,500 journals from at least 90 countries and is available by subscription through a number of interfaces, including the OVID interface that was used for the committee's searches. Citations cover all those indexed in Medline as well as more than 2,000 additional drug and pharmacy journals, which include journals published outside the United States, and 260,000 conference abstracts. The citations are fully indexed from 1947 to the present and selectively back from 1947 to 1902. This database is considered one of the most important databases for identifying studies typically associated with evidence-based practice, including meta-analyses, systematic reviews (such as those reviews by Cochrane), randomized controlled trials, cohort studies, case–control studies, case series, and other epidemiologic publications. Embase is also an extremely important database for identifying grey literature, such as reports from the Food and Drug Administration (FDA) and the National Institutes of Health.

Two supplemental databases of malaria-specific literature (the Malaria in Pregnancy Consortium library[2] and WWARN.org) were also searched using the generic and trade names for each antimalarial of interest. WWARN.org maintains a clinical trials publication library and a pharmacology publication database. Potentially relevant articles that were not captured by the search were also identified by searching the reference lists of relevant review and research articles.

Several types of publications were captured: epidemiologic studies, case reports and case series, clinical trials, laboratory animal studies, in vitro studies, reviews, meta-analyses, summaries of expert meetings, clinical and travel-based guidelines, conference abstracts, commentaries, and letters to the editor. Exact duplicate articles were deleted. An individual EndNote library was set up for each of the six drugs of interest. If an article examined multiple drugs, the article was placed into the library of each drug examined. For example, if a study examined mefloquine and atovaquone/proguanil, it was placed into both the mefloquine and atovaquone/proguanil libraries for further review. A study that reported on multiple drugs of interest was assessed for relevance in each of those chapters.

Use of Other Sources

In addition to carrying out the comprehensive literature search for studies that contained original data collection and analysis, the committee considered other sources of information in their deliberations, including review articles, national and foreign government reports, responses to committee-generated information

---

[2] See http://library.mip-consortium.org/index.php?home (accessed November 4, 2019).

requests, and information submitted by the public through invited presentations, comments, and data submissions.

Reviews and Other Non-Original Data Collection

Peer-reviewed studies with original data collection and analyses were preferred over studies that were re-analyses of a population (without the incorporation of additional information), pooled analyses or meta-analyses, reviews, and so on. Studies with original data were preferentially considered by the committee when assessing the strength of the association between an antimalarial of interest and a persistent or latent health outcome to draw its conclusions. These other types of studies and publications may be informative and may be discussed in conjunction with primary results or in synthesis sections on a given drug or health outcome.

Systematic reviews, such as those published by the Cochrane Collaboration, on topics of interest were also considered part of the evidentiary base. Although the committee did not assess review articles exhaustively, it did consider them for specific topics, such as the known biologic mechanisms of action and the pharmacokinetic and pharmacodynamic properties of the antimalarials of interest and their concurrent adverse events. Commentaries, opinions, letters to the editor, and author responses that referred to an included article were captured and considered along with the original article. National and global recommendations on malaria prophylaxis (by the Centers for Disease Control and Prevention [CDC], World Health Organization, European Union, etc.) were reviewed when they specifically reported on the rationale for changes to the recommendations for antimalarial prophylaxis. Data presented only in abstract form, such as from conferences, or in other unpublished formats were not included.

Grey Literature

Formal government reports on the drugs of interest from U.S. agencies or foreign governments were reviewed. Individual reports on adverse events from the FDA Adverse Event Reporting System (FAERS) were not requested or reviewed. However, if a publication used FAERS reports or the equivalent from other countries as part of its analysis, the committee considered it. The committee downloaded available drug labels and package inserts from FDA's website for each of the drugs of interest. These were used to provide information concerning specific changes and updates to the use of the drug or the warnings and contraindications associated with it. Package inserts are listed on the webpage with an action date, but the date provided in the downloaded package-insert document may occasionally differ from the action date posted on the webpage (e.g., a downloaded document listed as the 1989 mefloquine package insert was a July 2002 revision). Occasionally a downloaded document contained no date (e.g., the template's "month/year" placeholder is not filled). Additional requests for information were made to FDA, the Department of Defense (DoD), and the Department of Veterans Affairs (VA). Those requests and the received responses are part of the committee's public access file. The received information was integrated with the other evidence for drugs of interest.

Invited Presentations

As part of fulfilling its Statement of Task, the committee held two open sessions to assist in information gathering which served to inform the discussions throughout this report. The first presentation was made by representatives of VA to formally charge the committee with their Statement of Task and to answer clarifying questions related to the charge. The committee heard from presenters from DoD, the Department of State, and the Peace Corps with knowledge of malaria prophylaxis policies. In addition to presentations focused on the malaria prophylaxis policies of different government agencies, representatives from FDA gave an overview of the FDA's postmarketing pharmacovigilance system of adverse events and of how that information is used to monitor for signs of safety issues. A representative of CDC explained how the agency assembles and weighs data for making country-specific recommendations for malaria prophylaxis for U.S. travelers. Since those recommendations are based largely on the published literature, the second part of the CDC presentation reviewed some of the common strengths and limitations of pertinent literature. The committee heard from an advocacy organization that presented a hypothesis for the existence of a neuropsychiatric disease that the organization believes to be associated with the use of mefloquine prophylaxis in U.S. military service members. Finally, the committee heard a detailed presentation on the neurotoxic mechanisms of some antimalarials, particularly artemisinins. A more detailed summary of each invited presentation is found in Appendix B.

Public Comments

Each open session included time for attendees to make statements for the committee's consideration. Additionally, for the duration of the deliberation process, members of the public were encouraged to submit data and testimonials to the committee through the study email. Many of the public comments received and the in-person statements given described personal experiences of persistent effects following the use of mefloquine for malaria prophylaxis while the individual was serving in the military, the Department of State, or the Peace Corps or during personal travel. Several of those who testified on their experiences with mefloquine asked the committee to clearly communicate any limitations of the data used to base its conclusions, and to convey its thinking on research that may still be needed.

During the course of its work, the committee read and heard many moving personal accounts of individuals suffering from debilitating symptoms after using certain antimalarial drugs. The committee appreciated the opportunity to hear these accounts firsthand and understood the tremendous effort and strength that was required to speak publicly about these very personal experiences. Although the committee was not tasked with making judgments regarding specific cases in which individuals have claimed injury from use of an antimalarial drug, the reports from these individuals were welcomed, and the committee appreciated their desire to contribute in a positive way to the information gathering of the committee.

Submissions to the committee also included information on two planned postmarketing safety studies of tafenoquine (Arakoda™); statements that veterans' medical records submitted to FDA via MedWatch played a role in FDA's issuing of a boxed warning for mefloquine and that neurovestibular and neuro-ocular symptoms associated with mefloquine are not found in the published mefloquine literature; calls for examining the interactions of malaria-prophylactic drugs with other drugs when considering adverse effects; and requests that all sources of information be considered, including information from clinicians who diagnosed mefloquine-related disorders and medical records from the War-Related Illness and Injury clinics.

EVALUATION OF THE EVIDENCE

This section details the methods and two-step process used by the committee for screening the results of its searches to identify potentially relevant literature for full-text review. The first step involved screening for relevance by title and abstract, as available. The second step entailed a full-text review to determine the final set of studies that the committee considered, assessed, and synthesized. It was this final set of studies that provided the basis for the committee's conclusions on the relationships between the use of an antimalarial drug and specific categories of adverse health effects. The quantitative and qualitative procedures underlying the committee's literature evaluation have been made as explicit as possible, but ultimately the conclusions about associations expressed in this report are based on the committee's collective judgment. The committee has endeavored to express its judgments as clearly and precisely as the data allow.

Literature Screening

A total of approximately 11,700 titles and abstracts were captured in the literature search, covering all six drugs of interest. In step 1 of the process, article titles and abstracts were screened for relevance by the National Academies' Health and Medicine Division staff under the committee's direction to determine which articles should be considered for full-text retrieval. The screening criteria are outlined below. For each drug, two reviewers performed the initial screening. Titles and abstracts, where available, were reviewed to screen out articles that did not meet the committee's inclusion criteria. When the two primary reviewers were not in agreement, a third reviewer made the determination whether to include an article. Articles that did not have abstracts were generally passed to the full-text review stage unless the information included in the title clearly excluded the article. Staff reviewed reference lists of reviews and original articles for relevant articles or other information not picked up in the databases search and added these for consideration during full-text review. Another approximately 300 articles were identified in this way.

Because the committee's Statement of Task specified that persistent adverse events resulting from the prophylactic use of the antimalarials of interest in adults were of central concern, all publications that reported on a drug of interest used prophylactically were initially considered relevant when screening the literature. However, the committee also set additional criteria for final inclusion. Each article included in the final set must

- report an adverse event or effect (or if none were observed) or other health outcome when the drug was used as a prophylaxis, regardless of the timing of that event;
- have a comparison group;
- follow a population for more than 28 days (or reported as 4 weeks or 1 month); and
- in studies of humans, have study populations constrained to people 16 years or older. Studies of populations with mixed age groups, in which some of the individuals were less than 16 years old, were also included.

If any of this information was not clear from the title or abstract, the article was kept for review at the full-text stage.

Other areas were explored, although not exhaustively, using the human and animal literature. These areas included case reports of adverse events; studies of adherence to a drug of interest when used for malaria prophylaxis; the co-administration of an antimalarial for prophylaxis with sporozoite immunization; the co-administration of an antimalarial for prophylaxis with medications for other common conditions (e.g., antimalarial with warfarin, antihypertensives, insulin, etc.) that report on side effects or adverse events (or if none were observed); and interactions with nonmalarial drugs, supplements, and substances (e.g., food, alcohol, or nicotine). Studies of pharmacokinetics and pharmacodynamics, metabolism, and biologic mechanisms of action (e.g., system pathways, cell signaling, other biologic markers) were also included for drugs of interest or their metabolites. Articles that examined the drugs of interest for the treatment of malaria were considered only for tafenoquine because it was so recently approved by FDA for use, and such articles were considered only if the reported adverse events were not listed in the FDA package insert. For the other drugs of interest, the discussion of adverse events when the drugs were used for treatment was limited to review articles and discussed as background where relevant. Studies of pregnant women were limited to those who were taking antimalarial prophylaxis or intermittent preventive treatment in which adverse events are specified (either to the mother directly or to the fetus or newborn) or other reproductive outcomes were reported. The committee recognized that the risks of adverse events of the drugs under consideration can be influenced by a host of factors even if the specific mechanisms are not fully understood. Where the committee thought the evidence regarding risks to adult subpopulations with comorbid conditions (e.g., renal failure, cardiovascular conditions, immunosuppressed, human immunodeficiency virus positive status/acquired immunodeficiency syndrome [AIDS]) or having specific demographic features (such as women, older or younger age groups, race or ethnic background, etc.) was informative, these studies are briefly mentioned. However, most of the adverse events observed in these subpopulations are based on studies that reported concurrent use of the drug of interest and thus did not meet the inclusion criteria (described in the next section) to be considered a primary epidemiologic study.

Several types of articles were considered to be outside the committee's scope of work and were specifically excluded from consideration. These included studies of populations administered antimalarial drugs for a use other than malaria prophylaxis (e.g., for treatment of leishmaniasis, flukes, pneumonia, lupus, rheumatoid arthritis, cancer, or sexually transmitted infections) because studies of populations that use the antimalarial drugs of interest for reasons other than malaria prophylaxis were determined not to be comparable to or representative of the populations using the drugs for malaria prophylaxis; studies that exclusively examined antimalarial efficacy, effectiveness or sensitivity, or drug resistance without mentioning adverse effects (or the lack of them); trends of antimalarial prescriptions (no adverse events reported); studies that focused solely on the effects that an antimalarial of interest had on the malaria parasites or on the use of an antimalarial for the purpose of reducing transmission; and studies that focused on derivatives of the drugs of interest (such as for drug discovery) or drug-delivery systems (e.g., carriers, encapsulations). Additionally, studies that examined the simultaneous administration of an antimalarial drug of interest in combination with any other antimalarial drug that is not an FDA-approved combination (e.g., an artemisinin and mefloquine given at the same time or as a combination pill) were excluded.

In general, studies of recrudescence or relapse of malaria were excluded because they were focused on efficacy. An exception to this was for studies of primaquine and tafenoquine when they are used as presumptive anti-relapse therapy. For these two drugs, studies of malaria relapse were included and reviewed for other adverse events. Additionally, for these two drugs, combinations of prophylactic drugs were included (e.g., chloroquine followed by primaquine).

Approach to Evaluating and Assessing Individual Studies

In step 2 of the literature screening process, full text was obtained for any articles that were considered potentially relevant after applying the step 1 screening criteria for inclusion and exclusion. The committee began its assessment of the literature without regard to whether an association between prophylactic use of an antimalarial and any particular health outcome was suggested in the studies, focusing solely on its relevance to addressing that question. Similarly, because of the variability in the descriptions and diagnoses of the health conditions considered in this report, the committee made no a priori assumptions about the usefulness of any article or report, relying solely on the methods presented to assess the contribution of each study. Each study that met the inclusion criteria was reviewed and objectively evaluated for each health outcome it presented. If a study examined more than one drug or health outcome, it was considered separately for each drug and for each of those outcomes. After a review of more than 3,500 full-text articles, studies that were considered relevant were grouped and evaluated thoroughly. Full-text articles were grouped into categories of primary or supplemental evidence. Epidemiologic studies that presented original information in human populations were considered primary evidence. Supplemental or supporting literature included FDA labels and package inserts, reviews and meta-analyses, considerations of selected populations (such as pregnant women), case reports, additional information from the committee's information requests, and animal and mechanistic studies. The articles were then distributed among the committee members according to their areas of expertise, with at least two committee members reviewing each paper. All adverse events were considered regardless of severity.

Supplemental Evidence

Spontaneous reports of adverse events and case studies provide the least rigorous evidence of an effect. MedWatch, FDA's program for postmarketing surveillance, collects clinical information involving drugs from health care professionals and consumers through a variety of outlets, including mail, internet, and telephone, but the largest source of postmarketing information on adverse events is the drug companies themselves (IOM, 2007). Often reports of an adverse event lack important details such as the duration of the event or its effects, the tests performed, and if there was any follow-up. Moreover, the adverse event reported in case reports is associated with *use* of the drug; the drug has not necessarily been proven to be the *cause* of the adverse event.

Case reports and case series were considered when there was follow-up that lasted at least 28 days after drug cessation, but because these reports lack control groups, they contribute no meaningful information about the degree of risk in a population or even to other individuals who have the same underlying characteristics, and thus their contribution to the weight of the evidence was considered supportive rather than primary. Case reports of adverse events determined to be attributed to the use of a drug of interest were captured and are presented as supplemental information to the epidemiologic studies, specifically when evidence of a clinician-diagnosed outcome was presented. When case studies were reviewed, the EQUATOR consensus criteria for case studies aided in evaluating the strength of the evidence presented (Gagnier et al., n.d.; Rodgers et al., 2016). These criteria outline the elements that a high-quality case report should include. Reporting of de-identified patient-specific information, primary clinical concerns, and relevant history and previous treatments must be included, for example. Reported diagnostic information encompasses diagnostic methods, challenges, and reasoning. Detailed information about the intervention, follow-up, and outcomes, including adherence and tolerability, are required. Finally, an evaluation of the strengths and limitations, relevant medical literature, and rationale for conclusions are necessary.

Toxicologic studies in animal models and of in vitro cell cultures are included where appropriate to inform the understanding of pharmacokinetics and biologic plausibility through the toxicology of the drugs and their exposure pathways. Throughout the drug-specific chapters, pharmacokinetics refers to how the organism (human or experimental animal model) affects the drug, including via processes of absorption, metabolism, and excretion. Pharmacodynamic mechanisms are covered under the heading of "Biologic Plausibility" in that pharmacodynamics refers to how a drug affects an organism with particular emphasis on dose–response relationships. Because these studies were considered to provide supportive evidence, their results would not be enough to change the level of evidence for an association.

Primary Evidence

Studies that compared different groups of human populations based on the exposure to antimalarial drugs can be broadly classified as either observational studies or trials. The committee refers to both types of these comparative studies as "epidemiologic studies" throughout the report. The focus of the committee's assessment is on epidemiologic studies because epidemiology deals with the determinants, frequency, and distribution of disease in human populations rather than in individuals or in animal models, which have several limitations, as discussed below. Several types of epidemiologic studies were evaluated, including randomized controlled trials, cohort studies, case–control studies, and cross-sectional studies. Formal, well-designed, and well-conducted epidemiologic studies can serve to produce evidence of associations between an exposure and health outcomes.

For each full-text epidemiologic article that met the committee's screening inclusion, an additional criterion question was applied:

Does the study provide any empirical information about adverse effects that begin or persist, or indicate the lack of such events, following at least 28 days after cessation (final dose) of the drug of interest?

Although for step 1 of the screening process the population had to be followed for at least 28 days, during step 2 of the full-text review the inclusion was strengthened to require a follow-up of at least 28 days post-drug-cessation. As long as a study met the criteria, it was included, even if it had severe methodologic limitations. Studies that did not follow their populations for at least 28 days after the final dose of a drug of interest was administered or that did not distinguish the timing of the adverse events (e.g., the follow-up time was more than 28 days after drug cessation but the authors did not distinguish which adverse events occurred inside and outside of the 28-day window) are briefly mentioned but are not evaluated in depth. It is important to note that a study could be well designed and well conducted but have serious limitations in its ability to provide information that had direct bearing on the committee's work, such as by not distinguishing the timing of adverse events. The committee did not contact study authors for clarifications or additional data. For example, several studies included only a brief statement that "no serious adverse events were reported" without further explanation of what adverse events were examined, how "serious" was defined, or what the timing of those events was.

A total of 21 epidemiologic studies that reported on adverse events that were captured or persisted for more than 28 days are included in this report: Ackert et al., 2019; Andersen et al., 1998; DeSouza, 1983; Eick-Cost et al., 2017; Green et al., 2014; Laothavorn et al., 1992; Leary et al., 2009; Lee et al., 2013; Lege-Oguntoye et al., 1990; Meier et al., 2004; Miller et al., 2013; Nasveld et al., 2010; Rueangweerayut et al., 2017; Schlagenhauf et al., 1996; Schneider et al., 2013, 2014; Schneiderman et al., 2018; Schwartz and Regev-Yochay, 1999; Tan et al., 2017; Walsh et al., 2004; and Wells et al., 2006. A table that gives a high-level comparison (study design, population, exposure groups, and outcomes examined by body system) of each of these epidemiologic studies is presented in Appendix C. Although the committee considered using published tools to conduct risk-of-bias assessments for the studies, ultimately it was unable to identify an approach that addressed all of the committee's needs. Instead, the committee adopted selected components of these tools, primarily the Newcastle–Ottawa Scale (Wells et al., 2019), and applied them in its assessment of individual studies. The PICO (Participants, Interventions, Comparisons, and Outcomes) model is commonly used for characterizing clinical studies for formal systematic reviews and meta-analyses. As this assessment was neither a strict systematic review nor a meta-analysis, the committee used a modified PICO that characterized included studies according to their study design, population, study groups, and body systems examined (see next section on Methodologic Considerations). Based on the details of the study, the description of how adverse events were assessed or measured, and whether it distinguished between adverse events that began or persisted 28 days after cessation of the drug of interest, an epidemiologic study was classified either as a primary article, in which case it met the inclusion criteria and was thoroughly assessed, or as a secondary supporting article, in which case it did not meet inclusion criteria and was reviewed and more briefly described under the heading Other Identified Studies in Human Populations. Primary articles were assessed for quality based on the methods provided (e.g., adequate control for confounding variables, use of adequate diagnostic instruments, use of appropriate statistical tests; see next section, Methodologic Considerations) and the precision of the reported results. Effect estimates, data, and units of measure are presented as reported in the cited studies, except where otherwise noted. The responsible committee members then presented the information from each relevant study to the full committee for discussion, including the methods used for selecting the study populations and conducting the research (i.e., design, population, length of follow-up, sources of measurement for exposure and adverse events or health outcomes [such as self-reported information, medical records, claims data, validated tests and tools, etc.], the statistical analyses used, adjustment factors, etc.), the results, and a thorough assessment of the strengths, limitations, and potential biases and their implication.

The committee defined a health outcome as any recognized symptom, condition, or diagnosis. As the committee's Statement of Task specified that neurologic and psychiatric outcomes were to be addressed, and because these outcomes were not assessed consistently across studies, the committee adopted a rubric for categorizing the different outcomes. First, the committee considers all neurologic and psychiatric symptoms and disorders to be brain based. The committee recognizes that some of these experiences may not yet have empirically based neuroanatomical correlates, and it acknowledges that psychosocial factors play an etiologic role in psychiatric symptoms and disorders, but there is generally some functional overlap between "neurologic" and "psychiatric" symptoms and disorders. These categories were evaluated separately, rather than as a general "neuropsychiatric" category because of the specific charge in the Statement of Task. In that vein, some studies reported specific ICD-9-CM[3] diagnoses (e.g., Anxiety Disorders 300.0X, 300.2X, 300.3X) or broad categories of ICD-9-CM disorders (e.g., Mental Disorders 290-319), diagnosed by clinicians and coded in medical records. Outcomes in other studies were self-reported diagnoses or symptoms of constructs such as "anxiety," "depression," or "dizziness" that were not necessarily based on standardized self-report measures of symptoms. In studies that categorized and reported symptoms as "neuropsychiatric," the outcomes were separated into psychiatric or neurologic categories of disorders to the extent possible. Central and peripheral nervous system symptoms and disorders such as headaches, confusion, dizziness, vertigo, convulsions, and cognitive impairment were designated as neurologic symptoms. Symptoms, disorders, and diagnoses of depression, anxiety,

---

[3] ICD-9-CM: *International Classification of Diseases, 9th Revision, Clinical Modification.*

posttraumatic stress disorder (PTSD), psychosis, and insomnia were considered to be psychiatric outcomes.

Those epidemiologic studies that measured nonspecific outcomes, such as biologic markers of effect (e.g., changes in pathophysiology, cell signaling, or hormone levels and blood counts) are considered but are given less weight because of the uncertainty of their relevance to persistent adverse events as opposed to a recognized condition or disease. Several of the included studies assessed multiple outcomes, whereas others focused on a specific system (e.g., cardiovascular outcomes) or event (e.g., methemoglobin levels).

Methodologic Considerations

The human population studies that have been conducted on the persistent adverse effects of antimalarial drugs are quite diverse in both their methods and their quality. To assess their contribution to the overall weight of evidence concerning a given drug and health outcome, it is essential to consider the quality of the particular methods used to investigate the association because there is substantial unevenness in the rigor and informativeness of the specific studies. While there are textbooks that give general guidelines for epidemiologic study methods and randomized trials (Friedman, 2015; Gordis, 2004; Rothman et al., 2012), including those that address the interpretation of findings specifically (Savitz and Wellenius, 2016), the committee did not review these concepts in general but rather as they applied specifically to the question at hand, that is, the persistent or latent adverse events of antimalarial drugs.

In bringing in methodologic principles to appropriately weigh the evidence, the committee's intention was to do so objectively, based solely on the quality of the methods and not on the nature or implications of the findings. Some studies that met the inclusion criteria and are summarized in the following chapters had a rather high level of credibility based on the quality of the work, whereas others were virtually non-contributory based on their methods, and the committee provides the rationale by which such judgments were made. The committee sought to be as transparent as possible in indicating the underlying bases for its judgments. Before considering what substantive conclusions were justified based on the research for a given antimalarial drug and health outcome, the committee considered the overall quality of the body of available research.

In addition to the quality of individual studies, it is important to consider the number of such studies, which also tends to be quite limited, especially for certain antimalarial drugs. The need for replication is quite clear, and the evidence base should ideally consist of many studies with varying strengths and limitations to identify a pattern that can be discerned in a series of imperfect studies. To supplement the information provided by epidemiologic studies, the committee drew on knowledge of the biologic underpinnings of the phenomenon of interest, evaluating the degree to which the association of a specific drug and a specific adverse event is plausible based on the known biologic pathways by which such an impact could occur. This is another aspect of the search for convergent evidence, in this case not just across studies but across disciplines.

Given the small volume of distinct types of studies of markedly varying quality, the committee chose to summarize them by discussing each of the pertinent studies and integrating that assessment without formal weighting by quality or precision. Given how heterogeneous they are, the studies did not lend themselves to pooling, and there were too few of them for more formal methods of assessing the quality of information. Instead, for each study that met the inclusion criteria, the study methods are described, the implications of those methods on the results and inferences that can be made are discussed, and an assessment is presented of the contribution that the study makes individually and in the aggregate to the evidence base. The committee recognizes the challenges in traditional hypothesis testing and over-reliance on "statistically significant" p values that rely on arbitrary cutoffs. Throughout the report the findings and results of studies are reported as they appear in the published papers, but in drawing conclusions the committee weighted consistency of direction of associations over specific statistically significant findings, and the body of evidence was considered as a whole. In its examination and assessment of the available evidence, the committee was looking for signals of associations and it endeavored to be sensitive rather than specific, so that even isolated findings that may well reflect random error from making multiple comparisons, or those that have not been corroborated, are reported. Ultimately, replications of results were considered indications of stronger evidence for an association that the committee considered in its weighing but in assessing the rather limited literature, some of the indications may not be confirmed with further research. The committee notes that although most of the studies reported the results of two-sided tests, which formally assess only whether there is a difference between two groups (which could be in either direction), for simplicity and readability the committee generally discusses the results as "increased" or "decreased" based on the magnitude and precision of the point estimate; in doing so it does not mean to imply that a formal one-sided hypothesis test was done (which was never or rarely the case).

Study Design

Randomized controlled studies are considered the "gold standard" for evaluating the efficacy of drugs and other therapeutic interventions. With few exceptions, FDA requires having this type of evidence demonstrating both efficacy and safety before it approves a new drug for licensure. Typically licensing a new drug requires randomized controlled clinical trials in which there is a comparison with placebo. Such trials are often limited to healthy populations, may be too small to detect uncommon adverse events, and may be too short to detect delayed adverse events. In addition, clinical trials enroll volunteers who are often healthier than the populations that will eventually be exposed to the drugs; however, this requirement may help to enhance generalizability to the population of interest, since military populations also are comprised of selectively healthy individuals. Clinical trials also often exclude individuals with specific comorbidities or other exposures that could affect the response to the drug. Thus, large observational studies are important complements to trials, especially when assessing drug safety.

Most drug approvals require trials with placebo comparators and the masking of exposures to ensure unbiased reporting and an accurate assessment of symptoms specific to the drug compared with no drug. However, important adverse events may be missed in such placebo-controlled trials for a variety of reasons, including the presence of symptoms that are uncommon, that are more likely in volunteers excluded from participating (e.g., those with a history of mental illness), or that were not specifically assessed (such as many neuropsychiatric symptoms). When there is a specific indication for a drug, as exists for malaria prophylaxis, patients and prescribers find it useful to make comparisons between alternative drugs to help make the best choice of agent for individual patients. Observational studies have the advantage of using "real-world" populations, and often include larger numbers of exposed persons than clinical trials, but most lack a comparable non-exposed group. Observational studies of adverse events to a drug often compare users of one drug to those of another drug used for the same indication to help control for factors associated with receiving care for the specific indication and for being prescribed or filling a prescription for that indication. As such, the comparison is limited to relative rather than absolute risks of adverse events. The committee did not prioritize one type of exposure comparison over another (i.e., placebo versus another drug); instead, in its assessment, the committee used comparison groups as one factor to identify studies that were methodologically strong. The synthesis was based on the strength of the evidence including consistency between studies.

Although observational studies (cohort and case–control studies, among others) have the advantage of evaluating people who are using the drug of interest in real-world settings, a major challenge is identifying an appropriate comparison group. Ideally, the comparison group should consist of individuals who are similar to those taking the drug in both their eligibility to take the drug of interest and in their baseline risk of developing the outcomes of interest. To assess this, it is important to have information about both groups so that the baseline characteristics can be compared and important differences can be controlled for when assessing adverse events following exposure. This is a challenge since some factors associated with developing adverse events are unknown or known but not ascertained and, if they are distributed differently in exposed and comparison groups, can result in biased estimates of association.

Observational studies are also at risk for channeling bias. Channeling bias can occur when different drugs with similar indications are prescribed to individuals with different risks for potential adverse outcomes (independent of the drug). For example, those with a personal or family history of mental illness may avoid or not be prescribed mefloquine, and those who want to avoid gastrointestinal distress may avoid or not be prescribed doxycycline. There are analytic methods to help address such imbalances, but the reasons why people receive a specific drug are not always documented and may be difficult to account for.

Case reports and case series provide valuable information about the possibility of an adverse outcome due to a drug, but they rarely suffice to prove a causal association. Case reports may also be helpful in defining a new syndrome (e.g., eosinophilic myalgia syndrome and AIDS) (Vandenbroucke, 1999). Developing a specific case definition based on case reports may assist investigators to design studies that can address the specific drug–disease associations of interest. However, it is important to note that serious adverse events can also occur by chance following the introduction of any new drug or vaccine. A temporal relationship between exposure and outcome is necessary for making a causal inference, but given the lack of comparison to individuals without exposure to the drug, it is not sufficient. FDA may require drug labeling changes to include information from case reports if the outcomes reported are serious or if they are frequently reported following that drug exposure. However, further evidence, such as from randomized trials or rigorous non-experimental studies with carefully selected comparison groups, is usually needed to determine whether the drug is causally associated with a higher risk of experiencing the adverse event.

Thus, there are a number of potentially informative research strategies, such as large randomized trials with sufficiently long-term follow-up or observational studies that have comparison groups that are not strongly affected by bias or other insurmountable sources of likely confounding, with case reports supporting the findings of more rigorous designs.

Sample Size

In addition to the systematic biases and errors that may arise, random error and uncertainty in estimates are also important considerations. Data are rarely available on all of the possible people and outcomes for a given population, so statistical approaches are used to appropriately represent that uncertainty. The statistical power of a particular study is also an important consideration, especially when examining (sometimes rare) adverse events. Formally, statistical power refers to the probability that a particular statistical test (e.g., an effect estimate comparing outcomes between treatment and control groups in a randomized trial) will "reject" the null hypothesis (e.g., that there is no treatment effect) if in fact a specific alternative hypothesis (e.g., that there is an effect) is true. In lay terms, the statistical power refers to the ability of a study to detect a "true" effect when such an effect exists. A particularly relevant concern for the studies examined in this report is that if the statistical power is not sufficiently high, an apparent lack of association between some exposure (such as the use of a particular antimalarial drug) and an outcome could be the result of a sample size that is not large enough to allow the detection of an effect. Books such as Cohen (1988) and Kraemer and Blasey (2015) provide additional details on power analysis calculations.

Statistical power depends on many things, including the study design, the statistical analysis conducted, and how common the outcome of interest is. This is of particular relevance (and concern) when trying to study adverse events, which are often rare. As noted above, randomized controlled trials are considered the gold standard for internal validity due to their ability to provide unbiased effect estimates for the sample at hand. Many of the strongest study designs found in the reviewed literature involved the randomization of antimalarial drugs. However, those studies are generally designed—and powered—to provide sufficient sample size to detect a difference in efficacy of the drugs, which means that many do not have sufficient statistical power to detect rare safety-related outcomes related to taking the drug.

For example, consider a situation in which a malaria infection rate is 200 out of every 1,000 people (20%) and an antimalarial drug reduces risk of malaria by 50% (so that the resultant infection rate is 10%). A study that enrolls 200 individuals and randomly assigns each to receive the antimalarial drug or placebo would have about 80% power to detect that effect. However, if the outcome of interest was a rare adverse event, such as one experienced by only 1 in every 10,000 people taking the antimalarial (versus 1 in 100,000 people not exposed to the drug), the study would need to enroll approximately 200,000 people in order to have 80% power to detect that difference in outcome rates. (Note, too, that rare outcomes—such as one occurring in just 1 of every 100,000 people—may be particularly uncommon in the samples enrolled in typical randomized trials to establish efficacy, as those individuals are often healthier than the general population.) Thus, even randomized trials that are sufficiently powered to detect their primary outcomes of interest may have limited power to detect differences in rare adverse events unless that was part of the original design of the study, with large numbers of individuals randomized. This also implies that for studying rare adverse events, large non-experimental studies may be more useful in terms of statistical power, although confounding and other biases then become a concern.

Given the impact of power considerations, it was critical for the committee to distinguish between studies that were small and did not detect differences in adverse events between treatment arms and studies that appeared to have had sufficient power to detect differences in outcomes if such differences did exist. In other words, a lack of observed association does not necessarily imply a lack of true association, especially if the studies were small and not designed to examine the outcomes under consideration.

In summary, in evaluating the weight and quality of evidence, especially when null findings are reported, it is important to consider whether a study was sufficiently powered to detect the associations of interest. While the statistical power is a function of multiple features of the study, notably study size and the frequency of the outcome of interest, studies that have only sufficient power to detect very large effects (e.g., relative risks greater than 3) are of limited value, given that relative risks of smaller magnitude may have important implications.

Exposure Assessment

Whenever individuals' exposures to medications are measured in a study, there is the possibility of misclassification. To illustrate, people who experience an adverse health event may provide a more complete report of their current and past exposures to medicines. Similarly, people who receive a particular antimalarial believed to be associated with specific adverse events may be more likely to seek medical care for a given condition. There may also be important differences in the completeness and accuracy of the exposure data between various sources of information. Using only pharmacy claims or only dispensing records for determining exposure to a drug used to prevent a disease may lead to an overestimation of peoples' exposure to a given drug, particularly if there is reason to believe that the drug is associated with acute adverse events. Moreover, prescription and dispensing data are not surrogates of actual use or adherence to the approved regimen. These are examples of differential misclassification of exposure that can lead to an overestimation or an underestimation of effects. Misclassification can also be nondifferential, as would be the case when the degree of misclassification is similar for all exposure groups and outcomes. An example would be a situation in which all study participants have similar difficulties completing questionnaires or remembering past exposures. Nondifferential misclassification of exposure tends to bias the study results toward the null (i.e., attenuating the strength of an association between a drug and outcome). Obtaining data from more than one source or verifying data by examining pre-existing records (e.g., medical records or pharmacy records) may help to reduce the misclassification of exposures.

If studies of antimalarial drugs are to make meaningful contributions, there should be either documentation of drug prescriptions with a high likelihood—if not certainty—of adherence or else self-report based on carefully designed questionnaires. Even these methods are fallible, but in most cases they provide sufficient quality to be considered contributory evidence.

Outcome Assessment

Outcome misclassification occurs when individuals are placed into an incorrect category with respect to the outcome of interest. If the misclassification occurs differently for people with and without exposure to a drug, it is said to be differential misclassification, which may lead to an association between exposure to a drug of interest and an outcome being either exaggerated or underestimated. In nondifferential outcome misclassification, the misclassification is not related to exposure status (i.e., the use of a specific drug), and the effect estimates tend to underestimate the true effect. The outcomes reported in the epidemiologic literature for the antimalarial drugs of interest generally fall into six categories: neurologic, psychiatric, gastrointestinal, ocular, cardiovascular, and other (depending on the drug, this category may include such things as dermatologic or biochemical outcomes). The assessment and diagnosis of conditions in each of these categories is dependent on different criteria, measures, and tests, some more objective than others. For example, whereas electrocardiograms are tests based on objective biologic indicators that can be used to diagnose certain cardiovascular conditions, structured clinical interviews are needed to diagnose psychiatric conditions.

In part because some of these health outcomes do not have biologically based diagnostic tests, such as mental health diagnoses and symptoms and some neurologic symptoms such as cognitive impairment (e.g., problems with memory, attention, or concentration) and headaches, the committee discussed the strength and validity of these outcomes as reported in the included studies. PTSD, an outcome specified in the committee's Statement of Task, is a challenging condition to assess and report in epidemiologic studies. Clinically recorded diagnoses should be based on criteria from the *Diagnostic and Statistical Manual of Mental Disorders* (DSM) or the ICD, which require that a diagnosis should be made when trauma exposure is reported and that symptoms are in relation to a specific trauma. Self-reported diagnoses or symptom measurements do not usually have this requirement, making self-reported symptoms a less reliable measurement of PTSD. Generally, studies based on self-report measures fail to specifically connect PTSD symptoms to a specific traumatic event, as required by the DSM diagnostic formulation: Criterion A requires exposure to an event that was life-threatening or violent. Each of the subsequent symptom clusters (i.e., intrusion, avoidance, cognitive or emotional disturbance, or hyperarousal) must be experienced in relation to the traumatic event, and an exclusionary criterion is that the symptoms may not be due to medication. Because many studies do not link symptoms to an identified traumatic event, it is often difficult, if not impossible, to ascertain whether symptoms that are reported in the evaluated literature are the result of a medication-related experience, some other trauma, both, or neither, which lends uncertainty to the meaning of these outcomes when associations are found in populations of interest. Furthermore, because these symptoms and diagnoses are not linked directly to the experience of a specific traumatic event, it is unclear whether these symptoms or diagnoses are experienced in a timeframe that would make them likely to be related to the use of a particular medication.

An association between drug administration and other psychiatric outcomes, such as depression, suicidality, or psychotic experiences (e.g., hallucinations, delusions), is even harder to establish, for several different reasons. First, in the population of most relevance, service members, the age of exposure to antimalarials overlaps with the age of onset of many of the psychiatric symptoms of interest. Depression and symptoms of psychosis develop within the age window of the young adult population who are recruited to the military. The onset of psychiatric symptoms may be coincident to exposure to medication, but a causal relationship would be difficult to establish. Second, military-related confounders introduce powerful effects on the adverse health outcomes of interest (see Confounding section below). Additionally, the lack of understanding of the biologic mechanisms of risk and resilience in these psychiatric experiences presents multiple challenges to establishing causal relationships between most risk factors and psychiatric outcomes. Furthermore, because many of these psychiatric symptoms have variable courses, from presenting and remitting quickly to multiple episodes of relapse and remission to consistent persistence, it is unclear how any intervening risk factor would affect the natural course of these symptoms.

The committee defined "persistent" outcomes as those present at least 28 days following cessation of a drug, which is appropriate for the case of PTSD, as PTSD is not diagnosed until at least 1 month following a Criterion A traumatic event. However, if the symptoms of PTSD are assessed years after cessation of a drug, yet they are reported in the absence of a direct connection to the experience of taking the drug or any other traumatic event, it is difficult to determine the etiology of those symptoms. For other conditions reported in the literature, onset may be acute, but the condition may persist for more than 28 days post-drug-cessation and may not resolve without treatment. This would pertain, for example, to certain ophthalmic conditions, such as cataract.

The committee recognizes that it is difficult to achieve an optimal assessment of neuropsychiatric endpoints in this literature. Psychiatric and neurologic symptoms should be assessed and documented by a trained assessor, using structured and psychometrically sound assessment tools. For example, an optimal method is to include lifetime psychiatric diagnoses using structured clinical interviews based on DSM-5 criteria (e.g., Structured Clinical Interview for DSM-5, or SCID), administered by a trained assessor, with special attention to and documentation of symptom onset and remission and their relationship to medication exposure. A SCID would make it possible to connect the PTSD symptoms to a particular potentially traumatic event. Because previous diagnoses of PTSD significantly raise the risk for subsequent diagnoses, determining the lifetime diagnoses that occurred prior to medication exposure, rather than just the current diagnoses, would allow for a more reliable control for this variable.

Confounding

An important aspect of individual studies that must be considered when evaluating the quality of their methods is the attention paid to the potential for the results to reflect confounding bias rather than a true association. Part of an assessment of the potential for confounding is to examine any steps taken by the investigators to mitigate the impact of potential confounders. Confounding could occur, for example, if the use of antimalarial drugs for prophylaxis is associated with personal or situational attributes that may also predict the adverse outcome under study. These personal or situational attributes are said to "confound" the association between the antimalarial drug use and the adverse outcome of interest. For example, a history of psychiatric problems is a contraindication to the use of some of the antimalarials of interest. This personal characteristic (the presence or absence of psychiatric problems) is also likely to be a predictor of future adverse psychiatric outcomes. If the investigators do not take this into account, then the results of the study may suggest that individuals taking a particular antimalarial are less likely to develop adverse psychiatric outcomes than a comparison group whose members have not taken the drug because those with a history of psychiatric illness will have been excluded from the antimalarial group but not from the comparison group. Furthermore, as contraindications are introduced over time, studies will differ in their susceptibility to this bias in relation to the altered prescribing practices. This example highlights the importance of careful consideration of the comparison group, as discussed above. If, in this example, individuals with a history of psychiatric problems were excluded from the comparison group, then the potential for confounding by a history of psychiatric problems would be removed.

Another illustration relates specifically to use of antimalarials in the military. Service-related characteristics may act as confounders when assessing the association between antimalarial use and psychiatric outcomes. Specifically, a confounding factor could be whether individuals were deployed or assigned to duties outside of the United States. The stressors associated with living and working outside of the country may themselves increase risk for adverse health outcomes, especially psychiatric outcomes. Exposure to combat areas is also likely to increase the risk of negative health outcomes. Service members most likely to be prescribed antimalarials are those who are assigned to duty outside of the United States, and possibly even in combat areas, and these confounders can exert strong effects on the risk for negative health outcomes before considering antimalarial exposure. The potential for confounding in this hypothetical example could be addressed by adjusting for deployment location and combat exposure in the statistical analysis. As noted with regard to study design, one of the ways in which studies can be informative is to limit confounding where possible by choosing a suitable comparison group to compare those taking the drug with those in the comparison group having roughly similar levels of strong influences on outcome such as contraindications (e.g., psychiatric history), combat exposure, or selection for favorable health status. It is also possible to control for confounding to some extent by measuring the characteristics that may differ between the exposed and comparison group and making statistical adjustments.

Effect Modification

Effect modification, stemming from a potential presence of variables (known or unknown to the researcher) affecting the association between an exposure (e.g., drug) and an outcome (e.g., PTSD), is highly prevalent in epidemiologic studies. Effect modification occurs when an exposure has different effects among different subgroups or levels of the effect modifier. Consequently, the magnitude of the association may vary across studies, based on the level or presence of such variables. A common solution to addressing effect modification is to examine the association separately for each level of a third variable (e.g., the level of education of the subjects). While helpful, this solution is dependent on whether the data concerning such variables are collected (e.g., genetic markers are rarely examined in epidemiologic studies), and the statistical power (i.e., how many subjects at each level) for such an examination are at all sufficient. Such factors as a previous history of malaria treatment, mental health problems, exposure to concurrent drugs, adherence to drug dosing and schedule, and previous concurrent stressors may contribute to effect modification.

At present, there is not sufficiently compelling information to make the consideration of effect modifiers essential to having a meaningful study (i.e., it has not been established with any certainty that subgroups in the population are more or less vulnerable to any persistent adverse effects associated with antimalarial use). Where information on effect modification is provided, the results may suggest considering that possibility and therefore be of some value.

Biologic Plausibility

In assessing biologic plausibility—defined by the committee as the existence of mechanisms observed in studies of experimental animals, cell cultures, or pathophysiology assessments that could account for the various adverse events observed in humans using the various antimalarial drugs of interest for prophylaxis—the committee required that published articles include objective tests of the impact of these drugs on endpoints relevant to potential pathologic processes. Outcomes were not limited to any specific organ or system, and reviewed studies included the exposure of experimental animals, cell lines, and, in some cases, human tissue or blood samples to antimalarial drugs. In assessing biologic plausibility for a particular outcome, the number of papers describing the same mechanistic endpoints associated with drug exposure was considered as an indicator of the validity of findings. Although various biochemical and pathologic endpoints and outcomes were considered (and they are discussed in the individual antimalarial drug chapters as appropriate), the committee also notes any limitations of these types of studies with regard to applicability to prophylaxis, how analogous the models and time courses of observation used are to humans, and how closely the drug dosing and concentrations correspond to those experienced in humans using these drugs for malaria prophylaxis.

Types of Populations Considered

The studies evaluated for this report were conducted in different populations. Although U.S. service members and veterans are the target population of interest, studies of other populations were also considered as contributing to the evidence base for associations between antimalarial use and persistent adverse events.

Military and Veteran Populations

Because people who are currently serving or who have served in the U.S. military are the target population of the charge to this committee, studies of these populations were accorded considerable weight in the committees' deliberations and are presented first in the summaries of the identified literature for each drug. The committee reviewed all identified studies of U.S. and international service members and veterans that used any of the antimalarials of interest. In general, few studies included objective measures of drug chemical concentrations in the blood or tissue; those that are available were performed in small studies, usually to examine the pharmacokinetic and pharmacodynamic properties of a drug. Instead, the use of a particular antimalarial and its dosage for prophylaxis is based on self-report or, when observed by researchers or clinicians, as part of the study design. Often, full adherence to the drug regimen is assumed in estimating and quantifying the risk of specific adverse events and health outcomes related to the use of a particular drug, even though many studies have shown that individuals often fail to fully adhere to the regimen, especially when the drug is to be taken for long periods of time, introducing the potential for misclassification bias (Brisson and Brisson, 2012; Cunningham et al., 2014; Landman et al., 2014; Saunders et al., 2015). Consistent with other studies of health outcomes in military populations, when there are no actual measures of exposure to a specific chemical or group of toxicants, comparisons between deployed and nondeployed veterans are considered to be the next most relevant comparison. Since sending troops to known malaria-endemic areas without prevention measures when they are available would be unethical, several studies of military populations compare the effects of two or more different antimalarials. Because of the many other factors and stresses associated with deployed environments, including combat, specific effects attributable to the use of an antimalarial drug may be difficult to tease out.

Human Studies Among Non-Military or Veteran Populations

Although U.S. service members and veterans constitute the source population of interest, the committee has taken into account the potential for obtaining a more precise quantification and evaluation of the risks of adverse events and health outcomes associated with the antimalarial drugs of interest in better characterized cohorts. Such cohorts include occupationally exposed workers (such as Peace Corps volunteers, Department of State officials, etc.), travelers and expats, research volunteers, people with adverse events reported to national or manufacturer registries, and people living in malaria-endemic areas. These populations use antimalarial drugs but do not have some of the same potentially confounding stressors such as combat. Studies of short-term travelers who were followed for at least 28 days post-drug-cessation and of long-term travelers and expats who visited or moved to malaria-endemic areas and used antimalarial drugs for prophylaxis provide additional evidence of health outcomes following exposure to the antimalarial drugs of interest that can supplement the studies of service members and veterans. In addition, safety and tolerance studies performed in healthy residents of non-endemic areas who were followed for at least 28 days post-drug-cessation were reviewed. Finally, studies of adverse events associated with the prophylactic use of a drug in a population with a specific underlying condition (such as pregnancy, comorbid conditions) or demographic trait are described as appropriate.

Animal and Mechanistic Studies

The committee used animal and mechanistic studies to determine whether there is evidence of a pathophysiologic process or biologic mechanism that could provide reasonable evidence to support a relationship between exposure to an antimalarial drug and a persistent health effect, as seen in studies of humans using the antimalarial drugs for prophylaxis. A positive statistical association between an exposure and an outcome does not necessarily mean that the exposure is the cause of that outcome. Data from toxicology studies may support or conflict with a hypothesis that a specific drug or chemical can contribute to the occurrence of a particular condition or disease. Insights about biologic processes inform whether an observed pattern of statistical association might be interpreted as the product of more than error, bias, confounding, or chance. Discussions on biologic plausibility are presented after the evidence in humans is presented and before the synthesis of all the evidence. The degree of biologic plausibility itself influences whether the committee perceives positive findings in human studies to be indicative of a pattern or the product of bias or chance statistical associations. Ultimately, the results of the toxicology studies should be consistent with what is known about the human disease process if they are to support a conclusion that the development or persistence of a condition or disease was influenced by an exposure.

Studies of laboratory animals and other systems (such as studies using cell lines or in vitro human or other mammalian cell cultures) are essential to understanding possible health effects when experimental research in humans is not ethically or practically possible (NRC, 1991). These types of studies form the basis for much of what is known about the mechanisms behind the recognized biologic actions and effects of the drugs of interest. Studies in animal models can be used to characterize absorption, distribution, metabolism, elimination, and excretion of chemicals, and they may examine short-term or long-term exposures. Such studies permit a potentially toxic agent to be introduced under controlled conditions (with respect to dose, duration, and route of exposure) to probe the agent's physiologic and psychologic effects on various body systems and potentially to identify the mechanisms by which the effects are produced.

To be considered an acceptable surrogate for the study of a human physiology, an animal model must reproduce, with some degree of fidelity, the physiologic manifestations observed in humans. While most drug actions are similar across mammals, a given effect of an exposure in one animal species does not necessarily establish its occurrence in humans, nor does the apparent absence of a particular effect in a model animal mean that the effect could not occur in humans. But while animal models are not always ideal replicates of human conditions, there are enough similarities between human and animal responses to many toxicants that animal models can be used to examine mechanism-of-action hypotheses. There are numerous examples of the effective use of animal models to predict drug toxicity and efficacy and ample evidence that critical physiologic and psychological processes are conserved across mammalian evolution (Olson et al., 2000; Uhl and Warner, 2015). Animal studies are a valuable complement to human studies of genetic susceptibility or other biomarkers, and they can facilitate the study of chemical mixtures and their potential interactions. The most commonly used experimental animal models for testing the potential toxicity of antimalarial drugs are mice, rats, dogs, and rhesus monkeys.

Although animal and cell-culture studies provide important information for understanding the biochemical and molecular mechanisms associated with the toxicity induced by drugs and chemicals, many factors may lead to differences between the results of controlled animal studies and the effects observed in humans. These factors, which must be considered when extrapolating their results to human disease and disease progression, include the magnitude and duration of exposure, namely to prophylaxis in humans; the timing of exposure during development or differentiation; the route of exposure (e.g., injections in model organisms versus oral administration in humans); model-specific factors (such as sex, genetic background, and stress); and differences in pharmacokinetics and pharmacodynamics across species as well as different formulations of the drug being administered (e.g., pure compounds versus additives in tablets and pills). Another challenge of using animal data to study the persistent effects of antimalarial drugs in humans is that certain symptoms, such as headache, nausea, and muscle and joint pain—which have been reported by some people who have used particular antimalarial drugs—are difficult to study with standard tests in animals (OTA, 1990).

In Vitro Studies

Defined broadly, in vitro studies are tests or assessments of toxicologic phenomena in tissue slices, isolated organs, isolated primary cell cultures, cell lines, and subcellular fractions such as those of mitochondria, microsomes, and even membranes (Srivastava et al., 2018). In vitro methods are routinely used because correlating the findings with in vivo studies can help in understanding a specific in vivo response in a given species. Studies that use in vitro methods may be informative, but such data must be viewed with caution regarding their relationship to the human experience because in vitro test systems are an extremely simplified form of very complex in vivo systems. In addition, in vitro analyses generally lack mechanisms to metabolize drug present in the whole organism. Therefore, the ability to extrapolate in vitro data to in vivo results is limited.

APPROACH TO ASSESSING THE BODY OF EVIDENCE

To assess the assembled evidence, committee members first reviewed and discussed draft text on group calls and at in-person meetings until they reached a consensus on the description and assessment of the studies. Then, using all of the available information, the full committee came to a consensus regarding the conclusion and, based on the strength of the evidence, assigned a category of association (discussed below) between prophylactic use of an antimalarial of interest and persistent or latent health effects. The committee adopted a policy of giving the most evidentiary weight to inform its conclusions to peer-reviewed, published literature. Although the process of peer review by fellow professionals ensures high standards of quality, it does not guarantee the validity of a study or the generalizability of its results. Accordingly, committee members read each study critically and considered its relevance and quality.

When drafting language for a conclusion, the committee considered the timing and duration of the exposures, the nature of the specific adverse events or health outcomes, the populations exposed, and the quality, precision, and consistency of the evidence examined. The conclusion does not take into account any information regarding the benefit of the antimalarial to either population or individual health. Although both primary and supporting studies contributed to the committee's conclusion regarding the evidence of the prophylactic use of an antimalarial to be associated with a particular health condition or outcome, primary studies were given more weight. The committee did not use a formulaic approach to determining the number of primary or supporting studies that would be necessary to assign a specific category of association. Rather, the committee's review required a thoughtful and nuanced consideration of all the studies as well as expert judgment, as provided by the complement of expertise represented on the committee, and this could not be accomplished by adherence to a narrowly prescribed formula of what data would be required for each category of association or for a particular health outcome. The committee reviewed the data and made conclusions independently of other reports or author conclusions.

Categories of Association

A system of four categories of association to rate health outcomes according to the strength of the scientific evidence, which was adapted from those categories used by the International Agency for Research on Cancer, has gained wide acceptance by Congress, VA, researchers, and veterans groups and has been used in report series, including *Veterans and Agent Orange* (a 12-volume series) and *Gulf War and Health* (an 11-volume series), as well as several stand-alone reports on such topics as evaluations of vaccine safety and the adverse health outcomes of vaccines (IOM, 1991, 1994). The criteria for each of the four categories of association express a degree of confidence based on the extent to which bias and other sources of error could be reduced, and thus the quality of the evidence. The coherence of the full body of epidemiologic information, including supplemental evidence and biologic plausibility, was considered when the committee reached a judgment about association for a given outcome. As was the case with several committees that chose to use these categories of association, the Bradford Hill criteria for causality (Hill, 1965) was not applied as a checklist for strength-of-association assessments because those nine factors are not a definitive set of elements for assessing causality and they vary in the importance or weight that might be assigned to each. The committee discussed the evidence and reached consensus on the categorization of the evidence for persistent or latent health effects for each drug of interest, and these conclusions appear in the Synthesis and Conclusions section for each drug-specific chapter. If the evidence permitted, more specific conclusions were made regarding the use of an antimalarial and a particular outcome or group of outcomes. Implicit in these categories is that "the absence of evidence is not evidence of absence." That is, based on the currently available literature that met the committee's criteria for inclusion, a lack of informative data does not mean that there is no increased risk of a specific adverse event, only that the available evidence does not support claims of an increased risk. As the adverse events generally fall into six categories—neurologic, psychiatric, gastrointestinal, eye, cardiovascular, and other disorders—a conclusion is made for each category as appropriate. The four categories of association and the criteria for each follow. Each conclusion consists of two parts: the first sentence provides the category of association, and the second sentence offers a conclusion regarding whether further research in a particular area is merited based on any signals from all the currently available evidence reviewed for that outcome (assessed epidemiologic studies that reported outcomes at least 28 days post-drug-cessation, studies of concurrent adverse events, case reports, data from selected subpopulations, FDA labels, and biologic plausibility). For those health outcomes for which the committee concluded there is not a clear justification for additional research, the intention was to distinguish those issues for which there is presently an empirical basis for looking more closely and those for which such a basis is not present. As more research accumulates, the outcomes that warrant further research may change.

Sufficient Evidence of an Association

For effects to be classified as having "sufficient evidence of an association," a positive association between the prophylactic use of an antimalarial drug and the outcome must be observed in studies in which chance, bias, and confounding can be ruled out with reasonable confidence. For example, the committee might regard evidence from several small studies without known bias and confounding and that show an association that is consistent in magnitude and direction to be sufficient evidence of an association. Experimental data supporting the biologic plausibility of an association strengthen the likelihood of an association but are not a prerequisite and are not enough to establish an association without corresponding epidemiologic findings.

Limited or Suggestive Evidence of an Association

For health outcomes in the category of "limited or suggestive evidence of an association," the evidence must suggest an association between the prophylactic use of an antimalarial drug of interest and the outcome in studies of humans, but the evidence can be limited by an inability to confidently rule out chance, bias, or confounding. Typically, at least one high-quality study indicates a positive association, but the results of other studies could be inconsistent. Because there are a number of agents of concern whose toxicity profiles are not expected to be uniform—specifically, the antimalarial drugs of interest—apparent inconsistencies can be expected among study populations that have experienced different exposures. Even for a single exposure, a spectrum of results would be expected, depending on the power of the studies, the inherent biologic relationships, and other study design factors.

Inadequate or Insufficient Evidence to Determine an Association

By default, any health outcome is placed in the category of "inadequate or insufficient evidence to determine an association" before enough reliable scientific data have accumulated to promote it to the category of sufficient evidence or limited or suggestive evidence of an association or to move it to the category of limited or suggestive evidence of no association. In this category, the available human studies may have inconsistent findings or be of insufficient quality, validity, consistency, or statistical power to support a conclusion regarding the presence of an association. Such studies might have failed to control for confounding factors or might have had inadequate assessment of exposure. Because the committee could not possibly address every rare condition or disease, it does not draw explicit conclusions about outcomes that are not discussed, and thus, this category is the default or starting point for any health outcome. If a condition or outcome is not addressed specifically, then it will be in this category.

Limited or Suggestive Evidence of No Association

The category of "limited or suggestive evidence of no association" was originally defined for health outcomes for which several adequate studies covering the "full range of human exposure" were consistent in showing no association or reduced risk (not distinguished for the purposes of this evaluation, which was focused on the potential for adverse effects) with an exposure of interest at any concentration, with the studies having relatively narrow confidence intervals. A conclusion of "no association" is inevitably limited to the conditions, exposures, and observation periods covered by the available studies, and the possibility of a small increase in risk related to the magnitude of exposure studied can never be excluded. However, a change in classification from inadequate or insufficient evidence of an association to limited or suggestive evidence of no association would require new studies that correct for the methodologic problems of previous studies and that have samples large enough to limit the possible study results attributable to chance.

REFERENCES

Ackert, J., K. Mohamed, J. S. Slakter, S. El-Harazi, A. Berni, H. Gevorkyan, E. Hardaker, A. Hussaini, S. W. Jones, G. C. K. W. Koh, J. Patel, S. Rasmussen, D. S. Kelly, D. E. Baranano, J. T. Thompson, K. A. Warren, R. C. Sergott, J. Tonkyn, A. Wolstenholme, H. Coleman, A. Yuan, S. Duparc, and J. A. Green. 2019. Randomized placebo-controlled trial evaluating the ophthalmic safety of single-dose tafenoquine in healthy volunteers. *Drug Saf* 42(9):1103-1114.

Andersen, S. L., A. J. Oloo, D. M. Gordon, O. B. Ragama, G. M. Aleman, J. D. Berman, D. B. Tang, M. W. Dunne, and G. D. Shanks. 1998. Successful double-blinded, randomized, placebo-controlled field trial of azithromycin and doxycycline as prophylaxis for malaria in western Kenya. *Clin Infect Dis* 26(1):146-150.

Brisson, M., and P. Brisson. 2012. Compliance with antimalaria chemoprophylaxis in a combat zone. *Am J Trop Med Hyg* 86(4):587-590.

Cohen, J. 1988. *Statistical power analysis for the behavioral sciences.* 2nd ed. Hillsdale, NJ: Lawrence Erlbaum Associates.

Cunningham, J., J. Horsley, D. Patel, A. Tunbridge, and D. G. Lalloo. 2014. Compliance with long-term malaria prophylaxis in British expatriates. *Travel Med Infect Dis* 12(4):341-348.

DeSouza, J. M. 1983. Phase I clinical trial of mefloquine in Brazilian male subjects. *Bull World Health Organ* 61(5):809-814.

Eick-Cost, A. A., Z. Hu, P. Rohrbeck, and L. L. Clark. 2017. Neuropsychiatric outcomes after mefloquine exposure among U.S. military service members. *Am J Trop Med Hyg* 96(1):159-166.

Friedman, G. D. 2015. *Primer of epidemiology.* New York: McGraw-Hill.

Gagnier J. J., G. Kienle, D. G. Altman, D. Moher, H. Sox, D. Riley; and the CARE Group. n.d. The CARE guidelines: Consensus-based clinical case reporting guideline development. *Glob Advs Health Med* 2(5):38-43.

Gordis, L. 2004. *Epidemiology*. Philadelphia, PA: Elsevier Saunders.

Green, J. A., A. K. Patel, B. R. Patel, A. Hussaini, E. J. Harrell, M. J. McDonald, N. Carter, K. Mohamed, S. Duparc, and A. K. Miller. 2014. Tafenoquine at therapeutic concentrations does not prolong Fridericia-corrected QT interval in healthy subjects. *J Clin Pharmacol* 54:995-1005.

Hill, A. B. 1965. The environment and disease: Association or causation? *Proc J R Soc Med* 58:295-300.

IOM (Institute of Medicine). 1991. *Adverse effects of pertussis and rubella vaccines*. Washington, DC: National Academy Press.

IOM. 1994. *Adverse events associated with childhood vaccines: Evidence bearing on causality*. Washington, DC: National Academy Press.

IOM. 2007. *Adverse drug event reporting: The roles of consumers and health-care professionals: Workshop summary*. Washington, DC: The National Academies Press.

Kraemer, H. C., and C. Blasey. 2015. *How many subjects? Statistical power analysis in research*. Thousand Oaks, CA: SAGE Publications.

Landman, K. Z., K. R. Tan, P. M. Arguin, and Centers for Disease Control and Prevention. 2014. Knowledge, attitudes, and practices regarding antimalarial chemoprophylaxis in U.S. Peace Corps volunteers—Africa, 2013. *MMWR* 63(23):516-517.

Laothavorn, P., J. Karbwang, K. Na Bangchang, D. Bunnag and T. Harinasuta. 1992. Effect of mefloquine on electrocardiographic changes in uncomplicated falciparum malaria patients. *Southeast Asian J Trop Med Public Health* 23(1):51-54.

Leary, K. J., M. A. Riel, M. J. Roy, L. R. Cantilena, D. Bi, D. C. Brater, C. van de Pol, K. Pruett, C. Kerr, J. M. Veazey, Jr., R. Beboso, and C. Ohrt. 2009. A randomized, double-blind, safety and tolerability study to assess the ophthalmic and renal effects of tafenoquine 200 mg weekly versus placebo for 6 months in healthy volunteers. *Am J Trop Med Hyg* 81:356-362.

Lee, T. W., L. Russell, M. Deng, and P. R. Gibson. 2013. Association of doxycycline use with the development of gastroenteritis, irritable bowel syndrome and inflammatory bowel disease in Australians deployed abroad. *Intern Med J* 43(8):919-926.

Lege-Oguntoye, L., G. C. Onyemelukwe, B. B. Maiha, E. O. Udezue, and S. Eckerbom. 1990. The effect of short-term malaria chemoprophylaxis on the immune response of semi-immune adult volunteers. *East Afr Med J* 67(11):770-778.

Meier, C. R., K. Wilcock, and S. S. Jick. 2004. The risk of severe depression, psychosis or panic attacks with prophylactic antimalarials. *Drug Saf* 27(3):203-213.

Miller, A. K., E. Harrell, L. Ye, S. Baptiste-Brown, J. P. Kleim, C. Ohrt, S. Duparc, J. J. Möhrle, A. Webster, S. Stinnett, A. Hughes, S. Griffith, and A. P. Beelen. 2013. Pharmacokinetic interactions and safety evaluations of coadministered tafenoquine and chloroquine in healthy subjects. *Br J Clin Pharmacol* 76:858-867.

Nasveld, P. E., M. D. Edstein, M. Reid, L. Brennan, I. E. Harris, S. J. Kitchener, P. A. Leggat, P. Pickford, C. Kerr, C. Ohrt, W. Prescott, and the Tafenoquine Study Team. 2010. Randomized, double-blind study of the safety, tolerability, and efficacy of tafenoquine versus mefloquine for malaria prophylaxis in nonimmune subjects. *Antimicrob Agents Chemother* 54:792-798.

NRC (National Research Council). 1991. *Animals as sentinels of environmental health hazards*. Washington, DC: National Academy Press.

Olson, H., G. Betton, D. Robinson, K. Thomas, A. Monro, G. Kolaja, P. Lilly, J. Sanders, G. Sipes, W. Bracken, M. Dorato, K. Van Deun, P. Smith, B. Berger, and A. Heller. 2000. Concordance of the toxicity of pharmaceuticals in humans and in animals. *Regul Toxicol Pharmacol* 32(1):56-67.

OTA (Office of Technology Assessment). 1990. *Neurotoxicity: Identifying and controlling poisons of the nervous system*. Washington, DC: U.S. Government Printing Office.

Rodgers, M., S. Thomas, M. Harden, G. Parker, A. Street, and A. Eastwood. 2016. Developing a methodological framework for organisational case studies: A rapid review and consensus development process. *HS&DR* 4(1).

Rothman, K. J., S. Greenland, and T. L. Lash. 2012. *Modern epidemiology.* 3rd ed. Philadephia, PA: Lippincott Williams & Wilkins.

Rueangweerayut, R., G. Bancone, E. J. Harrell, A. P. Beelen, S. Kongpatanakul, J. J. Möhrle, V. Rousell, K. Mohamed, A. Qureshi, S. Narayan, N. Yubon, A. Miller, F. H. Nosten, L. Luzzatto, S. Duparc, J.-P. Kleim, and J. A. Green. 2017. Hemolytic potential of tafenoquine in female volunteers heterozygous for glucose-6-phosphate dehydrogenase (G6PD) deficiency (G6PD Mahidol variant) versus G6PD normal volunteers. *Am J 1443 Trop Med Hyg* 97(3):702-711.

Saunders, D. L., E. Garges, J. E. Manning, K. Bennett, S. Schaffer, A. J. Kosmowski, and A. J. Magill. 2015. Safety, tolerability, and compliance with long-term antimalarial chemoprophylaxis in American soldiers in Afghanistan. *Am J Trop Med Hyg* 93(3):584-590.

Savitz, D. A., and G. A. Wellenius. 2016. *Interpreting epidemiologic evidence.* New York: Oxford University Press.

Schlagenhauf, P., R. Steffen, H. Lobel, R. Johnson, R. Letz, A. Tschopp, N. Vranjes, Y. Bergqvist, O. Ericsson, U. Hellgren, L. Rombo, S. Mannino, J. Handschin, and D. Sturchler. 1996. Mefloquine tolerability during chemoprophylaxis: Focus on adverse event assessments, stereochemistry and compliance. *Trop Med Int Health* 1(4):485-494.

Schneider, C., M. Adamcova, S. S. Jick, P. Schlagenhauf, M. K. Miller, H. G. Rhein, and C. R. Meier. 2013. Antimalarial chemoprophylaxis and the risk of neuropsychiatric disorders. *Travel Med Infect Dis* 11(2):71-80.

Schneider, C., M. Adamcova, S. S. Jick, P. Schlagenhauf, M. K. Miller, H. G. Rhein, and C. R. Meier. 2014. Use of anti-malarial drugs and the risk of developing eye disorders. *Travel Med Infect Dis* 12(1):40-47.

Schneiderman, A. I., Y. S. Cypel, E. K. Dursa, and R. Bossarte. 2018. Associations between use of antimalarial medications and health among U. S. veterans of the wars in Iraq and Afghanistan. *Am J Trop Med Hyg* 99(3):638-648.

Schwartz, E., and G. Regev-Yochay. 1999. Primaquine as prophylaxis for malaria for nonimmune travelers: A 3062 comparison with mefloquine and doxycycline. *Clin Infect Dis* 29(6):1502-1506.

Srivastava, S., S. Mishra, J. Dewangan, A. Divakar, P. K. Pandey, and S. K. Rath. 2018. Chapter 2: Principles for in vitro toxicology. In A. Dhawan and S. Kwon (eds.), *In vitro toxicology.* New York: Academic Press. Pp. 21-44.

Tan, K. R., S. J. Henderson, J. Williamson, R. W. Ferguson, T. M. Wilkinson, P. Jung. and P. M. Arguin. 2017. Long term health outcomes among returned Peace Corps volunteers after malaria prophylaxis, 1995-2014. *Travel Med Infect Dis* 17:50-55.

Uhl, E. W., and N. J. Warner. 2015. Mouse models as predictors of human responses: Evolutionary medicine. *Curr Pathobiol Rep* 3(3):219-223.

Vandenbroucke, J. P. 1999. Case reports in an evidence-based world. *J R Soc Med* 92(4):159-163.

Walsh, D. S., C. Eamsila, T. Sasiprapha, S. Sangkharomya, P. Khaewsathien, P. Supakalin, D. B. Tang, P. Jarasrumgsichol, C. Cherdchu, M. D. Edstein, K. H. Rieckmann, and T. G. Brewer. 2004. Efficacy of monthly tafenoquine for prophylaxis of *Plasmodium vivax* and multidrug-resistant *P. falciparum* malaria. *J Infect Dis* 190(8):1456-1463.

Wells, G. A., B. Shea, D. O'Connell, J. Peterson, V. Welch, M. Losos, and P. Tugwell. 2019. *The Newcastle-Ottawa Scale (NOS) for assessing the quality of nonrandomized studies in meta-analyses.* http://www.ohri.ca/programs/clinical_epidemiology/oxford.asp (accessed October 29, 2019).

Wells, T. S., T. C. Smith, B. Smith, L. Z. Wang, C. J. Hansen, R. J. Reed, W. E. Goldfinger, T. E. Corbeil, C. N. Spooner, and M. A. Ryan. 2006. Mefloquine use and hospitalizations among US service members, 2002-2004. *Am J Trop Med Hyg* 74(5):744-749.

4

Mefloquine

In the late 1960s mefloquine hydrochloride—more commonly known simply as mefloquine—was developed by Walter Reed Army Institute as part of the U.S. Army Antimalarial Drug Development Project. Phase I human tolerance and safety testing for the treatment of malaria began in 1972, and the first trials for its use as a prophylactic occurred in 1976 (Shanks, 1994). In 1976 a collaboration was formed with the U.S. Army, the World Health Organization (WHO), and Hoffmann-La Roche (the manufacturer) to further develop mefloquine. Mefloquine (trade name Lariam®) was first introduced to the market in February 1984 (Adamcova et al., 2015) and became generally available for European travelers in 1985 (Heimgartner, 1986). A new drug application for it was submitted to the Food and Drug Administration (FDA) in 1986 and it was approved in 1989. The mefloquine dosing regimen for malaria prophylaxis begins with taking one tablet (250 mg salt in the United States or 228 mg base) once a week, starting two weeks prior to arriving in an endemic area, taking mefloquine weekly (allowing no more than 8 days to elapse) while in the endemic area, and continuing it for 4 weeks after leaving the endemic area (CDC, n.d.). The once-per-week regimen is perceived to be convenient and is preferred for many individuals, such as long-term travelers and military personnel, as it reduces the amount of medication people have to carry and may require less vigilance to correctly adhere to prescription guidelines than daily malaria prophylactic drugs (e.g., doxycycline, primaquine, atovaquone/proguanil [A/P]) (Adshead, 2014).

Soon after mefloquine entered the market, reports of associated adverse events, specifically neuropsychiatric in nature, began to be reported to FDA and coincided with increased attention from the media about possible side effects (Croft, 2007). This led to several reassessments that included more recent epidemiologic and toxicologic evidence and resulted in updates to the FDA label over time. Questions and concerns about mefloquine's short- and long-term safety combined with availability of newer prophylactic drugs that were reported to have fewer side effects likely contributed to a decline in the number of mefloquine prescriptions (Leggat, 2005; Leggat and Speare, 2003). Mefloquine continues to be available and recommended by national and global agencies for the prophylaxis of malaria in chloroquine-resistant areas because it is effective against all *Plasmodium* species (Schlagenhauf et al., 2019). Despite the cautions of adverse effects, the once-per-week mefloquine regimen has been preferred by some groups (Senn et al., 2007).

This chapter begins with a discussion of the changes that have been made to the mefloquine package insert since its approval in the United States in 1989, with particular emphasis on information in the Contraindications, Warnings, and Precautions sections. This is followed by summaries of findings and conclusions regarding the use of mefloquine in military forces reported by U.S. agencies and foreign governments. The known pharmacokinetics of mefloquine are then described, followed by a summary of the known short-term adverse events associated with use of mefloquine when used as directed for prophylaxis. Most of the chapter is dedicated to summarizing and assessing the 11 identified epidemiologic studies that contributed some information on persistent or latent health outcomes following the cessation of mefloquine. These are arranged by the type of population that was examined: first, studies of military and veterans (U.S. followed by international forces), then occupational groups (U.S. Peace Corps), travelers, and, finally, research volunteers. Where available, studies of U.S. participants are presented first. A table that gives a high-level comparison of each of the 11 epidemiologic studies that examined the use of mefloquine and that met the committee's inclusion criteria is presented in Appendix C. Supplemental supporting evidence is then presented, including other identified studies of health outcomes in populations that used mefloquine for prophylaxis but that did not meet the committee's inclusion criteria; case reports of persistent adverse events associated with mefloquine use; and information on adverse events associated with mefloquine use in selected subpopulations, such as women, women who are pregnant, people with low body mass index (BMI), those who have chronic health conditions, and those who concurrently use alcohol, marijuana, or illicit substances. After presenting the primary and supplemental evidence in humans, supporting literature from experimental animal and in vitro studies is then summarized. The chapter ends with a synthesis of the evidence presented and the inferences and conclusions the committee made from the available evidence.

FOOD AND DRUG ADMINISTRATION
PACKAGE INSERT FOR MEFLOQUINE

This section describes selected information that can be found on the FDA label or in the package insert for mefloquine. It begins with a summary of contraindications for its use based on the most recent FDA label and package insert. This is followed by a brief synopsis of drug interactions that are known or presumed to occur with concurrent mefloquine use. The final subsection provides a chronologic overview of changes to the label or package insert from its U.S. approval in 1989 to the most recent label, updated in 2016. The presented changes are specific to mefloquine when used for prophylaxis (not treatment) and in adults (not infants or children). The dates of the labels are based on the dates that appeared in the labels themselves (documents downloaded from Drugs@FDA Search or National Institutes of Health DailyMed websites) or, when no date appeared in the label, the action date listed on the website.

Contraindications

Mefloquine use is contraindicated in persons with a known hypersensitivity to mefloquine or related compounds (e.g., quinine and quinidine) and to drug-formulation excipients (FDA, 2016). It is also contraindicated for people with current depression, a recent history of depression, generalized anxiety disorder, psychosis, schizophrenia or other major psychiatric disorders, or with a history of convulsions (FDA, 2016).

Although policies are in place to prevent those with a contraindication from being prescribed mefloquine, in practice it still happens. For example, according to an analysis using the UK-based Clinical Practice Research Datalink, from January 2001 through June 2012, 165,218 people had a recorded prescription for an antimalarial for prophylaxis, of whom 25,294 (15.3%) were prescribed mefloquine. People with contraindications to mefloquine were twice as likely to be prescribed a different antimalarial drug, but occasionally people with contra-indications were prescribed mefloquine (Bloechliger et al., 2014). However, no additional follow-up or analyses of any reported adverse events were conducted to determine whether those with contraindications were at higher risk or experienced more severe adverse events.

Drug Interactions

The Warnings section of the package insert alerts against using halofantrine or ketoconazole concomitantly or within 15 weeks of the last dose of mefloquine due to risk of sudden cardiac death that can result from prolongation of the QTc interval (FDA, 2016). Co-administration of other drugs that affect cardiac conduction (e.g., anti-arrhythmic or beta-adrenergic blocking agents, calcium channel blockers, antihistamines or H_1-blocking agents, tricyclic antidepressants, and phenothiazines) might also contribute to a prolongation of the QTc interval (FDA, 2016). Administration of mefloquine with related antimalarials (e.g., quinine, quinidine, chloroquine) may produce electrocardiographic abnormalities and increase the risk of convulsions (FDA, 2016).

Taking mefloquine with an anticonvulsant (e.g., valproic acid, carbamazepine, phenobarbital, or phenytoin) may reduce seizure control, and the blood level of anti-seizure medication should be monitored. Moreover, concomitant administration of mefloquine with quinine or chloroquine in addition to an anticonvulsant can further increase the risk of seizures. Taking mefloquine concurrently with oral live typhoid vaccines may make the immunization ineffective. It is recommended that vaccination with live attenuated bacteria be completed at least 3 days before beginning mefloquine. Taking rifampin with mefloquine can decrease mefloquine concentration and elimination time. Mefloquine is metabolized by CYP3A4, and CYP3A4 inhibitors may modify the pharmacokinetics and metabolism of mefloquine and thus increase mefloquine plasma concentrations and the risk of adverse reactions. Similarly, CYP3A4 inducers may decrease mefloquine plasma concentrations and reduce mefloquine efficacy. Mefloquine is a substrate and an inhibitor of P-glycoprotein; thus drug–drug interactions could occur with drugs that are substrates or are known to modify the expression of this transporter, although the clinical relevance of these interactions is not known to date.

Changes to the Mefloquine Package Insert Over Time

There have been multiple important changes to the mefloquine package insert since the drug was first approved for prophylaxis and treatment of malaria in 1989. According to the FDA Center for Drug Evaluation and Research, for a drug to be approved by FDA, at a minimum it must be shown through submitted clinical trials, animal toxicology studies, and other evidence that the drug works as intended and that the health benefits outweigh the known risks (FDA, 2019a). Label changes may indicate that FDA has recognized potential problems with a drug but there may be other reasons for label changes, including approval for a new indication and expansion of the population for which the initial approval was obtained. Most safety-related label changes are the result of spontaneous adverse event reports that have been received during the postmarketing surveillance period, rather than well-designed epidemiologic studies, although if such epidemiologic studies are available they are considered along with new results from pharmacokinetic studies (Sekine et al., 2016). Moreover, the adverse event reports describe events that follow the reported use of the drug, and causality has not necessarily been proven.

Many of the labeling-update letters and package inserts for mefloquine listed on the Drugs@FDA Search website for the period 1989–2002 were unavailable for download. (The downloadable package insert listed with a May 1989 action date is actually a July 2002 revision.) In response to a request for the unavailable information, FDA provided a PDF of the original 1989 package insert as well as abbreviated extractions from editions of the *Physicians' Desk Reference* but noted that the committee might want to confirm the summary information.[1] In response to the committee's request for the specific information upon which FDA based mefloquine-labeling changes, FDA stated that it had performed "safety analyses" in 2007, 2013, 2015, and 2016 that supported labeling changes and that the committee could request redacted versions of these reviews via the Freedom of Information Act.[2] In response to the committee's request for the information that underlay the addition of the boxed warning to the mefloquine label, FDA referred the committee to the 2013 drug safety communication, a public announcement regarding the boxed warning (FDA, 2013a). The committee had quoted this document in its request to FDA, explaining that it sought more detail than the document provided. The 2013 drug safety communication states: "In conducting its assessment of vestibular adverse reactions associated with mefloquine use, FDA reviewed adverse event reports from the FDA Adverse Event Reporting System and the published literature, identifying patients that reported one or more vestibular symptoms such as dizziness, loss of balance, tinnitus, and vertigo." It notes further that "Patients who experienced vestibular symptoms usually had concomitant psychiatric symptoms such as anxiety, confusion, paranoia, and depression. Some of the psychiatric symptoms persisted for months to years after mefloquine was discontinued." As desired details were not provided about the evidence base for the labeling changes (e.g., quantification of adverse reactions reported, epidemiologic data), it was difficult for the committee to assess the implications of the changes.

A comparison of the 1989 package insert and the 2002 package inserts (July and December) showed numerous additions, many pertaining to neurologic and psychiatric adverse events, which were often grouped as "neuropsychiatric" (see Table 4-1 for a summary of the major changes to the package insert over time regarding neuropsychiatric adverse events). The 1989 version stated that "neuropsychiatric reactions have been reported during the use of Lariam" and warned that "if signs of unexplained anxiety, depression, restlessness or confusion are noticed, these may be considered prodromal to a more serious event" and the drug must be discontinued (FDA, 1989). The 2002 package insert added information on neuropsychiatric symptoms to the Contraindications and Warnings sections (FDA, 2002). Mefloquine used as prophylaxis was now contraindicated in persons with current psychiatric problems or a history of psychiatric disorders or convulsions. Symptoms that in 1989 had been listed in the Adverse Reactions' postmarketing surveillance section as "additional adverse reactions"—vertigo, visual disturbances, and central nervous system disturbances (e.g., psychotic manifestations, hallucinations, confusion, anxiety, and depression)—now appeared in

---

[1] Personal communication to the committee, Kelly Cao, Pharm.D., Safety Evaluator Team Leader, Division of Pharmacovigilance II, Office of Pharmacovigilance and Epidemiology, Office of Surveillance and Epidemiology, Center for Drug Evaluation and Research, March 20, 2019.

[2] Personal communication to the committee, Division of Drug Information, Center for Drug Evaluation and Research, FDA, April 30, 2019.

TABLE 4-1 Evolution of Neuropsychiatric Safety-Related Information in the FDA Mefloquine Package Insert and Medication Guide

Issue Date	Action
1989	FDA approval of Lariam; first package insert
2002	Additions to the *Contraindications, Warnings, Precautions,* and *Adverse Reactions* sections of package insert
2003	FDA requires Medication Guide be given to persons to whom drug is dispensed
2008	Additions to the *Precautions* section of package insert Additions to Medication Guide
2009	FDA requires manufacturer to submit a risk evaluation and mitigation strategy[a]
2011	Risk evaluation and mitigation strategy is no longer required
2013	Boxed warning ("black box"), the most serious kind of warning about potential problems, added to package insert Additions to *Warnings* and *Animal Toxicology* sections of package insert Additions to Medication Guide
2016	No substantive changes to package insert

[a] A risk evaluation and mitigation strategy (REMS) is a drug safety program that FDA requires for certain medications with serious safety concerns. They are designed to help reduce the occurrence and/or severity of certain serious risks and to ensure the benefits of the medication outweigh

Summary of Relevant Content in Package Insert, Medication Guide, or FDA Letters to Manufacturer
• Neuropsychiatric reactions have been reported
• Discontinue use if unexplained anxiety, depression, restlessness or confusion occur as it may be considered prodromal to a more serious event
• Exercise caution when driving, piloting airplanes, or operating machinery
• Contraindications added for those with current or past history of psychiatric disorders or convulsions and for those with hypersensitivity to mefloquine
• Symptoms previously listed in Adverse Reactions (postmarketing surveillance) are moved to Warnings section, with additional symptoms, including thoughts of suicide
• Text added that psychiatric symptoms may continue long after mefloquine use ceases
• Precautions expanded regarding performing activities requiring alertness and fine motor coordination
• Numerous symptoms are added to Adverse Reactions (postmarketing surveillance) section
• Lists contraindications and possible neuropsychiatric side effects, including thoughts of suicide
• Notes side effects may continue after drug is stopped
• Cautions to exercise care driving and performing activities requiring alertness and fine motor coordination
• Advised to consult health care provider if sudden onset of anxiety, depression, restlessness, or confusion occurs
• Vertigo added as side effect (package insert and medication guide)
• Dizziness or vertigo and loss of balance have been reported to continue for months after discontinuation of the drug (package insert and medication guide)
• Feeling restless added as side effect (medication guide)
• Assessment of REMS that should include an evaluation of:
– Patients' understanding of the serious risks of mefloquine
– A report on periodic assessments of the distribution and dispensing of the medication guide in accordance with 21 CFR 208.24
– A report on failures to adhere to distribution and dispensing requirements, and corrective actions taken to address noncompliance
• "The Medication Guide will continue to be part of the approved labeling."
• *Boxed warning*: "Mefloquine may cause neuropsychiatric adverse reactions that can persist after mefloquine has been discontinued. Mefloquine should not be prescribed for prophylaxis in patients with major psychiatric disorders. During prophylactic use, if psychiatric or neurologic symptoms occur, the drug should be discontinued and an alternative medication should be substituted."
• Neurologic symptoms such as dizziness or vertigo, tinnitus, and loss of balance may occur early in the course of mefloquine use and have been reported to continue for months or years after mefloquine has been stopped
• Dizziness or vertigo, tinnitus, and loss of balance have been reported to be permanent in some cases
• If the drug is to be administered for a prolonged period, periodic evaluations for neuropsychiatric effects should be performed
• Animal studies demonstrated that mefloquine daily for 22 days at equivalent human therapeutic concentration showed central nervous system penetration of mefloquine, with a 30- to 50-fold greater brain/plasma drug ratio up to 10 days after final dose

its risks. While all medications have labeling that provides information about medication risks, few medications require a REMS (FDA, 2019b).

the Warnings section. The Warnings section also stated that psychiatric symptoms "ranging from anxiety, paranoia, and depression to hallucinations and psychotic behavior" had been "reported to continue long after mefloquine has been stopped" (FDA, 1989, 2002). In addition, it noted, "Rare cases of suicidal ideation and suicide have been reported" (FDA, 2002). Cautions were expanded for mefloquine use while performing certain activities, specifically actions requiring alertness and fine motor coordination, "as dizziness, a loss of balance, or other disorders of the central or peripheral nervous system have been reported during and following the use of Lariam" (FDA, 2002). The Adverse Reactions' postmarketing surveillance section listed as among the most frequently reported adverse events dizziness or vertigo, loss of balance, and neuropsychiatric events such as headache, somnolence, and sleep disorders (insomnia, abnormal dreams) (FDA, 2002). This section also added a lengthy list of "more severe neuropsychiatric disorders" that had "occasionally" been reported (FDA, 2002).

The Precautions section now warned, "Hypersensitivity reactions ranging from mild cutaneous events to anaphylaxis cannot be predicted" (FDA, 2002). Users were also advised that contraception should be practiced for up to 3 months after drug cessation and that mefloquine use should be weighed carefully in patients aged ≥65 years since electrocardiographic abnormalities had been observed and cardiac disease is more prevalent in older patients (FDA, 2002).

Updates to information about other body systems included alerts that the concomitant administration of mefloquine and quinine or chloroquine may increase the risk of convulsions. Taking halofantrine after mefloquine might cause potentially fatal prolongation of the QTc interval on electrocardiograms (ECGs); theoretically, the co-administration of other drugs affecting cardiac conduction might also have that effect (FDA, 2002). Previously, users had been informed that if the drug was administered for a prolonged period, periodic evaluations, including liver function tests, should be performed; this language was strengthened to note that in those with impaired liver function, elimination of mefloquine may be prolonged, leading to higher plasma levels (FDA, 2002). The postmarketing surveillance section listed among "infrequent adverse events" cardiovascular, skin, and musculoskeletal disorders as well as "visual disturbances, vestibular disorders including tinnitus and hearing impairment, dyspnea, asthenia, malaise, fatigue, fever, sweating, chills, dyspepsia and loss of appetite." The two serious adverse reactions reported were cardiopulmonary arrest in one patient shortly after ingesting a single prophylactic dose of mefloquine while using propranolol and, second, encephalopathy of unknown etiology during prophylactic mefloquine administration.

In 2003 FDA required that pharmacists provide a medication guide—a paper handout that conveys risk information that is specific to a particular drug or drug class—to persons to whom mefloquine was dispensed (FDA, 2003a,b). The medication guide included labeled cautions and contraindications and advised users to consult a health care provider in the case of a sudden onset of anxiety, depression, restlessness, or confusion (FDA, 2003b). In 2008 the package insert's Precautions section added vertigo as a side effect and stated that "in a small number of patients, dizziness and loss of balance have been reported to continue for months after mefloquine has been stopped" (FDA, 2008). The medication guide warned users that they might suddenly experience severe anxiety, paranoia, hallucinations, depression, unusual behavior, and disorientation; "feeling restless" was added to possible side effects. The Adverse Reactions postmarketing surveillance section added respiratory disorders to "infrequent adverse events." In the 2009 package insert, the Warnings section alerted users against co-administration of halofantrine or ketoconazole with mefloquine; several additions were also made to the Drug Interactions section (FDA, 2009).

In 2013 FDA strengthened and updated warnings of previously included neurologic and psychiatric side effects, and it added a boxed warning, sometimes informally referred to as a "black box" (FDA, 2013b). This is FDA's most serious type of warning, and it appears on a prescription drug's label to call attention to serious or life-threatening risks (FDA, 2012). The boxed warning stated, "Mefloquine may cause neuropsychiatric adverse reactions that can persist after mefloquine has been discontinued," and it added that mefloquine should not be prescribed in patients with major psychiatric disorders and that if psychiatric or neurologic symptoms occur during prophylactic use, drug use should be halted (FDA, 2013b). The Warnings section now informed users that psychiatric symptoms "may occur early in the course of mefloquine use and that in some cases, symptoms have been reported to continue for months or years after mefloquine has been stopped" (FDA, 2013b). It also warned that neurologic effects, including dizziness, vertigo, loss of balance, and ringing in the ears, could occur soon after starting the drug and that they could persist or become permanent. It recommended that evaluations for "neuropsychiatric" effects be performed in persons using the drug long term. Prior language that stated that no relationship had been established between mefloquine and suicide or suicidal thoughts was deleted. Users with impaired liver function were now warned that this placed them at a higher risk of adverse reactions. The Toxicology section included a study in which rats given mefloquine daily for 22 days at levels equivalent to human therapeutic levels showed that mefloquine penetrated the central nervous system, with a 30- to 50-fold greater brain/plasma drug ratio up to 10 days after drug cessation. In the Adverse Reactions postmarketing surveillance section, hepatobiliary disorders, and blood and lymphatic system disorders were added to the "less frequently reported adverse reactions."

The most recent update to the package insert was made in 2016, and added ocular effects to the Warnings section (FDA, 2016). Regarding adverse events, the package insert states that the most frequently observed adverse event in clinical trials of malaria prophylaxis was vomiting (3%). Dizziness, syncope, extrasystoles, and other complaints were reported in less than 1% of users. Postmarketing surveillance has found that the most frequently reported adverse events are nausea, vomiting, loose stools or diarrhea, abdominal pain, dizziness or vertigo, loss of balance, and "neuropsychiatric" events such as headache, somnolence, and sleep disorders (insomnia, abnormal dreams). These adverse events are often reported without reference to a comparison group, and their duration is rarely detailed.

The Warnings section of the package insert includes several adverse events. It warns that psychiatric symptoms such as acute anxiety, depression, restlessness, or confusion should be viewed as potential precursors to more serious psychiatric or neurologic adverse reactions and that when they occur, mefloquine should be discontinued. More severe neurologic and psychiatric disorders have been reported, including sensory and motor neuropathies (including paresthesia, tremor, and ataxia), convulsions, agitation or restlessness, anxiety, depression, mood swings, panic attacks, memory impairment, confusion, hallucinations, aggression, psychotic or paranoid reactions, and encephalopathy. Suicidal thoughts and suicide have been also been reported. Neurologic symptoms including dizziness or vertigo, tinnitus, hearing loss, and loss of balance have been reported to occur after beginning the drug regimen and in some cases have continued for months, years, or even permanently after discontinuing mefloquine. Users are instructed to discontinue the drug if neurologic symptoms occur, and to use caution when performing activities requiring alertness and fine motor coordination (e.g., driving, piloting aircraft, operating machinery, and deep-sea diving) (FDA, 2016). Other short-term adverse events reported with the use of mefloquine have included transitory and clinically silent ECG alterations such as sinus bradycardia, sinus arrhythmia, first degree atrial–ventricular (AV) block, prolongation of the QTc interval, and abnormal T waves. Eye disorders, including optic neuropathy and retinal disorders, have also been reported during mefloquine use.

POLICIES AND INQUIRIES RELATED TO THE USE OF MEFLOQUINE BY MILITARY FORCES

This section reviews some of the policies regarding the use of mefloquine in U.S. and foreign militaries. When identified, the committee also considered issued reports by other countries (Australia, Canada, and the United Kingdom) on the use of mefloquine in their militaries, although this list is not meant to be exhaustive.

United States

Mefloquine was possibly used by the U.S. military as early as 1990[3] and by other military forces as early as 1986 (Croft and Geary, 2001). It was used as a first-line prophylactic agent only for deployments to high-malaria-risk areas in sub-Saharan Africa, such as for the Liberian Task Force in 2003, and it was

---

[3] Personal communication to the committee, COL Andrew Wiesen, M.D., M.P.H., Director, Preventive Medicine, Health Readiness Policy, and Oversight, Office of the Assistant Secretary of Defense (Health Affairs), DoD, April 16, 2019.

used as a second-line agent in Operation Enduring Freedom (OEF; 2001–2014), Operation Iraqi Freedom (OIF; 2003–2010), and Operation New Dawn (OND; 2010–2011).

In 2003 a Department of Defense (DoD) memorandum on antimalarials was issued by the Armed Forces Epidemiological Board (DoD, 2003). The authors note first that DoD is subject to Section 1107 of Title 10, United States Code, regarding the off-label use of force health protection medications. It then states that this would limit the prescription of Centers for Disease Control and Prevention (CDC)-recommended off-label prophylactic regimens (e.g., a loading dose of mefloquine for persons being deployed on short notice) to the context of a doctor–patient relationship or an investigational new-drug protocol, both of which could be problematic in a military setting. In its findings and recommendations, the board stated that it found the CDC consensus guidelines for malaria prevention "appropriate" for use by DoD and listed three options (A/P, mefloquine, and doxycycline) for areas with chloroquine-resistant *P. falciparum*. It noted that the contraindications for mefloquine were active depression and a history of psychosis or seizures and that it should be used cautiously in those with psychiatric disturbances. The board stated that mefloquine should continue to be available in the military drug armamentarium for malaria prophylaxis.

The committee reviewed a June 2004 "health information letter" that the U.S. Veterans Health Administration issued to clinicians caring for veterans who may have taken mefloquine as prophylaxis during OEF or OIF (VA, 2004). The Department of Veterans Affairs (VA) noted that mefloquine causes adverse events, possibly affecting adherence, and that anecdotal and media reports had suggested that the drug may cause serious neuropsychiatric effects. The letter also cited a DoD mefloquine "warning label" for clinicians that stated mefloquine should not be prescribed to persons "with a history of psychiatric or alcohol problems." The VA letter described a literature review that had been performed and noted that the literature (based on case reports, clinical trials, and epidemiologic studies with no separation of the timing of adverse events) suggested that "certain health effects of mefloquine may persist after the drug is stopped." It also stated that "clinical trials and epidemiological studies suggest that reported side effects are not common and are self-limiting" and that they included depression, panic attacks, anxiety, insomnia, vertigo, nausea and headache, and strange or vivid dreams. VA told the committee that such health information letters were used to provide information to VA staff and are not policy and that no record of additional information letters on the subject of mefloquine had been found.[4] The VA letter listed all of the published sources that were used in drawing its conclusions. The committee considered all of those case reports and studies captured by VA for its own assessment but found

---

[4] Personal communication to the committee, Peter D. Rumm, M.D., M.P.H., F.A.C.P.M., Director, Pre-9/11 Era Environmental Health Program, VA, June 6, 2019.

that most did not meet its criteria of reporting empirical data on adverse events that persist or occur at least 28 days post-cessation of mefloquine.

In response to the committee's request for further information on the DoD "warning label," VA could not provide it, and DoD responded that it does not issue warning labels.[5] DoD provided copies of information sheets for service members and their families (dated 2004) and for leaders (dated 2005) that had been available on the health.mil website (DoD, 2004, 2005a). These guides, in addition to warning against mefloquine use in those with a current or past history of psychiatric disorders, repeatedly warned against drinking alcohol while taking the drug because "alcohol may interfere with the medicine's effectiveness and cause more serious side effects." FDA mefloquine package inserts, including the most recent 2016 version, do not provide warnings or guidance on concurrent alcohol use (FDA, 2016).

In 2005 a DoD issuance outlined the U.S. Central Command deployment health protection policy (DoD, 2005b). It noted that component Combined Joint Task Force surgeons were authorized to modify malaria prophylaxis guidance for subordinate units based on latest intelligence, ground truth, and medical-risk assessment. The issuance stated that a mefloquine or doxycycline regimen must be used by personnel deploying to Central Asia, the Arabian Peninsula, and Africa; it stated further that mefloquine was not authorized for people on flight status.

A 2006 DoD policy memorandum directed that mefloquine be used by Coalition Forces Land Component Command personnel traveling to the Combined Joint Task Force–Horn of Africa area of operations; it instructed aviators and individuals unable to take mefloquine to take doxycycline (DoD, 2006).

The National Defense Authorization Act for Fiscal Year 2006 required the Secretary of Defense to conduct a study of adverse health events (including mental health) that may be associated with the use of antimalarial drugs, including mefloquine.[6] In response, the assistant secretary of defense for health affairs commissioned four scientific studies to assess the comparative rates of adverse events resulting from the use of antimalarial medications, including mefloquine, chloroquine, doxycycline, and A/P, in deployed service members (DoD, 2009a). One study associated with this charge was published (Wells et al., 2006), and it is summarized in the Post-Cessation Adverse Events section of this chapter. Another study was reported to have been completed but not published. This committee has no information on other studies that may have been commissioned in association with this charge.

---

[5] Personal communication to the committee, COL Andrew Wiesen, M.D., M.P.H., Director, Preventive Medicine, Health Readiness Policy, and Oversight, Office of the Assistant Secretary of Defense (Health Affairs), DoD, June 10, 2019.

[6] National Defense Authorization Act, Public Law 109-360, report on adverse health events associated with use of anti-malarial drugs, § 737, December 18, 2005.

In 2009 a DoD memorandum advised that in chloroquine-resistant areas where doxycycline and mefloquine are equally efficacious and when personnel have a history of neurobehavioral disorders, doxycycline should be the first-line agent, A/P should be the second-line agent, and, in those who cannot take doxycycline or A/P, mefloquine should be used very cautiously and with clinical follow-up (DoD, 2009b). The memo also stated, presumably regarding personnel with no history of neurobehavioral disorders, that mefloquine should only be used by those with contraindications to doxycycline and without contraindications to mefloquine. In a retrospective analysis of 11,725 active-duty U.S. military personnel who were assigned in support of combat and reconstruction operations in Afghanistan around 2007, DoD administrative databases were used to determine the number of personnel with medical or pharmacologic contraindications to mefloquine prior to their deployment (Nevin, 2010; Nevin et al., 2008). In this cohort, 4,505 (38.4%) service members received a prescription for mefloquine, including 155 (13.7%) of the 1,127 service members with an identified medical or pharmacologic contra-indication to mefloquine. A 2013 DoD memo stated that doxycycline and A/P were to be considered first-line agents in chloroquine-resistant areas, reserving meflo-quine for use by those intolerant to or with contraindications to both doxycycline and A/P (DoD, 2013a). The same year, a DoD issuance stated that U.S. Special Operations Command medical personnel were to immediately cease prescribing and using mefloquine for prophylaxis and that personnel currently taking meflo-quine were to transition to one of three alternative medications (DoD, 2013b). Total DoD mefloquine prescriptions fell from 23,889 in 2008 (18,942 active duty) to 263 (52 active duty) in 2017, representing a 99% reduction (99.8% among active duty) (Wiesen, 2019).

Australia

Although mefloquine continues to be recommended by WHO and CDC for malaria prophylaxis in civilians, several militaries have issued policies regarding its use in their members. Since 2015 the governments of Australia, Canada, and the United Kingdom have performed inquiries or investigations into the pos-sible association of mefloquine with adverse effects, particularly neurologic and psychiatric effects, when used for malaria prophylaxis by their military forces (Australia, 2018; Canada, 2017; UK, 2016). Both the Canadian and Australian governments performed a literature review as a part of their inquiry process (Aus-tralia, 2018; Canada, 2017). Concerns raised by veterans and commentary in the media contributed to the initiation of these inquiries. Military veterans of Canada, Ireland, and the United Kingdom have filed lawsuits against their governments, holding them responsible for adverse events they state were caused by mefloquine use during their military service, and a U.S. veteran has filed a lawsuit against Hoffman-La Roche, the manufacturer of Lariam® (BBC, 2016; Connolly, 2019; O'Faolain, 2019).

As part of its inquiry, the Australian Senate commissioned a literature review of mefloquine and a research study that involved a re-analysis of health study data on antimalarial use from the 2007–2008 Centre for Military and Veterans' Health deployment health studies (Australia, 2018). It heard or reviewed submitted testimony from government agencies (Department of Defence, Department of Health, Department of Veterans' Affairs, Australian Defence Force Malaria and Infectious Disease Institute, Indo-Pacific Centre for Health Security, Department of Foreign Affairs and Trade Repatriation Medical Authority), a malaria-control organization (Asia Pacific Leaders Malaria Alliance), professional medical associations (Australasian Society for Infectious Diseases, Australasian College of Tropical Medicine, Royal Australian College of General Practitioners), advocate organizations (Australian Quinoline Veterans and Families Association, Quinism Foundation, Defence Force Welfare Association, Royal Australian Regiment Corporation, RSL National), and product-development partnerships and pharmaceutical manufacturers (Medicines for Malaria Venture, National Health and Medical Research Council, GlaxoSmithKline, Biocelect, 60 Degrees Pharmaceuticals, Roche), as well as from roughly 25 individuals, includingphysicians, academics, and veterans. In submitted testimony, symptoms attributed to mefloquine use were referred to as "mefloquine poisoning" or an "acquired brain injury" by the Australian Quinoline Veterans and Families Association and as "chronic quinoline encephalopathy" or "neuropsychiatric quinism" by the U.S.-based Quinism Foundation (Australia, 2018). Some veterans attributed their symptoms to mefloquine use 15 or more years earlier. In the report summary, while the Australian Senate committee acknowledged that its members were not medical experts, it stated, "The weight of prevailing medical evidence provided to the committee in response to these claims is that long term problems as a result of taking mefloquine are rare," and it added that the committee had been informed that there was no definitive evidence to support the claim that mefloquine use results in acquired brain injury. It stated that while it believed that symptoms were being experienced by individuals, assigning a single cause to these illnesses did not take into account the multiple potential contributors to their health while they took the drug and in the years after. The committee recommended that the Australian Department of Veterans' Affairs expedite its investigation into antimalarial claims logged since September 2016 and that it offer assistance to claimants and facilitate their access to legal representation. That committee also made recommendations to ensure better access to care for sick veterans, including that the Australian Department of Veterans' Affairs prioritize developing a neurocognitive health program. It did not recommend that changes be made to military policy on antimalarial use, which currently allows mefloquine to be prescribed as a "third line agent" only when doxycycline or A/P are contraindicated. Few Australian Defence Force members have been prescribed mefloquine since 2010; in 2017 only two prescriptions were made (Australian Department of Defence, n.d.).

Canada

The Canadian Armed Forces recommends the use of A/P, doxycycline, and mefloquine for malaria prophylaxis in addition to other measures to prevent mosquito bites. The Canadian Armed Forces follows the guidance set forth by the Public Health Agency of Canada. Individual armed forces members, in consultation with their health care providers, make a personal and informed decision on which antimalarial drug they want to be prescribed (Canada, 2017). Similar to the U.S. and Australian military experiences, the number of mefloquine prescriptions has decreased since 2010; 20 prescriptions were made in 2016 (Canadian Forces Health Services Group, 2017). The Canadian Surgeon General report, which was developed by a task force of Canadian Armed Forces personnel and civilians from the Department of National Defence, examined the Canadian Armed Forces experience with mefloquine and conducted a systematic review and assessment of military-specific safety information compared with other available antimalarial drugs (Canada, 2017). Although the report concluded that mefloquine was not associated with an overall excess risk of adverse effects in force personnel and its use did not prevent personnel from being able to perform their occupational duties, the quality of the evidence of the available published literature on the long-term health effects of mefloquine compared with other available antimalarial drugs was weak and itself did not support a change to policy. However, based on a consideration of other factors, such as most members showing a preference for the other available agents (A/P and doxycycline), the fact that screening for potential contraindications was lacking (a medical chart audit showed that 12% of mefloquine prescriptions had been made to service members who had contraindications), the lack of evidence on long-term safety, a desire for consistency with allied militaries (such as the United States), and the desire to be responsive to defence force member and societal concerns, the report recommended that the military change its policy to limit mefloquine use to (1) persons for whom use of A/P, doxycycline, and chloroquine are inappropriate (e.g., due to contraindications or intolerance); and (2) persons who have previously used and tolerated mefloquine, indicate a preference for it, and do not have contraindications. The report further recommended that the Canadian Armed Forces develop policies or procedures to enhance screening (and screening documentation) of service members for contraindications to mefloquine and other antimalarials and that a formal audit process be implemented to enable monitoring of antimalarial screening and prescription practices (Canada, 2017).

United Kingdom

The UK Ministry of Defence amended its policy regarding the use of mefloquine and other antimalarials on September 12, 2016, and it was further revised in June 2017 in response to recommendations from the UK House of Commons

Defence Committee's report on mefloquine (UK, 2016). The inquiry by the House of Commons Defence Committee was more limited in scope than those undertaken by the Australian and Canadian governments. The committee did not perform a literature search, but testimony was heard and reviewed from government agencies (Surgeon General; Ministry for Defence Personnel, Welfare and Veterans; Defence Medical Services), the pharmaceutical manufacturer Roche Products Ltd., and roughly 15 individuals, including a research scientist, physicians, and veterans. That committee concluded that mefloquine should be considered as a drug of last resort in defense forces. The new policy restricts the use of mefloquine even more narrowly to military personnel who are unable to tolerate available alternatives, have been screened for safe use via a face-to-face assessment, and have been informed of and provided the option to take alternative agents. The other prophylactic drugs available to armed forces members are doxycycline, chloroquine, and A/P. Consistent with Australian and Canadian defense forces, few prescriptions for mefloquine are made; from April 2018 to March 2019, there were 31 mefloquine prescriptions (UK, 2019).

PHARMACOKINETICS

Mefloquine is a chiral antimalarial agent, available as the racemic combination of (+) and (–) enantiomers (Schlagenhauf, 1999). Five metabolites of mefloquine have been isolated (WHO, 1983). The pharmacokinetics of the mefloquine enantiomers have been found to be highly stereospecific (Gimenez et al., 1994). The plasma concentrations of the (–) enantiomer were shown to be significantly higher than those observed for the (+) enantiomer, and all major pharmacokinetic parameters, with the exception of T_{max}, were observed to be significantly different (Gimenez et al., 1994).

Mefloquine is primarily metabolized by CYP3A4 (Fontaine et al., 2000), and the major circulating metabolite is a 4-carboxylic acid derivative (Gimenez et al., 1994), which is inactive against *P. falciparum* (Ashley et al., 2006). Mefloquine appears to be excreted primarily in the bile and feces; urine excretion of the unchanged drug and of its acid metabolite amounted to 9% and 4.2% of the weekly dose, respectively (Schwartz et al., 1987; WHO, 1983).

Plasma protein binding of mefloquine is high, reportedly 98% (Karbwang and White, 1990; Palmer et al., 1993). Considerable interindividual variation in pharmacokinetic parameters has been reported (Gimenez et al., 1994; Karbwang and White, 1990; Karbwang et al., 1987; Palmer et al., 1993). The presence of food significantly increases the bioavailability of mefloquine (Schlagenhauf, 1999). In healthy volunteers, plasma concentrations peak 6–24 hours (mean 17.6 hours) after a single dose of mefloquine (Palmer et al., 1993). Clinical pharmacokinetic studies in male volunteers from Africa, Brazil, Europe, and the United States have shown that mefloquine has a long but variable plasma half-life of 6–23 days, with a mean value of around 14 days, but effective drug levels may persist for 30 days or more (WHO, 1983). Using a dosage of 250 mg weekly requires 7–10 weeks before a steady-state plasma concentration is achieved. Maximum blood concentrations appear to be two to three times higher in Asians than in non-Asians. In healthy adults, the terminal elimination half-life ranges from 14 to 28 (mean 18.1) days, indicating that mefloquine is distributed extensively in the tissues and is cleared slowly from the body (Palmer et al., 1993). Mefloquine blood concentrations in pregnant women are lower than those in nonpregnant adults (Thillainayagam and Ramaiah, 2016), but clearance may be increased during late pregnancy (Karbwang and White, 1990).

ADVERSE EVENTS

This section begins with a summary of known concurrent adverse events, such as those that occur immediately or within a few hours or days of taking a dose of mefloquine, from Cochrane systematic reviews. Epidemiologic studies of persistent adverse events in which information was available at least 28 days post-mefloquine-cessation are then summarized by population category (military or veterans, occupational groups, travelers, and research volunteers), with an emphasis placed on reported results of persistent or latent effects that were associated with the use of mefloquine (even if results on other antimalarial-drug comparison groups were presented).

Concurrent Adverse Events

Concurrent adverse events are well characterized for mefloquine. In general, mefloquine has a poorer reputation among the public and in military populations than the other available drugs for malaria prophylaxis. This is due mainly to the neurologic and psychiatric events associated with mefloquine, which are dose related, but that may occur at prophylactic doses (Stürchler et al., 1990; Weinke et al., 1991) and at a greater frequency than with other antimalarial prophylactics (Schlagenhauf et al., 2003, 2010). However, mefloquine-associated serious adverse events—defined as those that constitute a threat to life, require hospitalization, or result in severe disability—are rare, with estimated occurrences ranging from 1 in 10,000 to 1 in 20,000 depending on the population examined (Björkman et al., 1991; Schlagenhauf et al., 2003, 2010; Stürchler et al., 1990; Weinke et al., 1991; Wells et al., 2006). Instead of detailing every study that has reported concurrent adverse events that have been reported with use of mefloquine, the following paragraphs summarize the most common adverse events as well as those that are less commonly reported but still recognized as possibly related to the use of mefloquine for malaria prophylaxis using two identified Cochrane systematic reviews of the literature (Croft and Garner, 2000; Tickell-Painter et al., 2017a).

Results from analyses that compared mefloquine with placebo or no drug (as opposed to comparisons with another antimalarial drug) were of greatest interest to the committee because an observed lack of difference in effect between two drugs could occur because both drugs cause the (same) adverse events. Use of a placebo-controlled design helps provide information about the "base rate" of the adverse events, to understand if the rates observed among individuals taking the drug are higher than would be expected with no drug exposure.

The aim of the first published Cochrane review (Croft and Garner, 2000) was to determine the effects of mefloquine in nonimmune adult travelers compared with other antimalarial regimens in relation to episodes of malaria, withdrawal from prophylaxis, and adverse events. Ten randomized trials of adult travelers and non-traveling volunteers were considered as well as 516 case reports for adverse events analyses. More recently, Tickell-Painter et al. (2017a) conducted a systematic review to summarize the efficacy and safety of mefloquine used as prophylaxis for malaria in adults, children, and pregnant women travelers. This review included 20 randomized controlled trials (totaling 11,470 participants), 35 cohort studies (totaling 198,493 participants), and 4 large retrospective analyses of health records (800,652 participants). Although the aims of these two large reviews were slightly different, Tickell-Painter et al. included nearly all of the same randomized controlled trials as Croft and Garner.

Croft and Garner (2000) assessed the use of mefloquine in nonimmune adult travelers compared with other regimens; the analysis included a total of 2,750 participants. To compare tolerability, the authors reviewed data on neurologic and psychiatric symptoms (depression, abnormal dreams, fatigue, headache, insomnia), gastrointestinal symptoms (abdominal discomfort, anorexia, diarrhea, nausea, vomiting), and fever and pruritus; data were to have been collected "at first assessment." The authors identified five trials that compared outcomes with mefloquine versus placebo, and they reported that the tolerability outcome measures showed no statistically significant pattern relative to mefloquine or placebo, but that the numbers of study participants were generally small. Six trials were identified that compared mefloquine with other malaria-prophylactic drugs, but the comparator drugs were not named, except incidentally when specific comparisons were made. The authors calculated Peto odds ratios (used when pooling odds ratios) and found the overall incidence of adverse events with mefloquine to be no different from that of other antimalarials (OR = 1.00, 95%CI 0.80–1.27; 4 studies, 1,344 participants). There was no consistent pattern across the five neurologic and psychiatric symptoms analyzed (depression, dreams, fatigue, headache, insomnia), but mefloquine was shown to be more likely than other agents to cause insomnia (OR = 1.64, 95%CI 1.18–2.28; 4 studies, 1,344 participants) and fatigue (OR = 1.57, 95%CI 1.01–2.45; 4 studies, 1,344 participants). No consistent pattern was seen for the gastrointestinal symptoms analyzed, but abdominal discomfort was reported less frequently among users of mefloquine than among users of other antimalarials (OR = 0.57, 95%CI 0.42–0.77; 5 studies,

1,464 participants), as was the case with anorexia (OR = 0.64, 95%CI 0.43–0.95; 4 studies, 1,444 participants) and nausea (OR = 0.74, 95%CI 0.57–0.96; 6 studies, 1,717 participants). The authors noted the heterogeneity of the studies and stated that the overall effect regarding gastrointestinal symptoms appeared to be due to one study in which participants reported symptoms in the chloroquine-proguanil group more frequently than in the mefloquine group. Reports of fever and pruritus were similar in the mefloquine and comparator arms. The authors also noted that they had identified 328 case reports that involved mefloquine prophylaxis and adverse events (discussed later in this chapter under Case Reports and Case Series).

Tickell-Painter et al. (2017a) prespecified adverse events of interest to include these disorders: psychiatric (abnormal dreams, insomnia, anxiety, depression, psychosis); nervous system (dizziness, headache); ear and labyrinth (vertigo); eye (visual impairment); gastrointestinal tract (nausea, vomiting, abdominal pain, diarrhea, dyspepsia); and skin and subcutaneous tissues (pruritus, photosensitivity, vaginal candida). The assessment comparing the use of mefloquine for malaria prophylaxis with placebo or no treatment included 13 randomized controlled trials and 5 cohort studies. Dosages varied, as did methods of collecting adverse event data; eight of the trials were considered to be at high risk of bias from selective outcome reporting. The authors applied categories of certainty to the results based on the five GRADE considerations (risk of bias, consistency of effect, imprecision, indirectness, and publication bias) (Higgins et al., 2019).

Overall, among the six randomized controlled trials only one serious adverse event (death from septic shock after an emergency cesarean section for obstructed labor) was reported among study participants who used mefloquine (n = 592) compared with two that occurred among people using placebo (n = 629); none of these events were attributed to the drug regimen (Tickell-Painter et al., 2017a). In the cohort studies, seven serious adverse events (five were depression and two were dizziness, and all were attributed to the drug regimen) were reported among 913 mefloquine users, and none were reported in 254 travelers who did not use antimalarials. When analyses were performed to compare mefloquine with doxycycline (4 trials and 20 cohort studies), A/P (3 trials and 16 cohort studies), and chloroquine (6 trials and 15 cohort studies), no difference in the incidence of serious adverse events was found between mefloquine and doxycycline, A/P, or chloroquine. Participants receiving mefloquine were no more likely to discontinue their medication due to adverse events than were doxycycline users (RR = 1.08, 95%CI 0.41–2.87; 4 trials, 763 participants; low-certainty evidence), but mefloquine users were more likely to discontinue their medication due to adverse events than A/P users (RR = 2.86, 95%CI 1.53–5.31; 3 trials, 1,438 participants; high-certainty evidence) (Tickell-Painter et al., 2017a).

Regarding neurologic outcomes, people taking mefloquine were less likely than those taking placebo in trials to experience headache (RR = 0.84, 95%CI 0.71–0.99; 5 trials, 791 participants), but this was not observed in the one cohort study that reported on headache. Whereas mefloquine users in trials were no more likely than recipients who took a placebo or no drug to experience dizziness (RR = 1.03, 95%CI 0.90–1.17; 3 trials, 452 participants), in the cohort studies, participants who used mefloquine were statistically significantly more likely to experience dizziness (RR = 1.80, 95%CI 1.29–2.49; 3 studies, 1,901 participants) than those who used placebo or no drug. No differences were observed between mefloquine and placebo groups for vertigo in either trials or cohort studies. Cohort study comparisons between mefloquine and doxycycline users found no differences for headache or dizziness.

None of the randomized controlled trials reported on the psychiatric symptoms of abnormal dreams, insomnia, anxiety, depressed mood, or abnormal thoughts and perceptions (psychosis). Participants in cohort studies who received mefloquine were more likely than participants who did not take prophylaxis to experience abnormal dreams (RR = 2.35, 95%CI 1.15–4.80; 2 studies, 931 participants) and insomnia (RR = 1.46, 95%CI 1.06–2.02; 2 studies, 931 participants). Effects on anxiety (RR = 1.21, 95%CI 0.67–2.21; 2 studies, 931 participants), depressed mood (RR = 2.43, 95%CI 0.65–9.07; 3 studies, 1,901 participants), and abnormal thoughts or perceptions (RR = 5.77, 95%CI 0.79–42.06; 1 study, 970 participants) were not consistent across studies and did not reach standard levels of statistical significance. Findings from trials and cohort studies that used A/P as a comparator were similar, with mefloquine users statistically significantly more likely to report abnormal dreams, insomnia, anxiety, and depressed mood, although it should be noted that all of the effect estimates were quite imprecise. Using the six cohort studies that used doxycycline as a comparator, mefloquine users were more likely to report abnormal dreams (RR = 10.49, 95%CI 3.79–29.10; 4 studies, 2,588 participants), insomnia (RR = 4.14, 95%CI 1.19–14.44; 4 studies, 3,212 participants), anxiety (RR = 18.04, 95%CI 9.32–34.93; 3 studies, 2,559 participants), and depressed mood (RR = 11.43, 95%CI 5.21–25.07; 2 studies, 2,445 participants), but the pooled effect estimates were very imprecise. Additionally, 15 episodes of abnormal thoughts and perceptions were reported among mefloquine users and none among doxycycline users in the cohort studies reporting adverse events. In the single trial included and the large retrospective health care record analyses, there were either no differences between groups, or doxycycline users were more likely to experience psychiatric symptoms. Overall, the authors concluded that people taking mefloquine are more likely to have abnormal dreams, insomnia, anxiety, and depressed mood during travel than people who take A/P (moderate-certainty evidence) or doxycycline (very low-certainty evidence).

Mefloquine recipients were more likely to experience nausea than placebo recipients for both trials (RR = 1.35, 95%CI 1.05–1.73; 2 trials, 244 participants) and cohort studies (RR = 1.85, 95%CI 1.42–2.43; 3 studies, 1,901 participants), but there was no difference between groups for vomiting, abdominal pain, or diarrhea. For both trials and cohort studies, when mefloquine users were compared with A/P users, mefloquine users were statistically significantly more likely to experience nausea, but there was no statistically significant difference for vomiting, abdominal pain, or diarrhea. Based on data from cohort studies, mefloquine users were less likely than doxycycline users to report dyspepsia (RR = 0.26, 95%CI 0.09–0.74; 5 studies, 5,104 participants), vomiting (RR = 0.18, 95%CI 0.12–0.27; 4 studies, 5,071 participants), nausea (RR = 0.37, 95%CI 0.30–0.45; 5 studies, 2,683 participants), and diarrhea (RR = 0.28, 95%CI 0.11–0.73; 5 studies, 5,104 participants). No difference between mefloquine users and doxycycline users was found for abdominal pain (RR = 0.30, 95%CI 0.09–1.07; 4 studies, 2,569 participants). The authors stated that the estimates for dyspepsia and vomiting were given low or very low certainty of evidence. Other symptoms were also included when available. Based on one cohort study of 197 participants, mefloquine users were more likely than those who were given placebo to experience pruritus (RR = 6.71, 95%CI 1.58–28.55), although the estimate was imprecise. Pruritus was not statistically different between mefloquine users and placebo or non-drug users in trials (RR = 0.86, 95%CI 0.60–1.24; 3 trials, 609 participants). Based on the data from cohort studies, mefloquine users were less likely than doxycycline users to report photosensitivity (RR = 0.08, 95%CI 0.05–0.11) and vaginal thrush (RR = 0.10, 95%CI 0.06–0.16), but for both of these results the evidence was considered to be very low certainty. No differences were observed between mefloquine and placebo groups for visual impairment in either trials or cohort studies. Authors noted that comparisons of mefloquine with chloroquine added no new information and that subgroup analysis by study design, duration of travel, and military versus non-military participants provided no conclusive findings.

Post-Cessation Adverse Events

A total of 1,577 abstracts or titles were identified by the committee for inclusion for mefloquine. After screening, 489 abstracts and titles remained, and the full text for each was retrieved and reviewed to determine whether it met the committee's inclusion criteria, as defined in Chapter 3. The committee reviewed each article and identified 11 epidemiologic studies that included some mention of adverse events that occurred ≥28 days post-cessation of mefloquine (DeSouza, 1983; Eick-Cost et al., 2017; Laothavorn et al., 1992; Meier et al., 2004; Schlagenhauf et al., 1996; Schneider et al., 2013, 2014; Schneiderman et al., 2018; Schwartz and Regev-Yochay, 1999; Tan et al., 2017; Wells et al., 2006). A table that gives a high-level comparison (study design, population, exposure groups, and outcomes examined by body system) of each of the 11 epidemiologic studies that examined the use of mefloquine and that met the committee's inclusion criteria is presented in Appendix C. Other identified articles are cited in the background, case reports and selected subpopulations, and biologic plausibility sections as relevant.

Military and Veterans

Using DoD administrative databases, Eick-Cost et al. (2017) performed a retrospective cohort study among 367,840 active-duty service members who filled at least one prescription for an antimalarial drug for prophylaxis between 2008 and 2013: 36,538 were prescribed mefloquine, 318,421 doxycycline, and 12,881 A/P. The primary study objective was to assess and compare the risk of incident and recurrent *International Classification of Diseases, Ninth Revision, Clinical Modification* (ICD-9-CM)–coded neurologic and psychiatric outcomes (adjustment disorder, anxiety disorder, depressive disorder, posttraumatic stress disorder [PTSD], psychoses, suicide ideation, paranoia, confusion, tinnitus, vertigo, convulsions, hallucinations, insomnia, and suicide) that were reported at medical care visits during concurrent use plus 365 days after the end of the prescription for mefloquine, doxycycline, and A/P. Although the authors did not report results for the period of ≥28 days post-cessation of antimalarial drug use, they stated that they performed several sensitivity analyses, including one in which the risk period was restricted to 30 days post-prescription. The results of that analysis were summarized in the text as follows: "However, none of these analyses significantly changed the results of the study and are therefore not reported" (p. 161). This statement implies (but does not show directly) that similar findings to those reported would be seen if the data were restricted to the period of relevance to the committee's definition of persistence (i.e., ≥28 days after cessation of exposure). The committee was unsure how to interpret that sentence reporting that the results did not change significantly (statistical significance, precision of effect estimates, number of diagnoses, etc.), but given that the authors performed sensitivity analyses, the number of methodologic strengths, including strong measurement of relevant outcomes conducted in the target population, the committee chose to include it, despite the ambiguity in the language. If an individual had multiple prescriptions over the follow-up period, risk periods were merged. Doxycycline and A/P prescriptions were excluded if the service member previously or concurrently received mefloquine. Mefloquine risk periods were censored if an individual received a prescription for a different antimalarial. Analyses were stratified by deployment and psychiatric history. Models were adjusted for age, sex, service, grade, and year of prescription start; analyses of deployed service members also controlled for location and combat exposure. Mefloquine recipients had primarily served in the Air Force (58%), held a rank of senior enlisted (47%), and most had had prescriptions filled prior to 2010 (75%). Among the deployed service members, 29% of the individuals who had received mefloquine reported having had combat exposure (compared with 43% for doxycycline and 21% for A/P).

With few exceptions, adjusted incident rates were higher among the deployed than among the nondeployed for mefloquine as well as for the other antimalarial drugs considered. Effect estimates of neurologic and psychiatric outcomes for doxycycline and A/P are reported in those respective chapters. For mefloquine users the highest incident rates among both the deployed and nondeployed were for adjustment disorder (28.66 versus 18.75 per 1,000 person-years, respectively), followed by insomnia (15.78 versus 10.09 per 1,000 person-years, respectively) and anxiety disorder (14.51 versus 9.28 per 1,000 person-years, respectively). Incident depressive disorder (12.46 versus 8.59 per 1,000 person-years, respectively) and vertigo (12.19 versus 11.90 per 1,000 person-years, respectively) were also higher among the deployed group. The incidence of tinnitus, however, was higher among the nondeployed than among the deployed (14.02 versus 13.44 per 1,000 person-years, respectively) as was the case for convulsions, psychoses, suicide, and confusion. Among those prescribed mefloquine, the incidence rate of PTSD was 11.08 per 1,000 person-years in the deployed group and 5.05 per 1,000 person-years in the nondeployed group. Adjusted incidence rate ratios (IRRs) comparing mefloquine to doxycycline by deployment status found that among the deployed, the only statistically significant difference between the two drugs was for anxiety disorder (IRR = 1.12, 95%CI 1.01–1.24). When mefloquine and doxycycline users were compared among the nondeployed, the outcomes of adjustment disorder (IRR = 0.69, 95%CI 0.60–0.80), insomnia (IRR = 0.67, 95%CI 0.56–0.81), anxiety disorder (IRR = 0.70, 95%CI 0.57–0.86), depressive disorder (IRR = 0.68, 95%CI 0.55–0.84), vertigo (IRR = 0.52, 95%CI 0.31–0.88), and PTSD (IRR = 0.69, 95%CI 0.52–0.91) all showed a statistically significantly *lower* risk for mefloquine users but no differences were found for the other outcomes. Adjusted IRRs comparing mefloquine with A/P by deployment status found that the risk of tinnitus among both the deployed (IRR = 1.81, 95%CI 1.18–2.79) and the nondeployed (IRR = 1.51, 95%CI 1.13–2.03) was statistically significantly elevated among those taking mefloquine. No other outcomes were statistically significantly different between deployed mefloquine and A/P users. Among the nondeployed, the only other statistically significant difference between mefloquine and A/P users was for PTSD (IRR = 1.83, 95%CI 1.07–3.14). A subsequent analysis restricted the population to the first mefloquine or doxycycline prescription per individual and included individuals with a prior history of a neurologic or psychiatric diagnosis. Incidence rates and IRRs for each neurologic and psychiatric outcome were compared, stratified by those with and without a prior neurologic or psychiatric diagnosis. In total, 5.9% of those prescribed mefloquine and 9.2% of individuals prescribed doxycycline had had at least one neurologic or psychiatric diagnosis in the 365 days before the prescription, suggesting that those with a psychiatric disorder were less likely to be prescribed mefloquine, consistent with the contraindications of the drug. A diagnosis of PTSD was recorded for 131 (0.4%) individuals in the mefloquine group and for 2,671 (0.8%) individuals in the doxycycline group in the 365 days prior to the first antimalarial prescription. For both the mefloquine and doxycycline groups, individuals with a neurologic or psychiatric diagnosis in the year preceding the prescription had statistically significantly elevated risks for a subsequent diagnosis of the same condition for all conditions reported (adjustment disorder, anxiety, insomnia, depressive disorder, PTSD, tinnitus, vertigo, and convulsions) than individuals without a diagnosis in the prior year. However, when the IRRs contrasting mefloquine and doxycycline users were compared within strata of those with and without prior neurologic or psychiatric diagnoses, there were no statistically significant differences between mefloquine and doxycycline for any of the conditions, including PTSD (bootstrap RRR = 1.14, 95%CI 0.78–1.65).

The committee found this study to be well designed. Important factors that increased the study quality were the large sample size; the use of an administrative data source, which provides some degree of objectivity; and the careful consideration of potential confounding variables, including demographics, psychiatric history, and military characteristics of deployment and combat exposure. Because neurologic and psychiatric diagnoses occurring during current and recent use were analyzed together without distinguishing between events that occurred within 28 days of antimalarial use and those that occurred ≥28 days post-cessation, the study provides no quantitative information regarding the persistence of most events other than the notation in text that results did not change when restricted to the post-cessation period. The use of administrative data provided a standard, consistent method to capture filled prescriptions and medical diagnoses through the use of ICD-9-CM codes. However, filled prescriptions do not equate to adherence to the drug regimen. Moreover, if the antimalarials were provided to entire units as part of force health protection measures, the use of these drugs would not be coded in individual records. Whereas the use of medical diagnoses is likely to be more reliable for the outcomes than self-report, the data are dependent on the accuracy of the coding, and there was no validation of the diagnoses recorded in the administrative databases, and symptoms or events that did not result in a medical visit or diagnosis would have been missed. For PTSD diagnoses, there was no information about when the index trauma occurred. Given the largely decreased risks and null results reported for the study, this implies null results would be found for the period of interest, but the data were not presented to examine this directly.

Schneiderman et al. (2018) conducted a retrospective observational analysis of self-reported health outcomes associated with use of antimalarial drugs in a cohort of U.S. veterans who had responded to the 2009–2011 National Health Study for a New Generation of U.S. Veterans (referred to as the NewGen Study). The NewGen Study is a population-based survey that sampled 30,000 veterans who had been deployed to Iraq or Afghanistan between 2001 and 2008 and 30,000 nondeployed veterans who had served during the same time period; it included a 20% oversampling of women. The survey was conducted using mail, telephone, and web-based collection and yielded a response rate of only 34.3%. For this particular analysis, 19,487 participants were included who had self-reported their history of antimalarial medication use, and the use was grouped for the analysis by drug (mefloquine, chloroquine, doxycycline, primaquine, mefloquine in combination with other drugs, other antimalarials, and not specified) or no antimalarial use. Health outcomes were self-reported using standardized instruments: the Medical Outcomes Study 12-item Short Form (SF-12) for general health status,

PTSD Checklist–Civilian version (PCL-C), and the Patient Health Question-naire. These instruments yielded scores that were dichotomized for analysis on composite physical health, composite mental health (above or below the U.S. mean), PTSD (above or below screening cutoff), thoughts of death or self-harm, other anxiety disorders, and major depression. Potential confounders included in the multivariable analysis were the branch of service, sex, age, education, race/ethnicity, household income, employment status, marital status, and self-reported exposure to combat. Responses were weighted to account for survey non-response. Most veterans reported no antimalarial drug exposures (61.4%, n = 11,100), and these served as the referent group. Focusing first on those veterans who had been deployed (n = 12,456), of those who reported use of an antimalarial drug (n = 6,650), 307 (4.4% weighted) reported only using mefloquine, and 425 (6.0% weighted) reported using mefloquine and another antimalarial. Among the non-deployed (n = 7,031), 39 (2.2% weighted) used mefloquine alone, and 52 (2.8% weighted) used mefloquine and another antimalarial. The deployed mefloquine-plus-another-antimalarial users reported the highest prevalence of positive screens for PTSD (20.0%), other anxiety disorders (15.3%), and major depression (12.5%) compared with mefloquine alone and with the other antimalarial drug groups in the deployed and nondeployed strata. Descriptive statistics indicated that the deployed mefloquine users reported greater frequencies of mental health diagnoses than non-deployed mefloquine users—PTSD (14.2% versus 7.5%), other anxiety disorders (10.8% versus 5.7%), major depression (9.3% versus 3.3%), and thoughts of death or self-harm (14.0% versus 7.1%)—but no statistical inferences were presented. In the adjusted logistic regression models with all covariates considered (including demographics, deployment, and combat exposure), the use of mefloquine alone was not associated with an increased risk for any of the health outcomes when compared with nonuse of antimalarial drugs: composite mental health score (OR = 0.87, 95%CI 0.66–1.14), composite physical health score (OR = 0.96, 95%CI 0.73–1.26), PTSD (not adjusted for combat exposure) (OR = 0.86, 95%CI 0.58–1.27), thoughts of death or self-harm (OR = 1.21, 95%CI 0.80–1.82), other anxiety (OR = 0.77, 95%CI 0.49–1.22), and major depression (OR = 0.74, 95%CI 0.46–1.20). Results were similar and not statistically significant for mefloquine use in combination with other antimalarials for analyses restricted to the deployed subset of veterans. An additional analysis was performed on the six health indicators or outcomes stratified by antimalarial exposure and a four-level measure of combat exposure intensity. The weighted prevalence estimates seem to indicate an increasing prevalence of disorders with increasing combat exposure intensity, but it is challenging to interpret the results or to compare across antimalarial exposures given the small numbers in some cells and the lack of confidence intervals or hypothesis tests.

This analysis of the NewGen survey is highly relevant to the question of whether there are effects of mefloquine use that persist after the cessation of drug use. The study is large enough to generate moderately precise measures of association, the specific drugs were assessed, the outcomes were based on standardized instruments (although not face-to-face diagnostic interviews), important covariates of deployment and combat exposure were considered in addition to demographics and other military characteristics, and the data were appropriately analyzed. The number of mefloquine-only users in this sample was relatively small (346 of antimalarials users). It is noteworthy that adjustment for combat exposure consistently reduced the measures of association, potentially indicating the strong confounding that can exist due to combat exposure. Although the time period of drug use and the timing of health outcomes was not directly addressed, given that the populations were all veterans who had served between 2001 and 2008 and that the survey was not administered until 2009–2011, it is reasonable to assume that antimalarial drug use had ceased some time before. Nonetheless, the study could not address explicitly the health experiences during use and in specific time intervals following the cessation of use. There are a number of methodologic concerns that limit the strength of this study's findings. The low response rate of 34% raises concerns of non-response bias, but responses were weighted to account for non-response. Selective participation by both antimalarial drug use history and health status would be required to introduce bias. The accuracy of self-reported antimalarial drug use in this population is unknown. Although self-reported information has some advantages over studies based on prescriptions in that the individual recalls using the drug, validation of the reported drug and information on adherence is not captured. Self-reported health experience is subject to the usual disadvantages of recall bias and bias of reporting subjective experience without independent expert assessment; however, by using standardized assessment tools, these biases may have been circumvented to some extent.

The Wells et al. study was commissioned in 2004 by the assistant secretary of defense in response to concerns within DoD about adverse health outcomes associated with the use of mefloquine (DoD, 2009a). Wells et al. (2006) used DoD administrative databases and a retrospective observational design to examine U.S. active-duty service members who had been prescribed mefloquine (minimum seven tablets) and deployed at some time in calendar year 2002 (n = 8,858). Their health experience was compared with that of U.S. service personnel assigned to Europe or Japan (n = 156,203), who did not use antimalarials. This comparison group was intended to control for being healthy enough to be stationed overseas, but this group was not considered to be "deployed" in the same manner as to an operational theater or combat zone. A second control group consisted of active-duty service members who were deployed for 1 month or longer during 2002 but had not been prescribed mefloquine or other commonly used antimalarial drugs (n = 232,381). Although the use of two comparison groups can be helpful when results are consistent, it is important that both are similar to the exposed group. The demographic and military characteristics of the Europe- and Japan-stationed individuals differed substantially from those of the deployed individuals. Health outcomes were based on hospitalization records within the military health care system and the corresponding ICD-9-CM codes for diagnoses by body system, including a number of physical and mental health conditions. The use of hospitalizations indicates adverse events of a greater severity for reported disorders than may be experienced by other populations of mefloquine users. The association between mefloquine exposure and hospitalization was analyzed through Cox proportional hazards modeling, with the follow-up time beginning on return from deployment (with or without mefloquine exposure). Adjustment was made for sex, age, race/ethnicity, service branch, marital status, rank, occupation, and history of hospitalization in 2001. Compared with those nondeployed service members who were assigned to Europe or Japan, those prescribed mefloquine during their deployment had a statistically significantly lower risk of hospitalization for any cause (HR = 0.47, 95%CI 0.39–0.56) as well as for reasons specific to the digestive system (HR = 0.52, 95%CI 0.34–0.79), for reasons specific to the respiratory system (HR = 0.44, 95%CI 0.23–0.86), for musculoskeletal disorders (HR = 0.68, 95%CI 0.47–0.98), for ill-defined conditions (HR = 0.24, 95%CI 0.16–0.37), and for injury and poisoning (HR = 0.63, 95%CI 0.47–0.84). No statistically significant differences were found between mefloquine users and those assigned to Europe or Japan for hospitalizations related to mental disorders (HR = 0.76, 95%CI 0.55–1.07) or for disorders of the nervous system (HR = 0.58, 95%CI 0.26–1.32), the circulatory system (HR = 0.61, 95%CI 0.31–1.18), blood and blood-forming organs (HR = 0.51, 95%CI 0.19–1.36), or skin and subcutaneous tissues (HR = 0.88, 95%CI 0.43–1.80). The hazard ratios comparing mefloquine users with deployed nonusers of antimalarials yielded null results across the range of all outcomes reported, including hospitalization for any cause (HR = 0.94, 95%CI 0.79–1.12), mental disorders (HR = 1.23, 95%CI 0.87–1.72), or disorders of the nervous system (HR = 0.76, 95%CI 0.34–1.73), digestive system (HR = 0.90, 95%CI 0.60–1.37), circulatory system (HR = 0.69, 95%CI 0.35–1.34), blood and blood-forming organs (HR = 0.65, 95%CI 0.24–1.74), or skin and subcutaneous tissues (HR = 1.31, 95%CI 0.64–2.69). Hospitalizations related to categories of infections; neoplasms; disorders of endocrine, nutritional, or metabolism; and disorders of the genitourinary system were also examined between mefloquine users and the two reference groups but none reached statistical significance. A total of 37 hospitalizations for mental disorders as a category were reported for mefloquine users, and when hospitalizations due to specific psychiatric outcomes were considered, there were no cases of somatoform disorders, 6 cases each of mood disorders and anxiety disorders, 1 case of PTSD, 19 cases of substance use disorders, 7 cases of personality disorders, 13 cases of adjustment reactions, 4 cases of mixed syndromes, and 20 cases of "other disorders" among mefloquine users. A comparison of these rates with those of the two reference groups of service members resulted in imprecise and null estimates. Only six hospitalizations due to nervous system disorders were reported for mefloquine users, and comparisons with both reference groups showed that mefloquine users had no statistically significant difference in risk for nervous system disorders as a group. When hospitalizations due to specific neurologic outcomes were considered, among those receiving mefloquine there were no cases of nystagmus or dizziness and giddiness, one case of vertiginous syndromes, and three cases of migraine, which resulted in wide, imprecise, and null effect estimates when these rates were compared with those of the two reference groups of service members. Deployed mefloquine users had numerically higher rates than deployed nonusers, but no comparisons reached statistical significance, and all effect estimates of individual diagnoses had less precision than when reported by organ system. For example, only one diagnosis of PTSD was reported in the mefloquine user group, compared with 29 diagnoses in the deployed nonuser group (HR = 1.66, 95%CI 0.21–12.85) and 38 diagnoses in the Europe/Japan group (HR = 0.79, 95%CI 0.11–5.91). The only statistically significant difference found between mefloquine users and those assigned to Europe or Japan was for mood disorders (HR = 0.37, 95%CI 0.15–0.90).

Overall, this is a well-designed study that was likely adequately powered to detect moderate differences. Because the follow-up of the mefloquine users began at the time of their return from deployment, it is reasonable to assume that these results largely reflected their experiences following cessation of exposure of varying duration. Nonetheless, the results for varying time intervals following cessation of use (or time since return from deployment) were not presented. Although the use of two comparison groups can be helpful when the results are consistent, it is important that both be similar to the exposed group. The demographic and military characteristics of the Europe- and Japan-stationed individuals differed substantially from the deployed individuals, suggesting that this was not an appropriate comparison group. With regard to exposure, a prescription is not the same as having actually taken the drug or having taken it as indicated, creating the potential for misclassification. A reasonable set of covariates was used to adjust effect estimates, in particular the sociodemographic covariates. However, combat exposure was not specifically addressed, and although deployment may have been assumed to be a surrogate for combat, the lack of control for combat exposure itself is a limitation. The health outcomes were systematically and objectively ascertained but would reflect only the most severe experiences requiring hospitalization, and for this reason, the number of cases was generally small (i.e., 135 mefloquine users were hospitalized for any cause). Because the diagnoses were based on clinical encounters, the PTSD diagnoses are presumably linked to an index trauma criterion A event. Most people who experience mental health disorders would not be hospitalized, and the small number of specific neurologic and psychiatric cases reported further limits the generalizability of these results.

U.S. Peace Corps

Tan et al. (2017) conducted a retrospective observational Internet-based survey of 8,931 (11% response rate) returned Peace Corps volunteers (who had served during 1995–2014) to compare the prevalence of selected health conditions after

Peace Corps service between those who reported taking malaria prophylaxis (n = 5,055, 56.6%) and those who did not. The reported initial antimalarial prophylactic prescriptions were mefloquine (n = 2,981; 59.0%), A/P (n = 183; 3.6%), chloroquine (n = 674; 13.3%), doxycycline (n = 831; 16.4%), and 386 (7.6%) "other" prophylactic medications. In addition to questions on malaria prophylaxis (type, regimen, duration, and adherence), the survey included questions about the country of service, type of assignment, and whether malaria prophylaxis was required at the assigned site. Respondents were also asked to report medical diagnoses made by a health care provider before, during, and after service in the Peace Corps and to answer questions about medications used before, during, or after Peace Corps service; family history of disease and psychiatric illness; psychiatric history prior to exposure; and alcohol consumption. In total, more than 40 disease outcomes were examined for associations with each antimalarial, including derived outcomes of major depressive disorder, bipolar disorder, anxiety disorder, insomnia, psychoses, and cancers. Outcomes were grouped by system (neuropsychologic, cardiac, ophthalmologic, dermatologic, reproductive, and gastrointestinal) or class (infectious, hematologic/oncologic) and within each group several diagnoses were listed. "Any psychiatric outcome" included all reported psychiatric diagnoses both derived and those reported as individual diagnoses, including schizophrenia, obsessive-compulsive disorder, and "other." Neuropsychologic disorders were presented as a category that separately included dementia, migraines, seizures, tinnitus, vestibular disorder, "other" neurologic disorder, and "any" neurologic disorder. Among those who had reported any use of mefloquine, the prevalence of any psychiatric disease following Peace Corps service was 15.9%, which was lower than the prevalence for people who had not used mefloquine (18.8%). Among people with a prior psychiatric illness, fewer reported the use of mefloquine than among those without a prior psychiatric illness (16.2% versus 44.0%, respectively), which would be expected since prior psychiatric illness is a contraindication of mefloquine. Estimates adjusted for a prior history of psychiatric disease and a family history of psychiatric disease indicated that mefloquine users had a higher likelihood of having any psychiatric diagnosis post-service relative to individuals who did not take mefloquine (prevalence ratio = 1.15, 95%CI 1.07–1.23). When those with a prior psychiatric history were excluded from the analysis, there was no difference in the prevalence of any psychiatric outcomes between those who had used mefloquine and those who had not (prevalence ratio = 1.07, 95%CI 0.95–1.21), but the results were not presented separately for those with a prior psychiatric history. No difference in the prevalence of any psychiatric outcomes was found when comparing prolonged duration of mefloquine use with any other antimalarial. The authors reported that there were no differences in the prevalence of several diagnoses that have previously been reported as adverse events and feared adverse events associated with mefloquine use, including vestibular dysfunction, neurologic disorders, insomnia, arrhythmias, other cardiac diseases, and ophthalmologic disorders (a category that included macular degeneration, retinopathy, and "any" ophthalmologic disorder), although specific effect estimates were not shown. No other differences for other outcomes were reported.

The study had many limitations—primarily stemming from its design as an Internet-based survey of people with email addresses on file. The response rate was low (11%), the authors relied on self-report for both exposure and outcome information and the timing of each, and for some participants the time between exposure and the survey was many years. Most comparisons were between specific drug exposure (i.e., mefloquine, chloroquine, doxycycline, A/P, other) and no exposure to the drug of interest, so that the comparison group for each antimalarial was a mixture of those who did not report taking any antimalarials and those who reported taking antimalarial drugs other than the one being examined. Overall, there were few details of the limited analyses presented, making it difficult to understand the groups that were being compared, how they differed with respect to important covariates, and what variables were included in the models. The reliance on self-report, often years (range 2–20 years) after exposure, introduces several potential biases (selection bias, recall bias, and confounding bias), with inadequate information to determine the likely impact or direction of the potential biases acting in this study. While the use of self-reported diagnoses that were specified to be those made by a medical professional to ascertain health outcomes was arguably a better method than using a checklist of symptoms, the outcomes were not validated against any objective information. The results presented in this study do not support the presence of persistent or latent health effects, or incident neurologic or psychiatric effects specifically, post-cessation of mefloquine, but the design limitations of this study are such that any evidence provided by this study is weak.

Travelers

Three retrospective observational studies of travelers (Meier et al., 2004; Schneider et al., 2013, 2014) were conducted using data from the UK-based General Practice Research Database (GPRD)—which has since changed names to the Clinical Practice Research Datalink—to assess the incidence and compare the odds of developing first-time neurologic, psychiatric, or eye disorders in individuals using mefloquine compared with other antimalarial drugs for malaria prophylaxis. The Clinical Practice Research Datalink, which has been active for more than 30 years, collects de-identified patient data from a network of general practitioner practices across the United Kingdom for use in public health research and clinical studies, which have included investigations of drug safety, the use of medications, health care delivery, and disease risk factors (CPRD, 2019). While the specific outcomes examined (neurologic, psychiatric, and eye disorders) differed by study, the general methodology was the same. Using the GPRD, investigators identified individuals who had at least one prescription for mefloquine, A/P, doxycycline, or chloroquine and/or proguanil in the time period of interest and who had a pre-travel consultation within 1 week of the date of the prescription that included specific codes indicating that the prescription was for malaria prophylaxis. The start of follow-up was the date of receipt of the first prescription for an individual. *Current use* was defined as the period between the date a prescription was started and 1 week after the end of the prescription period. *Current exposure time* was calculated differently for each antimalarial drug because the regimen for each of the antimalarial drugs differs. Investigators based their assessment on the number of tablets recorded by the general practitioner and calculated the assumed exposure time for each of the antimalarial drugs being investigated. For mefloquine, the current exposure time (in days) was the number of tablets multiplied by 7 plus 28 days. Investigators added 90 days to each exposure to capture events that occurred during travel that came to the attention of the general practitioner after the traveler returned to the United Kingdom; this timeframe was termed "recent use" in Meier et al. (2004). Recent use included periods both relevant to the committee's charge (days 28–89) as well as time periods that the committee considered exclusionary (days 7–27). *Past use* started at day 90 (Meier et al., 2004) or day 91 (Schneider et al., 2013, 2014) and ended at a maximum of 540 days after the end of current exposure, reflecting a time period pertinent to the committee's assessment. Non-exposed people served as controls and had no antimalarial prescription during the study period or during 540 days after their pre-travel consultation, which also served as the date of the start of their follow-up. Participants were required to have at least 12 months of information on prescribed drugs and medical diagnoses before the first prescription date for an antimalarial or, for the non-exposed controls, before their travel consultation. An additional inclusion criterion required participants to have recorded medical activity (diagnoses or drug prescriptions) after receiving a prescription to ensure that only individuals who returned to the United Kingdom were included. A nested case–control analysis was also performed for a subset of the population in which up to six controls (who did not develop an outcome of interest during follow-up) were randomly selected per case; controls were matched to cases on age, sex, general practice, and calendar time (by assigning each control to the same index date as their matched case).

Overall, the design of these large, retrospective studies allowed for adequate power to detect differences in outcomes and for a uniform collection of exposures and outcomes that were not subject to recall bias. The nested case–control component allowed for the control of important covariates. Relying on recorded drug prescriptions to determine exposure ensured that the assessment was applied equally to all exposure groups; however, as with any study that relies on administrative databases, prescriptions are not a surrogate for adherence. Outcome assessment was uniform for all exposure groups and based on medical care visits coded in a database designed for both practice and research and with validated outcomes. Events that did not result in a medical care visit or that occurred outside of the national health care system would have been missed, and there may also have been some differences between the travelers who traveled to malaria-endemic areas versus areas that are not endemic for malaria, which could have led to some apparent differences in outcomes between the groups. However, it is unlikely that this would have resulted in differential selection bias. Additional strengths and limitations that are study specific are noted within each study summary.

Meier et al. (2004) used the GPRD to assess the incidence of depression (n = 505), psychosis (n = 16), panic attacks (n = 57), and death by suicide (n = 2) in recent users (90 days following current use) of mefloquine compared with both current users (during active use) of proguanil and/or chloroquine or doxycycline and past users (90–540 days) of any of these antimalarials. The study population encompassed 35,370 individuals aged 17–79 years who used antimalarials between January 1990 and December 1999: 16,491 mefloquine users, 16,129 chloroquine and/or proguanil users, and 4,574 doxycycline users (some individuals used multiple drugs). Investigators calculated the incidence of the four prespecified psychiatric outcomes during current, recent, and past use (people with prior diagnoses of the four psychiatric outcomes or alcoholism were excluded), and they also performed a nested case–control analysis in which both cases and controls had no history of the outcomes of interest prior to use of an antimalarial. The incidence rates of first-time diagnoses were calculated using person-years and were adjusted for age, gender, and calendar year. The incidence rate of first-time depression diagnosis did not differ between recent mefloquine users and all past users of antimalarials (RR = 1.0, 95%CI 0.7–1.4). In the nested case–control analysis, there was no difference in the odds of depression between recent mefloquine users and all other users combined after adjustment for age, gender, year, general practice, smoking status, and BMI (OR = 0.7, 95%CI 0.5–1.1). Only one case of incident psychosis was reported with recent mefloquine use, resulting in imprecise effect estimates in both the incident rate analysis and the nested case–control analysis. Regarding panic attacks, the incidence rate of a first-time diagnosis was not statistically significantly different between recent users of mefloquine and past users of antimalarials (RR = 2.4, 95%CI 1.0–5.7). This result remained nonstatistically significant in the nested case–control analysis after adjustment for smoking status and BMI (OR = 2.3, 95%CI 0.8–6.1). For current users of mefloquine compared with all past users of antimalarials and adjusted for smoking status and BMI, the odds of panic attack were statistically significantly elevated (OR = 2.7, 95%CI 1.1–6.5). The authors estimated that one psychosis episode and three panic attack events could be expected per 6,700 mefloquine courses. This was a large retrospective study that found no increase in depression associated with current or recent use of mefloquine compared with use of proguanil/chloroquine or all past users of antimalarials. The sample size was more limited for studying panic attacks and psychosis, leading to very imprecise estimates for those outcomes. Since current and recent use were analyzed separately, persistent outcomes were difficult to determine.

Schneider et al. (2013) used the GPRD to estimate the incidence of anxiety, stress-related disorders, or psychosis (n = 952); depression (n = 739); epilepsy (n = 86); or peripheral neuropathy (n = 56) in individuals (aged ≥ 1 year) with a pre-travel consultation and at least one prescription for mefloquine (n = 10,169), A/P (n = 28,502), or chloroquine and/or proguanil (n = 2,904) for malaria chemoprophylaxis, or no antimalarial prescription (but who had a travel consultation) (n = 41,573) between January 1, 2001, and October 1, 2009 (conducted approximately 10 years after Meier et al., 2004). Individuals were excluded if there was a record of a diagnosis of malaria prior to the start of antimalarial drug use; a history of cancer, alcoholism, or rheumatoid arthritis; or a diagnosis of an outcome of interest prior to a prescription for an antimalarial or, for the unexposed group, any of those diagnoses prior to the date of the pre-travel clinic visit. The date of the diagnosis of the first neurologic or psychiatric disorder was the index date for each case. Investigators estimated the incidence of the specified neurologic and psychiatric outcomes that occurred up to 540 days following current use of mefloquine compared with other antimalarials and with no use of antimalarials. Although 15.3% of the population was ≤18 years and the reported number of cases of each outcome was reported by age group, the authors presented only the associations between drugs and health outcomes for the total population (children and adults). Despite that limitation, the committee presents the results as reported because a relatively small proportion of the population was under age 18 years, and the results should approximate the associations that would have been found for adults only. The overall incidence rates for anxiety, stress-related disorders, or psychosis (presented as a group) and depression were lower for mefloquine users than for users of A/P, chloroquine and/or proguanil, or no antimalarial drug. A nested case–control analysis was also conducted in which investigators categorized subjects into current (use of drug plus 90 days post-cessation) or past-use (91–540 days post-cessation) exposure groups and controlled for age, sex, calendar time, general practice, smoking, and BMI. Individuals who did not develop the outcomes of interest during the follow-up period formed the control group, and six controls per case matched on sex, year of birth, general practice, and calendar time were selected. Over the study period, a total of 14 mefloquine users were diagnosed with incident epilepsy, 6 of whom were current users and 8 of whom were past users. Among the eight mefloquine users with incident neuropathies, five were current users and three were past users. A total of 99 mefloquine users (42 current users and 57 past users) were diagnosed with incident anxiety or stress-related disorders or psychosis, and 68 mefloquine users (16 current users and 52 past users) were diagnosed with incident depression. Comparing current users of mefloquine (which included a mixture of nonrelevant [during use to 27 days post-use] and relevant [days 28–90 post-use] time periods) with travelers who did not use any antimalarial prophylaxis, after adjustment for smoking and BMI, the odds of developing anxiety, stress-related disorders, or psychosis (OR = 0.76, 95%CI 0.53–1.08); epilepsy (OR = 0.85, 95%CI 0.32–2.20); or peripheral neuropathy (OR = 2.27, 95%CI 0.73–7.06) were no greater for current mefloquine users. Current mefloquine users had statistically significantly lower odds of developing depression than non-antimalarial users (OR = 0.32, 95%CI 0.19–0.54). The odds of developing anxiety, stress-related disorders, or psychosis (OR = 0.68, 95%CI 0.51–0.92) and depression (OR = 0.68, 95%CI 0.50–0.94) were statistically significantly lower in past users of mefloquine than in those who did not use an antimalarial, but the odds of epilepsy (OR = 0.61, 95%CI 0.27–1.40) and neuropathy (OR = 0.67, 95%CI 0.18–2.43) were no different. When anxiety, psychosis, phobia, and panic attack were analyzed as separate outcomes, the odds of anxiety were statistically significantly lower for mefloquine users (OR = 0.6, 95%CI 0.43–0.83) than for those who did not use antimalarials. Phobia and panic attack both showed decreased odds for mefloquine users compared with nonusers, but the findings were not statistically significant. Psychosis was elevated for mefloquine users compared with nonusers, but the effect was not statistically significant. However, these analyses were based on any use of mefloquine, and the use was not stratified on current or past exposure time.

This large, adequately powered study provides evidence of decreased odds of some neurologic and psychiatric adverse events in travelers prescribed mefloquine for malaria prophylaxis. However, the lower odds of anxiety and depression outcomes for mefloquine users versus the unexposed group suggests the possibility of uncontrolled confounding by contraindication. The comparison group consisted of travelers as well, but they may have traveled to non-malaria areas or had unmeasured risk factors that contraindicated antimalarial prophylaxis. The lower odds of adverse neurologic and psychiatric outcomes among mefloquine users in this study suggests that those prescribed mefloquine may have been screened more carefully for possible contraindications to mefloquine use. The 1-year medical history used to assess psychiatric conditions is unlikely to reflect a complete psychiatric history. Overall, this was a well-designed study that found no increase in anxiety, stress-related disorders, or psychosis (combined outcome), depression, epilepsy, or peripheral neuropathy associated with mefloquine use for malaria prophylaxis in travelers aged ≥1 year when assessing current use and 18 months following current use. The odds of developing anxiety, stress-related disorders, or psychosis (combined outcome) and the odds of developing depression were statistically significantly lower in past users of mefloquine than in those who did not use an antimalarial and the odds were not statistically significantly different among current users, suggesting that these psychiatric outcomes resolve and do not persist.

Using the same design and administrative database described by Schneider et al. (2013), Schneider et al. (2014) examined the incidence of clinical diagnoses of eye disorders (n = 652) in travelers aged ≥1 year with at least one prescription for mefloquine (n = 10,169), A/P (n = 28,502), or chloroquine and/or proguanil (n = 2,904) for malaria prophylaxis or no antimalarial prescription (but who had a pre-travel consultation) (n = 41,573) between January 1, 2001, and October 1, 2009. Individuals were excluded if they had a diagnosis of malaria prior to the start of antimalarial drug use; had cancer, alcoholism, or rheumatoid arthritis; or had been diagnosed with an eye disorder of interest (any eye disorder affecting the cornea, lens, retina, uvea, iris, or other parts of the eye, or glaucoma). Because only 20 of the total 652 eye disorders occurred among people ≤17 years, although the number of users of each drug was not stratified by age, the committee presents the results as reported, and it does not believe that the interpretation of findings and inferences that can be made are overly influenced by the inclusion of people ≤17 years. Among mefloquine users, a total of 85 incident eye disorders were identified (23 within 90 days of finishing the prescription and 62 between 91 and 540 days of the end of the prescription). The eye disorders were grouped as disorders of the cornea, cataract, glaucoma, disorders of the retina, impairment in visual acuity, vitreous detachment, disorders of the uvea, or neuro-ophthalmologic disorders, with the latter including optic neuritis, diplopia, trigeminal neuralgia, and other conditions. Incidence rates were estimated for each eye disorder category by antimalarial group, but statistical comparisons between antimalarial user groups were not made. A nested case–control analysis was performed in which BMI and a history of depression, diabetes, hypertension, sleep disorders, and use of corticosteroids and contraceptives were controlled for. Compared with travelers who did not use any antimalarial drugs, the odds of developing any of the eye disorders of interest were elevated for mefloquine users combined (OR = 1.33, 95%CI 1.01–1.75). However, when mefloquine use was stratified by current (defined as use of drug plus 90 days post-cessation) and past use (91–540 days post-cessation) and compared with the nonusers, current users had nonstatistically significantly different odds (OR = 0.92, 95%CI 0.57–1.48) whereas past users had statistically significantly higher odds (OR = 1.56, 95%CI 1.14–2.14) of any of the eye disorders of interest, suggesting that the overall finding was driven by the association with past exposure. When each of the individual eye disorder categories was examined, only cataract was statistically significantly related to mefloquine use (both current and past use combined) (OR = 1.93, 95%CI 1.11–3.36).

The strengths and limitations of this study mirror those discussed in Schneider et al. (2013) and Meier et al. (2004). Although "current use" likely captured some events within the 28-day post-cessation window, it was unlikely to result in selection bias. The large study population allowed for adequate power to assess incident eye disorders as a whole as well as eight specific categories of disorders in travelers using mefloquine for malaria prophylaxis. The finding of an increased risk of cataracts with mefloquine use was unexpected and would require confirmatory evidence. Other risk factors for cataracts, such as occupation and sun exposure, were not included in the analysis and may have differed between the groups. Overall, the study suggests an increased risk of developing eye disorders in past users of mefloquine—and, for cataracts specifically, for any users of mefloquine—relative to nonusers of antimalarials.

Schlagenhauf et al. (1996) conducted a prospective observational study of travelers to tropical Africa, all of whom had taken mefloquine for short-term malaria prophylaxis after visiting the Zurich University Vaccination Center between November 1992 and January 1994. The objective was to examine nonserious adverse events experienced during and following the use of mefloquine and to examine the association between adverse events and concentrations of racemic mefloquine, its enantiomers, and metabolite. Although study investigators did not make a traditional comparison between mefloquine exposed and unexposed groups, they did compare individuals who experienced adverse events with those who did not experience adverse events in the data analysis; thus, the committee included this study in their evaluation of the available scientific evidence. Of 420 recruited participants, complete data collection was available for 394 individuals. Participants were provided with mefloquine prophylaxis for the 2 weeks before travel, then during travel, and for 4 weeks after returning from their trips. Participants were interviewed and had blood drawn after beginning mefloquine prophylaxis but before travel and again after their return. As opposed to a list of symptoms, adverse events were reported in response to the interview question "How do you feel since you took the last tablet?" Only adverse events with some impact on activities were included in the study. Adverse events were classified as "neuropsychiatric" if they reflected sleep disturbances, dizziness/vertigo, headache, mood changes, unusual or vivid dreams, decreased concentration, or phobias. A total of 44 individuals experienced adverse events that affected activity, and 31 individuals (70.4% of those who experienced adverse events) experienced neuropsychiatric symptoms. Standardized instruments including computerized assessments of cognitive functioning (Neurobehavioral Evaluation System) and standardized self-report questionnaires assessing the severity of symptoms across body systems (Environmental Symptoms Questionnaire) and current mood state (Profile of Mood States) were administered to evaluate the neurologic and psychiatric adverse events. A subset of participants was assessed approximately 3 months after the last dose; it included only those participants who had experienced adverse events with some impact on activities along with a sex-, age-, and dosing-schedule-matched comparison group who had not experienced adverse events (controls). The results of the 3-month follow-up assessment are most relevant to the persistent effects of mefloquine since the other check points occurred while participants were still using the drug. Results from the Environmental Symptoms Questionnaire and the Profile of Mood States found greater though nonclinically significant symptoms of dizziness, light headedness, distress, restlessness, and sleep disturbance as well as more intense moods of tension, depression, fatigue, and confusion at baseline, but at follow-up there were no significant differences between controls and those who experienced adverse events. The majority of the adverse events were mild and transitory and did not result in statistically significant differences in performance on standardized neurobehavioral tests. When the plasma concentrations and ratios of the SR:RS enantiomers were analyzed, there was no statistically significant difference between participants with and without adverse events. Similarly, mean concentrations of mefloquine and its metabolite did not differ between mefloquine users who reported and who did not report adverse events. Overall, this study provides some information pertinent to the persistent neurologic and psychiatric effects of mefloquine, suggesting that although there are some mild neurologic or psychiatric adverse events upon initiation of mefloquine, these symptoms tend to resolve by 3 months. The use of objective measures (blood draws) and standardized, validated tests are strengths of the exposure and outcome assessment. Adherence was also specifically considered and found to be above 80% for all age groups. The study has several limitations, including that all study subjects received mefloquine so that the relationship of symptoms to the drug is unknown due to the lack of an unexposed comparison group, the fact that the comparison group at the start of the study was not followed for 3 months as was the subgroup who had experienced adverse events, and that the number people who reported adverse events (which were based on self-report) was small. Only adverse events with some impact on activities were included in the study. In addition, the groups of participants undergoing the standardized tests was both small in number and select (range 37% to 80% of those eligible). For the comparisons that were made, the matching was incomplete, making the control for covariates very limited. The authors postulated that the adverse events reported may have been the product of the stress of travel or even naturally occurring experiences.

Schwartz and Regev-Yochay (1999) performed a prospective observational study, and followed 158 Israeli male and female travelers aged 22–65 years who took part in rafting trips on the Omo River, Ethiopia, and who had visited a travel clinic to obtain malaria prophylaxis. Travelers were prescribed mefloquine (250 mg once weekly), primaquine, doxycycline, or hydroxychloroquine by travel group. The primary aim of the study was to assess incident malaria and to compare the effectiveness of these four antimalarial drugs against both *P. falciparum* and *P. vivax*. Travelers were followed from the time of their return to Israel for an average of 16.6 months (range 8–37 months) for incident malaria. Adherence to the prophylactic regimens and details about side effects were also collected by survey. The authors reported that "no severe side effects" were reported in any of the travelers and that no side effects or withdrawals were noted in the mefloquine users. The strengths of this study include its design and the long duration of follow-up (an average of 16.6 months after return from a malaria-endemic country). It is limited by its small sample size, nonrandomized design, and lack of details on adverse events beyond reporting that no severe events or withdrawals were reported among mefloquine users. As a result, this study provides limited information that can be used for inference.

Research Volunteers

DeSouza (1983) conducted a small clinical trial in a malaria-endemic area of Brazil. Healthy male volunteers were enrolled and administered a one-time dose of either 1,000 mg of mefloquine (n = 10) or 1,000 mg sulfadoxine and 50 mg pyrimethamine in a combined tablet (n = 10). Participants remained under surveillance in a hospital ward for the entire 66-day study period. A range of routine clinical assessments was conducted, including ECGs, measures of blood pressure and pulse rate, hematologic parameters and blood chemistry (red blood cell count, hemoglobin erythrocyte volume fraction, total and differential white blood cell counts, reticulocyte count, platelet count, cholesterol, triglycerides, glucose, urea, creatinine, etc.), and urine assays at varying intervals up to day 63 post-administration. Adverse events of headache, diarrhea, and dizziness were reported following mefloquine administration, but all resolved by day 4. The authors reported that no significant changes were observed over the study period for blood pressure, pulse rate, ECGs, or any of the hematologic or biochemical parameters for either drug group. Prior to drug administration, 8 individuals in the mefloquine group had enlarged liver (versus 5 individuals in the sulfadoxine/pyrimethamine group), and 3 individuals in both the mefloquine and sulfadoxine/pyrimethamine groups had enlarged spleen, but the enlargements reduced over the course of follow-up. Specific measures were grouped and reported as "day 14 onwards." Notably, the dose of mefloquine administered was four times higher than that used for prophylaxis, and few adverse events were reported and none persisted beyond 4 days following administration. This study is limited by the very small study population and the inability to isolate health outcomes for the period 28 days following administration of mefloquine.

Laothavorn et al. (1992) conducted a prospective observational study of ECG changes in a Thai population of 102 patients with malaria and 18 healthy male volunteers receiving mefloquine. As treatment is outside the scope of this report, only the information regarding the healthy volunteers was considered. The healthy volunteers were administered 750 mg of mefloquine (three times higher than the dose used for prophylaxis). ECGs were performed prior to mefloquine administration, daily for 1 week following mefloquine administration, and then weekly up to day 42. No significant changes were found for biochemical, hematologic, or cardiac parameters, specifically heart rate, standard cardiac intervals, sinus arrhythmias, sinus bradycardia, ventricular ectopic beats, atrial ectopic beats, or atrial–ventricular block at any time in the period following mefloquine administration. Given the small study size, the fact that the dose administered was three times higher than what is used for prophylaxis, the comparison of outcomes was with patients receiving treatment for malaria, and the inability to clearly isolate the time period of interest following cessation of drug exposure, this study provides limited evidence regarding persistent health effects from use of mefloquine.

OTHER IDENTIFIED STUDIES OF MEFLOQUINE PROPHYLAXIS IN HUMAN POPULATIONS

The committee reviewed several studies of mefloquine use in service members from the United States (Arthur et al., 1990; Boudreau et al., 1993; Nevin and Leoutsakos, 2017; Sanchez et al., 1993; Saunders et al., 2015; Wallace, 1996),

Australia (Kitchener et al., 2005; Rieckmann et al., 1993), France (Ollivier et al., 2004), Indonesia (Ohrt et al., 1997), Italy (Peragallo et al., 1999, 2001), the Netherlands (de Vries et al., 2000; Hopperus Buma et al., 1996), Sweden (Andersson et al., 2008), Thailand (Eamsila et al., 1993), Turkey (Sonmez et al., 2005), and the United Kingdom (Adshead, 2014; Croft et al., 1997; Terrell et al., 2015; Tuck and Williams, 2016). However, because the studies did not follow the military cohorts after mefloquine prophylaxis was complete or did not report on adverse events that occurred post-mefloquine-cessation (several studies followed the populations for cases of malaria only), these studies were not further considered.

Several of the studies that did not meet inclusion were designed to examine the safety or tolerability of mefloquine when used for long-term (>4 months) prophylaxis in different populations, but they did not report on adverse events or other outcomes post-cessation. These studies examined populations of U.S. soldiers (Saunders et al., 2015), Dutch marines (Hopperus Buma et al., 1996; Jaspers et al., 1996; Todd et al., 1997), members of the Japanese Self-Defense Forces (Fujii et al., 2007), Thai soldiers (Eamsila et al., 1993), Turkish soldiers (Sonmez et al., 2005), U.S. Peace Corps volunteers (Korhonen et al., 2007; Landman et al., 2014; Lobel et al., 1991, 1993), harbor workers in Columbia (Rombo et al., 1993), Chinese railway workers in Nigeria (Olanrewaju and Lin, 2000), semi-immune populations (Sossouhounto et al., 1995), Thai gem miners (Boudreau et al., 1991), and British expats (Cunningham et al., 2014). Additionally, an integrated safety analysis of tafenoquine was conducted using five studies in which mefloquine was the comparison in three of the studies, but the timing of adverse events (during use or post-cessation) was not reported (Novitt-Moreno et al., 2017). Nasveld et al. (2010) conducted a randomized double-blind controlled study to compare the safety and tolerability of tafenoquine with that of mefloquine (used for 26 weeks followed by primaquine for 2 weeks) for malaria prophylaxis in Australian soldiers; however, because the mefloquine comparison group also used primaquine, it was not considered to contribute evidence of persistent effects of mefloquine alone.

Studies of other populations were also excluded from the final set of studies evaluated in depth because the follow-up was not at least 28 days post-mefloquine-cessation or the follow-up was at least 28 days and adverse events were reported but the authors did not distinguish between the timing of those events (less than or at least 28 days post-cessation). Such studies included travelers from Australia (Phillips and Kass, 1996), Belgium (Peetermans and Van Wijngaerden, 2001), Denmark (Petersen et al., 2000), Finland (Vilkman et al., 2016), France (Carme et al., 1997), Germany (Huzly et al., 1996), Great Britain (Barrett et al., 1996; Bloechliger et al., 2014), Israel (Potasman et al., 2000, 2002; Schwartz et al., 2001), Italy (Laverone et al., 2006), Japan (Kato et al., 2013; Matsumura et al., 2005), the Netherlands (Hoebe et al., 1997; Sharafeldin et al., 2010; van Riemsdijk et al., 1997a, 2002a,b, 2004, 2005), and the United States (Hill, 2000; Kozarsky and Eaton, 1993; Lobel et al., 2001). Studies using combined populations of travelers who had visited clinics from several European countries, Canada, Israel, or

South Africa (Durrheim et al., 1999; Lobel et al., 2001; Overbosch et al., 2001; Reisinger et al., 1989; Schlagenhauf et al., 2003, 2009; Steffen et al., 1990, 1993; Waner et al., 1999) were also reviewed but did not meet inclusion. An analysis based on the Hoffman-La Roche global drug safety database was excluded from final consideration because the timing of events could not be distinguished (Adamcova et al., 2015), as were six studies that used research volunteers to examine the effects of mefloquine (Clyde et al., 1976; Davis et al., 1996; Hale et al., 2003; Hanboonkunupakarn et al., 2019; Rendi-Wagner et al., 2002; Vuurman et al., 1996). A small crossover study of Swissair trainee pilots was designed to determine the effects of steady-state mefloquine dosing on performance. Although participants who were first given mefloquine were followed for 4–6 months during the washout phase before being given a placebo, the authors did not report on adverse events that began or persisted during that time, and thus it was not further considered (Schlagenhauf et al., 1997).

Upon full text review and quality assessment, additional studies were excluded from further consideration. Bijker et al. (2014) conducted a double-blind randomized controlled trial of experimental infection 16 weeks following the administration of prophylactic doses of mefloquine (n = 10) or chloroquine (n = 5) in healthy volunteers in the Netherlands. Adverse events and corresponding severity were recorded over the duration of the study; all adverse events were reported to have resolved by the end of the study, but because the exact timing of the resolution was not provided, this study was not included in the primary epidemiologic studies. Bunnag et al. (1992) conducted a randomized double-blind study comparing the efficacy and tolerability of Fansimef®, mefloquine, Fansidar®, and chloroquine to placebo for malaria prophylaxis in 602 healthy adult males in Thailand who were followed for 4 weeks after the final dose. The timing of the adverse events was not specified, although blood measures were reported to remain stable throughout the study period, but because details were not presented the study did not meet inclusion criteria. Similar to Bunnag et al. (1992), Salako et al. (1992) conducted a randomized double-blind trial to assess the efficacy of Fansimef®, mefloquine, Fansidar®, and chloroquine compared with a placebo in semi-immune individuals. The follow-up extended for 4 weeks following the cessation of prophylaxis, but neither the details of what data were collected during those 4 weeks nor the timing of the adverse events were provided, and thus this study did not meet the criteria for inclusion as a primary epidemiologic study. In an early field trial conducted in 1977 to test the efficacy of three different doses and regimens of mefloquine against two regimens of sulfadoxine-pyrimethamine and a placebo, a semi-immune Thai population was administered the drug regimens for 26 weeks, with follow-up assessments conducted monthly for 3 months after the final dose. The authors stated that there was "no clinical evidence of drug toxicity" in any of the 990 participants and that no significant changes were found in the measured biochemical parameters, but no additional details of adverse events were reported in general or by regimen (Pearlman et al., 1980).

Case Reports and Case Series

Published case reports can offer detailed information about symptoms and their course, such as the timing of onset in relation to exposure to the drug, treatment, remission, and persistence of symptoms, but they rarely generate information for causative inference. To be considered, published case reports and case series had to report on a follow-up of at least 28 days post-mefloquine-cessation. Of the 56 case reports identified, many reported only acute symptoms that resolved within 28 days post-cessation. The committee closely reviewed the remaining 20 case reports (totaling 25 patients) that had been identified (Baker, 1996; Borruat et al., 2001; Chester and Sandroni, 2011; Dietz and Frolich, 2002; Eaton, 1996; Even et al., 2001; Jain et al., 2016; Javorsky et al., 2001; Jha et al., 2006; Katsenos et al., 2007; Lobel et al., 1998; McEvoy et al., 2015; Meszaros and Kasper, 1996; Nevin, 2012; Potasman and Seligmann, 1998; Tran et al., 2006; Udry et al., 2001; Walker and Colleaux, 2007; Watt-Smith et al., 2001; Whitworth and Aichhorn, 2005) as well as eight case series papers (Adamcova et al., 2015; Bem et al., 1992; Beny et al., 2001; Croft and Garner, 2000; Croft and Herxheimer, 2002; Ringqvist et al., 2015; Smith et al., 1999; van Riemsdijk et al., 1997b). Among the case reports, all patients had acute effects, and 16 patients had persistent neurologic or psychiatric effects for more than 28 days following their last dose of mefloquine. These symptoms included dizziness, anxiety, depression, insomnia/exhaustion, paranoia, hallucinations, visual illusions, mania, depersonalization, and suicidal ideation. Nevin (2012) published a detailed case of a patient who took mefloquine and acutely experienced anxiety, then developed fatigue, confusion, psychosis, dissociation, personality change, tinnitus, vertigo, dizziness, disequilibrium, and cognitive deficits, and he exhibited parasuicidal behavior. Objective testing discovered central vestibulopathy. The resultant diagnoses included vertigo of central origin, toxic encephalopathy, various psychiatric disorders, ataxic gait, and memory loss. Persistent findings (follow-up ended after 10 months of first symptom onset) following the resolution of symptoms of psychosis, were fatigue, vertigo, disequilibrium, visual illusions, photosensitivity, memory impairment, and personality changes.

One case of persistent retinopathy (Walker and Colleaux, 2007) and other ocular disturbances (Jain et al., 2016), one case of tinnitus resulting in hearing loss (Lobel et al., 1998), and one case of worsening psoriasis (Potasman and Seligmann, 1998) following mefloquine administration were reported. Additional cases reported neuropathy (Chester and Sandroni, 2011; Jha et al., 2006; Watt-Smith et al., 2001); paralysis, trouble breathing, heart palpitations (Eaton, 1996); eosinophilic pneumonia (Katsenos et al., 2007); weakness (Jha et al., 2006; Whitworth and Aichhorn, 2005); skin rash (Eaton, 1996; Jha et al., 2006); and pain in the face and extremities (Chester and Sandroni, 2011).

Five case series reported similar symptoms to those in the individual case reports. Beny et al. (2001) reported on 15 travelers who prematurely terminated their travel because of neurologic or psychiatric symptoms, and 7 of those had taken mefloquine. Of the mefloquine users, three had persistent anxiety and depression, although the timing of these symptoms relative to mefloquine use was unclear. In a review of adverse events reports submitted to the drug manufacturer, Bem et al. (1992) found 430 cases of adverse events when mefloquine was used prophylactically. More than half (56%) of these events were considered neurologic or psychiatric, as defined by WHO, and 59 of these individuals required hospitalization or resulted in severe disability. There were 26 reported cases of convulsions, and half of these cases had a neurologic or psychiatric history. All but one of the cases of convulsions resolved within 1 month of the last dose of mefloquine. Additionally, Bem reported 12 cases of depression or "manic-depression," and 9 of those cases had suicidal ideation or attempts, or both. Psychosis was reported in 20 cases, and 11 of those individuals recovered within 40 days (mean 21 days), while 2 recovered within 4–7 months. There was one case of toxic encephalopathy reported, but that person recovered within 3 months. Using postmarketing surveillance data of mefloquine in the Netherlands, van Riemsdijk et al. (1997b) reported on 132 cases with a range of symptoms including depression, anxiety, agitation, nightmares, insomnia, concentration impairment, psychosis, hallucinations, depersonalization, and paranoia. Of the 132 cases, 36 had persistent symptoms, 74 had complete recoveries following cessation of mefloquine, and the disposition of the remaining 22 people was unknown. Using reports of adverse events to the manufacturer's drug safety database between February 1984 and January 2011, Adamcova et al. (2015) performed an analysis of eye disorders associated with the prophylactic use of mefloquine. A total of 591 individuals were identified who experienced 695 eye disorder events, 223 of which were considered serious, that were subsequently categorized into visual acuity (to include blindness, reduced visual acuity, visual impairment, and blurred vison), events affecting the anatomical parts of the eye (retina, vitreous, lens, cornea, optic nerve and glaucoma, and other disorders), and neuro-ophthalmic disorders. The temporal relationship of mefloquine use to adverse events was considered. When available, risk factors such as relevant medical history, comedication, and associated conditions were also considered. The time of onset, which was available for only 70 of the events, ranged from 1 hour to 1,095 days (median 16.5 days). The duration of adverse events was known for only 5% of reports and, among those, ranged from 30 minutes to 270 days (median 10.5 days). Symptoms of optic neuropathy were reported for 48 individuals (53 events); 8 individuals (reporting 10 events) recovered, with sequelae that continued to affect visual acuity; and 3 individuals reported no complete recovery. Six events involving the cornea and five events involving the lens were reported, but eight of these had explanations other than mefloquine exposure and three of the reports did not contain sufficient information for a medical assessment. Of the 23 events involving retinal disorders, 9 were maculopathy, and most of these events were considered to be due to factors other than mefloquine.

Ringqvist et al. (2015) reported on 73 adults with mefloquine-associated adverse events (67 of them had used mefloquine for malaria prophylaxis) based on 95 reports to the Danish National Drug Authority Committee of Adverse Drug Reactions. Each person was contacted, and standardized instruments or interviews were used to elicit and categorize symptoms; these measures were completed 270–2,010 days following the adverse event. For 77% of cases, the individuals reported their symptoms as beginning in the first 3 weeks of mefloquine use, while 15% reported an onset of symptoms after 1–2 months of use, and 8% reported a symptom onset more than 8 weeks after the initiation of mefloquine. Of the 73 people, 45 reported physical symptoms, 27 reported signs of anxiety, 26 reported sleep disturbances including nightmares, 18 reported depression or feeling low, 11 reported signs of possible psychotic states (delusions/hallucinations), 9 reported cognitive problems, 3 reported confusion, and 1 reported mania; 40 individuals reported more than one complaint. Perceptual disturbances/hallucinations or delusional experiences were reported by 17 individuals following mefloquine use; all of these resolved within 9 months, and most within 3 weeks. Recurring nightmares were reported for 43 cases, and 9 individuals continued to have recurring nightmares for more than 3 years after mefloquine cessation. Cognitive dysfunction was reported in 42 cases and persisted for more than 3 years for 14 people. Included individuals reported significantly worse psychiatric symptoms than the matched controls in the Danish normative sample. Of the participants, 41% reported that they had obtained some treatment for their psychiatric adverse event. Although this case series provides some evidence supporting the development of persistent psychiatric problems after mefloquine use, the series was limited in that it was based on 73 cases of adverse events deemed severe enough to be reported to the Danish national registry. It is not known how complete the reporting to the Danish registry is, and there was no appropriate comparison group, only a comparison to Danish national norms for the self-report questionnaires administered after cases were reported to the registry. The investigators estimated that adverse events occurred at a rate of about 2 per 10,000 doses, suggesting that serious persistent events, if related to mefloquine, are rare.

A Cochrane review by Croft and Garner (2000) identified 136 published case studies totaling 516 nonimmune travelers who had experienced adverse events while using mefloquine. Of those 516 individuals, 328 were using mefloquine as malaria prophylaxis. Four case reports involved fatal reactions to mefloquine, but it is unclear whether the deaths were reported in cases involving mefloquine prophylaxis or treatment, and further details were not provided. The authors discussed the best measures of tolerability and the possible influence of differences among groups (e.g., gender, weight, age, ethnicity) on the occurrence of adverse events, but they did not provide analyses or conclusions regarding the case reports. It was not clear how many of these people had persistent symptoms, and, other than a listing of the citations, additional information was sparse. Croft and Herxheimer (2002) elaborated on these 516 cases, reporting that 328 of the individuals had taken mefloquine prophylactically, and the median duration of adverse events symptoms was 16 days (range 1–550). The authors postulated that the symptoms associated with taking mefloquine were primarily related to liver or thyroid pathology.

Smith et al. (1999) reviewed 74 published case reports of mefloquine use (prophylaxis or treatment) specific to dermatologic adverse events. Some of these cases were collected from outcomes of clinical trials, and nearly half had used mefloquine as treatment for malaria. The onset of the dermatologic effects was recorded in only 11 of the cases. The most common symptoms were pruritus and itching, which were reported in more than 40% of the cases, followed by rashes. The majority of effects were reported as mild or moderate in intensity and were usually self-limiting, although the timing was not specified. Other dermatologic adverse events included two reports of cutaneous vasculitis and one report each of Stevens-Johnson syndrome and toxic epidermal necrolysis.

Tickell-Painter et al. (2017b) performed a systematic review of reports of death or parasuicide (a suicide attempt not resulting in death) associated with mefloquine when used at various dosages for malaria prophylaxis. The literature search included all forms of prospective and retrospective studies of individual case reports or reviews of case reports that reported deaths or parasuicide up to July 11, 2017. Each case was reviewed using a formal causality assessment based on a causality assessment by WHO's Uppsala Monitoring Centre. When information was poor or conclusions could not be drawn, the event was categorized as "unclassifiable." Of the 527 articles identified and reviewed, 17 reported deaths or parasuicide, and only 8 had sufficient detail to be included in a causality assessment. Two deaths were identified as having a probable association with mefloquine. Both were in children and were characterized as "idiosyncratic drug reactions" (one involved pulmonary fibrosis and interstitial pneumonia; the other involved erythema, blistering, other complications, and eventually cardiac asystole). In the first case, symptoms began during mefloquine use, and death occurred 5 weeks after drug cessation; in the second, symptoms began during mefloquine use, but it is unclear when or even if the mefloquine use was stopped. Eight deaths were deemed "unlikely" to have been related to mefloquine or "unclassifiable" because of insufficient information. The authors identified one parasuicide with a "possible" causal association. A 22-year-old woman experienced episodes of crying, emotional detachment, and low mood 1 day after taking mefloquine 250 mg; her symptoms decreased on days 5 and 6; after an additional dose 1 week later, she experienced a relapse of symptoms, with ideas of guilt and death, and feelings of body transformation; and 5 days later she was hospitalized after a suicide attempt by drowning. Authors noted that the original source provided no information regarding the individual's past medical history, including her use of any other medications.

The authors concluded that the number of deaths that could be reliably attributed to the prophylactic use of mefloquine is very low (Tickell-Painter et al., 2017b). In their discussion, however, the authors stated that a limiting factor in their review was poor reporting in the literature; few reports, including those deriving from spontaneous adverse event reporting databases, provided sufficient detail to perform a critical assessment. Additionally, the cases represented different time points for the outcomes: some were concurrent and some were longer term, further limiting the contribution of this paper to this report.

In summary, there are published cases of persistent neurologic, psychiatric, and other adverse events following exposure to mefloquine. The majority of these case reports and case series presented individuals whose symptoms eventually resolved, even if they initially persisted beyond 28 days following the last dose of the medication. Although the case reports are compelling, without larger samples or comparison groups to establish base rates of disorders, it is difficult to establish a causal role for mefloquine in these cases.

Selected Subpopulations

In the course of its review of the literature on mefloquine, the committee identified and reviewed available studies that reported results stratified by demographic, medical, or behavioral factors to assess whether the risk for adverse events when using mefloquine for prophylaxis is associated with being part of or affiliated with a specific group. This was not done exhaustively, and the evidence included in this section is generally limited to adverse events observed with concurrent use of mefloquine. Many of these studies did not meet the inclusion criteria of following their population for at least 28 days post-mefloquine-cessation, but the committee considers these findings to be important indicators when considering the evidence as a whole. The following risk groups were specifically considered: females in general and pregnant women in particular, people with low weight or BMI, people with allergies and chronic conditions who may be taking concurrent medications, and people who use alcohol, marijuana, or illicit drugs.

Sex Differences

When studies of the prophylactic use of mefloquine have reported results stratified by sex, several have shown that women are significantly more likely than men to experience adverse events with mefloquine. This was observed in studies that examined any adverse event (Phillips and Kass, 1996; van Riemsdijk et al., 2002a) as well as for more specific outcomes including neurologic or psychiatric events (Huzly et al., 1996; Schlagenhauf et al., 1996, 2003; Schneider et al., 2013; van Riemsdijk et al., 1997a, 2002a, 2003, 2005) and gastrointestinal events (van Riemsdijk et al., 1997a) in several different types of populations and nationalities. In addition several studies found that women experience more severe adverse events that interfere with daily functioning than men (Rendi-Wagner et al., 2002; Schlagenhauf et al., 1996; Wernsdorfer et al., 2013), and that for women the time of onset of the adverse events is sooner and it takes longer for the symptoms to resolve (Rendi-Wagner et al., 2002; Wernsdorfer et al., 2013). Mefloquine is administered as a fixed-dose tablet of 250 mg salt in the United States or 228 mg base in other areas. While some studies that have measured serum levels of mefloquine or its metabolites have found that mean levels are statistically significantly higher in women than men, sometimes nearly double (Potasman et al., 2002; Wernsdorfer et al., 2013), other studies did not find significant differences in serum levels between men and women (Schwartz et al., 2001).

Possible explanations for sex-related differences may include reporting bias and greater adherence among women. Some of the observed differences between males and females might be due to females being more aware of neurologic and psychiatric disturbances than males and communicating symptoms more easily than males. For example, women report mental health problems at higher rates, particularly PTSD (Blanco et al., 2018; Breslau et al., 1997; Luxton et al., 2010; Norris et al., 2002) and depression (Breslau et al., 1995; Kessler et al., 1993; Luxton et al., 2010; Weissman and Klerman, 1977). However, several studies have adequately controlled for these factors, and sex-related differences in adverse event reporting continue to be observed.

It is also possible that biologic differences account for the heightened risk of PTSD and depression in women. These differences may include endocrine system differences, differences in neural connectivity in response to aversive stimuli, sex-by-genotype interactions, and sex differences in response to exposure to stress across the life span (see reviews by Eid et al., 2019, and Helpman et al., 2017). Sex differences of mefloquine distribution in cellular and fluid blood compartments, which may be related to the higher serum levels of mefloquine and its metabolites observed in women, may be associated with the occurrence of adverse events. However, Schwartz et al. (2001) found that although there was no difference in serum levels, women tended to be more susceptible than men to adverse events.

Pregnancy

In 2011 CDC recommended mefloquine for pregnant women both as a malaria treatment option and as an option to prevent malaria infection in all trimesters. For travel to areas where chloroquine resistance is present, mefloquine is the only medication recommended for malaria prophylaxis during pregnancy. Also in 2011, FDA reviewed available data for mefloquine use during pregnancy and reclassified it from category C (animal reproduction studies have shown an adverse effect on the fetus and there are no adequate and well-controlled studies in humans, but potential benefits may warrant use of the drug in pregnant women despite potential risks) to category B (animal reproduction studies have failed to demonstrate a risk to the fetus and there are no adequate and well-controlled studies in pregnant women) (CDC, 2019).

A 2018 Cochrane review concluded that mefloquine is safe in terms of adverse pregnancy outcomes, such as low birth weight, prematurity, stillbirths and abortions, and congenital malformations (González et al., 2018). That Cochrane review considered data from six trials conducted between 1987 and 2013 in Benin, Gabon, Kenya, Mozambique, Tanzania, and Thailand and included 8,192 pregnant women who met their inclusion criteria (Briand et al., 2009; Denoeud-Ndam et al., 2014; González et al., 2014a,b; Nosten et al., 1994). Initial concerns regarding the possible association between mefloquine and stillbirth were raised in a retrospective analysis in Thailand (Nosten et al., 1999) and a study of U.S. Army service women (Smoak et al., 1997) in which high rates of abortions were reported with mefloquine exposure in pregnancy. Smoak et al. posited that exposure to other stress factors could have increased the rate of abortions in the Army service women. These concerns about adverse reproductive outcomes have not been supported by studies of malaria prevention during pregnancy conducted in sub-Saharan Africa or Thailand (Briand et al., 2009; González et al., 2014b; Nosten et al., 1994; Schlagenhauf et al., 2012; Steketee et al., 1996). A postmarketing study of 1,627 spontaneous reports of women exposed to mefloquine before or during pregnancy estimated the birth prevalence of congenital malformations in women exposed to mefloquine to be 4%—no different from the prevalence observed in the general population (Vanhauwere et al., 1998). Mefloquine is not as well tolerated as other antimalarial drugs when used for intermittent preventive treatment in pregnancy (IPTp), but the dosage used is substantially higher than the dosage used for malaria prophylaxis. The 2018 Cochrane review reported that when it was used for IPTp, mefloquine was associated with higher risks of drug-related vomiting (RR = 4.76, 95%CI 4.13–5.49; 6,272 participants, 2 studies; high-certainty evidence) and dizziness (RR = 4.21, 95%CI 3.36–5.27; 6,272 participants, 2 studies; moderate-certainty evidence) in women without HIV. Briand et al. (2009) reported higher rates of vomiting, dizziness, tiredness, and nausea among mefloquine users for IPTp than among those using sulfadoxine-pyrimethamine (78% versus 32%), with all cases having resolved spontaneously within 3 days. They also reported that there were no neurologic symptoms reported among neonates born to women who had received mefloquine during pregnancy.

Rupérez et al. (2016) evaluated the safety of IPTp with mefloquine compared with sulfadoxine-pyrimethamine for key infant health and developmental outcomes at 1, 9, and 12 months of age. No significant differences were observed in the psychomotor development milestones assessed. Among infants born to women in the mefloquine group, there was an increased risk of being unable to stand without help (RR = 1.07, 95%CI 1.00–1.14), walk without support (RR = 1.10, 95%CI 1.01–1.21), and bring solid food to the mouth (RR = 1.32, 95%CI 1.03–1.70) at 9 months of age as compared with the children born to women in the sulfadoxine-pyrimethamine group, but these differences were not found at 1 or 12 months. No other statistically significant differences were observed in any of the other developmental, nutritional, or morbidity items assessed in the study visits, leading the authors to postulate that the differences could be the result of chance due to multiple comparison testing rather than true differences.

González et al. (2014b) reported no serious neurologic adverse events among the 4,749 pregnant women who were enrolled in an open-label randomized clinical trial conducted in Benin, Gabon, Mozambique, and Tanzania comparing mefloquine (n = 1,551 single dose, n = 1,562 split dose) with sulfadoxine-pyrimethamine (n = 1,561) for IPTp. They also found no difference in the prevalence of adverse pregnancy outcomes (including miscarriages, stillbirths, and congenital malformations) between groups.

Low Body Mass Index

Some studies of the prophylactic use of mefloquine have collected information on weight and BMI and have reported differences in the proportion or types of adverse events when results were stratified by these factors. For example, in a study of 169 French soldiers deployed to the Ivory Coast and randomly selected to take weekly mefloquine prophylaxis, those soldiers weighing the least (51–60 kg) reported the greatest number of adverse events (88.9% reported at least 1 adverse event, with a mean of 3.11 events per person) compared with the heaviest soldiers (81–115 kg; 52.9% reported at least one adverse event, with a mean of 0.94 events per person). Because mefloquine was administered as a fixed dose (the standard 250 mg pill), the concentrations of mefloquine as measured in urine were higher for lighter individuals (4.2–4.9 mg/kg among those weighing 51–60 kg versus 2.2–3.1 mg/kg for those weighing 81–115 kg), and the soldiers who reported adverse effects weighed less than those without any symptoms (p < 0.03) (Ollivier et al., 2004). In a study of 73 men and 78 women who were given mefloquine 3 weeks before their intended travel to malaria-endemic areas, those with the lowest BMI (≤20 kg/m^2) had the most impairment of mood state (particularly vigor and fatigue, measured using validated instruments) and a significantly increased reaction time; both effects were further modified by gender, with the most pronounced effects in women with the lowest BMI (van Riemsdijk et al., 2003). In a comparison of neurologic and psychiatric outcomes among mefloquine users (n = 58) and A/P users (n = 61) using the same validated tests as in van Riemsdijk et al. (2003), van Riemsdijk et al. (2002b) found that there were significant differences between people who took mefloquine and those who took A/P with respect to self-reported fatigue, vigor, and total mood disturbance, with those using mefloquine reporting worse scores. When stratified by BMI (≤25 versus >25 kg/m^2), those taking mefloquine reported worse psychiatric symptoms than those taking A/P in both strata.

Some of the observations of people of lower weight or BMI having more adverse effects may be related to sex, as women are generally smaller and weigh less than men. However, in a study of nonimmune Danish travelers in which mefloquine was compared with chloroquine and chloroquine plus proguanil, women reported depression more frequently than men (p = 0.005), but the frequency of adverse events was not associated with weight when stratified by gender (Huzly et al., 1996).

Chronic Health Conditions

Travelers who have allergies or other chronic health conditions and do not have contraindications for mefloquine have been found to report larger numbers of adverse events and experience them more frequently than people without these conditions (Huzly et al., 1996). Moreover, people with chronic disease report psychiatric reactions significantly more often than those without disease. People who take other drugs concomitantly (such as to treat their chronic conditions) with prophylaxis have been found to report more adverse reactions (Huzly et al., 1996).

Mefloquine elimination may be prolonged in those with impaired liver function, leading to higher plasma levels and a higher risk of adverse reactions. If the drug is administered for a prolonged period, periodic evaluations, including liver function tests and evaluations for "neuropsychiatric" effects, should be performed (FDA, 2016).

Using an existing database of self-administered questionnaires collected from travelers returning to Europe from Eastern Africa (between July 1988 and December 1991) and again 3 months after travel, Handschin et al. (1997) analyzed the association of adverse events experienced by travelers using four different prophylactic drug regimens (mefloquine, chloroquine, chloroquine plus proguanil, and no antimalarial drug) with and without concurrent use of other medications. Individual symptoms and comedications were grouped into categories for analysis. A total of 78,614 travelers were included in the analysis, and the majority used mefloquine (n = 48,264), followed by chloroquine plus proguanil (n = 19,727), chloroquine alone (n = 6,752; 300 mg or 600 mg doses), and no prophylactic drug (n = 3,871). Responses from both questionnaires were combined, so that the timing or persistence of adverse events could not be distinguished. Both the occurrence of adverse events (and the reported severity) and the use of any medications in addition to the antimalarials were self-reported. Among mefloquine users, 25,690 used a comedication, while 22,574 did not. Individuals comedicating had 1.5 times the risk of adverse events of any type or severity compared with individuals using only mefloquine. For severe adverse events, the relative risk was 2.2 times higher for comedication than for mefloquine alone (p < 0.01). Similarly increased risks with comedication use were found for the other prophylaxis (and no use of prophylaxis) groups as well. The number and severity of adverse events among mefloquine users correlated with the number of comedications taken and were statistically different from those in individuals who did not use comedication (p < 0.01). Drugs used to treat neurologic or psychiatric conditions were associated with the highest increases in risk for adverse events and severity, but the risk of adverse events was also statistically significant for analgesics, anti-infectives, and antidiarrheals compared with no comedication. No increase in the rate of adverse events or severity was observed with cardiovascular drugs such as beta blockers.

Concurrent Use of Alcohol, Marijuana, or Illicit Drugs

A number of factors may place travelers at increased risk of experiencing adverse events while using mefloquine, including stressful events during travel, interruptions of sleep cycles, and the use of alcohol, marijuana, and, in some cases, illicit drugs. In a study of 1,340 Israeli travelers to the tropics, mefloquine was used by 70.7%, and 151 of them (11%) reported neurologic or psychiatric problems (Potasman et al., 2000). A follow-up questionnaire was sent to the 151 people who reported neurologic or psychiatric problems to ascertain the symptoms, severity, and use of illicit drugs (reported as yes or no). A total of 26 travelers admitted to using recreational drugs during travel, but it is not known how many of these people also used mefloquine. In a case series of 15 Israeli travelers who had sought evaluation for psychiatric effects, 6 of them had used mefloquine for prophylaxis, and 8 had reported using marijuana, hashish, or charas; or LSD or Ecstasy (Beny et al., 2001). In three of these cases, the probable trigger of the psychiatric event was determined to be mefloquine or a combination of illicit drugs and mefloquine.

Although consuming large quantities of alcohol concurrently with taking mefloquine prophylactically has been reported to increase adverse events in at least one case report (Wittes and Saginur, 1995), mixed results have been reported in larger studies. In a comparison of the neurologic and psychiatric adverse events among users of mefloquine (n = 394) and proguanil (n = 493) with people who did not take any prophylactic drug (n = 340), van Riemsdijk et al. (1997a) found that in regular users of alcohol, nightmares were more frequent among those who used mefloquine than among those that did not use antimalarials, but the authors also noted that the number of people who reported using alcohol in the mefloquine group was statistically significantly higher than the group who did not use antimalarials (p = 0.01). To determine whether mefloquine affects psychomotor and actual driving performance when given at prophylactic levels, Vuurman et al. (1996) conducted a randomized double-blinded placebo-controlled study of 40 men and women. Alcohol was given to achieve a sustained blood-alcohol concentration of 0.35 mg/mL (for comparison, the legal driving limit in the United States in 0.8 mg/mL). The mefloquine group drove better than the placebo group with and without alcohol at all time points measured. At the low alcohol levels tested, mefloquine does not appear to potentiate adverse events of alcohol on driving performance and rather appears to have psychoactivating or provigilance properties rather than any that enhance maximum psychomotor ability.

BIOLOGIC PLAUSIBILITY

Weekly 250 mg oral doses of mefloquine used for prophylaxis result in plasma concentrations ranging from 0.25 to 1.7 µg/mL (0.66 to 4.5 µM) (Charles et al., 2007; Gimenez et al., 1994; Hellgren et al., 1990, 1997; Kollaritsch et al., 2000;

Looareesuwan et al., 1987; Mimica et al., 1983; Palmer et al., 1993; Pennie et al., 1993; Schlagenhauf et al., 1996). Given that 98% of a mefloquine dose is bound to plasma proteins, the free mefloquine concentration is ≤0.1 μM (Gribble et al., 2000). In two studies (Schlagenhauf et al., 1996; Schwartz et al., 2001), plasma levels of mefloquine did not correlate with adverse events, whereas in a more recent study (Tansley et al., 2010), plasma exposure of mefloquine as measured by C_{max} and area under the curve, especially the latter, did correlate with adverse events. In this same study, the global safety profile of (+) mefloquine was no better than that of racemic mefloquine; these data (Tansley et al., 2010) did not support the hypothesis that (+) mefloquine may have lower central nervous system liabilities than the (–) mefloquine.

As described in several reviews (Grabias and Kumar, 2016; McCarthy, 2015; Toovey, 2009), a number of mechanisms may be associated with concurrent adverse events observed in individuals using mefloquine for malaria prophylaxis. As a caveat, the committee does not discuss data from studies in which mefloquine concentrations substantially exceeded the highest plasma levels (4.5 μM) observed in pharmacokinetic studies of mefloquine prophylaxis. With respect to central nervous system adverse events, limited animal data indicate a 4- to 13-fold accumulation of mefloquine in the brain and central nervous system (Barraud de Lagerie et al., 2004; Baudry et al., 1997; Caridha et al., 2008). In two human cell lines, mefloquine inhibited the membrane efflux protein P-glycoprotein, also known as multidrug resistance protein 1 (MDR1) (Pham et al., 2000; Senarathna et al., 2016). One study showed that MDR1 polymorphisms seem to be associated with the "neuropsychiatric" adverse events of mefloquine during treatment, primarily in women (Aarnoudse et al., 2006).

A 1983 report published by United Nations Development Programme, World Bank and WHO indicated that mefloquine did not exhibit mutagenic, teratologic, or carcinogenic effects in rats or mice (WHO, 1983). Dow et al. (2006) explored directed behavioral effects of mefloquine on behavior and neurotoxicity using a comprehensive dosing regimen and plasma mefloquine measures in rats. The results suggest that 187 mg/kg doses of mefloquine enhance activity profiles and cause mild neurodegeneration, as reflected in silver staining in rat gracile, cuneate, and solitary tract nuclei. Behavioral and histologic abnormalities increased as doses exceeded the pharmacologic range. Of note, no pathologic changes were observed with lower "prophylactic" dosing (45 mg/kg), based on circulating mefloquine levels. All testing was performed 24–48 hours after dosing, and thus persistent or latent effects were not examined. In vitro studies provide evidence for potential actions of mefloquine on neurons. Mefloquine inhibited the growth of two rat neuronal cell lines with IC_{50} values ranging from 7 to 12 μM and produced changes in gene expression consistent with the hypothesis that the endoplasmic reticulum was the neuronal target (Dow et al., 2003, 2005). Similarly, mefloquine is neurotoxic at micromolar concentrations to cerebral cortical cultures from rat pups, possibly by an oxidative stress mechanism (Hood et al., 2010; Milatovic et al., 2011). However, it is difficult to extrapolate results from neuronal culture systems to in vivo action, owing to the inherent vulnerability of neurons lacking trophic support from other cell types normally present in nervous tissue (glia and extracellular matrix proteins).

Other mechanisms could contribute to mefloquine effects on brain function. These include enhanced weak inhibition of acetylcholinesterase (McArdle et al., 2005; Zhou et al., 2006) and induction of autophagy (Shin et al., 2012). Mefloquine inhibits coupling of GABAergic neurons in the cortex and nucleus accumbens, regions that are important in affect and cognition (Allison et al., 2011; Heshmati et al., 2016). Mefloquine is a potent adenosine A2A receptor antagonist (Weiss et al., 2003), so that it modulates an array of downstream physiologic actions and could modulate sleep (Grabias and Kumar, 2016).

Binding assays suggest that mefloquine has the capacity to bind to neurotransmitter receptors. Mefloquine is a partial 5-HT_{2A} agonist with an EC_{50} value of 1.9 µM (Janowsky et al., 2014), and it is also a 5-HT_{3A} and 5-HT_{3AB} antagonist with respective IC_{50} values of 0.66 and 2.7 µM (Thompson and Lummis, 2008). Though the studies were not performed in neuronal cells, the results suggest that there is a potential for in vivo action on serotonin signaling under some conditions, which are associated with but not causally linked to psychiatric conditions, including depression, suicidality, and low mood.

Mefloquine is an inhibitor of connexin 36 (Cx36) and connexin 50 (Cx50), which are gap junction proteins responsible for rapid, non-synaptic electrical coupling in neurons and other cells (enabling alterations of cellular excitation without actions at the membrane). Of particular relevance, Cx36 is present in the nervous system and has been implicated in numerous neuronal signaling processes, some of which are relevant to psychiatric or neurologic diseases (e.g., epilepsy, depression) (Cruikshank et al., 2004). The inhibition of the gap junction signaling has led to the use of mefloquine as a pharmacologic tool in studies exploring the biologic actions of gap junctions (Cruikshank et al., 2004). For example, mefloquine administration in rats can impair the processing of contextual fear, impairing retrieval and enhancing extinction of freezing responses to the fearful context via inhibition of connexins (Bissiere et al., 2011), suggesting a role for connexins (and perhaps mefloquine) in the modulation of emotional memory processing.

In one clinical trial, mefloquine led to mild hypoglycemia but did not alter calcium homeostasis (Davis et al., 1996). This mefloquine-induced hypoglycemia may result from the inhibition of potassium ion channels in pancreatic β-cells (Gribble et al., 2000), and it has the potential to affect metabolic function.

Cx50 is highly expressed in the lens, and Cx50 knockout mice exhibit visual impairments and lens defects (Cruikshank et al., 2004), which may be of relevance to the visual deficits reported following mefloquine (Adamcova et al., 2015; Martinez-Wittinghan, 2006; Schneider et al., 2014). In addition, mefloquine is photoreactive (Aloisi et al., 2004; Motten et al., 1999) and may be involved in retinopathies associated with the accumulation of mefloquine in the retina (binding to melanin in retinal photoreceptors) (Nencini et al., 2008).

Mefloquine inhibits several cardiac potassium channels (El Harchi et al., 2010; Kang et al., 2001; López-Izquierdo et al., 2011; Perez-Cortes et al., 2015). In addition, Coker et al. (2000) argued that the negative inotropic action of mefloquine is explained by the blockade of L-type calcium channels. In multiple cell types and in cardiac muscle, mefloquine perturbs calcium homeostasis, possibly by acting as an ionophore, similar to ionomycin (Adegunloye et al., 1993; Bissinger et al., 2015; Caridha et al., 2008; Coker et al., 2000; Unekwe et al., 2007). Caridha et al. (2008) argue that mefloquine has the requisite physicochemical properties of an ionophore, given its high affinity for membrane phospholipids (Chevli and Fitch, 1982; Go and Ngiam, 1997). Mefloquine also was found to inhibit sarcoendoplasmic reticulum calcium adenosine triphosphatase (SERCA) (Toovey et al., 2008) and calcium-activated chloride currents in a whole-cell patch clamp study (Maertens et al., 2000). The modulation of potassium and calcium signaling may be associated with but not causally linked to long-term actions of mefloquine on the heart.

Overall, these data suggest multiple mechanisms that could account for the adverse events associated with concurrent mefloquine use. However, these data do not definitively link mefloquine to adverse events in the context of the repeated dosing that occurs during prophylaxis. All of these studies have measured end-points immediately after mefloquine administration, making it difficult to assess or infer potential lasting or permanent pathologic changes.

SYNTHESIS AND CONCLUSIONS

In assessing all of the available, relevant evidence, the committee was struck by the few number of studies available that examined outcomes that occurred after or persisted for more than 28 days after use of mefloquine had ceased. Of the 11 epidemiologic studies that met the ≥28-day post-cessation criterion for inclusion, the methodologic quality of the studies varied greatly, as did the time periods in relation to cessation and when studies were published (1983 through 2018) and the range of adverse events and health outcomes that were considered or reported. For example, although seven studies collected and reported information that could be categorized as psychiatric outcomes, these ranged from nonspecific broad categories such as "neuropsychiatric" to specific symptoms, such as sleep disturbances or anxiety, or clinical diagnoses such as PTSD, depressive disorder, or psychosis, which made it difficult for the committee to make an integrated assessment. Given the inherently imperfect information generated by any one study, it would be desirable to have similar studies to assess consistency of findings, but the diversity of the methods makes it very difficult to combine information across the studies with confidence. Even when pertinent data appear to have been collected to meet the committee's inclusion criteria of reporting on an adverse event or health outcome (or if there were none reported) 28 days post-drug-cessation, not all of the information relevant to the committee's charge was presented because it was not a main objective or focus of the study (e.g., studies that were designed to examine long-term efficacy against clinical malaria). Only published information that was presented from the study was considered. In some cases, it was clear that the investigators collected more data than was reported, such as when the population was followed for months or even years after mefloquine cessation, but the only outcomes reported were incident cases of malaria or generic statements about all adverse events having resolved.

Given the diversity of the methodologic quality and the variety of outcomes examined, the summarized epidemiologic studies did not all contribute equally to the ultimate conclusion of the association between mefloquine and persistent events of a given health outcome, and, in particular, the inferences are based primarily on those few studies that had the following attributes:

- sound designs and analysis methods;
- documented exposure of mefloquine for malaria prophylaxis;
- documented health outcomes at least 28 days after cessation of mefloquine use;
- compared mefloquine users with similar people who did not use any antimalarial drug, were given a placebo, or who used other antimalarial drugs;
- large enough sample sizes to conduct informative analyses; and
- presented empirical information relevant to associations between adverse effects or events (or lack of any effects or events) ≥28 days after mefloquine use had ended.

In general, the post-cessation epidemiologic studies were not designed to examine the persistence of events in individuals, but rather they collected information on whether adverse events were detected at some time period at least 28 days after cessation of mefloquine. To avoid repetition for each outcome category, a short summary of the attributes of each study that were considered to be most contributory to the evidence base or that presented evidence germane to multiple body system categories is presented first. The evidence summaries for each outcome category refer back to these short assessment summaries.

For each body system category, supporting information from the FDA label and package insert, known concurrent adverse events, case studies, information on selected subpopulations, experimental animal and in vitro studies, and results from epidemiologic studies that were less methodologically sound is first summarized before the evidence from the assessed epidemiologic studies is presented. While the charge to the committee was to address persistent or latent adverse events, the occurrence of concurrent adverse events enhances the plausibility that problems may persist beyond the period after cessation of drug use. The synthesis of evidence is followed by a conclusion about the strength of evidence regarding an association between the use of mefloquine and persistent adverse events and whether the available evidence would support additional research into outcomes of that body system. The outcomes are presented in the following order: neurologic disorders, psychiatric disorders, gastrointestinal disorders, eye disorders, cardiovascular disorders, and other outcomes including dermatologic outcomes and disorders of other organ systems.

Epidemiologic Studies Presenting Contributory Evidence

Eick-Cost used DoD administrative databases to perform a large retrospective cohort study among active-duty service members who filled at least one prescription for mefloquine, doxycycline, or A/P between 2008 and 2013. The primary study objective was to assess and compare the risk of incident and recurrent ICD-9-CM-coded neurologic and psychiatric outcomes that were reported at medical care visits during concurrent antimalarial use plus 365 days after the end of a prescription. This was a well-designed study and included several important factors that increased its methodologic quality: a large sample size, an administrative data source for both exposure and outcomes, and careful consideration of potential confounders including demographics, psychiatric history, and the military characteristics of deployment and combat exposure. Because the neurologic and psychiatric diagnoses occurring during current and recent use were analyzed together without distinguishing between events that occurred within 28 days of antimalarial use and those that occurred ≥28 days post-cessation, it provides no quantitative information regarding the persistence of most events other than the notation in the text that the results did not change when restricted to a post-cessation period of 30 days. Whereas the use of medical diagnoses is likely to be more reliable for the outcomes than self-report, there was no validation of the diagnoses recorded in the administrative databases, and symptoms or events that did not result in a medical visit or diagnosis would have been missed. For PTSD diagnoses, there was no information concerning when the index trauma occurred.

Schneiderman et al. (2018) conducted an analysis of self-reported health outcomes associated with the use of antimalarials in a population-based cohort of deployed and nondeployed U.S. veterans, using information collected as part of the NewGen Study. Exposure and outcomes were systematically obtained, and psychiatric outcomes were measured by standardized assessment instruments. Antimalarial medication use was grouped by mefloquine, chloroquine, doxycycline, primaquine, mefloquine in combination with other drugs, other antimalarials, and not specified or no antimalarial drug exposures. Health outcomes were self-reported using standardized instruments: the SF-12 for general physical health status, PCL-C for PTSD, and the Patient Health Questionnaire. The overall sample was large, and the researchers used a reasonably thorough set of covariates in models estimating drug–outcome associations, including deployment and combat exposure. Although the time period of drug use and the timing of health outcomes were not directly addressed, given that the population consisted of veterans who had served between 2001 and 2008 and the survey was not administered until 2009–2011, it is reasonable to assume that antimalarial drug use had ceased some time before. The methodology and response rate (34% total; weighted 4.4% of deployed and weighted 2.2% of nondeployed individuals used mefloquine) for this study may have led to the introduction of non-response, recall, or selection biases; however, the committee believed that investigators used appropriate data analysis techniques to mitigate the effects of any biases that were present.

Wells et al. (2006) was a large, well-designed study that used DoD administrative databases to examine incident hospitalizations by body system among active-duty service members who had been prescribed mefloquine and deployed at some time in calendar year 2002. Because the follow-up of mefloquine users began at the time of their return from deployment, it is reasonable to assume that these results largely reflect experience following the cessation of exposures of varying duration. Nonetheless, the results for varying time intervals following the cessation of use (or time since return from deployment) were not presented. Two comparison groups who were not prescribed antimalarials (service members assigned to Europe or Japan and service members who were deployed for 1 month or longer) were used in the analysis, but the demographic and military characteristics of the Europe- or Japan-assigned individuals differed substantially from those of the deployed individuals, suggesting that this was not an appropriate comparison group. Several attributes of its design increase its methodologic quality: a large sample size, the use of an administrative data source for both exposure and ICD-9-CM-based outcomes, and the inclusion of a reasonable set of sociodemographic, psychiatric history, and military characteristic covariates in the analyses. However, combat exposure was not specifically addressed, and although deployment may have been assumed to be a surrogate for combat, the lack of control for combat exposure itself is a limitation. The health outcomes were systematically and objectively ascertained but would reflect only the most severe experiences requiring hospitalization, which would likely exclude most people who experienced mental health symptoms or disorders. The small number of specific diagnoses for certain outcomes further limits the generalizability of these results.

Three large, retrospective studies of travelers (Meier et al., 2004; Schneider et al., 2013, 2014) were conducted using data from the UK-based GPRD to assess the incidence and compare the odds of developing first-time neurologic, psychiatric, or eye disorders in individuals using mefloquine compared with other antimalarial drugs for malaria prophylaxis. While the specific outcomes examined differed by study, the general design and methodology were the same for all three. The use of GPRD data (a well-established platform designed for both clinical practice and research) allowed for adequate power to detect differences in outcomes and for a uniform collection of exposures (although recorded drug prescriptions do not equate to use or adherence) and outcomes (based on clinical diagnoses coded from medical care visits) that were not subject to recall bias. Events that did not result in a medical care visit or that occurred outside of the national health care system would have been missed; however, it is unlikely that this would result in differential selection bias. Diagnoses were defined a priori, which excluded other outcomes, including the potential to identify rare outcomes. The antimalarial-exposed populations were large, an appropriate comparison group of travelers not using any form of malaria prophylaxis was included, and health outcomes were reported in defined time periods, including current use through 90 days after a prescription ended (termed *current use* or *recent use* in analyses that included both irrelevant [7–27 days] and relevant [28–90 days] time periods) and 91–540 days following cessation of use (termed *past use* in analyses). Adjustments were made for several confounders, including age, sex, calendar time, practice, smoking status, and BMI using appropriate study design or analytic methods. Each study included a nested case–control component that allowed for control of important covariates.

The primary aim of Tan et al. (2017) was to assess the prevalence of several health conditions experienced by returned Peace Corps volunteers associated with the use of prophylactic antimalarial drugs. The number of participants was large (8,931 participants), and of those who used an antimalarial drug a majority (59%) had used mefloquine. A number of important covariates, such as psychiatric history and alcohol use, were collected, but the study had several methodologic issues. These limitations included its study design (self-report Internet-based survey), exposure characterization based on self-report (which introduces several potential biases such as recall bias, sampling bias, and confounding), outcome assessment (based on self-report of health provider-diagnosed conditions up to 20 years post-service), the use of mixed comparison groups, a lack of detail regarding the analysis methods, and a poor response rate (11%, which likely introduced selection bias). The evidence generated by this study was thus considered to contribute only weakly to the inferences of mefloquine and persistent adverse events or disorders.

Neurologic Disorders

There are recognized concurrent adverse neurologic events associated with mefloquine use, including dizziness, vertigo, loss of balance, headache, memory impairment, confusion, encephalopathy, sensory or motor neuropathies, convulsions, tinnitus, and hearing loss (FDA, 2016; Tickell-Painter et al., 2017a). In the epidemiologic studies examining persistent neurologic outcomes, these effects were not observed to occur at statistically different rates for mefloquine users compared with people who used other antimalarial drugs or who did not use any prophylaxis. However, persistent dizziness was found in a few case reports, and studies of mefloquine use in pregnant women showed an increased risk for dizziness that resolved spontaneously within a few days (Briand et al., 2009; Nosten et al., 1994). A recent Cochrane review of mefloquine use for prophylaxis in travelers also reported that current mefloquine use was associated with statistically significantly higher risks of dizziness than placebo or no prophylaxis in cohort studies, but in clinical trials no difference in experiencing dizziness was found between mefloquine users and those given a placebo. Other persistent neurologic symptoms and conditions of neuropathy, weakness, paralysis, convulsions, and concentration impairment were described in the case reports.

In addition to the data on neurologic outcomes in humans, animal and cell culture studies lend some support for plausible biologic mechanisms through which mefloquine may contribute to neurotoxic processes. These include the modulation of calcium homeostasis, the induction of oxidative stress, the inhibition of connexin signaling, and the modulation of neurotransmitter receptor binding.

The committee reviewed five epidemiologic studies that examined neurologic outcomes that occurred at least 28 days following the cessation of mefloquine (Eick-Cost et al., 2017; Schlagenhauf et al., 1996; Schneider et al., 2013; Tan et al., 2017; Wells et al., 2006). These outcomes were inconsistently identified and measured across studies: ICD-9-CM-coded disorders of the nervous system as a category, and specific neurologic outcomes of nystagmus, vertiginous syndromes, dizziness and giddiness, and migraine (Wells et al., 2006); ICD-9-CM-coded outcomes of confusion, tinnitus, vertigo, and convulsions (Eick-Cost et al., 2017); epilepsy and peripheral neuropathy (Schneider et al., 2013); "neuropsychologic" as a category and that separately included dementia, migraines, seizures, tinnitus, vestibular disorder, and "other" neurologic disorder (Tan et al., 2017); and "neuropsychiatric" adverse events that included dizziness/vertigo, headache, and decreased concentration (Schlagenhauf et al., 1996). While all five of these studies have methodologic limitations, the three that provided the most evidence for potential persistent or latent neurologic outcomes based on the strength of the methods used were Eick-Cost et al. (2017), Wells et al. (2006), and Schneider et al. (2013).

In their analysis of data from DoD administrative databases, Eick-Cost et al. (2017) examined neurologic outcomes, and analyses were stratified by deployment and, separately, by psychiatric history. Adjusted incident rates of tinnitus, convulsions, and confusion were higher among the nondeployed than among the deployed groups who used mefloquine. There were no statistically significant differences for any of the neurologic outcomes among the deployed mefloquine users compared with the doxycycline users. Among the nondeployed, only vertigo was statistically significantly different (decreased) for mefloquine versus doxycycline users. Adjusted IRRs comparing mefloquine with A/P by deployment status found that the risk of tinnitus was statistically significantly increased among both the deployed and the nondeployed groups. No other outcomes were statistically significantly different between deployed mefloquine and A/P users. For both the mefloquine and doxycycline groups, there were no statistically significant differences between drugs when adjusting for history of psychiatric disorder. In a second study of U.S. service members, Wells et al. (2006) presented hospitalizations from nervous system disorders as a single category. Only six hospitalizations due to nervous system disorders were reported for mefloquine users, and comparisons with both reference groups showed that mefloquine users had no statistically significant different risk for nervous system disorders as a group. When hospitalizations due to specific neurologic outcomes were considered, among those receiving mefloquine there were no cases of nystagmus or dizziness and giddiness, one case of vertiginous syndromes, and three cases of migraine, which resulted in wide, imprecise, and null effect estimates when these rates were compared with those of the two reference groups of service members. Schneider et al. (2013) assessed incident diagnoses of epilepsy and peripheral neuropathy among travelers who had been prescribed mefloquine and compared them with those given another antimalarial and, separately, with travelers who had a travel consult but were not prescribed antimalarial drugs; the analysis was stratified by time since cessation. Over the approximately 8.5-year period of data examined, a total of 14 mefloquine users were diagnosed with incident epilepsy, 6 of whom were current use and 8 of whom were past use. Among the eight mefloquine users with incident neuropathies, five were current users and three were past users. In the nested case–control analysis, after adjusting for smoking and BMI, the odds of developing epilepsy were decreased, and the odds of developing peripheral neuropathies were elevated for mefloquine users, but neither of these results reached statistical significance. Similarly, when stratified by current use or past use, the adjusted odds of epilepsy for mefloquine users compared with non-antimalarial users were not statistically significantly different. The FDA package insert warns individuals with epilepsy that taking mefloquine may increase the risk for convulsions, and people who had previously been diagnosed with epilepsy were excluded from the study. Compared with nonusers of antimalarials, current users of mefloquine had increased odds of neuropathy, while past users had decreased odds of neuropathy but neither of these estimates was statistically significant. In sum, this was a well-designed study, and the stratification of past use in particular provides some evidence for an absence of increased persistent neurologic effects of epilepsy and peripheral neuropathy following the use of mefloquine. Overall, these three well-designed studies provide some evidence for an absence of persistent neurologic events following the use of mefloquine, but the number of neurologic disorders was small, making these results far from definitive.

The two other epidemiologic studies with post-cessation follow-up (Schlagenhauf et al., 1996; Tan et al., 2017) that presented some information on neurologic outcomes were not as methodologically robust as Eick-Cost et al. (2017), Wells et al. (2006), or Schneider et al. (2013), and their results lend additional weak support for an absence of increased persistent neurologic effects.

Based on the available evidence, the committee concludes that there is insufficient or inadequate evidence of an association between the use of mefloquine for malaria prophylaxis and persistent or latent neurologic events. Current evidence suggests further study of such an association is warranted, given the evidence regarding biologic plausibility, adverse events associated with concurrent use, or data from the existing epidemiologic studies.

Psychiatric Disorders

The evidence supporting concurrent adverse psychiatric effects of mefloquine is compelling. These effects include anxiety, depression, mood swings, panic attacks, abnormal dreams, insomnia, hallucinations, aggression, and psychotic or paranoid reactions. Suicidal thoughts and death by suicide have been also been reported with concurrent use of mefloquine. While the charge to the committee was to address persistent or latent adverse events, the occurrence of concurrent adverse events enhances the plausibility that problems may persist beyond the period of drug use. The FDA package insert warns that psychiatric symptoms such as acute anxiety, depression, and restlessness should be viewed as potential precursors to more serious psychiatric or neurologic adverse events and that mefloquine should be discontinued if they occur. In addition, the FDA labeling has increasingly invoked the potential for persistent adverse psychiatric events, suggesting reports received warranted these changes, although no research is cited as the basis for these changes. Two Cochrane reviews examined concurrent adverse events of mefloquine use in travelers. Croft and Garner (2000) reported on psychiatric symptoms in six trials comparing the tolerability of mefloquine to other antimalarials and found that the only outcomes with increased odds associated with mefloquine use were insomnia and fatigue. Tickell-Painter et al. (2017a) found that mefloquine users were more likely than users of doxycycline and users of A/P to experience insomnia, anxiety, abnormal dreams, and depressed mood. In cohort studies mefloquine users were more likely than participants who did not take prophylaxis to experience abnormal dreams and insomnia. However, this review included concurrent adverse events, and several outcomes had imprecise effect estimates because of the small numbers of adverse events (e.g., serious adverse effects, depressed mood, abnormal thoughts or perceptions). Additional studies of selected subpopulations of concurrent mefloquine use lend some evidence for a relationship with psychiatric outcomes. Mefloquine users who use another medication for a chronic illness (Handschin et al., 1997; Huzly et al., 1996) or who drink alcohol while taking mefloquine (van Riemsdijk et al., 1997a) appear to have an increased risk for adverse events. Furthermore, women (Rendi-Wagner et al., 2002; Schlagenhauf et al., 1996; Wernsdorfer et al., 2013) and individuals with low BMI (van Riemsdijk et al., 2002b, 2003) may be at increased risk for adverse psychiatric symptoms when taking mefloquine. A number of published case reports suggest that persistent psychiatric symptoms (including anxiety, depression, insomnia/exhaustion, paranoia, hallucinations, visual illusions, mania, depersonalization, or suicidal ideation) may be associated with mefloquine use and continue beyond the period after drug exposure has ended. Again, these findings support the plausibility of persistent adverse events, but they are inherently limited in the quality of scientific evidence that they can provide. However, a recent Cochrane review concluded that mefloquine is safe during pregnancy (González et al., 2018).

Animal and in vitro studies indicate that mefloquine may negatively affect processes relevant to psychiatric conditions. Mefloquine can affect processes that may in turn interfere with brain circuits regulating mood and cognition, including calcium homestasis (synaptic signaling), oxidative stress (managing energetic challenge), and connexins (intercellular communication). In particular, mefloquine's binding to serotonin receptors suggests possible interactions with signaling processes relevant to mood regulation. However, the data from these experimental studies do not definitively explore mefloquine exposures relevant to prophylaxis doses or use. Moreover, the studies have measured endpoints immediately after mefloquine administration, making it difficult to address persistent or latent pathologic changes.

The most weight for evidence of an association between use of mefloquine and persistent or latent psychiatric adverse events comes from the seven epidemiologic studies that examined psychiatric outcomes that occurred at least 28 days following cessation of mefloquine (Eick-Cost et al., 2017; Meier et al., 2004; Schlagenhauf et al., 1996; Schneider et al., 2013; Schneiderman et al., 2018; Tan et al., 2017; Wells et al., 2006). The seven studies each used different methods for measuring outcomes, and the psychiatric outcomes of interest varied across studies. Considering the studies of U.S. military or veteran populations, Eick-Cost et al. (2017) examined adjustment disorder, anxiety disorder, depressive disorder, PTSD, psychoses, suicide ideation, paranoia, hallucinations, insomnia, and death by suicide using clinical diagnoses coded in DoD administrative databases. Wells et al. (2006) also used clinical diagnoses coded in DoD administrative databases to examine "mental disorders" as a diagnostic category and specific psychiatric diagnoses of somatoform disorder, mood disorder, anxiety disorder, PTSD, substance use disorders, personality disorder, adjustment reaction, "mixed syndromes," and "other disorders." And Schneiderman et al. (2018) used standardized self-report instruments to examine outcomes of PTSD, thoughts of death or self-harm, other anxiety disorders, and major depression. Both studies of UK travelers used clinical diagnoses coded in a health care administrative database to examine incident psychiatric outcomes. Meier et al. (2004) included depression, psychoses, panic attacks, and death by suicide among people aged 17–79 years, and Schneider et al. (2013) examined depression and anxiety, stress-related disorders, and psychoses as a group in individuals aged ≥1 year (Schneider et al., 2013). Schlagenhauf et al. (1996) used standardized self-report instruments to examine sleep disturbances, mood changes, unusual or vivid dreams, and phobias in travelers who had taken mefloquine for short-term malaria prophylaxis after visiting a Swiss vaccination center.

In their analysis of returned U.S. Peace Corps volunteers, Tan et al. (2017) used unverified self-reported symptoms of depression, anxiety, and insomnia to derive clinical diagnoses of major depressive disorder, bipolar disorder, anxiety disorder, schizophrenia, obsessive-compulsive disorder, and "other." Findings related to PTSD are considered separately, below.

While all seven of these studies have methodologic limitations, the five that, based on their methodologic quality, provided the strongest evidence for examining the presence of persistent psychiatric outcomes are Eick-Cost et al. (2017), Meier et al. (2004), Schneider et al. (2013), Schneiderman et al. (2018), and Wells et al. (2006). Four of the studies (Eick-Cost et al., 2017; Meier et al., 2004; Schneider et al., 2013; Wells et al., 2006) evaluated data from administrative databases with clinically diagnosed outcomes, included at least two comparison groups in the analyses, applied a reasonably thorough set of covariates to the analyses of effect estimates, and measured the psychiatric outcomes of interest systematically and objectively, based on medical care visits and coded in the database. Although both Eick-Cost et al. and Wells et al. used data from DoD administrative databases, they used different years, and Wells et al. limited diagnoses to hospitalizations, which would suggest that the outcomes reported in Wells et al. were of greater severity than those in the Eick-Cost et al. sample, limiting the cross-study. The Schneiderman et al. (2018) study was somewhat less rigorous as the researchers based their exposure and outcome assessments on self-report. Both exposure and outcomes were systematically obtained, and psychiatric outcomes were measured by standardized psychometric instruments. The sample was large and adequately powered, and the investigators used a reasonably thorough set of covariates in analyses of effect estimates. Again, the difference in ascertainment of data limits comparison of data across studies.

In their analysis of active-duty service members, Eick-Cost et al. (2017) found that with the exception of psychoses and death by suicide, the adjusted incident rates for psychiatric outcomes were higher among the deployed groups who used mefloquine than among the nondeployed groups who used mefloquine. When comparisons between mefloquine and doxycycline use were stratified by deployment, the only statistically significant difference for any of the psychiatric outcomes for the deployed was a slight increased risk for anxiety disorders among mefloquine users. Among the nondeployed, mefloquine users had statistically significantly decreased risks of adjustment disorder, insomnia, anxiety disorder, depressive disorder, and PTSD compared with doxycycline users, but no differences were found for the other five psychiatric outcomes. In comparisons of mefloquine users and A/P users by deployment status, no outcomes were statistically significantly different for the deployed, but in the nondeployed group, mefloquine users had an increased risk of PTSD, although no other psychiatric outcomes showed differences in risk between mefloquine and A/P users. For both the mefloquine and doxycycline groups, individuals with a psychiatric diagnosis in the year preceding the prescription had statistically significantly elevated risks for a subsequent diagnosis of the same condition for all conditions reported (adjustment disorder, anxiety, insomnia, depressive disorder, and PTSD) compared with individuals without a diagnosis in the prior year. However, when the IRRs comparing mefloquine and doxycycline users were stratified by those with and without prior psychiatric diagnoses, there were no statistically significant differences between mefloquine and doxycycline for any of the conditions. The results of a sensitivity analysis in which the risk period was restricted to 30 days post-prescription were not reported, although the authors stated that the results were similar to the primary analyses. Similarly, in their analysis of service member hospitalizations Wells et al. (2006) reported a total of 37 hospitalizations for mental disorders as a category for mefloquine users, and the rate of hospitalizations was not statistically significantly different from the two comparison groups. When hospitalizations due to specific psychiatric outcomes were considered, there were no cases of somatoform disorders, 6 cases each of mood disorders and anxiety disorders, 1 case of PTSD, 19 cases of substance use disorders, 7 cases of personality disorders, 13 cases of adjustment reactions, 4 cases of mixed syndromes, and 20 cases of "other disorders" among mefloquine users, which resulted in imprecise and null effect estimates when these rates were compared with those of the two reference groups of service members. Using a large population-based cohort of deployed and nondeployed U.S. veterans, Schneiderman et al. (2018) found that, like Eick-Cost et al., deployed mefloquine users had higher frequencies of mental health diagnoses than nondeployed mefloquine users for the four psychiatric outcomes examined. However, in the adjusted logistic regression models with all covariates considered (including demographics, deployment, and combat exposure), mefloquine was not associated with any of the psychiatric outcomes examined: composite mental health score, thoughts of death or self-harm, other anxiety, and major depression. It is noteworthy that adjusting for combat exposure consistently reduced the measures of association, but when combat exposure intensity was specifically considered, the weighted prevalence estimates indicated that the prevalence of disorders increased with greater combat exposure intensity. This study could not address explicitly the health experiences during use and in specific time intervals following the cessation of use. Overall, the studies in military service members and veterans were well designed and provide some evidence for an absence of increased risk of persistent or latent psychiatric outcomes in mefloquine users.

Factors that may be present in groups of military or veterans that may confound associations between the use of mefloquine and adverse psychiatric events, such as deployment and combat exposure, are rarely encountered with leisure travelers. The results of Meier et al. (2004) and Schneider et al. (2013), who used UK travelers and stratified by time post-cessation corroborated the findings of Eick-Cost et al. (2017) and Schneiderman et al. (2018) in that the use of mefloquine was not associated with an increased risk of depression diagnoses in either the cohort analysis or the nested case–control studies. Schneider et al. (2013) found that in the adjusted analyses, the odds of developing an incident diagnosis of depression was statistically significantly decreased in both current and past mefloquine users compared with nonusers. Meier et al. (2004) also found no difference in the risk of developing depression for recent mefloquine users versus all past users of other antimalarials. Schneider et al. (2013) found that when the data were stratified by current use or past use, the adjusted odds of anxiety, stress-related disorders, or psychosis as a group were no different in current users but were statistically significantly reduced in the past users of mefloquine compared with nonusers. When anxiety, psychosis, phobia, and panic attack were analyzed as separate outcomes with no timing stratifications, compared with nonusers of antimalarials, only the odds of anxiety were statistically significantly decreased for mefloquine users (which was consistent with the findings of Eick-Cost et al.). Meier et al. (2004) found that first-time diagnoses of panic attacks and psychosis were not statistically significantly different for recent users of mefloquine compared with all past users of antimalarials, but the odds of panic attacks were statistically significantly increased in the adjusted nested case–control analysis. Both Meier et al. and Schneider et al. excluded people who had previously been diagnosed with the psychiatric outcomes of interest from their study populations. In sum, the studies of travelers corroborate the findings of studies of service members and veterans, and the use of stratification of post-cessation time, particularly past use, provides some evidence for an absence in—and possibly even a reduction in—persistent psychiatric effects of anxiety, stress-related disorders, or psychoses as a group, depression, and panic disorder following the use of mefloquine, but the small number of incident diagnoses for these psychiatric disorders does not provide definitive evidence of no effect.

The two other studies considered by the committee that presented some information on psychiatric outcomes (Schlagenhauf et al., 1996; Tan et al., 2017) were not as methodologically robust as Eick-Cost et al. (2017), Wells et al. (2006), Schneider et al. (2013), Meier et al. (2004), or Schneiderman et al. (2018), and therefore their findings were given less weight. However, the results of these two studies overall lend additional weak support for an absence of persistent or latent psychiatric events.

PTSD

Three studies—all conducted using active-duty U.S. military or veteran populations—reported PTSD diagnoses (based on ICD-9-CM codes) or PTSD symptoms (based on validated instruments). Each of these studies adjusted for deployment and combat in the analysis of PTSD and other psychiatric outcomes. Adjusted effect estimates showed attenuated associations between mefloquine exposure and diagnoses or symptoms of PTSD. In an analysis of active-duty service members, Eick-Cost et al. (2017) presented adjusted effect estimates of

PTSD stratified by deployment status. Among the nondeployed, those who were prescribed mefloquine were found to have a statistically significant decrease in PTSD diagnoses relative to those prescribed doxycycline, but the risk of PTSD diagnoses for those prescribed mefloquine was statistically significantly increased relative to individuals who were prescribed A/P. There was no difference in PTSD diagnoses for deployed service members prescribed mefloquine compared with those prescribed doxycycline or A/P. When service members were stratified by prior psychiatric history, no statistically significant differences between mefloquine and doxycycline use were found for PTSD diagnosis. However, Eick-Cost et al. did not present the data in a manner that allowed a separation of concurrent from persistent (≥28 days) psychiatric outcomes, although the authors stated that they performed a sensitivity analysis that restricted the risk period to 30 days post-cessation and that the results of those analyses were similar to what was presented.

In their analysis of hospitalizations of active-duty service members, Wells et al. (2006) reported no statistically significant differences for PTSD diagnoses for deployed service members who were prescribed mefloquine versus deployed service members who did not use an antimalarial drug or who were assigned to Europe or Japan. In this study, only one diagnosis of PTSD was reported in the mefloquine group compared with 29 diagnoses in the deployed nonuser group and 38 diagnoses in the assigned-to-other-locations group. Likewise, in their study of U.S. veterans, Schneiderman et al. (2018) also found no difference in PTSD symptoms using a standardized instrument between mefloquine users and nonusers of antimalarials after controlling for demographics and deployment. No difference in PTSD was found between veterans who reported using mefloquine and another antimalarial and those with no antimalarial use after adjusting for demographics, deployment, and combat. In sum, most of the findings with respect to risk for PTSD in mefloquine users show no difference or a lower risk when they are compared with nonusers of antimalarials and those who received other drugs, after adjusting for deployment status. However, one analysis showed an increased risk of PTSD in mefloquine users relative to A/P users but only among those who were nondeployed; the implications of this are unclear.

Based on the available evidence, the committee concludes that there is insufficient or inadequate evidence of an association between the use of mefloquine for malaria prophylaxis and persistent or latent psychiatric events, including PTSD. Current evidence suggests further study of such an association is warranted, given the evidence regarding biologic plausibility, adverse events associated with concurrent use, or data from the existing epidemiologic studies.

Gastrointestinal Disorders

The most recent FDA package insert for mefloquine states that the most frequently observed adverse event in clinical trials of malaria prophylaxis was vomiting (3%), while postmarketing surveillance found the most frequently reported gastrointestinal adverse events to be nausea, vomiting, loose stools or diarrhea, and abdominal pain, but the duration of such symptoms is not detailed. Systematic reviews of adverse events in travelers who used mefloquine compared with other regimens, placebo, or no antimalarial drug included concurrent gastrointestinal symptoms (abdominal discomfort or pain, anorexia, diarrhea, nausea, vomiting, dyspepsia). In the systematic review by Croft and Garner (2000), no consistent pattern was seen for the gastrointestinal symptoms analyzed, due in part to the heterogeneity of studies, but abdominal discomfort was reported statistically less frequently with other antimalarial drugs, as were anorexia and nausea. In a second systematic review examining the adverse events of mefloquine prophylaxis among travelers that included two randomized controlled trials and three cohort studies, mefloquine recipients were statistically significantly more likely to experience nausea than placebo recipients, but there was no difference between groups for vomiting, abdominal pain, or diarrhea. Based on cohort studies that compared mefloquine users with doxycycline users, mefloquine users were statistically significantly less likely to report dyspepsia and vomiting, but these results were given low or very low certainty of evidence, respectively. However, among pregnant women using mefloquine for intermittent preventive treatment in pregnancy, for which the dosage used is substantially higher than the dosage used for malaria prophylaxis, mefloquine was associated with a statistically significantly higher risk of drug-related vomiting and higher rates of nausea compared with use of sulfadoxine-pyrimethamine, but these symptoms all were reported to resolve spontaneously within 3 days.

Published individual case reports that had follow-up of at least 28 days post-mefloquine-cessation did not report on gastrointestinal disorders. The FDA package insert warns that mefloquine elimination may be prolonged in people who have impaired liver function, which may lead to higher plasma levels and a higher risk of adverse events. In a small study, DeSouza (1983) found that liver and spleen enlargement was reduced among the mefloquine participants (and sulfadoxine/pyrimethamine participants) over the course of follow-up. In one case series (Croft and Herxheimer, 2002) that reviewed case reports of adverse event reports associated with the use of mefloquine, the researchers hypothesized that adverse events may be due to liver or thyroid pathology; however, no objective validation of the adverse events reported by the cases or other follow-up was conducted, among other limitations of this analysis.

Biologic plausibility data on gastrointestinal effects are lacking. While there is some evidence of mefloquine action on β-cells, no experimental studies have provided data on mechanisms to support the potential for observed gastrointestinal disorders to become persistent.

The committee reviewed several epidemiologic studies that examined gastrointestinal disorders and outcomes that occurred during or immediately after (within 28 days of) mefloquine use, but because they did not follow or report on these adverse events 28 days post-cessation, the results are not considered to contribute to the evidence base of persistent gastrointestinal events post-mefloquine-use. Only Wells et al. (2006), based on the strength of the methods used in that analysis, was considered to provide robust evidence for gastrointestinal disorders that occurred or persisted at least 28 days following the cessation of mefloquine. Using ICD-9-CM codes, Wells et al. grouped disorders of the digestive system and found that 23 mefloquine users were hospitalized for these disorders. When mefloquine users were compared with deployed service members who were not prescribed an antimalarial, there was no difference in the risk of digestive system disorders, but compared with those service members who were assigned to Europe or Japan, deployed mefloquine users had a statistically significantly lower risk of hospitalization for digestive system disorders. This study provides some evidence for an absence of increased risk for serious persistent digestive system disorders following the use of mefloquine, but it is unclear if some of these concurrent adverse events persisted or if concurrent events preceded persistent outcomes that may not resolve without additional treatment. Tan et al. (2017) lends additional weak support (given its serious methodologic limitations) to an absence of increased risk of persistent gastrointestinal disorders following use of mefloquine.

Based on the available evidence, the committee concludes that there is insufficient or inadequate evidence of an association between the use of mefloquine for malaria prophylaxis and persistent or latent gastrointestinal events. Current evidence does not suggest further study of such an association is warranted, given the lack of evidence regarding biologic plausibility, adverse events associated with concurrent use, or findings from the existing epidemiologic studies.

Eye Disorders

Although there are reports of concurrent visual disturbance including optic neuropathy and retinal disorders associated with mefloquine use (FDA, 2016; Tickell-Painter et al., 2017a), in the epidemiologic studies that examined persistent eye disorders, these effects were not observed to occur at statistically different rates for mefloquine users than for people who used other antimalarial drugs or who did not use any prophylaxis. Among the case reports, concurrent adverse events included visual illusions and one case of persistent retinopathy. A large analysis of eye disorders associated with mefloquine use reported to the manufacturer's drug safety database provides additional indirect support for adverse events of visual acuity and disorders affecting the retina or cornea (Adamcova et al., 2015). In addition to the available data on eye disorders in humans, experimental data may support plausible biologic mechanisms for mefloquine affecting ocular components, acting via a disruption of connexin signaling in the lens and possible phototoxic changes in the retina.

Of the 11 epidemiologic studies on persistent adverse events, 2 made a mention of eye disorders that occurred at least 28 days following the cessation of mefloquine (Schneider et al., 2014; Tan et al., 2017). Given the serious methodologic limitations of Tan et al. (2017), only Schneider et al. (2014) was considered, based on the strength of the methods used in that analysis, to provide robust evidence for persistent ophthalmic outcomes. Schneider et al. (2014) assessed incident diagnoses of eye disorders among travelers aged ≥1 year who had been prescribed mefloquine and compared them with two other groups of travelers: travelers who had been prescribed another antimalarial and travelers who had a travel consult but were not prescribed antimalarial drugs. Eye disorders were grouped into eight categories, some specific (such as cataract, glaucoma, and vitreous detachment) and others a compilation of disorders of the cornea, retina, visual acuity, uvea, and neuro-ophthamology. The timing of incident diagnoses was stratified into "current use," which mixed irrelevant (7–28 days post-cessation) and relevant (28–90 days post-cessation) time periods, and "past use" (91–540 days post-cessation), all of which was relevant. Over the approximately 8.5-year period of data examined, a total of 85 people who had used mefloquine were diagnosed with an incident eye disorder of interest; 23 incident eye disorders were found for current users, and 62 were found for past users. A nested case–control analysis found that the odds of developing any of the eye disorders of interest were statistically significantly elevated for mefloquine users compared with travelers who did not use any antimalarial drugs. However, when mefloquine use was stratified by current use and past use and the users compared with the nonusers, there was no statistically significant difference for current users, although past users had statistically significantly increased odds of experiencing any eye disorder when all were grouped as a single category. When each of the individual eye disorders was examined without timing stratification, only cataract was statistically significantly related to mefloquine use compared with no use of antimalarials. Other risk factors for cataracts, such as occupation and sun exposure, were not included in the analysis and may have differed between the groups. Overall, this was a well-designed study, and the stratification of past use in particular provides some evidence for an absence of increased risk of persistent eye disorder diagnoses following the use of mefloquine. The findings of no differences in risk of ophthalmologic disorders of macular degeneration, retinopathy, and "any" ophthalmologic disorder by Tan et al. (2017) provide additional weak supportive evidence of an absence of increased risk of eye disorders. However, the finding of increased risk of cataracts with mefloquine use in Schneider et al. (2014) requires confirmatory evidence.

Based on the available evidence, the committee concludes that there is insufficient or inadequate evidence of an association between the use of mefloquine for malaria prophylaxis and persistent or latent eye disorders, including cataract. Current evidence suggests further study of such an association is warranted, given the evidence regarding biologic plausibility, adverse events associated with concurrent use, or findings from the existing epidemiologic studies.

Cardiovascular Disorders

The most recent FDA package insert for mefloquine states that syncope and extrasystoles were reported in less than 1% of mefloquine users participating in clinical trials of malaria prophylaxis. Other concurrent adverse events reported with the use of mefloquine have included transitory and clinically silent ECG alterations such as sinus bradycardia, sinus arrhythmia, first degree AV block, prolongation of the QTc interval, and abnormal T-waves. Among the case reports that followed outcomes at least 28 days post-cessation of mefloquine, heart palpitations were reported in one case in which concurrent symptoms of paralysis and trouble breathing were also reported (Eaton, 1996). The available biologic plausibility data on cardiovascular effects are limited, but some data suggest that mefloquine may induce cardiovascular effects through the inhibition of several cardiac potassium channels. Mefloquine may also affect intracellular calcium homeostasis in cardiac myocytes, suggesting some potential for cardiac indications, although this was not tested in the context of persistent or latent actions.

The committee reviewed four epidemiologic studies that examined cardiovascular or circulatory system outcomes that occurred at least 28 days following the cessation of mefloquine (DeSouza, 1983; Laothavorn et al., 1992; Tan et al., 2017; Wells et al., 2006). Similar to the other body system outcome categories, cardiovascular and circulatory system outcomes were inconsistently identified and measured across studies. DeSouza (1983) used ECGs and measured blood pressure and pulse rate, as well as hematologic parameters of red blood cell count, hemoglobin erythrocyte volume fraction, total and differential white blood cell counts, reticulocyte count, and platelet count. Measurements of other biochemical parameters (including cholesterol, triglycerides, glucose, urea, creatinine, etc.) in sera were also performed. Laothavorn et al. (1992) also used ECGs to measure heart rate and different cardiac intervals and to diagnose abnormalities of sinus bradycardia, sinus arrhythmia, ventricular ectopic beats, atrial ectopic beats, atrial–ventricular block, and heart rate; they also performed weekly blood count tests. The two other studies (Tan et al., 2017; Wells et al., 2006) grouped cardiovascular outcomes. In Tan et al. the cardiac category included arrhythmia, congestive heart failure, myocardial infarction, and "any" cardiac disorder, while Wells et al. grouped outcomes by ICD-9-CM code into disorders of the blood and blood-forming organs and a separate category of disorders of the circulatory system.

While none of these studies is without methodologic limitations, Wells et al. (2006) provided the most robust evidence regarding persistent cardiovascular and circulatory system outcomes. In short, only four hospitalizations related to blood and blood-forming organs (ICD-9-CM: 280–289) and nine hospitalizations from circulatory system disorders (ICD-9-CM: 390–459) were reported for mefloquine users. Comparisons with both reference groups showed that mefloquine users had no difference in risk for both groups of disorders, providing some evidence for an absence of increased risk of persistent disorders of blood or blood-forming organs or the cardiovascular system following use of mefloquine. The results from the three other epidemiologic studies lend additional support, although of less weight, for an absence of increased persistent cardiovascular events. Tan et al. (2017) reported that there were no statistically significant differences in cardiac outcomes between users of mefloquine and of the other antimalarial drugs for prophylaxis, but they did not provide frequencies of the events or effect estimates. Although both DeSouza (1983) and Laothavorn et al. (1992) used objective tests (ECGs) and standard hematologic and laboratory measures in their investigations, the presented results are not readily comparable between studies and were sometimes vague. DeSouza stated that blood pressure, pulse rate, and ECG remained normal throughout the study period (63 days after mefloquine administration), but no other details regarding the ECG results were provided. Hematologic tests were conducted several times throughout the study, but only those taken on days 28 and 63 post-administration were relevant to the committee's work. No significant adverse changes were reported for any of the collected parameters for the group administered mefloquine. Laothavorn et al. performed ECGs on healthy volunteers prior to mefloquine administration, daily for 1 week post-administration, and then weekly until day 42 post-administration. All ECG parameters were reported to be within normal limits, and no changes in biochemical or hematologic measures were found following mefloquine administration. Although the results from the DeSouza and Laothavorn studies appear to be consistent with an absence in increased persistent events of cardiovascular or circulatory disorders following use of mefloquine—especially considering that the administered doses of mefloquine were 3–4 times higher than the dose used for prophylaxis—both of these studies were small and underpowered and were limited in the information reported. The concurrent events listed in the FDA package insert were not found to occur in the epidemiologic studies that measured them.

Based on the available evidence, the committee concludes that there is insufficient or inadequate evidence of an association between the use of mefloquine for malaria prophylaxis and persistent or latent cardiovascular events. Current evidence does not suggest further study of such an association is warranted, given the lack of evidence regarding biologic plausibility, adverse events associated with concurrent use, or findings from the existing epidemiologic studies.

Other Outcomes and Disorders

In addition to those outcomes synthesized above, two of the epidemiologic studies examined other outcomes and disorders that occurred at least 28 days following the cessation of mefloquine. Tan et al. (2017) included dermatologic outcomes as a group that included allergic dermatitis, eczema, psoriasis, "other" and "any" dermatologic conditions and reported that there were no statistically significant differences between users of mefloquine and those of the other antimalarial drugs for prophylaxis, but neither the frequencies of such events nor effect estimates were provided. Wells et al. (2006) reported nine hospitalizations from skin and subcutaneous tissues (ICD-9-CM: 680–709) among mefloquine users in their study of U.S. service members, but no difference in risk was found between deployed service members who were prescribed mefloquine and those who were not prescribed an antimalarial. In one systematic review, reports of fever and pruritus were similar in the mefloquine and comparator arms (Croft and Garner, 2000). In a second systematic review, skin and subcutaneous tissues outcomes (pruritus, photosensitivity, vaginal candida) were examined, and based on data from cohort studies, mefloquine users were statistically significantly less likely than doxycycline users to report photosensitivity or vaginal thrush, but both findings were based on very low-certainty evidence. In the case reports, one case of worsening psoriasis was reported (Potasman and Seligmann, 1998). In a case series (Smith et al., 1999) of 74 published case reports of mefloquine use (pro-phylaxis or treatment) specific to dermatologic adverse events, the timing of onset of dermatologic effects was only recorded in 11 of the cases; pruritus and itching were reported in more than 40% of all the cases. Most effects were reported as mild or moderate in intensity and usually self-limiting, although the timing was not specified. Other dermatologic adverse events in this case series included two reports of cutaneous vasculitis and one report each of Stevens-Johnson syndrome and toxic epidermal necrolysis. In sum, several studies of varying quality have examined skin disorders associated with the use of mefloquine, but taken as a whole there is some evidence for an absence of increased risk of persistent skin and subcutaneous tissue disorders following use of mefloquine.

Wells et al. (2006) also reported hospitalizations for other system disorders among active-duty U.S. service members. In total, 135 hospitalizations for any cause were reported among mefloquine users, but there was no statistical differ-ence in the risk compared with deployed service members who were not prescribed an antimalarial. Hospitalizations related to categories of infections; neoplasms; disorders of endocrine, nutritional, or metabolism; disorders of the respiratory system; disorders of the genitourinary system; disorders of musculoskeletal and connective tissue; ill-defined conditions; and injury and poisoning were also examined and compared between mefloquine users and the two reference groups. Comparisons of mefloquine users with deployed service members who were not prescribed an antimalarial resulted in a mix of increased and decreased effect estimates for categories of neoplasms; disorders of endocrine, nutritional, or metabolism; disorders of the respiratory system; disorders of the genitourinary system; disorders of musculoskeletal and connective tissue; ill-defined condi-tions; and injury and poisoning, but none reached statistical significance. Although methodologically limited, Tan et al. (2017) reported that reproductive outcomes (miscarriage), infections (amebiasis, giardia, "other" and "any" gastrointestinal infection), and hematologic/oncologic disorders (breast cancer, gastric cancer, leukemia, liver cancer, lymphoma, prostate cancer, "other" and "any" cancers) were not statistically significantly different between users of mefloquine and the other antimalarial drugs for prophylaxis, but frequencies of such events or effect estimates were not provided. In sum, several categories of other outcomes were examined for differences in risk associated with use of mefloquine, and there is some limited evidence for an absence of increased risk of persistent adverse events for any of those categories of disorders following the use of mefloquine.

REFERENCES

Aarnoudse, A. L., R. H. van Schaik, J. Dieleman, M. Molokhia, M. M. van Riemsdijk, R. J. Ligthelm, D. Overbosch, I. P. van der Heiden, and B. H. Stricker. 2006. MDR1 gene polymorphisms are associated with neuropsychiatric adverse effects of mefloquine. *Clin Pharmacol Ther* 80(4):367-374.

Adamcova, M., M. T. Schaerer, I. Bercaru, I. Cockburn, H. G. Rhein, and P. Schlagenhauf. 2015. Eye disorders reported with the use of mefloquine (Lariam®) chemoprophylaxis—A drug safety database analysis. *Travel Med Infect Dis* 13(5):400-408.

Adegunloye, B. J., O. A. Sofola, and H. A. Coker. 1993. Relaxant effects of mefloquine on vascular smooth muscle in vitro. *Eur J Clin Pharmacol* 45(1):85-88.

Adshead, S. 2014. The adverse effects of mefloquine in deployed military personnel. *J R Nav Med Serv* 100(3):232-237.

Allison, D. W., R. S. Wilcox, K. L. Ellefsen, C. E. Askew, D. M. Hansen, J. D. Wilcox, S. S. Sandoval, D. L. Eggett, Y., Yanagawa, and S. C. Steffensen. 2011. Mefloquine effects on ventral tegmental area dopamine and GABA neuron inhibition: A physiologic role for connexin-36 GAP junctions. *Synapse* 65(8):804-813.

Aloisi, G. G., A. Barbafina, M. Canton, F. Dall'Acqua, F. Elisei, L. Facciolo, L. Latterini, and G. Viola. 2004. Photophysical and photobiological behavior of antimalarial drugs in aqueous solutions. *Photochem Photobiol* 79(3):248-258.

Andersson, H., H. H. Askling, B. Falck, and L. Rombo. 2008. Well-tolerated chemoprophylaxis uniformly prevented Swedish soldiers from *Plasmodium falciparum* malaria in Liberia, 2004-2006. *Mil Med* 173(12):1194-1198.

Arthur, J. D., P. Echeverria, G. D. Shanks, J. Karwacki, and L. Bodhidatta. 1990. Comparative study of gastrointestinal infections in United States soldiers receiving doxycycline or mefloquine for malaria prophylaxis. (Reannouncement with new availability information.) *Am J Trop Med Hyg* 43(6):608-613.

Ashley, E. A., K. Stepniewska, N. Lindegardh, R. McGready, R. Hutagalung, R. Hae, P. Singha-sivanon, N. J. White, and F. Nosten. 2006. Population pharmacokinetic assessment of a new regimen of mefloquine used in combination treatment of uncomplicated falciparum malaria. *Antimicrob Agents Chemother* 50(7):2281-2285.

Australia. 2018. *The use of the quinoline anti-malarial drugs mefloquine and tafenoquine in the Australian Defence Force.* December 2018. https://www.aph.gov.au/Parliamentary_Business/Committees/Senate/Foreign_Affairs_Defence_and_Trade/Mefloquine (accessed November 13, 2019).

Australian Department of Defence. n.d. *Mefloquine FAQs.* http://www.defence.gov.au/Health/HealthPortal/Malaria/Anti-malarial_medications/Mefloquine/FAQs.asp (accessed July 24, 2019).

Baker, P. G. 1996. An antimalarial malady. *Aust Fam Physician* 25(5):791.

Barraud de Lagerie, S., E. Comets, C. Gautrand, C. Fernandez, D. Auchere, E. Singlas, F. Mentre, and F. Gimenez. 2004. Cerebral uptake of mefloquine enantiomers with and without the P-gp inhibitor elacridar (GF1210918) in mice. *Br J Pharmacol* 141(7):1214-1222.

Barrett, P. J., P. D. Emmins, P. D. Clarke, and D. J. Bradley. 1996. Comparison of adverse events associated with use of mefloquine and combination of chloroquine and proguanil as antimalarial prophylaxis: Postal and telephone survey of travellers. *BMJ* 313(7056):525-528.

Baudry, S., Y. T. Pham, B. Baune, S. Vidrequin, C. Crevoisier, F. Gimenez, and R. Farinotti. 1997. Stereoselective passage of mefloquine through the blood–brain barrier in the rat. *J Pharm Pharmacol* 49(11):1086-1090.

BBC (British Broadcasting Corporation). 2016. *Ministry of Defence faces legal claims over malaria drug.* May 11. https://www.bbc.com/news/uk-36267818 (accessed November 13, 2019).

Bem, J. L., L. Kerr, and D. Stuerchler. 1992. Mefloquine prophylaxis: an overview of spontaneous reports of severe psychiatric reactions and convulsions. *J Trop Med Hyg* 95(3):167-179.

Beny, A., A. Paz, and I. Potasman. 2001. Psychiatric problems in returning travelers: Features and associations. *J Travel Med* 8(5):243-246.

Bijker, E. M., R. Schats, J. M. Obiero, M. C. Behet, G. J. Van Gemert, M. Van De Vegte-Bolmer, W. Graumans, L. Van Lieshout, G. J. H. Bastiaens, K. Teelen, C. C. Hermsen, A. Scholzen, L. G. Visser, and R. W. Sauerwein. 2014. Sporozoite immunization of human volunteers under mefloquine prophylaxis is safe, immunogenic and protective: A double-blind randomized controlled clinical trial. *PLOS ONE* 9(11):e112910.

Bissiere, S., M. Zelikowsky, R. Ponnusamy, N. S. Jacobs, H. T. Blair, and M. S. Fanselow. 2011. Electrical synapses control hippocampal contributions to fear learning and memory. *Science* 331(6013):87-91.

Bissinger, R., S. Barking, K. Alzoubi, G. Liu, G. Liu, and F. Lang. 2015. Stimulation of suicidal erythrocyte death by the antimalarial drug mefloquine. *Cell Physiol Biochem* 36(4):1395-1405.

Björkman, A., R. Steffan, M. Armengaud, N. Picot, and S. Piccoli. 1991. Malaria chemoprophylaxis with mefloquine. *Lancet* 337:1479-1480.

Blanco, C., N. Hoertel, M. M. Wall, S. Franco, H. Peyre, Y. Neria, L. Helpman, and F. Limosin. 2018. Toward understanding sex differences in the prevalence of posttraumatic stress disorder: Results from the National Epidemiologic Survey on Alcohol and Related Conditions. *J Clin Psychiatry* 79(2):16m11364.

Bloechliger, M., P. Schlagenhauf, S. Toovey, G. Schnetzler, I. Tatt, D. Tomianovic, S. S. Jick, and C. R. Meier. 2014. Malaria chemoprophylaxis regimens: A descriptive drug utilization study. *Travel Med Infect Dis* 12(6):718-725.

Borruat, F. X., B. Nater, L. Robyn, and B. Genton. 2001. Prolonged visual illusions induced by mefloquine (Lariam): A case report. *J Travel Med* 8(3):148-149.

Boudreau, E. F., L. W. Pang, S. Chaikummao, and C. Witayarut. 1991. Comparison of mefloquine, chloroquine plus pyrimethamine-sulfadoxine (Fansidar), and chloroquine as malarial prophylaxis in eastern Thailand. *Southeast Asian J Trop Med Public Health* 22(2):183-189.

Boudreau, E., B. Schuster, J. Sanchez, W. Novakowski, R. Johnson, D. Redmond, R. Hanson, and L. Dausel. 1993. Tolerability of prophylactic Lariam regimens. *Trop Med Parasitol* 44(3):257-265.

Breslau, N., L. Schultz, and E. Peterson. 1995. Sex differences in depression: A role for preexisting anxiety. *Psychiatry Res* 58(1):1-12.

Breslau, N., G. C. Davis, P. Andreski, E. L. Peterson, and L. R. Schultz. 1997. Sex differences in posttraumatic stress disorder. *Arch Gen Psychiatry* 54(11):1044-1048.

Briand, V., J. Bottero, H. Noel, V. Masse, H. Cordel, J. Guerra, H. Kossou, B. Fayomi, P. Ayemonna, N. Fievet, A. Massougbodji, and M. Cot. 2009. Intermittent treatment for the prevention of malaria during pregnancy in Benin: A randomized, open-label equivalence trial comparing sulfadoxine-pyrimethamine with mefloquine. *J Infect Dis* 200(6):991-1001.

Bunnag, D., S. Malikul, S. Chittamas, D. Chindanond, T. Harinasuta, M. Fernex, M. L. Mittelholzer, S. Kristiansen, and D. Sturchler. 1992. Fansimef for prophylaxis of malaria: A double-blind randomized placebo controlled trial. *Southeast Asian J Trop Med Public Health* 23(4):777-782.

Canada. 2017. *Surgeon General task force report on mefloquine.* June 1, 2017. https://www.canada.
ca/en/department-national-defence/corporate/reports-publications/health/surgeon-general-task-
force-report-on-mefloquine.html (accessed November 13, 2019).

Canadian Forces Health Services Group. 2017. *Mefloquine use in the Canadian Armed Forces.* https://
www.veterans.gc.ca/eng/about-vac/what-we-do/stakeholder-engagement/advisory-groups/men-
tal-health-advisory-group/06-29-2017 (accessed July 24, 2019).

Caridha, D., D. Yourick, M. Cabezas, L. Wolf, T. H. Hudson, and G. S. Dow. 2008. Mefloquine-
induced disruption of calcium homeostatis in mammalian cells is similar to that induced by
ionomycin. *Antimicrob Agents Chemother* 52(2):684-693.

Carme, B., C. Peguet, and G. Nevez. 1997. Compliance with and tolerance of mefloquine and
chloroquine + proguanil malaria chemoprophylaxis in French short-term travellers to sub-
Saharan Africa. *Trop Med Int Health* 2(10):953-956.

CDC (Centers for Disease Control and Prevention). 2019. *Malaria.* https://wwwnc.cdc.gov/travel/
yellowbook/2018/infectious-diseases-related-to-travel/malaria#1939 (accessed July 12, 2019).

CDC. n.d. *Medicines for the prevention of malaria while traveling: Mefloquine.* https://www.cdc.gov/
malaria/resources/pdf/fsp/drugs/mefloquine.pdf (accessed November 11, 2019).

Charles, B. G., A. Blomgren, P. E. Nasveld, S. J. Kitchener, A. Jensen, R. M. Gregory, B. Robertson,
I. E. Harris, M. P. Reid, and M. D. Edstein. 2007. Population pharmacokinetics of mefloquine
in military personnel for prophylaxis against malaria infection during field deployment. *Eur J
Clin Pharmacol* 63(3):271-278.

Chester, A. C., and P. Sandroni. 2011. Case report: Peripheral polyneuropathy and mefloquine
prophylaxis. *Am J Trop Med Hyg* 85(6):1008-1009.

Chevli, R., and C. D. Fitch. 1982. The antimalarial drug mefloquine binds to membrane phospholipids.
Antimicrob Agents Chemother 21(4):581-586.

Clyde, D. F., V. C. McCarthy, R. M. Miller, and R. B. Hornick. 1976. Suppressive activity of
mefloquine in sporozoite-induced human malaria. *Antimicrob Agents Chemother* 9(3):384-386.

Coker, S. J., A. J. Batey, I. D. Lightbown, M. E. Diaz, and D. A. Eisner. 2000. Effects of mefloquine
on cardiac contractility and electrical activity in vivo, in isolated cardiac preparations, and in
single ventricular myocytes. *Br J Pharmacol* 129(2):323-330.

Connolly, A. 2019. *Mefloquine lawsuits against federal government filed in court for military use
of drug.* https://globalnews.ca/news/5226181/mefloquine-lawsuits-canadian-forces (accessed
July 18, 2019).

CPRD (Clinical Practice Research Datalink). 2019. https://www.cprd.com (accessed October 16,
2019).

Croft, A. M. 2007. A lesson learnt: The rise and fall of Lariam and Halfan. *J R Soc Med* 100(4):170-174.

Croft, A. M., and P. Garner. 2000. Mefloquine for preventing malaria in non-immune adult travellers.
Cochrane Database Syst Rev 4(4):CD000138.

Croft, A. M., and K. G. Geary. 2001. The malaria threat. *Med Trop (Mars)* 61(1):63-66.

Croft, A. M., and A. Herxheimer. 2002. Adverse effects of the antimalaria drug, mefloquine: Due to
primary liver damage with secondary thyroid involvement? *BMC Public Health* 2:6.

Croft, A. M., T. C. Clayton, and M. J. World. 1997. Side effects of mefloquine prophylaxis for malaria:
An independent randomized controlled trial. *Trans R Soc Trop Med Hyg* 91(2):199-203.

Cruikshank, S. J., M. Hopperstad, M. Younger, B. W. Connors, D. C. Spray, and M. Srinivas. 2004.
Potent block of Cx36 and Cx50 gap junction channels by mefloquine. *Proc Natl Acad Sci USA*
101(33):12364-12369.

Cunningham, J., J. Horsley, D. Patel, A. Tunbridge, and D. G. Lalloo. 2014. Compliance with long-
term malaria prophylaxis in British expatriates. *Travel Med Infect Dis* 12(4):341-348.

Davis, T. M., L. G. Dembo, S. A. Kaye-Eddie, B. J. Hewitt, R. G. Hislop, and K. T. Batty. 1996.
Neurological, cardiovascular and metabolic effects of mefloquine in healthy volunteers:
A double-blind, placebo-controlled trial. *Br J Clin Pharmacol* 42(4):415-421.

de Vries, M., P. M. Soetekouw, D. M. J. W. Van, and G. Bleijenberg. 2000. Fatigue in Cambodia veterans. *QJM: Mon J Assoc Phys* 93(5):283-289.

Denoeud-Ndam, L., D. M. Zannou, C. Fourcade, C. Taron-Brocard, R. Porcher, F. Atadokpede, D. G. Komongui, L. Dossou-Gbete, A. Afangnihoun, N. T. Ndam, P. M. Girard, and M. Cot. 2014. Cotrimoxazole prophylaxis versus mefloquine intermittent preventive treatment to prevent malaria in HIV-infected pregnant women: Two randomized controlled trials. *J Acquir Immune Defic Syndr* 65(2):198-206.

DeSouza, J. M. 1983. Phase I clinical trial of mefloquine in Brazilian male subjects. *Bull WHO* 61(5):809-814.

Dietz, A., and L. Frolich. 2002. Mefloquine-induced paranoid psychosis and subsequent major depression in a 25-year-old student. *Pharmacopsychiatry* 35(5):200-202.

DoD (Department of Defense). 2003. *Memorandum on antimalarials and current practice in the military (July 31, 2003)*. Provided by COL Andrew Wiesen, M.D., M.P.H., director, preventive medicine, health readiness policy, and oversight, Office of the Assistant Secretary of Defense (Health Affairs), DoD, on August 22, 2019.

DoD. 2004. Mefloquine (Lariam®) information for military service members and their families (September 1, 2004). Provided by COL. Andrew Wiesen, M.D., M.P.H., director, preventive medicine, health readiness policy, and oversight, Office of the Assistant Secretary of Defense (Health Affairs), DoD, on June 10, 2019.

DoD. 2005a. Mefloquine (Lariam®) for leaders. Provided by COL Andrew Wiesen, M.D., M.P.H., director, preventive medicine, health readiness policy, and oversight, Office of the Assistant Secretary of Defense (Health Affairs), DoD, on June 10, 2019.

DoD. 2005b. Mod 7 to USCENTCOM individual protection and individual/unit deployment policy (January 1, 2005). Provided by COL Andrew Wiesen, M.D., M.P.H., director, preventive medicine, health readiness policy, and oversight, Office of the Assistant Secretary of Defense (Health Affairs), DoD, on June 10, 2019.

DoD. 2006. Third U.S. Army/USARCENT/CFLCC policy memorandum on malaria chemoprophylaxis (February 18, 2006; #SUR-01AFRD-SURG). Provided by COL Andrew Wiesen, M.D., M.P.H., director, preventive medicine, health readiness policy, and oversight, Office of the Assistant Secretary of Defense (Health Affairs), DoD, on August 22, 2019.

DoD. 2009a. Final report to congress. Adverse health events associated with use of anti-malarial drugs (October 2009). https://health.mil/Reference-Center/Reports/2010/07/08/Adverse-Health-Events-Associated-with-Use-of-AntiMalarial-Drugs (accessed November 25, 2019).

DoD. 2009b. Policy memorandum on the use of mefloquine (Lariam®) in malaria prophylaxis (September 4, 2009, #HA 09-017). Provided by COL Andrew Wiesen, M.D., M.P.H., director, preventive medicine, health readiness policy, and oversight, Office of the Assistant Secretary of Defense (Health Affairs), DoD, on January 25, 2019.

DoD. 2013a. Memorandum on guidance on medications for prophylaxis of malaria (April 15, 2013). Provided by COL Andrew Wiesen, M.D., M.P.H., director, preventive medicine, health readiness policy, and oversight, Office of the Assistant Secretary of Defense (Health Affairs), DoD, on January 25, 2019.

DoD. 2013b. Ceasing use of mefloquine in U.S. army special operations command units (September 13, 2013). Provided by COL Andrew Wiesen, M.D., M.P.H., director, preventive medicine, health readiness policy, and oversight, Office of the Assistant Secretary of Defense (Health Affairs), DoD, on August 22, 2019.

Dow, G. S., T. H. Hudson, M. Vahey, and M. L. Koenig. 2003. The acute neurotoxicity of mefloquine may be mediated through a disruption of calcium homeostasis and ER function in vitro. *Malar J* 2:14.

Dow, G. S., D. Caridha, M. Goldberg, L. Wolf, M. L. Koenig, D. L. Yourick, and Z. Wang. 2005. Transcriptional profiling of mefloquine-induced disruption of calcium homeostasis in neurons in vitro. *Genomics* 86(5):539-550.

Dow, G., R. Bauman, D. Caridha, M. Cabezas, F. Du, R. Gomez-Lobo, M. Park, K. Smith, and K. Cannard. 2006. Mefloquine induces dose-related neurological effects in a rat model. *Antimicrob Agents Chemother* 50(3):1045-1053.

Durrheim, D. N., S. Gammon, S. Waner, and L. E. Braack. 1999. Antimalarial prophylaxis—use and adverse events in visitors to the Kruger National Park. *S Afr Med J. Suid-Afrikaanse Tydskrif Vir Geneeskunde* 89(2):170-175.

Eamsila, C., P. Singharaj, P. Yooyen, P. Chatnugrob, A. Nopavong Na Ayuthya, H. K. Webster, R. Lasserre, M. L. Mittelholzer, and D. Sturchler. 1993. Prevention of *Plasmodium falciparum* malaria by Fansimef and Lariam in the northeastern part of Thailand. *Southeast Asian J Trop Med Public Health* 24(4):672-676.

Eaton, L. 1996. Adverse reactions. *Nurs Times* 92(24):16-17.

Eick-Cost, A. A., Z. Hu, P. Rohrbeck, and L. L. Clark. 2017. Neuropsychiatric outcomes after mefloquine exposure among U.S. military service members. *Am J Trop Med Hyg* 96(1):159-166.

Eid, R. S., A. R. Gobinath, and L. A. M. Galea. 2019. Sex differences in depression: Insights from clinical and preclinical studies. *Prog Neurobio* 176(2019):86-102.

El Harchi, A., M. J. McPate, Y. H. Zhang, H. Zhang, and J. C. Hancox. 2010. Action potential clamp and mefloquine sensitivity of recombinant "I KS" channels incorporating the V307L KCNQ1 mutation. *J Physiol Pharmacol* 61(2):123-131.

Even, C., S. Friedman, and K. Lanouar. 2001. Bipolar disorder after mefloquine treatment. *J Psychiatry Neurosci* 26(3):252-253.

FDA (Food and Drug Administration). 1989. Package insert for Lariam® (mefloquine hydrochloride) tablets. Provided by Kelly Cao, Pharm.D., safety evaluator team leader, Division of Pharmacovigilance II, Office of Pharmacovigilance and Epidemiology, Office of Surveillance and Epidemiology, Center for Drug Evaluation and Research, FDA, on March 20, 2019.

FDA. 2002. Package insert for Lariam® brand of mefloquine hydrochloride tablets. https://www.accessdata.fda.gov/scripts/cder/daf/index.cfm?event=BasicSearch.process (accessed June 13, 2019).

FDA. 2003a. Letter regarding Lariam® (mefloquine hydrochloride) tablets, 250 mg. https://www.accessdata.fda.gov/scripts/cder/daf/index.cfm?event=BasicSearch.process (accessed November 13, 2019).

FDA. 2003b. Package insert for Lariam® brand of mefloquine hydrochloride tablets. https://www.accessdata.fda.gov/scripts/cder/daf/index.cfm?event=BasicSearch.process (accessed June 13, 2019).

FDA. 2008. Package insert for Lariam® brand of mefloquine hydrochloride tablets. https://www.accessdata.fda.gov/scripts/cder/daf/index.cfm?event=BasicSearch.process (accessed June 13, 2019).

FDA. 2009. Package insert for Lariam® brand of mefloquine hydrochloride tablets. https://www.accessdata.fda.gov/scripts/cder/daf/index.cfm?event=BasicSearch.process (accessed June 13, 2019).

FDA. 2012. *A guide to drug safety terms at FDA*. https://www.fda.gov/media/74382/download (accessed July 8, 2019).

FDA. 2013a. FDA drug safety communication: FDA approves label changes for antimalarial drug mefloquine hydrochloride due to risk of serious psychiatric and nerve side effects. https://www.fda.gov/drugs/drug-safety-and-availability/fda-drug-safety-communication-fda-approves-label-changes-antimalarial-drug-mefloquine-hydrochloride (accessed November 25, 2019).

FDA. 2013b. Package insert for mefloquine hydrochloride tablets USP. https://www.accessdata.fda.gov/scripts/cder/daf/index.cfm?event=overview.process&ApplNo=076392 (accessed November 12, 2019).

FDA. 2016. Package insert for mefloquine hydrochloride tablets USP. https://dailymed.nlm.nih.gov/dailymed/drugInfo.cfm?setid=43fde257-36ee-49ea-a03c-01a1a4e1da3d (accessed June 25, 2019).

FDA. 2019a. Development & approval process: Drugs. https://www.fda.gov/drugs/development-approval-process-drugs (accessed November 12, 2019).

FDA. 2019b. Risk evaluation and mitigation strategies. https://www.fda.gov/drugs/drug-safety-and-availability/risk-evaluation-and-mitigation-strategies-rems (accessed December 3, 2019).

Fontaine, F., G. de Sousa, P. C. Burcham, P. Duchene, and R. Rahmani. 2000. Role of cytochrome P450 3A in the metabolism of mefloquine in human and animal hepatocytes. *Life Sci* 66(22):2193-2212.

Fujii, T., K. Kaku, T. Jelinek, and M. Kimura. 2007. Malaria and mefloquine prophylaxis use among Japan ground self-defense force personnel deployed in East Timor. *J Travel Med* 14(4):226-232.

Gimenez, F., R. A. Pennie, G. Koren, C. Crevoisier, I. W. Wainer, and R. Farinotti. 1994. Stereoselective pharmacokinetics of mefloquine in healthy Caucasians after multiple doses. *J Pharm Sci* 83(6):824-827.

Go, M. L., and T. L. Ngiam. 1997. Thermodynamics of partitioning of the antimalarial drug mefloquine in phospholipid bilayers and bulk solvents. *Chem Pharm Bull (Tokyo)* 45(12):20552060.

González, R., U. Hellgren, B. Greenwood, and C. Menéndez. 2014a. Mefloquine safety and tolerability in pregnancy: A systematic literature review. *Malar J* 13:75.

González, R., G. Mombo-Ngoma, S. Ouédraogo, M. A. Kakolwa, S. Abdulla, M. Accrombessi, J. J. Aponte, D. Akerey-Diop, A. Basra, V. Briand, M. Capan, M. Cot, A. M. Kabanywanyi, C. Kleine, P. G. Kremsner, E. Macete, J. R. Mackanga, A. Massougbodgi, A. Mayor, A. Nhacolo, G. Pahlavan, M. Ramharter, M. Rupérez, E. Sevene, A. Vala, R. Zoleko-Manego, and C. Menéndez. 2014b. Intermittent preventive treatment of malaria in pregnancy with mefloquine in HIV-negative women: A multicentre randomized controlled trial. *PLOS Med* 11(9):e1001733.

González, R., C. Pons-Duran, M. Piqueras, J. J. Aponte, F. O. Ter Kuile, and C. Menendez. 2018. Mefloquine for preventing malaria in pregnant women. *Cochrane Database Syst Rev* 3:CD011444.

Grabias, B., and S. Kumar. 2016. Adverse neuropsychiatric effects of antimalarial drugs. *Expert Opin Drug Saf* 15(7):903-910.

Gribble, F. M., T. M. Davis, C. E. Higham, A. Clark, and F. M. Ashcroft. 2000. The antimalarial agent mefloquine inhibits ATP-sensitive K-channels. *Br J Pharmacol* 131(4):756-760.

Hale, B. R., S. Owusu-Agyei, D. J. Fryauff, K. A. Koram, M. Adjuik, A. R. Oduro, W. R. Prescott, J. K. Baird, F. Nkrumah, T., L. Ritchie, E. D. Franke, F. N. Binka, J. Horton, and S. L. Hoffman. 2003. A randomized, double-blind, placebo-controlled, dose-ranging trial of tafenoquine for weekly prophylaxis against *Plasmodium falciparum*. *Clin Infect Dis* 36(5):541-549.

Hanboonkunupakarn, B., R. W. van der Pluijm, R. Hoglund, S. Pukrittayakamee, M. Winterberg, M. Mukaka, N. Waithira, K. Chotivanich, P. Singhasivanon, N. J. White, A. M. Dondorp, J. Tarning, and P. Jittamala. 2019. Sequential open-label study of the safety, tolerability, and pharmacokinetic interactions between dihydroartemisinin-piperaquine and mefloquine in healthy Thai adults. *Antimicrob Agents Chemother* 63(8).

Handschin, J. C., M. Wall, R. Steffen, and D. Sturchler. 1997. Tolerability and effectiveness of malaria chemoprophylaxis with mefloquine or chloroquine with or without co-medication. *Journal of Travel Medicine* 4(3):121-127.

Heimgartner, E. 1986. Practical experience with mefloquine as an antimalarial. *Schweiz Rundsch Med Prax* 75(16):459-462.

Hellgren, U., V. H. Angel, Y. Bergqvist, A. Arvidsson, J. S. Forero-Gomez, and L. Rombo. 1990. Plasma concentrations of sulfadoxine-pyrimethamine and of mefloquine during regular long term malaria prophylaxis. *Trans R Soc Trop Med Hyg* 84(1):46-49.

Hellgren, U., I. Berggren-Palme, Y. Bergqvist, and M. Jerling. 1997. Enantioselective pharmacokinetics of mefloquine during long-term intake of the prophylactic dose. *Br J Clin Pharmacol* 44(2):119-124.

Helpman, L., X. Zhu, B. Suarez-Jimenez, A. Lazarov, C. Monk, and Y. Neria. 2017. Sex differences in trauma-related psychopathology: A critical review of neuroimaging literature (2014-2017). *Curr Psychiatry Rep* 19(12):104.

Heshmati, M., S. A. Golden, M. L. Pfau, D. J. Christoffel, E. L. Seeley, M. E. Cahill, L. A. Khibnik, and S. J. Russo. 2016. Mefloquine in the nucleus accumbens promotes social avoidance and anxiety-like behavior in mice. *Neuropharmacology* 101:351-357.

Higgins, J. P. T., T. Lasserson, J. Chandler, D. Tovey, and R. Churchill. 2019. Standards for the conduct of new Cochrane Intervention Reviews. In J. P. T. Higgins, T. Lasserson, J. Chandler, D. Tovey, and R. Churchill (eds.), *Methodological expectations of Cochrane intervention reviews*. London: Cochrane. Pp. C1-C75.

Hill, D. R. 2000. Health problems in a large cohort of Americans traveling to developing countries. *Journal of Travel Medicine* 7(5):259-266.

Hoebe, C., J. de Munter, and C. Thijs. 1997. Adverse effects and compliance with mefloquine or proguanil antimalarial chemoprophylaxis. *Eur J Clin Pharmacol* 52(4):269-275.

Hood, J. E., J. W. Jenkins, D. Milatovic, L. Rongzhu, and M. Aschner. 2010. Mefloquine induces oxidative stress and neurodegeneration in primary rat cortical neurons. *Neurotoxicology* 31(5):518-523.

Hopperus Buma, A. P., P. P. van Thiel, H. O. Lobel, C. Ohrt, E. J. van Ameijden, R. L. Veltink, D. C. Tendeloo, T. van Gool, M. D. Green, G. D. Todd, D. E. Kyle, and P. A. Kager. 1996. Long-term malaria chemoprophylaxis with mefloquine in Dutch marines in Cambodia. *J Infect Dis* 173(6):1506-1509.

Huzly, D., C. Schonfeld, W. Beuerle, and U. Bienzle. 1996. Malaria chemoprophylaxis in German tourists: A prospective study on compliance and adverse reactions. *J Travel Med* 3(3):148-155.

Jain, M., R. L. Nevin, and I. Ahmed. 2016. Mefloquine-associated dizziness, diplopia, and central serous chorioretinopathy: A case report. *J Med Case Rep* 10(1):305.

Janowsky, A., A. J. Eshleman, R. A. Johnson, K. M. Wolfrum, D. J. Hinrichs, J. Yang, T. M. Zabriskie, M. J. Smilkstein, and M. K. Riscoe. 2014. Mefloquine and psychotomimetics share neurotransmitter receptor and transporter interactions in vitro. *Psychopharmacology* 231(14):2771-2783.

Jaspers, C. A., A. P. Hopperus Buma, P. P. van Thiel, R. A. van Hulst, and P. A. Kager. 1996. Tolerance of mefloquine chemoprophylaxis in Dutch military personnel. *Am J Trop Med* Hyg 55(2):230-234.

Javorsky, D. J., G. Tremont, G. I. Keitner, and A. H. Parmentier. 2001. Cognitive and neuropsychiatric side effects of mefloquine. *J Neuropsychiatry Clin Neurosci* 13(2):302.

Jha, S., R. Kumar, and R. Kumar. 2006. Mefloquine toxicity presenting with polyneuropathy— A report of two cases in India. *Trans R Soc Trop Med Hyg* 100(6):594-596.

Kang, J., X. L. Chen, L. Wang, and D. Rampe. 2001. Interactions of the antimalarial drug mefloquine with the human cardiac potassium channels KvLQT1/minK and HERG. *J Pharmacol Exp Ther* 299(1):290-296.

Karbwang, J., and N. J. White. 1990. Clinical pharmacokinetics of mefloquine. *Clin Pharmacokinet* 19(4):264-279.

Karbwang, J., D. Bunnag, A. M. Breckenridge, and D. J. Back. 1987. The pharmacokinetics of mefloquine when given alone or in combination with sulphadoxine and pyrimethamine in Thai male and female subjects. *Eur J Clin Pharm* 32(2):173-177.

Kato, T., J. Okuda, D. Ide, K. Amano, Y. Takei, and Y. Yamaguchi. 2013. Questionnaire-based analysis of atovaquone-proguanil compared with mefloquine in the chemoprophylaxis of malaria in nonimmune Japanese travelers. *J Infect Chemother* 19(1):20-23.

Katsenos, S., K. Psathakis, M. I. Nikolopoulou, and S. H. Constantopoulos. 2007. Mefloquine-induced eosinophilic pneumonia. *Pharmacotherapy* 27(12 I):1767-1771.

Kessler, R. C., K. A. McGonagle, M. Swartz, D. G. Blazer, and C. B. Nelson. 1993. Sex and depression in the National Comorbidity Survey. I: Lifetime prevalence, chronicity and recurrence. *J Affect Disord* 29(2-3):85-96.

Kitchener, S., P. Nasveld, S. Bennett, and J. Torresi. 2005. Adequate primaquine for vivax malaria. *J Travel Med* 12(3):133-135.

Kollaritsch, H., J. Karbwang, G. Wiedermann, A. Mikolasek, K. Na-Bangchang, and W. H. Wernsdorfer. 2000. Mefloquine concentration profiles during prophylactic dose regimens. *Wien Klin Wochenschr* 112(10):441-447.

Korhonen, C., K. Peterson, C. Bruder, and P. Jung. 2007. Self-reported adverse events associated with antimalarial chemoprophylaxis in Peace Corps volunteers. *Am J Prev Med* 33(3):194-199.

Kozarsky, P., and M. Eaton. 1993. Use of mefloquine for malarial chemoprophylaxis in its first year of availability in the United States. *Clin Infect Dis* 16(1):185-186.

Landman, K. Z., K. R. Tan, and P. M. Arguin. 2014. Adherence to malaria prophylaxis among Peace Corps volunteers in the Africa region, 2013. *Travel Med Infect Dis* 13:61-68.

Laothavorn, P., J. Karbwang, K. Na Bangchang, D. Bunnag, and T. Harinasuta. 1992. Effect of mefloquine on electrocardiographic changes in uncomplicated falciparum malaria patients. *Southeast Asian J Trop Med Public Health* 23(1):51-54.

Laverone, E., S. Boccalini, A. Bechini, S. Belli, M. G. Santini, S. Baretti, G. Circelli, F. Taras, S. Banchi, and P. Bonanni. 2006. Travelers' compliance to prophylactic measures and behavior during stay abroad: Results of a retrospective study of subjects returning to a travel medicine center in Italy. *J Travel Med* 13(6):338-344.

Leggat, P. A. 2005. Trends in antimalarial prescriptions in Australia from 1998 to 2002. *J Travel Med* 12(6):338-342.

Leggat, P. A., and R. Speare. 2003. Trends in antimalarial drugs prescribed in Australia 1992 to 1998. *J Travel Med* 10(3):189-191.

Lobel, H. O., K. W. Bernard, S. L. Williams, A. W. Hightower, L. C. Patchen, and C. C. Campbell. 1991. Effectiveness and tolerance of long-term malaria prophylaxis with mefloquine. Need for a better dosing regimen. *JAMA* 265(3):361-364.

Lobel, H. O., M. Miani, T. Eng, K. W. Bernard, A. W. Hightower, and C. C. Campbell. 1993. Long-term malaria prophylaxis with weekly mefloquine. *Lancet* 341(8849):848-851.

Lobel, H. O., P. E. Coyne, and P. J. Rosenthal. 1998. Drug overdoses with antimalarial agents: Prescribing and dispensing errors. *JAMA* 280(17):1483.

Lobel, H. O., M. A. Baker, F. A. Gras, G. M. Stennies, P. Meerburg, E. Hiemstra, M. Parise, M. Odero, and P. Waiyaki. 2001. Use of malaria prevention measures by North American and European travelers to East Africa. *J Travel Med* 8(4):167-172.

Looareesuwan, S., N. J. White, D. A. Warrell, I. Forgo, U. G. Dubach, U. B. Ranalder, and D. E. Schwartz. 1987. Studies of mefloquine bioavailability and kinetics using a stable isotope technique: Comparison of Thai patients with falciparum malaria and healthy Caucasian volunteers. *Br J Clin Pharmacol* 24:37-42.

López-Izquierdo, A., D. Ponce-Balbuena, E. G. Moreno-Galindo, I. A. Aréchiga-Figueroa, M. Rodríguez-Martínez, T. Ferrer, A. A. Rodríguez-Menchaca, and J. A. Sánchez-Chapula. 2011. The antimalarial drug mefloquine inhibits cardiac inward rectifier K+ channels: Evidence for interference in PIP2-channel interaction. *J Cardiovasc Pharmacol* 57(4):407-415.

Luxton, D. D., N. A. Skopp, and S. Maguen. 2010. Gender differences in depression and PTSD symptoms following combat exposure. *Depress Anxiety* 27(11):1027-1033.

Maertens, C., L. Wei, G. Droogmans, and B. Nilius. 2000. Inhibition of volume-regulated and calcium-activated chloride channels by the antimalarial mefloquine. *J Pharmacol Exp Ther* 295(1):29-36.

Martinez-Wittinghan, F. J., M. Srinivas, C. Sellitto, T. W. White, and R. T. Mathias. 2006. Mefloquine effects on the lens suggest cooperative gating of gap junction channels. *J Membr Biol* 211(3):163-171.

Matsumura, T., T. Fujii, T. Miura, T. Koibuchi, T. Endo, H. Nakamura, T. Odawara, A. Iwamoto, and T. Nakamura. 2005. Questionnaire-based analysis of mefloquine chemoprophylaxis for malaria in a Japanese population. *J Infect Chemother* 11(4):196-198.

McArdle, J. J., L. C. Sellin, K. M. Coakley, J. G. Potian, M. C. Quinones-Lopez, C. A. Rosenfeld, L. G. Sultatos, and K. Hognason. 2005. Mefloquine inhibits cholinesterases at the mouse neuromuscular junction. *Neuropharmacology* 49(8):1132-1139.

McCarthy, S. 2015. Malaria prevention, mefloquine neurotoxicity, neuropsychiatric illness, and risk–benefit analysis in the Australian Defence Force. *J Parasitol Res* 2015:287651.

McEvoy, K., B. Anton, and M. S. Chisolm. 2015. Depersonalization/derealization disorder after exposure to mefloquine. *Psychosomatics* 56(1):98-102.

Meier, C. R., K. Wilcock and S. S. Jick. 2004. The risk of severe depression, psychosis or panic attacks with prophylactic antimalarials. *Drug Saf* 27(3):203-213.

Meszaros, K., and S. Kasper. 1996. Psychopathological phenomena in long-term follow-up of acute psychosis after preventive mefloquine (Lariam) administration. *Nervenarzt* 67(5):404-406.

Milatovic, D., J. W. Jenkins, J. E. Hood, Y. Yu, L. Rongzhu, and M. Aschner. 2011. Mefloquine neurotoxicity is mediated by non-receptor tyrosine kinase. *Neurotoxicology* 32(5):578-585.

Mimica, I., W. Fry, G. Eckert, and D. E. Schwartz. 1983. Multiple-dose kinetic study of mefloquine in healthy male volunteers. *Chemotherapy* 29(3):184-187.

Motten, A. G., L. J. Martinez, N. Holt, R. H. Sik, K. Reszka, C. F. Chignell, H. H. Tonnesen, and J. E. Roberts. 1999. Photophysical studies on antimalarial drugs. *Photochem Photobiol* 69(3):282-287.

Nasveld, P. E., M. D. Edstein, M. Reid, L. Brennan, I. E. Harris, S. J. Kitchener, P. A. Leggat, P. Pickford, C. Kerr, C. Ohrt, W. Prescott, and the Tafenoquine Study Team. 2010. Randomized, double-blind study of the safety, tolerability, and efficacy of tafenoquine versus mefloquine for malaria prophylaxis in nonimmune subjects. *Antimicrob Agents Chemother* 54(2):792-798.

Nencini, C., L. Barberi, F. M. Runci, and L. Micheli. 2008. Retinopathy induced by drugs and herbal medicines. *Eur Rev Med Pharmacol Sci* 12(5):293-298.

Nevin, R. L. 2010. Mefloquine prescriptions in the presence of contraindications: Prevalence among U.S. military personnel deployed to Afghanistan, 2007. *Pharmacoepidemiol Drug Saf* 19(2):206-210.

Nevin, R. L. 2012. Limbic encephalopathy and central vestibulopathy caused by mefloquine: A case report. *Travel Med Infect Dis* 10(3):144-151.

Nevin, R. L., and J. M. Leoutsakos. 2017. Identification of a syndrome class of neuropsychiatric adverse reactions to mefloquine from latent class modeling of FDA adverse event reporting system data. *Drugs R&D* 17(1):199-210.

Nevin, R. L., P. P. Pietrusiak, and J. B. Caci. 2008. Prevalence of contraindications to mefloquine use among USA military personnel deployed to Afghanistan. *Malar J* 7:30.

Norris, F. H., M. J. Friedman, P. J. Watson, C. M. Byrne, E. Diaz, K. Kaniasty. 2002. 60,000 disaster victims speak: Part I. An empirical review of the empirical literature, 1981-2001. *Psychiatry* 65(3):207-239.

Nosten, F., F. ter Kuile, L. Maelankiri, T. Chongsuphajaisiddhi, L. Nopdonrattakoon, S. Tangkitchot, E. Boudreau, D. Bunnaq, and N. J. White. 1994. Mefloquine prophylaxis prevents malaria during pregnancy: A double blind, placebo-controlled study. *J Infect Dis* 69 (3):595-603.

Nosten, F., M. Vincenti, J. Simpson, P. Yei, K. L. Thwai, A. de Vries, T. Chongsuphajaisiddhi, and N. J. White. 1999. The effects of mefloquine treatment in pregnancy. *Clin Infect Dis* 28(4):808-815.

Novitt-Moreno, A., J. Ransom, G. Dow, B. Smith, L. T. Read, and S. Toovey. 2017. Tafenoquine for malaria prophylaxis in adults: An integrated safety analysis. *Travel Med Infect Dis* 17:19-27.

O'Faolain, A. 2019. *Retired solider sues over alleged impact of anti-malaria drug.* https://www.irishtimes.com/news/crime-and-law/courts/high-court/retired-soldier-sues-over-alleged-impact-of-anti-malaria-drug-1.3933560 (accessed July 18, 2019).

Ohrt, C., T. L. Richie, H. Widjaja, G. D. Shanks, J. Fitriadi, D. J. Fryauff, J. Handschin, D. Tang, B. Sandjaja, E. Tjitra, L. Hadiarso, G. Watt, and F. S. Wignall. 1997. Mefloquine compared with doxycycline for the prophylaxis of malaria in Indonesian soldiers: A randomized, double-blind, placebo-controlled trial. *Ann Intern Med* 126(12):963-972.

Olanrewaju, I. W., and L. Lin. 2000. Mefloquine chemoprophylaxis in Chinese railway workers on contract in Nigeria. *J Travel Med* 7(3):116-119.

Ollivier, L., K. Tifratene, R. Josse, A. Keundjian, and J. P. Boutin, 2004. The relationship between body weight and tolerance to mefloquine prophylaxis in non-immune adults: Results of a questionnaire-based study. *Ann Trop Med Parasit* 98(6):639-641.

Overbosch, D., H. Schilthuis, U. Bienzle, R. H. Behrens, K. C. Kain, P. D. Clarke, S. Toovey, J. Knobloch, H. D. Nothdurft, D. Shaw, N. S. Roskell, J. D. Chulay, and the Malarone International Study Team. 2001. Atovaquone-proguanil versus mefloquine for malaria prophylaxis in nonimmune travelers: Results from a randomized, double-blind study. *Clin Infect Dis* 33(7):1015-1021.

Palmer, K. J., S. M. Holliday, and R. N. Brogden. 1993. Mefloquine. A review of its antimalarial activity, pharmacokinetic properties and therapeutic efficacy. *Drugs* 45(3):430-475.

Pearlman, E. J., E. B. Doberstyn, S. Sudsok, W. Thiemanun, R. S. Kennedy, and C. J. Canfield. 1980. Chemosuppressive field trials in Thailand. IV. The suppression of *Plasmodium falciparum* and *Plasmodium vivax* parasitemias by mefloquine (WR 142,490, A 4-quinolinemethanol). *Am J Trop Med Hyg* 29(6):1131-1137.

Peetermans, W. E., and E. Van Wijngaerden. 2001. Implementation of pretravel advice: Good for malaria, bad for diarrhea. *Acta Clin Belg* 56(5):284-288.

Pennie, R. A., G. Koren, and C. Crevoisier. 1993. Steady state pharmacokinetics of mefloquine in long-term travellers. *Trans R Soc Trop Med Hyg* 87(4):459-462.

Peragallo, M. S., G. Sabatinelli, and G. Sarnicola. 1999. Compliance and tolerability of mefloquine and chloroquine plus proguanil for long-term malaria chemoprophylaxis in groups at particular risk (the military). *Trans R Soc Trop Med Hyg* 93(1):73-77.

Peragallo, M. S. 2001. The Italian army standpoint on malaria chemoprophylaxis. *Med Trop (Mars)* 61(1):59-62.

Perez-Cortes, E. J., A. A. Islas, J. P. Arevalo, C. Mancilla, E. Monjaraz, and E. M. Salinas-Stefanon. 2015. Modulation of the transient outward current (Ito) in rat cardiac myocytes and human Kv4.3 channels by mefloquine. *Toxicol Appl Pharmacol* 288(2):203-212.

Petersen, E., T. Ronne, A. Ronn, I. Bygbjerg, and S. O. Larsen. 2000. Reported side effects to chloroquine, chloroquine plus proguanil, and mefloquine as chemoprophylaxis against malaria in Danish travelers. *J Travel Med* 7(2):79-84.

Pham, Y. T., A. Regina, R. Farinotti, P. Couraud, I. W. Wainer, F. Roux, and F. Gimenez. 2000. Interactions of racemic mefloquine and its enantiomers with P-glycoprotein in an immortalised rat brain capillary endothelial cell line, GPNT. *Biochim Biophys Acta* 1524(2-3):212-219.

Phillips, M. A., and R. B. Kass. 1996. User acceptability patterns for mefloquine and doxycycline malaria chemoprophylaxis. *J Travel Med* 3(1):40-45.

Potasman, I., and H. Seligmann. 1998. A unique case of mefloquine-induced psoriasis. *J Travel Med* 5(3):156.

Potasman, I., A. Beny, and H. Seligmann. 2000. Neuropsychiatric problems in 2,500 long-term young travelers to the tropics. *J Travel Med* 7(1):5-9.

Potasman, I., Y. Juven, B. Weller, and E. Schwartz. 2002. Does mefloquine prophylaxis affect electroencephalographic patterns? *Am J Med* 112(2):147-149.

Reisinger, E. C., R. D. Horstmann, and M. Dietrich. 1989. Tolerance of mefloquine alone and in combination with sulfadoxine-pyrimethamine in the prophylaxis of malaria. *Trans R Soc Trop Med Hyg* 83(4):474-477.

Rendi-Wagner, P., H. Noedl, W. H. Wernsdorfer, G. Wiedermann, A. Mikolasek, and H. Kollaritsch. 2002. Unexpected frequency, duration and spectrum of adverse events after therapeutic dose of mefloquine in healthy adults. *Acta Trop* 81(2):167-173.

Rieckmann, K. H., A. E. Yeo, D. R. Davis, D. C. Hutton, P. F. Wheatley, and R. Simpson. 1993. Recent military experience with malaria chemoprophylaxis. *Med J Aust* 158(7):446-449.

Ringqvist, A., P. Bech, B. Glenthoj, and E. Petersen. 2015. Acute and long-term psychiatric side effects of mefloquine: A follow-up on Danish adverse event reports. *Travel Med Infect Dis* 13(1):80-88.

Rombo, L., V. H. Angel, G. Friman, U. Hellgren, M. L. Mittelholzer, and D. Sturchler. 1993. Comparative tolerability and kinetics during long-term intake of Lariam and Fansidar for malaria prophylaxis in nonimmune volunteers. *Trop Med Parasitol* 44(3):254-256.

Rupérez, M., R. González, G. Mombo-Ngoma, A. M. Kabanywanyi, E. Sevene, S. Ouédraogo, M. A. Kakolwa, A. Vala, M. Accrombessi, V. Briand, J. J. Aponte, Z. R. Manego, A. A. Adegnika, M. Cot, P. G. Kremsner, A. Massougbodji, S. Abdulla, M. Ramharter, E. Macete, and C. Menéndez. 2016. Mortality, morbidity, and developmental outcomes in infants born to women who received either mefloquine or sulfadoxine-pyrimethamine as intermittent preventive treatment of malaria in pregnancy: A cohort study. *PLOS Med* 13(2):e1001964.

Salako, L. A., R. A. Adio, O. Walker, A. Sowunmi, D. Sturchler, M. L. Mittelholzer, R. Reber-Liske, and U. Dickschat. 1992. Mefloquine-sulphadoxine-pyrimethamine (fansimef, roche) in the prophylaxis of *Plasmodium falciparum* malaria: A double-blind, comparative, placebo-controlled study. *Ann Trop Med Parasitol* 86(6):575-581.

Sanchez, J. L., R. F. DeFraites, T. W. Sharp, and R. K. Hanson. 1993. Mefloquine or doxycycline prophylaxis in U.S. troops in Somalia. *Lancet* 341:1021-1022.

Saunders, D. L., E. Garges, J. E. Manning, K. Bennett, S. Schaffer, A. J. Kosmowski, and A. J. Magill. 2015. Safety, tolerability, and compliance with long-term antimalarial chemoprophylaxis in American soldiers in Afghanistan. *Am J Trop Med Hyg* 93(3):584-590.

Schlagenhauf, P. 1999. Mefloquine for malaria chemoprophylaxis, 1992–1998: A review. *J Travel Med* 6(2):122-133.

Schlagenhauf, P., R. Steffen, H. Lobel, R. Johnson, R. Letz, A. Tschopp, N. Vranjes, Y. Bergqvist, O. Ericsson, U. Hellgren, L. Rombo, S. Mannino, J. Handschin, and D. Sturchler. 1996. Mefloquine tolerability during chemoprophylaxis: Focus on adverse event assessments, stereochemistry and compliance. *Trop Med Int Health* 1(4):485-494.

Schlagenhauf, P., H. Lobel, R. Steffen, R. Johnson, K. Popp, A. Tschopp, R. Letz, and C. Crevoisier. 1997. Tolerance of mefloquine by Swiss Air trainee pilots. *Am J Trop Med Hyg* 56(2):235-240.

Schlagenhauf, P., A. Tschopp, R. Johnson, H. D. Nothdurft, B. Beck, E. Schwartz, M. Herold, B. Krebs, O. Veit, R. Allwinn, and R. Steffen. 2003. Tolerability of malaria chemoprophylaxis in non-immune travellers to sub-Saharan Africa: Multicentre, randomised, double blind, four arm study. *BMJ* 327(7423):1078.

Schlagenhauf, P., R. Johnson, E. Schwartz, H. D. Nothdurft, and R. Steffen. 2009. Evaluation of mood profiles during malaria chemoprophylaxis: A randomized, double-blind, four-arm study. *J Travel Med* 16(1):42-45.

Schlagenhauf, P., M. Adamcova, L. Regep, M. T. Schaerer, and H. G. Rhein. 2010. The position of mefloquine as a 21st century malaria chemoprophylaxis. *Malar J* 9:357.

Schlagenhauf, P., W. A. Blumentals, P. Suter, L. Regep, G. Vital-Durand, M. T. Schaerer, M. S. Boutros, H. G. Rhein, and M. Adamcova. 2012. Pregnancy and fetal outcomes after exposure to mefloquine in the pre- and periconception period and during pregnancy. *Clin Infect Dis* 54(11):e124-e131.

Schlagenhauf, P., M. E. Wilson, A. Petersen, A. McCarthy, L. H. Chen, J. S. Keystone, P. E. Kozarsky, B. A. Connor, H. D. Nothdurft, M. Mendelson, and K. Leder. 2019. Malaria chemoprophylaxis. *J Travel Med* 4(15):145-167.

Schneider, C., M. Adamcova, S. S. Jick, P. Schlagenhauf, M. K. Miller, H. G. Rhein, and C. R. Meier. 2013. Antimalarial chemoprophylaxis and the risk of neuropsychiatric disorders. *Travel Med Infect Dis* 11(2):71-80.

Schneider, C., M. Adamcova, S. S. Jick, P. Schlagenhauf, M. K. Miller, H. G. Rhein, and C. R. Meier. 2014. Use of anti-malarial drugs and the risk of developing eye disorders. *Travel Med Infect Dis* 12(1):40-47.

Schneiderman, A. I., Y. S. Cypel, E. K. Dursa, and R. Bossarte. 2018. Associations between use of antimalarial medications and health among U.S. veterans of the wars in Iraq and Afghanistan. *Am J Trop Med Hyg* 99(3):638-648.

Schwartz, E., and G. Regev-Yochay. 1999. Primaquine as prophylaxis for malaria for nonimmune travelers: A comparison with mefloquine and doxycycline. *Clin Infect Dis* 29(6):1502-1506.

Schwartz, D. E., G. Eckert, and J. M. Ekue. 1987. Urinary excretion of mefloquine and some of its metabolites in African volunteers at steady state. *Chemother* 33(5):305-308.

Schwartz, E., F. Paul, H. Pener, S. Almog, M. Rotenberg, and J. Golenser. 2001. Malaria antibodies and mefloquine levels among United Nations troops in Angola. *J Travel Med* 8(3):113-116.

Sekine, S., E. E. Pinnow, E. Wu, R. Kurtzig, M. Hall, and G. J. Dal Pan. 2016. Assessment of the impact of scheduled postmarketing safety summary analyses on regulatory actions. *Clin Pharmacol Ther* 100(1):102-108.

Senarathna, S. M., M. Page-Sharp, and A. Crowe. 2016. The interactions of P-glycoprotein with antimalarial drugs, including substrate affinity, inhibition, and regulation. *PLOS ONE* 11(4):e0152677.

Senn, N., V. DAcremont, P. Landry, and B. Genton. 2007. Malaria chemoprophylaxis: What do the travelers choose, and how does pretravel consultation influence their final decision. *Am J Trop Med Hyg* 77(6):1010-1014.

Shanks, G. D. 1994. 1993 Sir Henry Wellcome Medal and Prize recipient. The rise and fall of mefloquine as an antimalarial drug in South East Asia. *Mil Med* 159(4):275-281.

Sharafeldin, E., D. Soonawala, J. P. Vandenbroucke, E. Hack, and L. G. Visser. 2010. Health risks encountered by dutch medical students during an elective in the tropics and the quality and comprehensiveness of pre-and post-travel care. *BMC Med Educ* 10:89.

Shin, J. H., S. J. Park, Y. K. Jo, E. S. Kim, H. Kang, J. H. Park, E. H. Lee, and D. H. Cho. 2012. Suppression of autophagy exacerbates mefloquine-mediated cell death. *Neurosci Lett* 515(2):162-167.

Smith, H. R., A. M. Croft, and M. M. Black. 1999. Dermatological adverse effects with the antimalarial drug mefloquine: A review of 74 published case reports. *Clin Exp Dermatol* 24(4):249-254.

Smoak, B. L., J. V. Writer, L. W. Keep, J. Cowan, and J. L. Chantelois. 1997. The effects of inadvertent exposure of mefloquine chemoprophylaxis on pregnancy outcomes and infants of US Army servicewomen. *J Infect Dis* 176(3):831-833.

Sonmez, A., A. Harlak, S. Kilic, Z. Polat, L. Hayat, O. Keskin, T. Dogru, M. I. Yilmaz, C. H. Acikel, and I. H. Kocar. 2005. The efficacy and tolerability of doxycycline and mefloquine in malaria prophylaxis of the ISAF troops in Afghanistan. *J Inf* 51(3):253-258.

Sossouhounto, R. T., B. N. Soro, A. Coulibaly, M. L. Mittelholzer, D. Stuerchler, and L. Haller. 1995. Mefloquine in the prophylaxis of *P. falciparum* malaria. *J Travel Med* 2(4):221-224.

Steffen, R., R. Heusser, R. Machler, R. Bruppacher, U. Naef, D. Chen, A. M. Hofmann, and B. Somaini. 1990. Malaria chemoprophylaxis among European tourists in tropical Africa: Use, adverse reactions, and efficacy. *Bull WHO* 68(3):313-322.

Steffen, R., E. Fuchs, J. Schildknecht, U. Naef, M. Funk, P. Schlagenhauf, P. Phillips-Howard, C. Nevill, and D. Sturchler. 1993. Mefloquine compared with other malaria chemoprophylactic regimens in tourists visiting east Africa. *Lancet* 341(8856):1299-1303.

Steketee, R. W., J. J. Wirima, W. L. Slutsker, C. O. Khoromana, J. G. Breman, and D. L. Heymann. 1996. Objectives and methodology in a study of malaria treatment and prevention in pregnancy in rural Malawi: The Mangochi Malaria Research Project. *Am J Trop Med Hyg* 55(1 Suppl):8-16.

Stürchler, D., J. Handschin, D. Kaiser, L. Kerr, M. L. Mittelholzer, R. Reber, and M. Fernex. 1990. Neuropsychiatric side effects of mefloquine. *N Engl J Med* 322(24):1752-1753.

Tan, K. R., S. J. Henderson, J. Williamson, R. W. Ferguson, T. M. Wilkinson, P. Jung, and P. M. Arguin. 2017. Long term health outcomes among returned Peace Corps volunteers after malaria prophylaxis, 19952014. *Travel Med Infect Dis* 17:50-55.

Tansley, R., J. Lotharius, A. Priestley, F. Bull, S. Duparc, and J. Mohrle. 2010. A randomized, double-blind, placebo-controlled study to investigate the safety, tolerability, and pharmacokinetics of single enantiomer (+)-mefloquine compared with racemic mefloquine in healthy persons. *Am J Trop Med Hyg* 83(6):1195-1201.

Terrell, A. G., M. E. Forde, R. Firth, and D. A. Ross. 2015. Malaria chemoprophylaxis and self-reported impact on ability to work: Mefloquine versus doxycycline. *J Travel Med* 22(6):383-388.

Thillainayagam, M., and S. Ramaiah. 2016. Mosquito, malaria and medicines—A review. *Res J Pharm Tech* 9(8):1268-1276.

Thompson, A. J., and S. C. Lummis. 2008. Antimalarial drugs inhibit human 5-HT(3) and GABA(A) but not GABA(C) receptors. *Br J Pharmacol* 153(8):1686-1696.

Tickell-Painter, M., N. Maayan, R. Saunders, C. Pace, and D. Sinclair. 2017a. Mefloquine for preventing malaria during travel to endemic areas. *Cochrane Database Syst Rev* 10:CD006491.

Tickell-Painter, M., R. Saunders, N. Maayan, V. Lutje, A. Mateo-Urdiales, and P. Garner. 2017b. Deaths and parasuicides associated with mefloquine chemoprophylaxis: A systematic review. *Travel Med Infect Dis* 20:5-14.

Todd, G. D., A. P. Hopperus Buma, M. D. Green, C. A. Jaspers, and H. O. Lobel. 1997. Comparison of whole blood and serum levels of mefloquine and its carboxylic acid metabolite. *Am J Trop Med Hyg* 57(4):399-402.

Toovey, S. 2009. Mefloquine neurotoxicity: A literature review. *Travel Med Infect Dis* 7(1):2-6.

Toovey, S., L. Y. Bustamante, A. C. Uhlemann, J. M. East, and S. Krishna. 2008. Effect of artemisinins and amino alcohol partner antimalarials on mammalian sarcoendoplasmic reticulum calcium adenosine triphosphatase activity. *Basic Clin Pharmacol Toxicol* 103(3):209-213.

Tran, T. M., J. Browning, and M. L. Dell. 2006. Psychosis with paranoid delusions after a therapeutic dose of mefloquine: A case report. *Malar J* 5:74.

Tuck, J., and J. Williams. 2016. Malaria protection in Sierra Leone during the Ebola outbreak 2014/15; The UK military experience with malaria chemoprophylaxis Sep 14–Feb 15. *Travel Med Infect Dis* 14(5):471-474.

Udry, E., F. Bailly, M. Dusmet, P. Schnyder, R. Lemoine, and J. W. Fitting. 2001. Pulmonary toxicity with mefloquine. *Eur Respir J* 18(5):890-892.

UK (United Kingdom). 2016. *An acceptable risk? The use of Lariam for military personnel. Fourth report of session 2015–16.* https://publications.parliament.uk (accessed November 13, 2019).

UK. 2019. *Mefloquine prescribing in the UK Armed Forces, 12 September–March 2019.* https://assets.publishing.service.gov.uk/government/uploads/system/uploads/attachment_data/file/801417/20190502-Official_Statistic_Mefloquine_Prescribing_in_the_UK_Armed_Forces.pdf (accessed November 13, 2019).

Unekwe, P. C., J. O. Ogamba, K. C. Chilaka, and J. C. Okonkwo. 2007. Effect of mefloquine on the mechanical activity of the mouse isolated rectal smooth muscle. *Niger J Physiol Sci* 22(1-2):43-47.

VA (Department of Veterans Affairs). 2004. Veterans Health Administration information letter on possible long-term health effects from the malarial prophylaxis mefloquine (Lariam) (June 23, 2004, Letter 10-2004-007). Provided by Peter D. Rumm, M.D., M.P.H., F.A.C.P.M., director, Pre-9/11 Era Environmental Health Program, on May 7, 2019.

van Riemsdijk, M. M., M. M. van der Klauw, J. A. van Heest, F. R. Reedeker, R. J. Ligthelm, R. M. Herings, and B. H. Stricker. 1997a. Neuro-psychiatric effects of antimalarials. *European Journal of Clinical Pharmacology* 52(1):1-6.

van Riemsdijk, M. M., M. M. van der Klauw, L. Pepplinkhuizen, and B. H. Stricker. 1997b. Spontaneous reports of psychiatric adverse effects to mefloquine in the Netherlands. *Br J Clin Pharmacol* 44(1):105-106.

van Riemsdijk, M. M., J. M. Ditters, M. C. Sturkenboom, J. H. Tulen, R. J. Ligthelm, D. Overbosch, and B. H. Stricker. 2002a. Neuropsychiatric events during prophylactic use of mefloquine before travelling. *European Journal of Clinical Pharmacology* 58(6):441-445.

van Riemsdijk, M. M., M. C. Sturkenboom, J. M. Ditters, R. J. Ligthelm, D. Overbosch, and B. H. Stricker. 2002b. Atovaquone plus chloroguanide versus mefloquine for malaria prophylaxis: A focus on neuropsychiatric adverse events. *Clin Pharm Ther* 72(3):294-301.

van Riemsdijk, M. M., M. C. Sturkenboom, J. M. Ditters, J. H. Tulen, R. J. Ligthelm, D. Overbosch, and B. H. Stricker. 2003. Low body mass index is associated with an increased risk of neuropsychiatric adverse events and concentration impairment in women on mefloquine. *Br J Clin Pharmacol* 57(4):506-512.

van Riemsdijk, M. M., M. C. Sturkenboom, J. M. Ditters, J. H. Tulen, R. J. Ligthelm, D. Overbosch, and B. H. Stricker. 2004. Low body mass index is associated with an increased risk of neuropsychiatric adverse events and concentration impairment in women on mefloquine. *Br J Clin Phar* 57(4):506-512.

van Riemsdijk, M. M., M. C. Sturkenboom, L. Pepplinkhuizen, and B. H. Stricker. 2005. Mefloquine increases the risk of serious psychiatric events during travel abroad: a nationwide case-control study in the Netherlands. *J Clin Psychiatry* 66(2):199-204.

Vanhauwere, B., H. Maradit, and L. Kerr. 1998. Post-marketing surveillance of prophylactic mefloquine (Lariam) use in pregnancy. *Am J Trop Med Hyg* 58(1):17-21.

Vilkman, K., S. H. Pakkanen, T. Laaveri, H. Siikamaki, and A. Kantele. 2016. Travelers' health problems and behavior: Prospective study with post-travel follow-up. *BMC Infectious Diseases* 16(1):328.

Vuurman, E. F., N. D. Muntjewerff, M. M. Uiterwijk, L. M. van Veggel, C. Crevoisier, L. Haglund, M. Kinzig, and J. F.O'Hanlon. 1996. Effects of mefloquine alone and with alcohol on psychomotor and driving performance. *Eur J Clin Pharmacol* 50(6):475-482.

Walker, R. A., and K. M. Colleaux. 2007. Maculopathy associated with mefloquine (Lariam) therapy for malaria prophylaxis. *Can J Ophthalmol* 42(1):125-126.

Wallace, M. R. 1996. Malaria among United States troops in Somalia. *Am J Med* 100(1):49-55.

Waner, S., D. Durrhiem, L. E. Braack, and S. Gammon. 1999. Malaria protection measures used by in-flight travelers to South African game parks. *J Travel Med* 6(4):254-257.

Watt-Smith, S., K. Mehta, and C. Scully. 2001. Mefloquine-induced trigeminal sensory neuropathy. *Oral Surg Oral Med Oral Pathol Oral Radiol Endod* 92(2):163-165.

Weinke, T., M. Trautmann, T. Held, G. Weber, D. Eichenlaub, K. Fleischer, W. Kern, and H. D. Pohle. 1991. Neuropsychiatric side effects after the use of mefloquine. *Am J Trop Med Hyg* 45(1):86-91.

Weiss, S. M., K. Benwell, I. A. Cliffe, R. J. Gillespie, A. R. Knight, J. Lerpiniere, A. Misra, R. M. Pratt, D. Revell, R. Upton, and C. T. Dourish. 2003. Discovery of nonxanthine adenosine A2A receptor antagonists for the treatment of Parkinson's disease. *Neurology* 61(11 Suppl 6):S101-S106.

Weissman, M. M., and G. L. Klerman. 1977. Sex differences and the epidemiology of depression. *Arch Gen Psychiatry* 34(1):98-111.

Wells, T. S., T. C. Smith, B. Smith, L. Z. Wang, C. J. Hansen, R. J. Reed, W. E. Goldfinger, T. E. Corbeil, C. N. Spooner, and M. A. Ryan. 2006. Mefloquine use and hospitalizations among U.S. service members, 2002–2004. *Am J Trop Med Hyg* 74(5):744-749.

Wernsdorfer, W. H., H. Noedl, P. Rendi-Wagner, H. Kollaritsch, G. Wiedermann, A. Mikolasek, J. Karbwang, and K. Na-Bangchang. 2013. Gender-specific distribution of mefloquine in the blood following the administration of therapeutic doses. *Malar J* 12:443.

Whitworth, A. B., and W. Aichhorn. 2005. First-time diagnosis of severe depression: Induced by mefloquine? *J Clin Psychopharmacol* 25(4):399-400.

WHO (World Health Organization). 1983. Development of mefloquine as an antimalarial drug. *Bull WHO* 61(2):169-178.

Wiesen, A. 2019. Overview of DoD antimalarial use policies. Presentation to the Committee to Review Long-Term Health Effects of Antimalarial Drugs on January 28, 2019.

Wittes, R. C., and R. Saginur. 1995. Adverse reaction to mefloquine associated with ethanol ingestion. *CMAJ* 152(4):515-517.

Zhou, C., C. Xiao, J. J. McArdle, and J. H. Ye. 2006. Mefloquine enhances nigral gamma-aminobutyric acid release via inhibition of cholinesterase. *J Pharmacol Exp Ther* 317(3):1155-1160.

5

Tafenoquine

Tafenoquine, an 8-aminoquinoline, was discovered in 1978 by the Walter Reed Army Institute of Research during a search for a safer, more effective, and longer-acting drug than primaquine (Ebstie et al., 2016; Shanks and Edstein, 2005). The institute partnered with GlaxoSmithKline and Medicines for Malaria Venture to develop the drug (Ebstie et al., 2016). In July 2018 the Food and Drug Administration (FDA) new drug application for Krintafel™ (tafenoquine 150 mg tablet) submitted by GlaxoSmithKline was approved for the radical cure (prevention of relapse) of *Plasmodium vivax* malaria in people receiving therapy for acute *P. vivax* infection (FDA, 2018a). In August 2018 FDA approved the new drug application submitted by 60 Degrees Pharmaceuticals for Arakoda™ (tafenoquine 100 mg tablet) for malaria prophylaxis for up to 6 months of continuous use in people aged 18 years and older (FDA, 2018b). The Arakoda™ approval was granted under FDA's priority review, an accelerated evaluation process for drugs that potentially offer significant improvements in the safety or effectiveness of a treatment or preventive agent when compared with standard applications (FDA, 2018c). The two drugs have the same composition but different formulations and indications; as malaria prophylaxis is the focus of the committee's assessment, its focus is on only Arakoda™. The three-decade lag between the drug's discovery and FDA approval has been attributed to tafenoquine being discovered at a time when less attention was paid to antimalarial drug development; in recent years, recognition of the global health implications of malaria has spurred development efforts (Baird, 2018).

Tafenoquine has activity against all pre-erythrocytic (liver) and erythrocytic (blood) stages of the *Plasmodium* species, including *P. falciparum* and *P. vivax*. Thus, like primaquine, it can be used as primary prophylaxis while in an endemic region, and it is also effective post-exposure (toward the end of or after a stay in an endemic region) for prophylactic presumptive anti-relapse therapy (PART), also called "terminal prophylaxis," owing to its ability to eliminate the hypnozoites of *P. falciparum* and *P. vivax* (FDA, 2018c). Hypnozoites, which are undetectable by diagnostic tests, can lie dormant in the liver for months to years and then differentiate, causing clinical malaria and enabling malaria transmission (Ackert et al., 2019; Rishikesh and Sarava, 2016). The FDA-approved malaria-prophylaxis regimen for tafenoquine is a loading dose of 200 mg (2 × 100 mg tablet) once daily for 3 days before travel to a malaria-endemic area, followed by a maintenance dose of 200 mg once weekly while in the malaria area, followed by one 200 mg dose 7 days after the last maintenance dose (FDA, 2018d); this dosage is also recommended by the Centers for Disease Control and Prevention (Haston et al., 2019). Studies of other drugs for malaria prophylaxis in U.S. soldiers suggest that antimalarials with a weekly regimen may yield higher adherence rates than regimens requiring more frequent dosing (Sánchez et al., 1993; Saunders et al., 2015).

Because tafenoquine is a newly approved drug, published data containing information on adverse effects are limited compared with what is available for drugs that have been in use longer. In an effort to include any data that might inform its understanding of adverse effects that could be associated with the use of tafenoquine, the committee reviewed certain types of evidence that were not included in other drug chapters; the reasoning for each inclusion will be addressed in the section in which the evidence appears. This chapter begins with information from the tafenoquine package insert and label, with emphasis on the Contraindications and Warnings, Precautions, and Drug Interactions sections. This is followed by summaries of findings and conclusions regarding the use of tafenoquine in military forces as reported by U.S. and foreign governments. The pharmacokinetic properties of tafenoquine are then described before a summary of the known concurrent adverse events associated with use of tafenoquine when used as directed for prophylaxis. Most of the chapter is dedicated to summarizing and assessing the seven identified epidemiologic studies that contributed some information on persistent or latent health outcomes following cessation of tafenoquine. These are ordered by population, with studies of military and veterans first, followed by studies with research volunteers. A table that gives a high-level comparison of each of the seven epidemiologic studies that examined the use of tafenoquine and that met the committee's inclusion criteria is presented in Appendix C. Supplemental supporting evidence is then presented, beginning with other identified studies of health outcomes in populations that used tafenoquine for prophylaxis but that did not meet the committee's inclusion criteria regarding the timing of follow-up, followed by case reports of persistent adverse events associated with tafenoquine use and adverse events findings from treatment trials. Information on adverse events associated with tafenoquine use in specific groups, including women and women who are pregnant, is presented. After the primary and supplemental evidence in humans has been presented, supporting literature from experimental animal and in vitro studies is then summarized. The chapter ends with a synthesis of all of the evidence presented along with the inferences and conclusions that the committee made from the available evidence, organized by health outcome category.

FOOD AND DRUG ADMINISTRATION PACKAGE INSERT FOR TAFENOQUINE

This section describes selected information found in the FDA label or package insert for tafenoquine (Arakoda™); since tafenoquine was approved in 2018, FDA has issued only one label. The information from the insert is followed by a brief synopsis of drug interactions known or presumed to occur with concurrent tafenoquine use.

Contraindications, Warnings, and Precautions

The FDA package insert states that in five clinical prophylaxis trials in which participants received the FDA-approved tafenoquine loading and maintenance dosing regimen (200 mg for 3 days, followed by 200 mg weekly) (n = 825), the most common "selected" adverse reactions (incidence $\geq 1\%$) were headache, dizziness, back pain, diarrhea, nausea, vomiting, increased alanine aminotransferase, motion sickness, insomnia, depression, abnormal dreams, and anxiety (FDA, 2018d). These five clinical trials are referred to in this section as the "safety set."

According to the FDA package insert, contraindications to tafenoquine include glucose-6-phosphate dehydrogenase (G6PD) deficiency (see Chapter 2) or unknown G6PD status, due to the risk of hemolytic anemia, and breastfeeding by a lactating woman when the infant is found to be G6PD deficient or if the G6PD status of the infant is unknown (FDA, 2018d). Tafenoquine should be administered only to those with a safe level of G6PD activity (see Chapter 2). If severe hemolytic anemia is not treated or controlled, it can lead to serious complications, including arrhythmias, cardiomyopathy, heart failure, and death (Baird, 2019; NIH, n.d.). Qualitative G6PD tests are sufficient to diagnose G6PD deficiency in males, but quantitative G6PD testing is necessary to differentiate G6PD statuses (deficient, intermediate, normal) in females (Chu et al., 2018). Testing for G6PD deficiency is mandatory before prescribing tafenoquine (FDA, 2018d). Because tafenoquine is contraindicated with G6PD deficiency, the committee did not review this adverse event in depth.

A history of psychotic disorders or current psychotic symptoms (i.e., hallucinations, delusions, or grossly disorganized behavior) is a contraindication for tafenoquine (FDA, 2018d). Users are also warned that because of the long half-life of tafenoquine (approximately 17 days), the signs or symptoms of psychiatric adverse reactions could be delayed in onset or duration. The FDA package insert states, "If psychotic symptoms (hallucinations, delusions, or grossly disorganized thinking or behavior) occur, consider discontinuation of Arakoda™ and prompt evaluation by a mental health professional as soon as possible. Other psychiatric symptoms, such as changes in mood, anxiety, insomnia, and nightmares, should be promptly evaluated by a medical professional if they are moderate and last more than three days or are severe." The package insert notes that psychiatric adverse reactions in participants receiving tafenoquine in clinical trials included sleep disturbances (2.5%), depression/depressed mood (0.3%), and anxiety (0.2%), and that tafenoquine was discontinued in one participant who attempted suicide (0.1%); however, the source of these data is not cited.

Known hypersensitivity reactions to tafenoquine, other 8-aminoquinolines, or any component of tafenoquine (FDA, 2018d) are also a contraindication. The FDA package insert's Warnings and Precautions section alerts against contraindication-associated conditions and disorders as well as methemoglobinemia and further warns that because of tafenoquine's long half-life, hemolytic anemia, methemoglobinemia, and signs or symptoms of hypersensitivity reactions that may occur could be delayed in onset or duration.

Tafenoquine is associated with methemoglobinemia; persons with nicotinamide adenine dinucleotide (NADH)-dependent methemoglobin reductase deficiency should be monitored and should stop the drug and seek medical attention if signs of methemoglobinemia occur (FDA, 2018d). Methemoglobinemia results from increased levels of methemoglobin (>1%) in red blood cells, which can result in decreased availability of oxygen to tissues (Denshaw-Burke et al., 2018). High levels of methemoglobin (>15%) can lead to complications, including abnormal cardiac rhythms, altered mental status, delirium, seizures, coma, and profound acidosis; if the levels exceed 70%, death can occur.

Methemoglobinemia, which is usually mild and reversible, is a well-characterized feature in recipients of 8-aminoquinolines at therapeutic dosing (Baird, 2019). Tafenoquine is associated with decreases in hemoglobin, and decreases ≥3 g/dL were observed in 2.3% of tafenoquine recipients in the safety set (FDA, 2018d). The package insert notes that in the safety set, symptomatic elevations in methemoglobin occurred in 13% of tafenoquine recipients and hemoglobin decreases ≥3 g/dL occurred in 2.3%. However, no additional information is provided on what the starting or ending hemoglobin values were or whether they were outside of the normal hemoglobin ranges.

The "hypersensitivity reactions" referred to in the FDA package insert's Contraindications and Warnings/Precautions sections are not defined other than by referring to urticaria and angioedema as two examples and directing the reader to the "6.1. Clinical Trials Experience" section (FDA, 2018d). Section 6.1 provides data based on six trials: the safety set trials and one additional trial (NCT #01290601) in which participants received 400 mg of tafenoquine for 3 days to treat *P. vivax* (NIH, 2018). No adverse events are characterized as "hypersensitivity reactions"; "hypersensitivity" is listed as an adverse reaction within the category "Immune system disorders" among adverse reactions reported by <1% in the five prophylaxis trials.

The FDA package insert reported that in a pooled analysis of four of the five safety set trials (Hale et al., 2003; Leary et al., 2009; Shanks et al., 2001; Study 030, unpublished), the incidence of diarrhea was 5% in tafenoquine recipients, compared with 1% in mefloquine recipients and 3% in placebo recipients (FDA, 2018d). Serious gastrointestinal adverse events included one participant each with abdominal pain, diarrhea, upper abdominal pain, and irritable bowel syndrome.

The package insert (FDA, 2018d) states that vortex keratopathy[1] was reported in 21–93% of tafenoquine recipients in three trials that included ophthalmic evaluations (Leary et al., 2009; Nasveld et al., 2010; NCT #0129060, a malaria treatment trial). The label notes further that the vortex keratopathy did not result in functional visual changes and resolved within 1 year of drug cessation, that retinal abnormalities occurred in less than 1% of the tafenoquine recipients, and that seven serious ocular adverse reactions were reported (five vortex keratopathy; two retinal disorders).

The FDA package insert also mentions other adverse events. It states that, based on a study of healthy adults who were administered 400 mg tafenoquine (twice the recommended dose for prophylaxis) for 3 days, the mean increase in the QTcF[2] interval for tafenoquine is less than 20 ms (FDA, 2018d). It states that the effects of tafenoquine have not been studied in people with renal or hepatic impairment (FDA, 2018d).

In addition, FDA required that pharmacists provide a medication guide—a paper handout that conveys risk information that is specific to a particular drug or drug class—to persons to whom tafenoquine is dispensed (FDA, 2012, 2018b). The medication guide alerts consumers to the most important information about a drug, including serious side effects. For tafenoquine (Arakoda™), these serious side effects include hemolytic anemia, methemoglobinemia, and mental health symptoms (FDA, 2018d).

---

[1] Vortex keratopathy manifests as a whorl-like pattern of deposits in the inferior interpalpebral portion of the cornea. Certain medications bind with the cellular lipids of the basal epithelial layer of the cornea due to their cationic, amphiphilic properties. It is rare for these deposits to result in a reduction in visual acuity or ocular symptoms, although this has occurred. The deposits typically resolve with discontinuation of the medications (AAO, 2019).

[2] The QT interval is a measure of the duration of ventricular repolarization, approximating the time interval between the start and end of repolarization of the ventricular myocardium. QT prolongation is associated with a risk for cardiac arrhythmias because it can lead to early-after depolarizations, provoke Torsades des Pointes, and lead to ventricular fibrillation, resulting in sudden cardiac death. A corrected QT is QTc. QTcF refers to a QT interval corrected using the Fridericia formula (Vandenberk et al., 2016).

Drug Interactions

Tafenoquine inhibited metformin transport via human organic cation transporter-2 (OCT2), multidrug and toxin extrusion-1 (MATE1), and MATE2-K transporters (FDA, 2018d). The effect of co-administration of tafenoquine on the pharmacokinetics of OCT2 and MATE1 substrates in humans is unknown (FDA, 2018c). In vitro studies show a potential for increased concentrations of OCT2 and MATE substrates that may increase the risk of toxicity of these drugs. Co-administration with OCT2 and MATE substrates should be avoided. Among these drugs are the antidiabetic metformin; gastroesophageal proton-pump inhibitors (e.g., cimetidine, ranitidine); antivirals (e.g., lamivudine); the antiarrhythmic, dofetilide; and chemotherapeutics (e.g., cisplatin, oxaliplatin).

POLICIES AND INQUIRIES RELATED TO THE USE OF TAFENOQUINE BY MILITARY FORCES

A December 2019 Department of Defense (DoD) Defense Health Agency document outlines policy for the force health protection use of tafenoquine for malaria prophylaxis in U.S. service members (DoD, 2019). The issuance states that tafenoquine "is an acceptable alternative medication" for primary prophylaxis in areas where chloroquine-sensitive malaria is present if intolerance or contraindications to chloroquine, atovaquone/proguanil (A/P), and doxycycline are documented; similarly, "it may be considered" in areas where chloroquine-resistant malaria is present for those with contraindications or intolerance to A/P and doxycycline. The dosage is 200 mg once daily for 3 days before entering a malaria-endemic area, 200 mg weekly as a maintenance regimen, and one 200 mg dose 7 days after the last maintenance dose. The policy instructs that testing for G6PD deficiency is mandatory for personnel deploying to areas requiring tafenoquine or primaquine. As tafenoquine is an FDA-approved drug, military health-system providers are permitted to prescribe it to service members on an individualized basis.[3] In addition to being effective against all stages of all *Plasmodium* species, an effective hypnozoiticide is of particular value to the U.S. military because *P. vivax* is endemic in Southeast Asia (CDC, 2019; Howes et al., 2016), where military operations occur. Examples include Afghanistan, where *P. vivax* represents 95% of malaria cases, and Iraq, where the 1991 Gulf War led to a years-long resurgence of *P. vivax* (CDC, 2019; Schlagenhauf, 2003).

The Australian Senate performed an investigation into the possible association of tafenoquine with adverse effects, particularly neuropsychiatric effects, when used for malaria prophylaxis by its military forces (Australia, 2018). Because

---

[3] Personal communications to the committee, COL Andrew Wiesen, M.D., M.P.H., Director, Preventive Medicine, Health Readiness Policy, and Oversight, Office of the Assistant Secretary of Defense (Health Affairs), April 16, 2019, and December 11, 2019.

tafenoquine was not approved for use as malaria prophylaxis by the Australian Therapeutic Goods Administration until September 2018 (ATGA, 2019), studies of tafenoquine were conducted as clinical trials in Australian military service members from as early as 1998 (Nasveld et al., 2002). As part of its inquiry, the Australian Senate commissioned a literature review on the impact of quinoline antimalarials and a research study that involved a re-analysis of health study data on antimalarial use from the 2007–2008 Centre for Military and Veterans' Health deployment-health studies (Australia, 2018). It heard or reviewed submitted testimony from government agencies (Department of Defence, Department of Health, Department of Veterans' Affairs, Australian Defence Force Malaria and Infectious Disease Institute, Indo-Pacific Centre for Health Security, Department of Foreign Affairs and Trade Repatriation Medical Authority); malaria-control organizations (Asia Pacific Leaders Malaria Alliance); professional medical associations (Australasian Society for Infectious Diseases, Australasian College of Tropical Medicine, Royal Australian College of General Practitioners); advocate organizations (Australian Quinoline Veterans and Families Association, Quinism Foundation, Defence Force Welfare Association, Royal Australian Regiment Corporation, RSL National); product development partnerships, pharmaceutical manufacturers, and their partner organizations (Medicines for Malaria Venture, National Health and Medical Research Council, Biocelect, GlaxoSmithKline, 60 Degrees Pharmaceuticals, Roche); and roughly 25 individuals, including physicians, academics, and veterans. In submitted testimony, a collection of adverse events (psychiatric disorders, cognitive impairments, hearing problems, vestibular disorders, neurologic disorders) reported to be due to the use of tafenoquine was referred to as "quinoline poisoning" and "an acquired brain injury" by the Australian Quinoline Veterans and Families Association, and as "chronic quinoline encephalopathy" or "neuropsychiatric quinism" by the U.S.-based Quinism Foundation. Some veterans attributed their symptoms to tafenoquine use that had occurred 15 or more years before (Australia, 2018). In the report summary, however, the Senate committee did not agree with these claims. While the committee acknowledged that its members were not medical experts, it stated, "The weight of prevailing medical evidence provided to the committee in response to these claims is that … there is no compelling evidence that tafenoquine causes long term effects" and explained that the committee had been informed that there was no definitive evidence to support the claim that tafenoquine use results in acquired brain injury. It stated that while it believed that the symptoms were being experienced by individuals, assigning a single cause to these illnesses did not take into account the multiple possible contributors to their health while they took the drug and in the years after. The committee recommended that the Australian Department of Veterans' Affairs expedite its investigation into antimalarial claims logged since September 2016 and that it offer assistance to claimants and facilitate their access to legal representation. The Australian Senate committee also made recommendations to ensure better access to care for sick veterans, including that the Australian Department of Veterans' Affairs prioritize developing a neurocognitive health program. It did not recommend that changes be made to military policy on antimalarial use. Tafenoquine can be prescribed for malaria prevention (under the name Kodatef™) to Australian service members (Australia, n.d.).

PHARMACOKINETICS

Tafenoquine is an antimalarial drug of the 8-aminoquinoline class, a synthetic analog of primaquine (Brueckner et al., 1998). It is a prodrug that requires activation through metabolism by CYP2D6 (Marcsisin et al., 2014). However, little metabolism was observed in vitro in human liver microsomes and hepatocytes (FDA, 2018d). The major route(s) of excretion of tafenoquine in humans is unknown. In healthy adults taking tafenoquine once daily for 3 days, unchanged tafenoquine was the only notable drug-related component observed in plasma at approximately 3 days after the first dose.

In a population pharmacokinetics study (Charles et al., 2007), tafenoquine concentrations were 321 ± 63 ng/mL when measured within 5% of the time of the estimated mean population T_{max} of 21.4 h in individuals given the clinically recommended 200 mg weekly dose of tafenoquine. The elimination half-life is approximately 14–17 days (Castelli et al., 2010; Edstein et al., 2001a,b; FDA, 2018d). Food appears to increase the amount but not the rate of tafenoquine absorption, and it has been suggested that the bioavailability of tafenoquine increases with a high-fat meal (Edstein et al., 2001b). In the majority of the clinical trials reviewed for FDA drug approval, tafenoquine was administered under fed conditions (FDA, 2018c). The FDA package insert states that the pharmacokinetics of tafenoquine were not significantly affected by age, sex, ethnicity, or body weight (FDA, 2018d). The effect of renal or hepatic impairment on tafenoquine pharmacokinetics is not known.

ADVERSE EVENTS

This section begins with a summary of the known concurrent adverse effects, such as those that occur immediately or within a few hours or days of taking a dose of tafenoquine. This information is derived from the FDA package insert, the FDA briefing document on tafenoquine, and an integrated safety analysis. Epidemiologic studies of persistent or latent health effects in which information was available at least 28 days post-tafenoquine-cessation are then summarized by population category (military or veterans, and research populations recruited for safety studies) with the emphasis of reported results being on those persistent or latent effects that were associated with use of tafenoquine (even if results on other antimalarial drug comparison groups were presented).

Concurrent Adverse Events

The committee was unable to identify any Cochrane reviews examining concurrent adverse events associated with tafenoquine when used for malaria prophylaxis. In an effort to include useful data, the committee reviewed and summarized information from the FDA briefing document on tafenoquine, which was prepared by FDA for panel members of the Antimicrobial Drugs Advisory Committee (FDA, 2018c) and contained a safety summary. In addition, an integrated safety analysis is summarized.

FDA Briefing Document

Data from five clinical trials in which tafenoquine recipients received FDA-approved prophylactic loading and maintenance dosages are presented both in the FDA package insert and in the FDA briefing document (FDA, 2018c,d). As before, this data set will be referred to as the safety set. The safety set included Nasveld et al. (2010), which compared tafenoquine with mefloquine in deployed Australian soldiers; Hale et al. (2003) and Study 030 (unpublished), which compared tafenoquine with mefloquine and placebo in residents of Ghana and Kenya, respectively; and Leary et al. (2009) and Shanks et al. (2001), which compared tafenoquine with placebo in U.S. and UK residents, and in residents of malaria-endemic Kenya, respectively (FDA, 2018c,d). For the analyses of the safety set, no formal hypothesis testing was noted, and no statistical comparisons were provided. Neither the package insert nor the FDA briefing document specify the timing of the adverse events summarized below.

The FDA briefing document noted that systematic monitoring for neurologic symptoms, such as actively asking participants about symptoms, was not performed for the safety set trials. In an analysis of the safety set (tafenoquine group, n = 825), the incidence of headache and lethargy, respectively, were similar between the tafenoquine group (29% and 3%) and the mefloquine group (30% and 4%), and the incidence of dizziness and vertigo/tinnitus, respectively, were lower in the tafenoquine group (3% and 5%) than in the mefloquine group (6% and 7%) (FDA, 2018c). One study in the safety set, which included deployed Australian soldiers (Nasveld et al., 2010), reported the incidence of dizziness, myalgia, and deafness to be similar in the tafenoquine (1.4%, 0.6%, and 0%, respectively) and mefloquine (1.2%, 0.6%, and 0.6%) groups. In the same study, incidence was reported to be lower in the tafenoquine group than in the mefloquine group for headache (14.6% versus 18.5%), fatigue and lethargy (5.7% versus 6.8%), and vertigo/tinnitus (4.9% versus 6.8%) (FDA, 2018c).

In a pooled analysis (the methods of which were not specified) of three studies from the safety set that had a similar duration of exposure (12–15 weeks) and that included tafenoquine (n = 252), mefloquine (n = 147), and placebo (n = 256) groups, there was a higher incidence of the grouped outcomes of falls, dizziness, and lightheadedness with tafenoquine (5.2%) and mefloquine (10.2%) than with placebo (3.1%); the incidence of myalgia, however, was higher with placebo (12.1%) than with tafenoquine or mefloquine (both 9.5%) (FDA, 2018c). In the same analysis, the incidence of headache was found to be 30.5% for placebo, 33.3% for tafenoquine, and 46.3% for mefloquine; the incidence of vertigo and tinnitus was 0% for placebo and tafenoquine, and 1.4% for mefloquine; and the incidence of fatigue/lethargy and visual disturbance was similar among the three groups. In an additional study (Leary et al., 2009) that compared tafenoquine with placebo, the incidence of myalgia in the tafenoquine group was higher than in the placebo group (7.4% versus 0%), while headache, fatigue, lethargy, and visual disturbance as well as the category of falls, dizziness, and lightheadedness were "numerically higher" for placebo than tafenoquine. The one case of tinnitus reported in the tafenoquine group remained unresolved at study end.

Three studies in the safety set had a mefloquine comparator arm, and people with a history of psychiatric disorders were excluded; another study in the set excluded those with a history of drug or alcohol abuse (FDA, 2018c). The FDA briefing document states that there was no systematic monitoring of psychiatric symptoms, such as actively asking participants about symptoms or using a rating scale for psychiatric symptoms, in the trials in the safety set and that "this may result in an underestimation of the actual incidence of neurologic adverse events" (FDA, 2018c). In the safety set, psychiatric adverse reactions were reported in 3.9% (32/825) of participants receiving tafenoquine, 3.2% (10/309) of the participants receiving mefloquine, and 0.8% (3/396) of the participants receiving placebo. Insomnia was reported in 1.2% (10/825) of the participants in the tafenoquine group, 0.8% (3/396) in the placebo group, and 0.3% (1/309) in the mefloquine group. Psychiatric adverse events led to discontinuation of the drug in two participants taking tafenoquine (one suicide attempt; one case of depression), one taking mefloquine (severe anxiety), and none taking placebo. In a study within the safety set that included deployed Australian soldiers (Nasveld et al., 2010), the incidence of any kind of adverse sleep symptom (insomnia, abnormal dreams, nightmares, sleep disorder, somnambulism) was similar between the tafenoquine (3.5%) and mefloquine groups (3.7%) (FDA, 2018c). Anxiety was reported in 0.8% (4/492) of the tafenoquine group versus no reports in the mefloquine group (0/162); depression was reported in 0.2% (1/492) of the tafenoquine group and 0.6% (1/162) of the mefloquine group; and euphoric mood and agitation were each reported in 0.4% (2/492) of the tafenoquine group compared with no reports in the mefloquine group.

Use of the approved prophylactic loading and maintenance dosages of tafenoquine is associated with adverse gastrointestinal events of abdominal pain, diarrhea, nausea, and vomiting (FDA, 2018c). The safety profile of tafenoquine when administered without food was not assessed in the drug-development program (FDA, 2018c). In a pooled analysis of the safety set, gastrointestinal adverse reactions with an incidence ≥1% were abdominal pain, upper abdominal pain, constipation, diarrhea, dyspepsia, gastritis, nausea, and vomiting (FDA, 2018c). Diarrhea (12.7%) and vomiting (3.8%) occurred at a higher incidence in the tafenoquine group than in the placebo group (5.8% and 1.5%, respectively) and the mefloquine group (10.7% and 3.6%, respectively) (FDA, 2018c). Two withdrawals due to gastrointestinal effects occurred among tafenoquine recipients (one with upper abdominal pain; one with irritable bowel syndrome) (FDA, 2018c). However, in the study of deployed Australian soldiers (Nasveld et al., 2010), the incidence of gastrointestinal adverse events (≥1%) was lower in the tafenoquine group than in the mefloquine group: diarrhea, 18.1% versus 19.8%; nausea, 6.9% versus 9.3%; vomiting, 4.9% versus 5.6%; and abdominal pain, 4.9% versus 7.4% (FDA, 2018c).

Regarding tafenoquine-associated eye disorders, the FDA briefing document, referring to the study in deployed Australian soldiers, notes that baseline retinal photography was not performed and that the incidence of reported retinal disorders was similar in the tafenoquine (1.4% [7/492]) and mefloquine (1.9% [3/162]) groups (FDA, 2018c). In a malaria treatment trial (not part of the safety set) that assessed ophthalmic measures, retinal pigmentation was observed on day 28 in 19.6% (9/46) of tafenoquine recipients and was still present in eight people at day 90, compared with only 4.2% (1/24) of chloroquine/primaquine recipients who had developed retinal findings; no retinal findings were associated with vision changes. In summarizing, the FDA briefing document notes that tafenoquine is associated with reversible vortex keratopathy and that the risk of adverse effects on vision and the retina cannot be adequately ascertained based on the data available.

The FDA briefing document notes that there were no serious cardiac events in tafenoquine recipients in the safety set and that no cardiac adverse events occurred at an incidence ≥1% (FDA, 2018c). No information on comparators was provided.

Taking FDA-approved loading/maintenance dosages of tafenoquine is associated with a decrease in hemoglobin levels, hemolytic anemia, and methemoglobinemia (FDA, 2018c). In a pooled analysis of the safety set, 0.4% (3/825) of tafenoquine recipients withdrew because of decreased hemoglobin, compared with 0.3% (1/396) of the placebo recipients and none (0/309) of the mefloquine recipients.

In the safety set, mild, transient glomerular filtration rate decreases led two participants (0.2%) in one study to leave the study (Leary et al., 2009); the individuals' serum creatinine remained within normal range (FDA, 2018c). In the safety set, five participants (0.6%) in the tafenoquine group and two (0.5%) in the placebo group experienced glomerular filtration rate decreases, compared with none in the mefloquine group; these were classified as serious adverse events. Creatinine changes also occurred in three (0.4%) participants in the tafenoquine group, one (0.3%) in the placebo group, and three (1%) in the mefloquine group. In one study from the safety set (Nasveld et al., 2010), mean serum creatinine increases from baseline in the tafenoquine and mefloquine groups were not clinically significant (FDA, 2018c). In this study, a long-term renal follow-up study was conducted in a cohort (tafenoquine, n = 147; mefloquine, n = 36) with serum creatinine concentrations ≥0.23 mg/dL greater than baseline at the end of the prophylactic phase or at follow-up (FDA, 2018c). In the published study (Nasveld et al., 2010), the authors noted that at follow-up, 6–8% of participants in both groups had creatinine values that were still 25% above baseline, but few values were outside the normal range, and no values were considered clinically significant.

Other Reviews

Novitt-Moreno et al. (2017) performed an integrated safety analysis of the same five malaria-prophylaxis trials referred to as the safety set above. The authors stratified the study population by deployment status (Australian National Defence soldiers taking tafenoquine [n = 492] and non-military residents taking tafenoquine [n = 333] or placebo [n = 295]) and reported that several adverse events occurred in both tafenoquine-deployed and tafenoquine-resident groups at a higher incidence than in the placebo resident group: diarrhea, nausea, vomiting, ringworm, gastroenteritis, nasopharyngitis, sinusitis, tonsillitis, laceration, ligament sprain, back pain, neck pain, and rash. The frequency of adverse events reported by the placebo-resident (64.1%) and tafenoquine-resident (67.6%) groups were generally similar. However, several adverse events, including ear and labyrinth disorders, psychiatric disorders, eye disorders, gastrointestinal disorders, immune system disorders, infections and infestations, musculoskeletal and connective tissue disorders, and skin and subcutaneous tissue disorders were reported at higher rates in the tafenoquine-deployed group than in either of the resident groups, suggesting that deployment contributed to occurrence of some of the adverse events. The adverse events that occurred in the tafenoquine-deployed group with an incidence of at least 10% more than in the tafenoquine-resident group or the placebo-resident group were, respectively, diarrhea (18.1% versus 4.8% versus 3.1%), gastroenteritis (37.2% versus 7.8% versus 5.8%), and nasopharyngitis (19.7% versus 3.3% versus 2.4%) (Novitt-Moreno et al., 2017). When the authors compared psychiatric adverse events in the tafenoquine-deployed group with the tafenoquine-resident group and the placebo-resident group, the number of cases was 25 (5.1%) versus 7 (2.1%) and 3 (1.0%), respectively, for all psychiatric disorders. Only comparisons between the tafenoquine-deployed group and the tafenoquine-resident group were reported for specific psychiatric adverse events; 18 (3.7%) versus 3 (0.9%) for psychiatric disorders affecting sleep; 8 (1.6%) versus 2 (0.6%) for insomnia; 5 (1%) versus 0 for abnormal dreams; and <1% (for both groups) for any other itemized psychiatric disorders. After reviewing medical histories and adjusting for confounding illnesses or events for individuals with insomnia or sleep-related disorders, similar percentages (0.3–0.4%) of the two groups experienced insomnia or sleep-related disorders.

Eye disorders were reported in 17% of tafenoquine-deployed users versus 10.2% of the tafenoquine-resident users, and 10.5% of the placebo-resident users (Novitt-Moreno et al., 2017). However, ophthalmologic assessments were done in a cohort of the deployed tafenoquine users (Nasveld et al., 2010), enabling identification of vortex keratopathy, which was reported in 13.8% of the subgroup and accounted for the majority of eye disorders in deployed users. The vortex keratopathy was determined to be reversible and cause no functional vision changes (Novitt-Moreno et al., 2017). No breakdown of the remaining eye disorders in the tafenoquine-deployed group or of the eye disorders in the tafenoquine-resident group or the placebo group was provided.

Post-Cessation Adverse Events

A total of 423 abstracts or article titles were identified by the committee for inclusion for tafenoquine. After screening, 116 abstracts and titles remained, and the full text for each was retrieved and reviewed to determine whether it met the committee's inclusion criteria, as defined in Chapter 3. The committee reviewed each article and identified seven epidemiologic studies that met its inclusion criteria (Ackert et al., 2019; Green et al., 2014; Leary et al., 2009; Miller et al., 2013; Nasveld et al., 2010; Rueangweerayut et al., 2017; Walsh et al., 2004). These studies were reviewed comprehensively and are summarized below. A table that gives a high-level comparison (study design, population, exposure groups, and outcomes examined by body system) of each of the seven epidemiologic studies that examined the use of tafenoquine and that met the committee's inclusion criteria is presented in Appendix C. Five studies (Ackert et al., 2019; Green et al., 2014; Miller et al., 2013; Rueangweerayut et al., 2017; Walsh et al., 2004) used off-label dosages of tafenoquine.

Military and Veterans

Nasveld et al. (2010) conducted a randomized double-blind controlled study to compare the safety and tolerability of tafenoquine for 26 weeks followed by placebo for 2 weeks (n = 492) or mefloquine for 26 weeks followed by primaquine for 2 weeks (n = 162) for malaria prophylaxis in male and female Australian soldiers aged 18–55 years. The soldiers were deployed on United Nations peacekeeping duties to East Timor. They were predominantly young, Caucasian men and were judged to be healthy by a medical history and physical examination with normal hematologic and biochemical values and to be G6PD normal. Participants with a history of psychiatric disorders or seizures were excluded, as were women who were pregnant, lactating, or unwilling or unable to comply with contraception. A subset of 98 participants (77 from the tafenoquine group and 21 from the mefloquine group) underwent extra safety assessments at baseline and at the end of the prophylactic phase to investigate drug-induced phospholipidosis and methemoglobinemia as well as ophthalmic and cardiac safety. Safety and tolerability assessments occurred at weeks 2 and 12 during the follow-up phase after the last dose of study medication, and there was additional telephone follow-up at weeks 18 and 24. Adverse-event monitoring was supplemented by a review of the subjects' medical records. In the safety subgroup, vortex keratopathy (corneal deposits) was found in 69 of 74 (93.2%) tafenoquine recipients and 0 of 21 mefloquine recipients. The changes were not associated with visual disturbances; 10% persisted at 6 months, but complete resolution occurred in all by 1 year. Mean methoglobin levels increased by 1.8% in the tafenoquine group (compared with 0.1% in the mefloquine group), but the increase resolved by week 12 of follow-up. A small reduction in mean QT interval was also seen in tafenoquine recipients (compared with a small increase in QT interval in the mefloquine group); whether the change in interval resolved with time is not stated, but none of these findings were considered to be clinically significant by the authors. The authors stated that during the relapse follow-up phase, 203 (41.3%) tafenoquine/placebo subjects and 53 (33.9%) mefloquine/primaquine subjects reported adverse events, but no notable difference between the groups in the incidence or nature of events was observed. The adverse events are not named nor is their timing specified. Authors do state that at follow-up, 6–8% of participants in both arms had creatinine values that were 25% above the baseline, but few had values outside the normal range, and none were considered clinically significant.

The overall study design was rigorous, with randomization to medications, temporal ordering of exposures and outcomes, systematic data collection, high adherence to assigned medications, and little attrition from the study (94% of subjects in both arms completed the trial), and the study was conducted in a highly relevant population for the committee's task. However, it is limited in the information it provides with respect to persistent adverse events for tafenoquine because of the small number of subjects (n = 77) who underwent detailed safety evaluation as well as the use of mefloquine as a comparison exposure rather than a placebo or no antimalarial exposure. Exposure assessment was fairly strong, owing to consistent measurements across the arms of the study and the use of medication logs to measure adherence prospectively. However, all exposure was self-reported, with no direct observation or biologic measures. Most adverse events were not assessed in a systematic way, limiting the quality of these measures. In addition, with the exception of few measures (ophthalmic, cardiac, and methoglobin levels) in the safety evaluation subset, the timing of adverse events was not clearly specified beyond the prophylaxis phase, and therefore the persistence of adverse events could not be ascertained. While the statistical power was sufficient for the primary goal of the study, which was to assess the antimalarial efficacy, the sample size was insufficient for the study of most persistent or latent adverse events. The study reported persistent vortex keratopathy that resolved by 1 year and had no effect on vision. There were no persistent increases in methemoglobin or cardiac outcomes.

Walsh et al. (2004) conducted a randomized double-blind placebo-controlled study in 205 healthy Thai soldiers aged 18–55 years (median 23 years). The primary objective was to assess tafenoquine's efficacy as malaria prophylaxis; secondary outcomes were safety and tolerability. Laboratory tests were conducted monthly during drug administration and then for up to 2 months after the last medication dose. Participants were screened for G6PD deficiency and had not received antimalarial treatment within the prior 2 weeks (5 weeks for mefloquine). Volunteers were examined for malaria and received a 7-day course of artesunate and doxycycline, administered concurrently, to eliminate subpatent[4] blood stages of malaria if needed. In any case of patent parasitemia, parasite clearance was confirmed at the end of presumptive therapy. After the presumptive therapy, soldiers received a loading dose of tafenoquine 400 mg (base) daily for 3 days, followed by 400 mg monthly (n = 104) or placebo (n = 101) for up to 5 consecutive months. The tafenoquine dosage is not within FDA-approved labeling for prophylaxis. Monthly doses were administered under direct observation, within a window of 25–31 days after a previous dose, and within 2 hours of a meal or light snack, for better gastrointestinal tolerance and bioavailability. Volunteers who developed parasitemia while receiving the medication and who were classified as having had treatment failure received the presumptive therapy regimen and were given the option of no further prophylaxis, doxycycline at 100 mg daily, or open-label tafenoquine administered at a loading dose of 400 mg for 3 days and then 400 mg weekly. Adverse events were recorded daily during the 3-day loading dose and then at approximately 24 hours after each dose, according to a predefined coded checklist of the most commonly expected adverse events. Serious adverse events were defined as those requiring hospital admission. All volunteers who had received at least one dose of tafenoquine or placebo medication were included in the safety and tolerability analysis. The follow-up time was measured from the first dose of tafenoquine (day 0) until the date of drug failure, withdrawal from the study (non-malaria-related), loss to follow-up, or study completion (6 months for most volunteers). A total of 17 participants (8.3%) were lost to follow-up; in the placebo group, 5 were reassigned to distant posts and 4 left the service, while in the tafenoquine group, 6 were reassigned and 2 left the service. Methemoglobin levels were monitored in a manner that did not affect blinding. Monthly hematologic and biochemical laboratory values were recorded. Complete blood counts and hepatic and renal function tests were conducted monthly and for up to 2 months after the last drug dose. Group treatment means (95%CIs) were computed and compared by use of Student's t test (unpaired and paired if appropriate). No differences were reported between the treatment arms for hepatic and renal function outcomes, and the authors note, "For [complete blood counts], there were no significant differences between the mean monthly values of the tafenoquine and placebo recipients for any parameter throughout the study or any significant changes from baseline values in either group." Adverse events were summarized by the two treatment arms, but the study was not designed to reliably estimate adverse event rates with a low incidence or powered to detect differences in those events between the two groups.

---

[4] Infections in persons who tested negative for *Plasmodium* parasitemia by rapid malaria diagnostic test but tested positive by polymerase chain reaction (Kobayashi et al., 2019).

The overall study design was rigorous, with randomization, double blinding, and a placebo control. There was also temporal ordering of exposures and outcomes, systematic data collection, medication-adherence monitoring, and relatively little attrition from the study. The population of Thai soldiers is also relevant for the population of interest, and there were few exclusion criteria beyond prior antimalarial treatment and age >55 years; participants had only to be "in good general health" and have normal G6PD screens. Exposure assessment was strong, with direct observation of dosing. In terms of persistent or latent events, a major limitation is that, with the exception of complete blood counts and hepatic and renal function tests conducted monthly, data collection was not systematic. In addition, the study was powered for the primary outcome (an 85% reduction in the 6-month cumulative incidence of slide-proven malaria), which resulted in approximately 90 subjects per arm; as the authors acknowledge, this provides insufficient power to detect differences in rare adverse safety between the two treatment arms. All serious adverse events reported were during the prophylaxis period. It is unknown whether no serious adverse events occurred after that time or the post-drug-cessation data were not collected or reported. In summary, the study reported persistent adverse hematologic, hepatic, and renal outcomes, but the study was insufficient to examine a broad set of persistent or latent adverse events.

Research Volunteers

Ackert et al. (2019) conducted a randomized single-blind controlled trial to compare the ophthalmic safety of a single dose of tafenoquine (300 mg) (n = 306) with that of placebo (n = 161) in adults at three U.S. study centers. The tafenoquine dose is not within FDA-approved labeling for prophylaxis. Participants were men and women aged 18–45 years, weighing 35–100 kg, and deemed healthy by an investigator, with normal hematology and chemistry values. Exclusion criteria included current or chronic history of liver disease, known hepatic or biliary abnormalities, hemoglobin values outside the lower limit of normal range, G6PD deficiency, and a QTcF interval of >450 ms. Participants with reproductive potential had to be capable of adherence to contraception. Pregnant and lactating females were excluded. Key ophthalmic exclusion criteria were a bilateral best-corrected visual acuity of ≤72 letters; eye disease that could compromise ophthalmic assessments; an intraocular surgery or laser photocoagulation within 3 months of dosing; high myopia (equal to or worse than −6.00 diopters); anterior, intermediate, or posterior uveitis or history of significant intraocular infectious disease or another active inflammatory disease; spectral domain optical coherence tomography (SD-OCT) central subfield thickness <250 μm or >290 μm; presence of significant abnormal patterns on fundus autofluorescence (FAF) or ocular abnormalities on fundus photography at screening; or uncontrolled intraocular pressure >22 mmHg. Outcomes were compared among tafenoquine group members and placebo group members, with an adverse event assessment performed over the telephone at approximately 30 and 60 days post-cessation and with full ophthalmic exams, including visual field examination, slit-lamp evaluation of anterior segment structures, and SD-OCT and FAF, carried out at baseline and on approximately day 90. One participant in each group met the composite endpoint for retinal changes identified with SD-OCT or FAF. Both subjects had unilateral focal ellipsoid zone disruption at day 90, although it was determined that the tafenoquine-treated subject actually had this anomaly at baseline and was enrolled in error. There were no subjects with bilateral retinal changes. Additional secondary endpoints for ophthalmic safety were also examined; there were no treatment differences in central subfield thickness, central retinal/lesion thickness, macular cube volume, subretinal fluid thickness, or best-corrected visual acuity. There were no clinically important changes from baseline to day 90 in intraocular pressure. One subject in the tafenoquine group was reported to have vortex keratopathy; however, it was later determined to be a Lasik scar with calcium deposits. General safety events were also collected, in particular, the frequency of adverse events and serious adverse events. The frequency of adverse events was similar between groups, and no serious or severe adverse events were reported during the study, although the timing of the adverse events was not clear. The study design was strong, with randomization and a blinding of the outcome assessment, sufficient power for the study questions, high follow-up rates (93% in the tafenoquine group and 96% in the placebo group), treatment administration directly observed, and systematic measurement of ophthalmic outcomes. Systematic measurement of ophthalmic endpoints was performed.

Green et al. (2014) conducted a Phase I single-blind randomized placebo- and active-controlled parallel-group study at two U.S. sites to investigate whether tafenoquine at supratherapeutic and therapeutic concentrations prolonged cardiac repolarization in healthy volunteers aged 18–65 years. The primary objective was to demonstrate a lack of effect of supratherapeutic tafenoquine (1,200 mg) on QTcF as determined by the baseline-adjusted maximum time-matched QTcF effect as compared with placebo ($\Delta\Delta$QTcF). Secondary objectives included demonstrating a lack of effect of tafenoquine therapeutic doses (300 and 600 mg) on $\Delta\Delta$QTcF, describing tafenoquine pharmacokinetics, and characterizing the pharmacokinetic/pharmacodynamic relationship between tafenoquine concentrations and any change in QTcF. The tafenoquine doses are not within the FDA-approved labeling for prophylaxis. Participants (n = 52 per arm) returned for follow-up at 5, 10, 24, and 60 days after the last dose of study medication. Safety was evaluated by physical examination, vital signs, clinical laboratory tests (hematology, biochemistry, and urinalysis) and adverse event monitoring. While mild, dose-related elevations in methemoglobin levels occurred, levels returned to normal by the final follow-up visit, and there were no signs or symptoms of methemoglobinemia. Resting single 12-lead electrocardiograms (ECGs) were performed at screening and at days –2, 1, 2, 3, 4, 5, 6, 27, and 63. No clinically significant abnormalities were reported from the ECGs. The strengths of the study include a randomized design, multiple tafenoquine-dose arms, and a placebo control arm. The study also included a moxifloxacin (positive [active] control) arm, but moxifloxacin is not FDA approved for malaria prophylaxis, and those results are not reported here. The temporality of exposure before the outcomes was guaranteed by the design, and there was low attrition from the study arms. While the study was sufficiently powered for the main comparisons of interest, a design limitation for the committee's purposes is that each study arm had only 52 participants, limiting the power to detect persistent adverse events. Drug exposure was conducted in a supervised clinical laboratory setting and thus is very strong. Outcome assessment for the outcomes of interest was systematic, and cardiac-related safety was evaluated in standardized ways, including a physical examination (including ECGs), vital signs, clinical laboratory tests, and adverse event monitoring 24 and 60 days after the final drug exposure. However, a broader set of potential adverse events was not collected in a systematic way, and the results presented did not differentiate their timing. The study reported no persistent adverse methemoglobin or cardiac outcomes, but the study was insufficient to examine a broad set of persistent or latent adverse events.

Leary et al. (2009) conducted a randomized double-blind study to assess the ophthalmic and renal effects of tafenoquine 200 mg weekly versus placebo for 24 weeks in 120 healthy men and women between the ages of 15 and 55 years (mean age 33.9 years) recruited from the United States and the United Kingdom. Exclusion criteria included a history of eye surgery, corneal or retinal abnormalities, current use of eye drops, participation in activities that could affect vision (e.g., scuba diving, exposure to high altitude, or excessive sunlight), a history of drug or alcohol abuse, and the use of prescription medications within 30 days of the study's start. The 120 participants were randomized in a 2:1 ratio: 81 were assigned to tafenoquine 200 mg once daily for 3 consecutive days (600 mg loading dose), followed by 200 mg once weekly for 23 weeks (24 weeks of drug administration); 39 were assigned to placebo. In addition to regular screening during the prophylactic phase, participants were followed for 24 weeks, with data collected at weeks 12 and 24 after drug cessation. The primary ophthalmic endpoint was the proportion of persons with impaired night vision as measured by the forward light scatter test, a test that is sensitive to the presence of scatter secondary to corneal deposits. Secondary ophthalmic endpoints included further assessment of night vision, assessment of macular function, visual acuity, color vision, corneal deposits, and changes in retinal morphology. For ophthalmic measures, there were no meaningful differences between the study groups in changes to high-contrast visual acuity and measured color vision; the majority of people (>98% in the tafenoquine group, >96% in the placebo group) had normal test results throughout the study. At screening, corneal deposits were reported in 10 of 70 (14.3%) and 7 of 32 (21.9%) in the tafenoquine and placebo groups, respectively. Treatment-emergent corneal deposits occurred in 15 of 60 (25%) of the tafenoquine group and 4 of 25 (16%) of the placebo group, with no observed pattern for time to onset. In 14 tafenoquine-dosed participants, new-onset corneal deposits resolved within 12 weeks of onset, in most cases during active use; in the one remaining person, the deposits resolved by 24 weeks after drug cessation. Another tafenoquine recipient showed retinal abnormalities during the follow-up period, but this was not associated with a decrement in visual acuity, foveal sensitivity, or visual field up to 11 months after drug cessation. The primary renal endpoint was tafenoquine's effect on the mean change in the glomerular filtration rate (GFR) compared with placebo. Secondary renal endpoints included the number of participants with significant changes in GFR, serum creatinine, or urinalysis findings at any time after drug administration. Of those with urinalysis results at week 24, clinically important findings were found in 3.6% and 11.5% of participants in the tafenoquine and placebo groups, respectively. Two tafenoquine recipients showed hematuria greater than trace. None of these cases were associated with a significant change in glomerular filtration rate or serum creatinine concentration; all resolved without treatment. One tafenoquine recipient displayed hemolytic anemia at week 3, with a 17% decrease in hemoglobin and a 23% decrease in haptoglobin. After ceasing tafenoquine therapy, hematology values returned to normal within 12 weeks. Another tafenoquine recipient showed creatinine phosphokinase values outside the normal range during the follow-up period; further information was not provided.

Strengths of this study include a randomized design and a placebo control group. The temporality of the exposure before outcomes was ensured by the design. A weakness is that attrition was relatively high, with only 58 of 81 (71.6%) tafenoquine recipients and 29 of 39 (74.3%) placebo recipients completing the 24-week visit post-drug-cessation. A design limitation for the committee's purposes is that, while powered for the primary outcome of interest, the number of participants (79 in the tafenoquine arm; 39 in the placebo arm) provided limited power for detecting persistent adverse events (and insufficient power for even the secondary endpoints). Exposure assessment was considered to be strong, with the drug administration supervised directly in some weeks and confirmed by telephone in others. The outcome assessment for the primary and secondary outcomes of interest (ophthalmic and renal) was systematic; ophthalmic tests and hematologic and biochemical measures were obtained at 12 and 24 weeks post-drug-cessation. Most outcomes examined showed no abnormal results at any time point, and in nearly all individuals the concurrent ophthalmic or renal problems resolved by 24 weeks post-dosing. However, a broader set of potential adverse events was not collected in a systematic way, and the reported data did not distinguish their timing, so the information was insufficient for examining a broad set of persistent or latent adverse events.

Miller et al. (2013) conducted a small randomized double-blind three-arm study to examine the effect of tafenoquine in healthy men and women in the United States aged 18–55 years. This was designed as a safety trial for malaria treatment, but since one arm was tafenoquine alone, the healthy participants did not have malaria, and the follow-up was 56 days, the committee believed it might be informative. The tafenoquine 450 mg dose is not within FDA-approved labeling for prophylaxis. Participants were administered 600 mg chloroquine on days 1 and 2 (n = 20); or 450 mg tafenoquine on days 2 and 3 (n = 20); or 600 mg chloroquine on day 1, 600 mg chloroquine plus 450 mg tafenoquine on day 2, and 300 mg chloroquine plus 450 mg tafenoquine on day 3 (n = 20). The exclusion criteria included cardiac conduction abnormalities on 12-lead ECGs; a history of cardiovascular disease or clinically significant arrhythmia; aspartate aminotransferase, alanine aminotransferase, or alkaline phosphatase >1.5 times the upper limit of normal or total bilirubin outside the normal range at screening; documented G6PD deficiency as determined by a quantitative enzyme activity assay; a history of hemoglobinopathy or methemoglobinemia or a methemo-globin percentage above the reference range at screening; or a history of retinal eye surgery, Lasik surgery within 90 days, or retinal or corneal abnormalities. Participants were also excluded if they had taken prescription or non-prescription drugs in the previous 7 (or 14, for enzyme inducers) days. While adverse events were reported only through day 7, clinical laboratory tests and methemoglobin and ophthalmic assessments were performed at screening or at day –1, multiple times throughout the study, and then again at day 56. As the committee's focus is tafenoquine used for malaria prophylaxis, the findings for the tafenoquine-alone arm are emphasized here. Changes in vital signs and clinical laboratory values were similar across treatment groups and were reported to be clinically insignificant. A trend for mild declines (1.5–2.5 g dl^{-1}) in hemoglobin was noted in a greater proportion of tafenoquine-treated subjects than in those treated with chloroquine alone (tafenoquine 22%, tafenoquine/chloroquine 17%, and chloro-quine 4%). Two African American females who received tafenoquine experienced a decrease in hemoglobin >2.5 g dl^{-1} (2.8 and 3.0 g dl^{-1}) on day 10, but those values returned to baseline by day 56. No clinically significant changes from baseline were found in macular function across treatment groups. A trend of minor declines of visual acuity was seen in the tafenoquine-treated group; how-ever, the study was not powered to compare differences between treatments. One tafenoquine recipient showed a clinically significant reduction from baseline in visual acuity at day 28 that spontaneously resolved by day 56 (logMAR scores of −0.1, 0.3, and 0, at baseline, day 28, and day 56, respectively). The subject had no retinal abnormalities, eye-related adverse events, or vortex keratopathy. Mean percentage methemoglobin measures increased slightly from baseline in the groups that received a regimen containing tafenoquine. Maximal mean changes from baseline were observed on day 14 (<1% chloroquine, 4% tafenoquine, and 6% chloroquine/tafenoquine), and elevations in three women in the tafenoquine/chloroquine group were greater than 10%, but mean methemoglobin values for the three women returned to baseline by day 28 and for all others by day 56.

The overall study design was strong, as it was randomized and had double blinding. There was also a clear temporal ordering of exposures and outcomes, direct observation of medication adherence, and relatively low attrition. A design limitation for the committee's purposes is that, while sufficiently powered for the primary pharmacokinetic outcome of interest, the number of participants was very small (58 across three treatment arms) and thus provided limited power for detecting potentially rare persistent or latent adverse events. Clinical laboratory values and vital signs, methemoglobin levels, and ophthalmic measures were evaluated 1 and 2 months post-drug-cessation. Beyond these few specific assessments, the evaluation of general persistent adverse events was limited, with a collection of adverse events and serious adverse events performed only during the 7-day confinement period. In summary, the very small size of this study and the lack of assessment of a broad set of adverse outcomes makes the study minimally informative for this review.

Rueangweerayut et al. (2017) used a prospective observational study design to examine the tolerability of tafenoquine (100, 200, or 300 mg, single-dose) compared with primaquine (15 mg for 14 days) in a total of 51 healthy Thai females who were heterozygous for Mahidol-variant G6PD deficiency (40–60% of adjusted site defined median value for G6PD-normal males) (n = 6 for each tafenoquine dosage arm; n = 5 for primaquine) or G6PD normal ($\geq$90% of adjusted site median normal value) (n = 6 for each tafenoquine dosage arm; n = 6 for primaquine). Two additional cohorts of G6PD-deficient participants with greater G6PD activity (61–80% and >80% of site median normal value; n = 2 and n = 5, respectively) were administered 200 mg of tafenoquine. The 300 mg tafenoquine dose is not within FDA-approved labeling for prophylaxis. The primary outcome was the maximum absolute decrease in hemoglobin or hematocrit from pre-treatment up to day 14 following treatment. The subsequent outpatient follow-up visits were at days 21, 28, and 56. The safety assessments included adverse event monitoring, vital signs, 12-lead ECGs, clinical biochemistry, hematology (including methemoglobin determined by oximetry), and urinalysis. The tafenoquine dose escalation was halted when hemoglobin decreased by $\geq$2.5 g/dL or the hematocrit declined $\geq$7.5% versus pretreatment values. In the G6PD-deficient arms, dose-limiting effects were reported to occur in 3 of 3 of the 300 mg dose tafenoquine arm and 3 of 5 of the primaquine arm; of these, two recipients of each drug experienced both a decrease $\geq$2.5 g/dL in hemoglobin and a decrease $\geq$7.5% in hematocrit versus pre-treatment, with the greatest decrease in hemoglobin with tafenoquine being –2.95 g/dL. No tafenoquine recipient showed methemoglobin levels >5.0%. Among the primaquine recipients, 4 of 6 of the G6PD-normal group showed sustained elevations in methemoglobin (maximum values 5.5–13.1%); in the G6PD-deficient group, values did not exceed 3.9%. The authors reported that there were no accompanying clinical symptoms associated with hemolysis or increased methemoglobin levels, no other clinically important changes in laboratory measures, and no notable ECG changes. The study was limited by the very small sample size and the narrow range of enzyme activities examined, making it minimally informative for this review.

OTHER IDENTIFIED STUDIES OF TAFENOQUINE IN HUMAN POPULATIONS

The committee reviewed five additional studies on malaria prophylaxis involving tafenoquine, but they were excluded because they did not distinguish between adverse events that occurred ≥28 days post-cessation of tafenoquine and adverse events that occurred during tafenoquine use or shortly after cessation (Brueckner et al., 1998; Hale et al., 2003; Lell et al., 2000; Nasveld et al., 2002; Shanks et al., 2001). In addition to those epidemiologic studies that did not meet criteria for inclusion, the committee also reviewed case reports, studies of tafenoquine used for the treatment of malaria, and studies of tafenoquine that considered demographic differences.

In its approval letter, FDA stated that it had determined that an analysis of the spontaneous postmarketing adverse events reported would not be sufficient to assess a signal of serious risks of ophthalmic, psychiatric, and hematologic adverse reactions, nor would the pharmacovigilance system that FDA is required to establish (FDA, 2018b). Therefore, FDA has required the manufacturer to conduct two studies. One will be an observational study to evaluate safety, including neurologic, hypersensitivity, psychiatric, and hematologic adverse reactions, in people taking tafenoquine for the prophylaxis of malaria. The study, which will compare tafenoquine with atovaquone/proguanil in travelers (>10,000 participants), is in the planning stages.[5] The second required study, which is currently recruiting participants (NCT #03320174), is a randomized double-blind placebo-controlled study that will enroll 600 healthy G6PD-normal volunteers. Participants who meet the eligibility criteria will be randomized (ratio 1:1) to receive a loading dose of tafenoquine 200 mg (2 × 100 mg tablets) or placebo daily for 3 days, followed by the study treatment (tafenoquine 200 mg or placebo) once weekly for 51 weeks, with safety follow-up visits at weeks 4, 12, 24, and 52. Participants will return to the clinic at week 64 for an end-of-study visit. A participant who has an ongoing adverse event at the week 64 visit will be assessed up to three more times at approximately 12-week intervals or until resolution or stabilization of the adverse event, whichever is earlier.

Treatment Studies and Case Report

While the use of antimalarial drugs for the treatment of malaria falls outside the scope of the committee's task, because tafenoquine is so new to the market the committee wanted to ensure that it captured any adverse event from such studies that might raise concern. A Cochrane review published in 2015 included a meta-analysis of three randomized controlled treatment trials that compared tafenoquine

---

[5] Personal communication to the committee, Geoffrey Dow, M.B.A., Ph.D., Chairman and Chief Executive Officer, 60 Degrees Pharmaceuticals, LLC, on January 28, 2019.

plus chloroquine to chloroquine alone in some arms and to primaquine plus chloroquine in other arms in persons with *P. vivax* (Rajapaske et al., 2015). Persons with G6PD deficiency were excluded, and all participants received chloroquine therapy. The participants in these trials took higher doses of tafenoquine, 300–600 mg per day for up to 3 days versus the approved prophylactic dosage of 200 mg daily for 3 days followed by 200 mg weekly. In the comparison of tafenoquine plus chloroquine to chloroquine alone, there was no difference in serious adverse events (three trials, 358 participants) and no difference for any reported adverse events (one trial, 272 participants). There was a dose-dependent rise in methemoglobin in tafenoquine-treated groups that was asymptomatic. There was also no difference in serious or total adverse events in tafenoquine versus primaquine groups (two trials, 323 participants). Three additional treatment trials published after the Cochrane review and one case report are summarized below.

Fukuda et al. (2017) studied men and women 20–60 years of age with malaria and no prior ophthalmic conditions who received 400 mg of tafenoquine daily for 3 days (n = 46) compared with those who received chloroquine followed by primaquine for 14 days (n = 24). Participants were followed up to day 120. The adverse events that occurred in tafenoquine recipients more frequently than in chloroquine/primaquine recipients were methemoglobinemia (defined as methoglobin level $\geq 8.5\%$) (47.8% versus 0); vortex keratopathy (31.8% versus 0); upper respiratory tract infection (30.4% versus 20.8%); headache (30.4% versus 16.7%); dizziness (26.1% versus 12.6%); retinopathy/retinal disorder (22.7% versus 4.2%); thrombocytopenia (13% versus 0); nausea (13% versus 12.5%); aesthenia (8.7% versus 8.3%); and dyspepsia, diarrhea, hepatomegaly, hypokalemia, and myalgia (6.5% each versus 4.2%, 0, 0, 4.2%, 4.2%, respectively). There were no clinically relevant changes in visual acuity or the results of macular function tests and no evidence of clinically relevant ocular toxicity, although early retinal morphologic changes could not be ruled out in one case.

Lacerda et al. (2019) enrolled 522 men and women ≥ 16 years of age, all of whom received a 3-day course of chloroquine (total dose of 1,500 mg) to treat malaria. In addition, participants were assigned to receive a single 300 mg dose of tafenoquine on day 1 or day 2 (n = 260), or placebo (n = 133), or primaquine for 14 days (n = 129). Participants were followed up for 180 days. Adverse events occurring at any point during the 6-month study in tafenoquine recipients with a greater frequency than placebo were dizziness (8.5% versus 3%), vomiting (5.8% versus 5.3%), diarrhea (3.8% versus 3.0%), and a decline in hemoglobin (5.4% versus 1.5%). No adverse event led to withdrawal from the trial.

In Llanos-Cuentas (2019), 251 male and female participants with malaria aged 16 years and older received a 3-day course of chloroquine. In addition, participants received a single 300 mg dose of tafenoquine on day 1 or day 2 (n = 166) or primaquine for 14 days starting on day 1 or day 2 (n = 85). The follow-up period was 180 days. The frequency of adverse events occurring throughout the study period (days 1–180) that were more common in tafenoquine than in primaquine recipients included dizziness (16.3% versus 15.3%), vomiting (6.6% versus 5.9%), upper abdominal pain (4.8% versus 1.2%), diarrhea (3.6% versus 3.5%), hemoglobin decline (2.4% versus 1.2%), insomnia (1.2% versus 0), urinary tract infection (3.6% versus 3.5%), nasopharyngitis (3.6% versus 2.4%), and fever (1.8% versus 1.2%). All adverse events resolved spontaneously; none led to discontinuation of treatment.

A case study (Cannon et al., 2015) reported a 38-year-old man who had been referred to a physician following two incidents of severe rhinitis, wheezing, and breathlessness after airborne exposure to powdered tafenoquine in a tablet-manufacturing plant. Exposure to a control dust (lactose) for 15 minutes provoked no symptoms and no changes in forced expiratory volume in one second. Exposure for the same duration to 1% tafenoquine in 250 mg of lactose provoked a 19% fall in forced expiratory volume in one second 10 minutes after challenge and a maximum fall of 32% at 8 hours. Changes in lung function were accompanied by severe rhinitis, which persisted for several days.

Selected Subpopulations

To date there have been no studies of tafenoquine prophylaxis that have focused on people with comorbid conditions. Pregnant women have been excluded from clinical trials of tafenoquine because of concerns about the potential for G6PD deficiency in the fetus.

Sex Differences

A difference between women and men in the incidence of gastrointestinal adverse events has been reported. An open-label randomized study in Australian Defence Force members was designed to compare tafenoquine with primaquine as a post-deployment malaria prophylaxis regimen (Nasveld et al., 2002). When a higher-than-anticipated number of early participants taking tafenoquine (400 mg daily for 3 days) experienced nausea and vomiting, the authors theorized that the "routine doxycycline prophylaxis" participants were also taking might have increased the likelihood of gastrointestinal effects, so an additional cohort of participants was added, which was discussed in a separate paper (Edstein et al., 2007). This cohort ceased taking doxycycline 1 day before receiving tafenoquine, either in a single daily dose (400 mg for 3 days) or in a split dose (200 mg twice daily for 3 days) (Edstein et al., 2007). This dose is not within FDA-approved labeling. The frequency of nausea and abdominal distress in women was more than double that in men in both the once-daily group (76 men, 11 women) and the split-dose group (73 men, 13 women). Reports of gastrointestinal disturbances (e.g., nausea, vomiting, diarrhea, abdominal distress) differed significantly between males and females in the once-daily group but not in the split-dose group. In volunteers who experienced gastrointestinal disturbances, the mean plasma tafenoquine concentrations 12 hours after the last dose were approximately 1.3-fold higher in women than in men (mean±SD: 737±118 ng/mL versus 581±113 ng/mL, respectively). The average body weight of the women was lower than that of the men (66.5 kg versus 81.6 kg, respectively; p < 0.001). Statistical analyses indicated that women weighing less than 78 kg in the once-daily group and 64 kg in the split-dose group were likely to experience gastrointestinal effects. The authors noted the small numbers of women in the study but hypothesized that the increased chance of gastrointestinal effects among those of lower weight was related to the higher drug concentrations achieved in these women.

BIOLOGIC PLAUSIBILITY

Studies of the use of tafenoquine in supratherapeutic doses conducted in rats (single-dose) and rhesus monkeys found no signs of neurologic toxicity. In a single-dose study in adult rats, doses up to the minimum lethal dose (500 mg/kg) did not result in any evidence of brainstem neuropathology 7 days after administration (the longest time point tested) (60 Degrees Pharmaceuticals, 2018; Dow et al., 2017). In rhesus monkeys, doses at least 27-fold higher than those determined to be clinically relevant for radical cure were not associated with clinical neurologic signs or neurodegeneration (60 Degrees Pharmaceuticals, 2018). Berman et al. (2018) reviewed rhesus monkey literature and reported that tafenoquine (unlike the older 8-aminoquinolines pentaquine, pamaquine, and plasmocid) does not cause neuro-pathologic changes in the brainstem. Overall, on the basis of these studies, the committee believes that the probability for neurotoxic actions of tafenoquine is low. No data associated with either concurrent or persistent adverse events are reported linking tafenoquine to known mechanisms associated with neuropathology.

The committee did not find evidence of biologic plausibility for eye disorders in animal models. No tafenoquine-related ophthalmic pathologies are reported in dogs (Levine et al., 1997a,b). A 6-month toxicity study in rats showed no treatment-related ophthalmic lesions at week 13 or week 26 (Levine, 1996).

Like primaquine and other 8-aminoquinolines, tafenoquine causes hemo-lytic toxicity (Baird, 2019). A study in dogs of five different 8-aminoquinoline compounds, including tafenoquine, corroborates reversible methemoglobinemia following administration (Anders et al., 1988). When the methemoglobin-forming properties of tafenoquine were studied in vitro, tafenoquine was found to cause methemoglobin formation at a rate of 140 ± 2 pmol/min, which is a greater rate than that observed with primaquine. In mice, tafenoquine blunts platelet response to calcium ions, and it increases measures of platelet aggregation, especially with concurrent thrombin exposure (Cao et al., 2017). However, the authors concluded that their results "do not allow any safe conclusions as to the mechanisms underlying the effect of tafenoquine on platelet apoptosis." In vivo studies would be required to test whether tafenoquine can alter subtle measures of coagulation in mice—and potentially in humans. In a study in rats, supertherapeutic doses (400–700 mg/kg) had negative impact on red blood cell parameters and increased liver enzymes (Dow et al., 2017).

Again, as is the case with other 8-aminoquinolines, tafenoquine-induced hemolysis and toxicity are enhanced in individuals with G6PD deficiency (Melariri et al., 2015). In an in vitro study (Bhuyan et al., 2016), human erythrocytes from healthy volunteers were exposed to tafenoquine at a clinically relevant dose for 48 hours. Results showed that tafenoquine triggers suicidal erythrocyte death or eryptosis. In a study of tafenoquine in G6PD-normal women and women with heterozygous G6PD deficiency, a single dose of tafenoquine (100–300 mg) in the G6PD-deficient women decreased hemoglobin and hematocrit measures, although not to dangerous levels; the highest dose of tafenoquine lowered hemoglobin to around –3.0 g/dL (–2.65 to –2.95 g/dL in three participants) (Rueangweerayut et al., 2017). The hemolytic potential was dose dependent, and hemolysis was greater in G6PD-heterozygous females with lower G6PD-enzyme activity levels.

Tafenoquine tested negative in cell-based assays for point mutations and chromosomal aberrations (Levine, 1998). The developmental toxicity of tafenoquine was studied in female rats (maternal and fetal no-observable-effect level was 3 and 30 mg/kg/day, respectively) and rabbits (maternal and fetal no-observable-effect level was 7 and 25 mg/kg/day, respectively) by dosing during gestation days (Levine, 1998). The observed outcomes in rats included a decrease in body weight and food consumption, and enlarged spleen; the observed outcomes in rabbits included a decrease in body weight and food consumption, decrease in viable fetuses, premature delivery, and abortion. The reproductive toxicity of tafenoquine was investigated by the administration of daily doses of the drug to male rats for 67 days and to pregnant female rats for 23–47 days, which included 29 days of dosing prior to cohabitation in males and 15 days of dosing prior to cohabitation in females (Levine, 1998). The 15 mg/kg daily dose of tafenoquine affected oocyte maturation but not ovulation, mating behavior, implantation, or embryonic development. The no-observable-effect level for reproductive capability in males and females was 15 and 5 mg/kg/day, respectively. There was no evidence that toxicokinetic data were generated in any of these studies. The authors also did not discuss putative mechanisms for the observed toxicities. Manifestations of tafenoquine neurotoxicity seemed to be rare in these studies. The extensive preclinical toxicity data described in these reports do not provide many mechanistic clues to help explain potential persistent or latent adverse effects of tafenoquine in humans.

SYNTHESIS AND CONCLUSIONS

Tafenoquine was approved by FDA in 2018 for malaria prophylaxis. Seven epidemiologic studies were identified that included some mention of adverse events or data collection that occurred ≥28 days post-cessation of tafenoquine that provided directly relevant information for assessing persistent adverse events (Ackert et al., 2019; Green et al., 2014; Leary et al., 2009; Miller et al., 2013; Nasveld et al., 2010; Rueangweerayut et al., 2017; Walsh et al., 2004). The studies varied in the amount of usable information, so their findings are not weighted equally in drawing conclusions, and epidemiologic evidence was given more weight than supportive information. As described in Chapter 3, the committee considered several methodologic issues in assessing each study's contribution to the evidence base on persistent or latent adverse events, including the overall study design, the quality of exposure and health outcome assessment, the ability to address confounding and other potential biases, sample size, and the extent to which the post-cessation health experience was effectively isolated. Six of the studies had strong designs with randomization of participants; four of these were double blinded (Leary et al., 2009; Miller et al., 2013; Nasveld et al., 2010; Walsh et al., 2004), and two (Ackert et al., 2019; Green et al., 2014) were single blinded. Four studies used a placebo-control arm (Ackert et al., 2019; Green et al., 2014; Leary et al., 2009; Walsh et al., 2004). All were considered high-quality studies that contributed to the evidence for the outcomes addressed in the syntheses. The studies are heterogeneous in the populations that were used (active military or veterans, and research volunteers), the numbers of participants (range 51–654), the modes of data collection (administrative records, researcher collected, self-report) on drug exposure, health outcomes and covariates, the type of prophylactic regimen and dosages used (five studies used off-label dosages of tafenoquine), and, particularly, the nature of the health outcomes that were considered. The relevant studies were also notably inconsistent in the reporting of results, covering different time periods in relation to the cessation of drug exposure. Given the inherently imperfect information generated by any one study, it would be desirable to have similar studies in order to assess the consistency of findings, but the diversity of the studies' methods makes it very difficult to combine information across the studies with confidence.

For each health outcome category, supporting information from FDA; known concurrent adverse events, including data from selected treatment trials with long-term follow-up; and experimental animal and in vitro studies are first summarized, after which the evidence from the post-cessation epidemiologic studies is described. While the charge to the committee was to address persistent and latent adverse events, the occurrence of concurrent adverse events enhances the plausibility that problems may persist beyond the period after cessation of drug use. The synthesis of the evidence is followed by a conclusion about the strength of the evidence regarding an association between the use of tafenoquine and persistent or latent adverse events and whether the available evidence would support additional research into those outcomes. The outcomes are presented in the following order: neurologic disorders, psychiatric disorders, gastrointestinal disorders, eye disorders, cardiovascular disorders, and other outcomes, which includes renal, hepatic, and hematologic parameters as well as nasopharyngitis.

The committee believes it is pertinent that FDA is requiring the manufacturer of tafenoquine to conduct two post-approval studies. The first, which is still in its planning stages, is an observational study to evaluate safety, including neurologic, hypersensitivity, psychiatric, and hematologic adverse reactions, in participants taking tafenoquine compared with atovaquone/proguanil. The second, which is currently recruiting participants (NCT #03320174), is a randomized double-blind placebo-controlled study that will administer a loading dose of tafenoquine and 51 weeks of prophylaxis, with long-term follow-up to monitor adverse events.

Neurologic Disorders

The sources of supporting information that contributed to the evidence base to assess tafenoquine and neurologic disorders were the FDA package insert and briefing document, three malaria-treatment studies, and biologic plausibility studies. The FDA package insert and the FDA briefing document both referred to a safety set of data comprising five studies (FDA, 2018c,d). In a pooled analysis of the safety set, the most common concurrent neurologic adverse reactions (incidence ≥1%) with tafenoquine use were headache, dizziness, and motion sickness, although the studies did not conduct systematic monitoring for neurologic symptoms (FDA, 2018c,d). The incidence of headache and lethargy was similar between the tafenoquine group and the mefloquine group, and the incidence of dizziness and vertigo/tinnitus was lower in the tafenoquine group than in the mefloquine group (FDA, 2018c). In a pooled analysis of three studies from the safety set (all with 12–15 weeks of exposure), the incidence of the grouped outcomes of falls, dizziness, and lightheadedness with tafenoquine was higher than for placebo but lower than for mefloquine (FDA, 2018c). In the same analysis, the incidence of headache was found to be similar in the tafenoquine and placebo groups but higher for mefloquine; the incidence of vertigo and tinnitus was 0% for placebo and tafenoquine, and 1.4% for mefloquine. Three malaria-treatment trials (Fukuda et al., 2017; Lacerda et al., 2019; Llanos-Cuentas, 2019) used higher-than-prophylactic dosages for 1–3 days and had follow-up periods of 120–180 days (including the dosage period), although the timing of the adverse events was not distinguished. One study (Fukuda et al., 2017) reported greater frequencies of headache and dizziness with tafenoquine (400 mg for 3 days) than with chloroquine/primaquine. The other two studies (Lacerda et al., 2019; Llanos-Cuentas, 2019) used a single 300 mg tafenoquine dose following chloroquine; one reported a higher frequency of dizziness with chloroquine/tafenoquine versus chloroquine/placebo, and the other an only slightly higher frequency of dizziness with chloroquine/tafenoquine versus chloroquine/primaquine.

Biologic plausibility studies of tafenoquine did not support signs of clinical neurologic effects or neurodegeneration or mechanisms of neurologic toxicity or neuropathology, even when supratherapeutic doses were given to rats and rhesus monkeys.

None of the seven epidemiologic studies included data for neurologic adverse events for which timing post-drug-cessation was specified.

Based on the available evidence, the committee concludes that there is insufficient or inadequate evidence of an association between the use of tafenoquine for malaria prophylaxis and persistent or latent neurologic events. Current evidence does not suggest further study of such an association is warranted, given the lack of evidence regarding biologic plausibility, adverse events associated with concurrent use, or findings from the existing epidemiologic studies.

Psychiatric Disorders

Tafenoquine is contraindicated in persons with a history of psychotic disorders or who have current psychotic symptoms. The FDA package insert and the FDA briefing document both referred to a safety set of data comprising five studies (FDA, 2018c,d). In an analysis of the safety set, the most common concurrent psychiatric adverse reactions (incidence ≥1%) were insomnia, depression, abnormal dreams, and anxiety (FDA, 2018d). Individuals with a history of psychiatric disorders were excluded from three of the five studies; those with a history of drug or alcohol abuse were excluded from a fourth. In the safety set, the reported incidences of psychiatric adverse reactions for tafenoquine and mefloquine were similar, but both were higher than with placebo (FDA, 2018c). The incidence of insomnia was higher with tafenoquine than with placebo, which in turn was higher than with mefloquine, although the incidence among the three groups was similar. Psychiatric adverse events led to study discontinuation by two participants taking tafenoquine (one suicide attempt; one depression), one taking mefloquine (depression), and none taking placebo. A study in the safety set that included deployed Australian soldiers (Nasveld et al., 2010) reported the incidence of any kind of sleep symptom (insomnia, abnormal dreams, sleep disorder, somnambulism) to be similar in the tafenoquine and mefloquine groups (FDA, 2018c), as was the incidence for anxiety, depression, euphoric mood, and agitation. In a different analysis of the same five studies (Novitt-Moreno et al., 2017), after stratifying for deployed or resident status, the occurrence of any psychiatric adverse events was higher in the tafenoquine-deployed group (5.1%) than in the tafenoquine-resident group (2.1%) and the placebo-resident group (1.0%). Only comparisons between the tafenoquine-deployed group and the tafenoquine-resident group were reported for specific psychiatric adverse events, and the tafenoquine-deployed group had a higher incidence of all psychiatric disorders than the tafenoquine-resident group, suggesting a deployment effect on the occurrence of these types of adverse events. A malaria-treatment study reported a slightly higher frequency of insomnia in participants given chloroquine/tafenoquine than in those given chloroquine/primaquine, but the chloroquine/tafenoquine incidence was only 1.2% (Llanos-Cuentas, 2019).

Studies of the use of tafenoquine in supratherapeutic doses conducted in rats and rhesus monkeys found no signs of neurologic toxicity. Animal studies with tafenoquine do not show the classic brain stem pathology found with earlier 8-aminoquinolines in rhesus monkeys, even with high doses, but the available data are limited (60 Degrees Pharmaceuticals, 2018; Berman et al., 2018; Dow et al., 2017).

None of the seven epidemiologic studies included data for psychiatric adverse events for which the timing post-drug-cessation was specified.

Based on the available evidence, the committee concludes that there is insufficient or inadequate evidence of an association between the use of tafenoquine for malaria prophylaxis and persistent or latent psychiatric events. Current evidence suggests further study of such an association is warranted, given the evidence regarding biologic plausibility, adverse events associated with concurrent use, or findings from the existing epidemiologic studies.

Gastrointestinal Disorders

The FDA package insert and the FDA briefing document both referred to a safety set of data comprising five studies (FDA, 2018c,d). In a pooled analysis of the safety set, concurrent gastrointestinal adverse reactions with an incidence ≥1% were abdominal pain, upper abdominal pain, constipation, diarrhea, dyspepsia, gastritis, nausea, and vomiting (FDA, 2018c). The incidence of diarrhea and vomiting was higher with tafenoquine than with mefloquine or placebo (FDA, 2018c). However, in one of the studies in the safety set, carried out in deployed Australian soldiers (Nasveld et al., 2010), the reported incidence of diarrhea, nausea, vomiting, and abdominal pain was lower with tafenoquine than with mefloquine (FDA, 2018c). In a different analysis of the same five studies (Novitt-Moreno et al., 2017), after stratifying for deployed or resident status, concurrent adverse events that occurred in both deployed and resident tafenoquine recipients at an incidence ≥1% and at a higher incidence than the placebo-resident group included diarrhea, nausea, vomiting, and gastroenteritis. In comparisons among the tafenoquine-deployed group, the tafenoquine-resident group, and the placebo-resident group, diarrhea (18.1% versus 4.8% versus 3.1%) and gastroenteritis (37.2% versus 7.8% versus 5.8%) were highest in the tafenoquine-deployed group, again suggesting a deployment effect on the occurrence of these types of adverse events.

Three malaria-treatment trials (Fukuda et al., 2017; Lacerda et al., 2019; Llanos-Cuentas, 2019) used higher-than-prophylactic dosages for 1–3 days and had follow-up periods of 120–180 days (including dosage period), although timing of the adverse events was not distinguished. One study (Fukuda et al., 2017) reported a greater frequency of nausea, dyspepsia, and diarrhea in tafenoquine-alone recipients than in chloroquine/primaquine recipients. In a second study (Lacerda et al., 2019), vomiting and diarrhea occurred more frequently in the chloroquine/tafenoquine group than in the chloroquine/placebo group. In a third study (Llanos-Cuentas, 2019), vomiting, upper abdominal pain, and diarrhea occurred more frequently in the chloroquine/tafenoquine group than in the chloroquine/primaquine group. Edstein et al. (2007) found that women who took a 3-day course of tafenoquine 400 mg daily (as a single or split dose) following a course of doxycycline experienced nausea and abdominal distress more than twice as often as men; the difference was statistically significant for the once-daily comparison. Among those who experienced gastrointestinal symptoms, women had higher concentrations of drug 12 hours after the last dose and a significantly lower average body weight than the men. Statistical analysis indicated that women weighing <78 kg in the once-daily group and <64 kg in the split-dose group were likely to experience gastrointestinal effects. No studies were identified that provided information on biologic plausibility for gastrointestinal disorders.

None of the seven epidemiologic studies that the committee reviewed included data for gastrointestinal adverse events for which timing post-drug-cessation was specified.

Based on the available evidence, the committee concludes that there is insufficient or inadequate evidence of an association between the use of tafenoquine for malaria prophylaxis and persistent or latent gastrointestinal events. Current evidence does not suggest further study of such an association is warranted, given the lack of evidence regarding biologic plausibility, adverse events associated with concurrent use, or findings from the existing epidemiologic studies.

Eye Disorders

The FDA package insert states that vortex keratopathy was reported in 21–93% of tafenoquine recipients in three trials that included ophthalmic evaluations (Leary et al., 2009; Nasveld et al., 2010; a malaria-treatment trial [NCT #0129060]), but the condition caused no functional visual changes and resolved within 1 year of drug cessation (FDA, 2018d). Retinal abnormalities occurred in less than 1% of tafenoquine recipients. The FDA briefing document noted that while tafenoquine is associated with reversible vortex keratopathy, the risk of adverse effects on vision and the retina cannot be adequately ascertained based on available data (FDA, 2018c). In an integrated safety study of five clinical trials (Novitt-Moreno et al., 2017), after stratifying by deployment or resident status, eye disorders were reported to have occurred in 17% of the tafenoquine-deployed group, 10.2% of the tafenoquine-resident group, and 10.5% of the placebo-resident group. Vortex keratopathy represented the majority of the deployed group's eye disorders; these reversed after drug cessation and caused no functional vision changes. The identification of the remainder of eye disorders in the deployed group and all eye disorders in the resident groups was not provided. A malaria-treatment trial (Fukuda et al., 2017) of tafenoquine (400 mg for 3 days) versus a chloroquine/primaquine regimen reported vortex keratopathy in 31.8% and retinopathy/retinal disorder in 22.7% of tafenoquine recipients, compared with 0% and 4.2%, respectively, of the chloroquine/primaquine recipients. While there were no clinically relevant effects, possible early retinal morphologic changes were reported in one tafenoquine participant.

In experimental studies, no tafenoquine-related ophthalmic pathologies have been reported in dogs (Levine, 1997a,b). A 6-month toxicity study in rats showed no treatment-related ophthalmic lesions at week 13 or week 26 (Levine, 1996).

Of the seven epidemiologic studies that met inclusion criteria, four studies (Ackert et al., 2019; Leary et al., 2009; Miller et al., 2013; Nasveld et al., 2010) included data for eye-disorder adverse events for which the timing post-drug-cessation was specified. Two studies (Leary et al., 2009; Nasveld et al., 2010) reported a high rate of mild reversible vortex keratopathy (corneal deposits) and no related visual disturbances. All cases resolved while taking the drug or within 3 to 12 months after drug cessation; retinal abnormalities were reported in one case but were not associated with a decrement in visual acuity, foveal sensitivity, or visual field up to 11 months after drug cessation. A study that compared oph-thalmic outcomes in participants taking a single 300 mg dose of tafenoquine or placebo (Ackert et al., 2010) reported no difference in ophthalmic safety between groups. A fourth, small study (Miller et al., 2013) reported a clinically significant reduction in visual acuity in one tafenoquine recipient (450 mg for 2 days) that resolved by day 56.

Based on the available evidence, the committee concludes that there is sufficient evidence of an association between the use of tafenoquine for malaria prophylaxis and vortex keratopathy, but with unclear clinical significance.

There is insufficient or inadequate evidence of an association between the use of tafenoquine for malaria prophylaxis and other persistent or latent eye disorders. Current evidence suggests further study of such an association is warranted, given evidence regarding biologic plausibility, adverse events associated with concurrent use, or data from the existing epidemiologic studies.

Cardiovascular Disorders

The FDA package insert states that based on a study of healthy adults who were administered 400 mg tafenoquine (twice the recommended dose) for 3 days, the mean increase in the QTcF interval for tafenoquine was less than 20 ms (FDA, 2018d). The FDA briefing document reports that there were no serious cardiac events reported in tafenoquine recipients in a data set of five trials, and no car-diac adverse events occurred at an incidence $\geq 1\%$ (FDA, 2018c). Cardiovascular adverse events were not examined or were not reported by sources of supporting evidence (reviews, treatment studies, case report, biologic plausibility studies).

Two epidemiologic studies that met the inclusion criteria—a long-term pro-phylaxis trial (Nasveld et al., 2010) and a dose-ranging safety trial (Green et al., 2014)—assessed cardiac events as primary outcomes, measuring the effects of tafenoquine on QT interval and QTcF, respectively, and reported no evidence of persistent adverse cardiac events.

Based on the available evidence, the committee concludes that there is insufficient or inadequate evidence of an association between the use of tafenoquine for malaria prophylaxis and persistent or latent cardiovascular events. Current evidence does not suggest further study of such an association is warranted, given the lack of evidence regarding biologic plausibility, adverse events associated with concurrent use, or findings from the existing epidemiologic studies.

Other Outcomes and Disorders

Renal

In the safety set of five clinical trials referred to by the FDA package insert and FDA briefing document, 0.6% of the tafenoquine group and 0.5% of the placebo group experienced GFR decreases compared with none in the mefloquine group (FDA, 2018c). Creatinine changes occurred in 0.4% of the tafenoquine group, 0.3% of the placebo group, and 1% of the mefloquine group. Mild GFR decreases led to study discontinuation by 0.2% of tafenoquine recipients in one of the safety set studies (Leary et al., 2009), although serum creatinine remained within normal range (FDA, 2018c). A malaria treatment trial (Fukuda et al., 2017) reported that hypokalemia occurred more frequently in tafenoquine-alone recipients (6.5%) than in chloroquine/primaquine recipients (4.2%).

Three epidemiologic studies met the inclusion criteria and included data for renal adverse events for which the timing post-drug-cessation was specified (Leary et al., 2009; Nasveld et al., 2010; Walsh et al., 2004). A study in Thai soldiers (Walsh et al., 2004) comparing tafenoquine (400 mg, loading dose and weekly) and placebo reported no differences in renal function between the treatment arms. A study in Australian soldiers (Nasveld et al., 2010) reported that at follow-up, 6–8% of participants in the tafenoquine and mefloquine arms had creatinine values that were 25% above baseline, but few were outside the normal range, and none were clinically significant. In a third study (Leary et al., 2009), clinically important renal findings were reported in the tafenoquine arm (3.6%) and placebo arm (11.5%), but no cases were associated with a significant change in GFR or serum creatinine concentration, and all resolved without treatment. One tafenoquine recipient showed creatinine phosphokinase values outside the normal range during the follow-up, but further information was not provided.

Hepatic

In the package insert, in a pooled analysis of a safety set of five trials, increased alanine aminotransferase incidence was reported in ≥1% of tafenoquine recipients (FDA, 2018d). A malaria-treatment trial (Fukuda et al., 2017) reported hepatomegaly more frequently in tafenoquine recipients (6.5%) than in chloroquine/primaquine recipients (0%). Supertherapeutic doses (400–700 mg/kg) in rats were reported to increase liver enzymes (Dow et al., 2017). One epidemiologic study included data for hepatic outcomes for which timing post-drug-cessation was specified (Walsh et al., 2004) and found no differences in hepatic function between Thai soldiers who used tafenoquine 400 mg (loading dose, and weekly for up to 5 months) and those on placebo.

Nasopharyngitis

An integrated safety analysis of five clinical trials (Novitt-Moreno et al., 2017), after stratifying by deployment and resident status, reported that nasopharyngitis occurred in both the deployed and resident tafenoquine groups at an incidence ≥1% and at a higher incidence than in the placebo-resident group. Further analysis showed a higher incidence of nasopharyngitis in the tafenoquine-deployed group (19.7%) than in the tafenoquine-resident group (3.3%). A malaria-treatment trial (Llanos-Cuentas, 2019) reported nasopharyngitis to occur with greater frequency in the chloroquine/tafenoquine group than in the chloroquine/primaquine group (3.6% versus 2.4%). A case study (Cannon et al., 2015) reported that an individual exposed to airborne powdered tafenoquine in a factory experienced severe rhinitis, wheezing, and breathlessness that persisted for several days. Nasopharyngeal adverse events were not examined or not reported in biologic plausibility studies. None of the seven post-cessation epidemiologic studies reported nasopharyngitis as a persistent or latent adverse event.

Hematologic

Tafenoquine is contraindicated in individuals with G6PD deficiency and in those whose G6PD status is unknown, in breastfeeding women when the infant is G6PD deficient or G6PD status is unknown, and in pregnant women if the status of the fetus is unknown (FDA, 2018d). G6PD testing must be performed before prescribing tafenoquine. The danger of hemolysis and hemolytic anemia in G6PD-deficient persons who use 8-aminoquinolines is well known.

Methemoglobinemia, usually mild and reversible, is another well-characterized feature of the use of 8-aminoquinolines. The package insert states that tafenoquine is associated with methemoglobinemia and that persons with NADH-dependent methemoglobin reductase deficiency should be monitored during use (FDA, 2018d). Referring to a safety set of five clinical trials, the package insert reports that asymptomatic elevations in methemoglobin occurred in 13% of tafenoquine recipients. Tafenoquine is also associated with decreases in hemoglobin, and decreases ≥3 g/dL were observed in 2.3% of tafenoquine recipients in the safety set. One malaria treatment study reported a greater frequency of methemoglobinemia and thrombocytopenia with a tafenoquine regimen than with a chloroquine/primaquine regimen (Fukuda et al., 2017); other treatment studies reported a greater frequency of a decline in hemoglobin with a chloroquine/

tafenoquine regimen than with a chloroquine/placebo regimen (5.4% versus 1.5%) (Lacerda et al., 2019) and a chloroquine/primaquine regimen (2.4% versus 1.2%) (Llanos-Cuentas, 2019). A Cochrane review of three earlier malaria treatment trials reported a dose-dependent asymptomatic rise in methemoglobin in tafenoquine-treated groups (Rajapaske et al., 2015).

The biologic plausibility of tafenoquine causing reversible methemoglobinemia is supported by studies in dogs (Anders et al., 1988). Tafenoquine was shown in vitro to cause methemoglobin formation at a greater rate than primaquine. In mice, tafenoquine blunted platelet response to calcium ions and it increased platelet aggregation, especially with concurrent thrombin exposure (Cao et al., 2017). However, no conclusions were made as to the mechanisms underlying the drug's effects on platelet apoptosis, and further study is needed of its effects on coagulation. In a study in rats, supertherapeutic doses negatively affected red blood cell parameters (Dow et al., 2017). As an 8-aminoquinoline, tafenoquine-induced hemolysis and toxicity is enhanced in people with G6PD deficiency (Melariri et al., 2015). In an in vitro study, human erythrocytes from healthy volunteers were exposed to tafenoquine at a clinically relevant dose for 48 hours, and tafenoquine was shown to trigger suicidal erythrocyte death (eryptosis).

Five epidemiologic studies that met the inclusion criteria included data for hematologic adverse events for which the timing post-drug-cessation was specified. Nasveld et al. (2010) reported that mean methemoglobin levels increased by 1.8% in the tafenoquine group compared with 0.1% in the mefloquine group, but the increases resolved by week 12 of follow-up. Green et al. (2014) reported that tafenoquine at supratherapeutic and therapeutic concentrations prolonged elevations in methemoglobin levels, but without signs or symptoms, and the levels returned to normal by day 63 of follow-up. In Miller et al. (2013), mean methemoglobin measures increased slightly from baseline in the tafenoquine and chloroquine/tafenoquine groups; the greatest increases (>10%) occurred in the chloroquine/tafenoquine group, but these values returned to normal by day 28 and in all cases by day 56. A trend for mild declines (1.5 to 2.5 g dl^{-1}) in hemoglobin was noted in a greater proportion of tafenoquine-treated subjects than in those treated with chloroquine alone; the greatest decreases (2.8 and 3.0 g dl^{-1} on day 10) were seen in two African American women but values returned to baseline by day 56. Walsh et al. (2004) reported that for complete blood counts, there were no significant differences between the mean monthly values of the tafenoquine and placebo groups and no significant changes from baseline values in either group. In a study in women with normal G6PD activity and with heterozygous G6PD deficiency, a single dose of tafenoquine (100–300 mg) in the G6PD-deficient group decreased hemoglobin and hematocrit measures but not to dangerous levels; the highest dose of tafenoquine lowered hemoglobin to approximately −3.0 g/dL (Rueangweerayut et al., 2017). The hemolytic potential was dose dependent, and hemolysis was greater in G6PD-heterozygous females with lower G6PD-enzyme activity levels.

If severe hemolytic anemia is not treated or controlled, it can lead to serious complications, including arrhythmias, cardiomyopathy, heart failure, and death (Baird, 2019; NIH, n.d.). Methemoglobinemia can result in decreased availability of oxygen to tissues, and more severe methemoglobinemia can lead to complications, including abnormal cardiac rhythms, altered mental status, delirium, seizures, coma, and profound acidosis and death (Denshaw-Burke et al., 2018). Drug-associated hemolysis and methemoglobinemia resolve with withdrawal of exposure to tafenoquine. Although the above effects are possible and could cause sequelae that endure beyond the time of exposure, the committee did not identify any published cases of persistent or latent effects resulting from prophylactic doses of tafenoquine.

REFERENCES

60 Degrees Pharmaceuticals, LLC. 2018. *Arakoda™ (tafenoquine succinate) tablets for the prevention of malaria in adults*. NDA 210607. Briefing document for the Antimicrobial Drugs Advisory Committee, July 26, 2018.

AAO (American Academy of Ophthalmology). 2019. Corneal verticillata. https://www.aao.org/bcscs-nippetdetail.aspx?id=27980840-6807-4c45-aaae-b8652b087987 (accessed December 11, 2019).

Ackert, J., K., Mohamed, J. S. Slakter, S. El-Harazi, A. Berni, H. Gevorkyan, E. Hardaker, A. Hussaini, S. W. Jones, G. C. K. W. Koh, J. Patel, S. Rasmussen, D. S. Kelly, D. E. Baranano, J. T. Thompson, K. A. Warren, R. C. Sergott, J. Tonkyn, A. Wolstenholme, H. Coleman, A. Yuan, S. Duparc, and J. A. Green. 2019. Randomized placebo-controlled trial evaluating the ophthalmic safety of single-dose tafenoquine in healthy volunteers. *Drug Saf* 42(9):1103-1114.

Anders, J. C., Chung, H., and Theoharides. A. D. 1988. Methemoglobin formation resulting from administration of candidate 8-aminoquinoline antiparasitic drugs in the dog. *Fundam Appl Toxicol* 10(2):270-275.

ATGA (Australian Therapeutic Goods Administration). 2019. Australian public assessment report for tafenoquine succinate. https://www.tga.gov.au/sites/default/files/auspar-tafenoquine-succi-nate-190408.docx (accessed December 17, 2019).

Australia. 2018. The use of the quinoline anti-malarial drugs mefloquine and tafenoquine in the Australian Defence Force. December. https://www.aph.gov.au/Parliamentary_Business/Committees/Senate/Foreign_Affairs_Defence_and_Trade/Mefloquine (accessed November 13, 2019).

Australia. n.d. Department of Defence. Tafenoquine FAQs. https://www.defence.gov.au/Health/HealthPortal/Malaria/AMI_research/tafenoquine-trials/FAQs.asp (accessed November 14, 2019).

Baird, J. K. 2018. Tafenoquine for travelers' malaria: Evidence, rationale and recommendations. *J Travel Med* 25(1):tay110.

Baird, J. K. 2019. 8-aminoquinoline therapy for latent malaria. *Clin Microbiol Rev* 32(4):e00011-19.

Berman, J., T. Brown, G. Dow, and S. Toovey. 2018. Tafenoquine and primaquine do not exhibit clinical neurologic signs associated with central nervous system lesions in the same manner as earlier 8-aminoquinolines. *Malar J* 17(1):407.

Bhuyan, A.A.M, R. Bissinger, K. Stockingera, and F. Lang, 2016. Stimulation of suicidal erythrocyte death by tafenoquine. *Cell Physiol Biochem* 39:2464-2476.

Brueckner, R. P., K. C. Lasseter, E. T. Lin, and B. G. Schuster. 1998. First-time-in-humans safety and pharmacokinetics of WR 238605, a new antimalarial. *Am J Trop Med Hyg* 58:645-649.

Cannon, J., B. Fitzgerald, M. Seed, R. Agius, A. Jiwany, and P. Cullinan. 2015. Occupational asthma from tafenoquine in the pharmaceutical industry: Implications for QSAR. *Occup Med (Lond)* 65(3):256-258.

Cao, H., R. Bissinger, A. T. Umbach, A. Al Mamun Bhuyan, F. Lang, and M. Gawaz. 2017. Effects of antimalarial tafenoquine on blood platelet activity and survival. *Cell Physiol Biochem* 41(1):369-380.

Castelli, F., S. Odolini, B. Autino, E. Foca, and R. Russo. 2010. Malaria prophylaxis: A comprehensive review. 2010. *Pharmaceuticals* 3:3212-3239.

CDC (Centers for Disease Control and Prevention). 2019. *Malaria information and prophylaxis by country*. https://www.cdc.gov/malaria/travelers/country_table/a.html (accessed August 29, 2019).

Charles, B. G., A. K. Miller, P. E. Nasveld, M. G. Reid, I. E. Harris, and M. D. Edstein. 2007. Population pharmacokinetics of tafenoquine during malaria prophylaxis in healthy subjects. *Antimicrob Agents Chemother* 51(8):2709-2715.

Chu, C. S., G. Bancone, F. Nosten, N. J. White, and L. Luzzatto. 2018. Primaquine-induced haemolysis in females heterozygous for G6PD deficiency. *Malar J* 17(1):101.

Denshaw-Burke, M., A. L. Curran, D. C. Savior, and M. Kumar. 2018. Methemoglobinemia. Medscape. https://webcache.googleusercontent.com/search?q=cache:MoqV2XjOJHIJ:https://emedicine.medscape.com/article/204178-overview+&cd=1&hl=en&ct=clnk&gl=us (accessed December 23, 2019).

DoD (Department of Defense). 2019. Defense Health Agency procedural instruction (December 17, 2019, #6490.03). Deployment health procedures. Provided by COL Andrew Wiesen, M.D., M.P.H., Director, Preventive Medicine, Health Readiness Policy, and Oversight, Office of the Assistant Secretary of Defense (Health Affairs), DoD, December 19, 2019.

Dow, G. S., T. Brown, M. Reid, B. Smith, and S. Toovey. 2017. Tafenoquine is not neurotoxic following supertherapeutic dosing in rats. *Travel Med Infect Dis* 17:28-34.

Ebstie, Y. A., S. M. Abay, W. T. Tadesse, and D. A. Ejigu. 2016. Tafenoquine and its potential in the treatment and relapse prevention of *Plasmodium vivax* malaria: The evidence to date. *Drug Des Devel Ther* 10:2387-2399.

Edstein, M. D., D. S. Walsh, C. Eamsila, T. Sasipraphа, P. E. Nasveld, S. Kitchener, and K. H. Rieckmann. 2001a. Malaria prophylaxis/radical cure: Recent experiences of the Australian Defence Force. *Med Trop (Mars)* 61(1):56-58.

Edstein, M. D., D. A. Kocisko, T. G. Brewer, D. S. Walsh, C. Eamsila, and B. G. Charles. 2001b. Population pharmacokinetics of the new antimalarial agent tafenoquine in Thai soldiers. *Br J Clin Pharmacol* 52(6):663-670.

Edstein, M. D., P. E. Nasveld, D. A. Kocisko, S. J. Kitchener, M. L. Gatton, and K. H. Rieckmann. 2007. Gender differences in gastrointestinal disturbances and plasma concentrations of tafenoquine in healthy volunteers after tafenoquine administration for post-exposure *vivax* malaria prophylaxis. *Trans R Soc Trop Med Hyg* 101(3):226-230.

FDA (U.S. Food and Drug Administration). 2012. *A guide to drug safety terms at FDA*. https://www.fda.gov/media/74382/download (accessed July 8, 2019).

FDA. 2018a. Letter regarding Krintafel (tafenoquine) tablets package insert. https://www.accessdata.fda.gov/scripts/cder/daf/index.cfm?event=overview.process&ApplNo=210795 (accessed November 8, 2019).

FDA. 2018b. Letter regarding Arakoda (tafenoquine) tablets package insert. https://www.accessdata.fda.gov/scripts/cder/daf/index.cfm?event=overview.process&ApplNo=210607 (accessed October 29, 2019).

FDA. 2018c. FDA briefing document. Tafenoquine tablet, 100 mg. Meeting of the Antimicrobial Drugs Advisory Committee (AMDAC). July 26, 2018. https://www.fda.gov/media/114753/download (accessed November 11, 2019).

FDA. 2018d. Package insert for Arakoda™ (tafenoquine) tablets. https://www.accessdata.fda.gov/scripts/cder/daf/index.cfm?event=overview.process&ApplNo=210607 (accessed October 29, 2019).

Fukuda, M. M., S. Krudsood, K. Mohamed, J. A. Green, S. Warrasak, H. Noedl, A. Euswas, M. Ittiverakul, N. Buathong, S. Sriwichai, R. S. Miller, and C. Ohrt. 2017. A randomized, double-blind, active-control trial to evaluate the efficacy and safety of a three day course of tafenoquine monotherapy for the treatment of *Plasmodium vivax* malaria. *PLOS ONE* 12(11):e0187376.

Green, J. A., A. K. Patel, B. R. Patel, A. Hussaini, E. J. Harrell, M. J. McDonald, N. Carter, K. Mohamed, S. Duparc, and A. K. Miller. 2014. Tafenoquine at therapeutic concentrations does not prolong Fridericia-corrected QT interval in healthy subjects. *J Clin Pharamacol* 54(9):995-1005.

Hale, B. R., S. Owusu-Agyei, D. J. Fryauff, K. A. Koram, M. Adjuik, A. R. Oduro, W. R. Prescott, J. K. Baird, F. Nkrumah, T. L. Ritchie, E. D. Franke, F. N. Binka, J. Horton, and S. L. Hoffman. 2003. A randomized, double-blind, placebo-controlled, dose-ranging trial of tafenoquine for weekly prophylaxis against *Plasmodium falciparum*. *Clin Infect Dis* 36(5):541-549.

Haston, J. C., J. Hwang, and K. R. Tan. 2019. Guidance for using tafenoquine for prevention and antirelapse therapy for malaria - United States, 2019. *MMWR* 68(46):1062-1068.

Howes, R. E., K. Battle, K. N. Mendis, D. L. Smith, R. E. Cibulskis, J. K. Baird, and S. I. Hay. 2016. Global epidemiology of *Plasmodium vivax*. *Am J Trop Med Hyg* 95(6 Suppl):15-34.

Kobayashi, T., M. Kanyangarara , N. M. Laban, M. Phiri, H. Hamapumbu, K. M. Searle, J. C. Stevenson, P. E. Thuma, and W. J. Moss. 2019. Characteristics of subpatent malaria in a pre-elimination setting in southern Zambia. *Am J Trop Med Hyg* 100(2):280-286.

Lacerda, M. V. G., A. Llanos-Cuentas, S. Krudsood, C. Lon, D. L. Saunders, R. Mohammed, D. Yilma, D. Batista Pereira, F. E. J. Espino, R. Z. Mia, R. Chuquiyauri, F. Val, M. Casapia, W. M. Monteiro, M. A. M. Brito, M. R. F. Costa, N. Buathong, H. Noedl, E. Diro, S. Getie, K. M. Wubie, A. Abdissa, A. Zeynudin, C. Abebe, M. S. Tada, F. Brand, H. P. Beck, B. Angus, S. Duparc, J. P. Kleim, L. M. Kellam, V. M. Rousell, S. W. Jones, E. Hardaker, K. Mohamed, D. D. Clover, K. Fletcher, J. J. Breton, C. O. Ugwuegbulam, J. A. Green, and G. Koh. 2019. Single-dose tafenoquine to prevent relapse of *Plasmodium vivax* malaria. *N Engl J Med* 380(3):215-228.

Leary, K. J., M. A. Riel, M. J. Roy, L. R. Cantilena, D. Bi, D. C. Brater, K. van de Pol, K. Pruett, C. Kerr, J. M. Veazey, Jr., R. Beboso, and C. Ohrt. 2009. A randomized, double-blind, safety and tolerability study to assess the ophthalmic and renal effects of tafenoquine 200 mg weekly versus placebo for 6 months in healthy volunteers. *Am J Trop Med Hyg* 81:356-362.

Lell, B., J. F. Faucher, M. A. Missinou, S. Borrmann, O. Dangelmaier, J. Horton, and P. G. Kremsner. 2000. Malaria chemoprophylaxis with tafenoquine: A randomised study. *Lancet (London, England)*. 355:2041-2045.

Levine, B. S. 1996. *Six month oral toxicity study of WR238605 succinate in rats, volume 2*. Defense Technical Information Center. https://apps.dtic.mil/dtic/tr/fulltext/u2/a640549.pdf (accessed January 6, 2020).

Levine, B. 1998. *Preclinical toxicology studies for new drugs and vaccines*. NTIS Technical Report 280(37). https://apps.dtic.mil/docs/citations/ADA640543 (accessed November 30, 2019).

Levine, B. S., A. P. Brown, and R. L. Morrissey. 1997a. *One year oral toxicity study of WR238605 succinate in dogs, volume 1*. Defense Technical Information Center. https://archive.org/details/DTIC_ADA640544/page/n1 (accessed November 30, 2019).

Levine, B. S., A. P. Brown, and R. L. Morrissey. 1997b. *One year oral toxicity study of WR238605 succinate in dogs, volume 2*. Defense Technical Information Center. https://apps.dtic.mil/dtic/tr/fulltext/u2/a640543.pdf (accessed January 6, 2020).

Llanos-Cuentas, A. 2019. Tafenoquine versus primaquine to prevent relapse of *Plasmodium vivax* malaria. *N Engl J Med* 380:229-241.

Marcsisin, S. R., J. C. Sousa, G. A. Reichard, D. Caridha, Q. Zeng, N. Roncal, R. McNulty, J. Careagabarja, R. J. Sciotti, J. W. Bennett, V. E. Zottig, G. Deye, Q. Li, L. Read, M. Hickman, N. P. Dhammika Nanayakkara, L. A. Walker, B. Smith, V. Melendez, and B. S. Pybus. 2014. Tafenoquine and NPC-1161B require CYP 2D metabolism for anti-malarial activity: Implications for the 8-aminoquinoline class of anti-malarial compounds. *Malar J* 13(2):2.

Melariri, P., L., Kalombo, P., Nkuna, A. Dube, R. Hayeshi, B. Ogutu, L. Gibhard, C. deKock, P. Smith, L. Wiesner, and H. Swai. 2015. Oral lipid-based nanoformulation of tafenoquine enhanced bioavailability and blood stage antimalarial efficacy and led to a reduction in human red blood cell loss in mice. *Int J Nanomed* 10:1493-1503.

Miller, A. K., E. Harrell, L. Ye, S. Baptiste-Brown, J. P. Kleim, C. Ohrt, S. Duparc, J. J. Möhrle, A. Webster, S. Stinnett, A. Hughes, S. Griffith, and A. P. Beelen. 2013. Pharmacokinetic interactions and safety evaluations of coadministered tafenoquine and chloroquine in healthy subjects. *Br J Clin Pharmacol* 76:858-867.

Nasveld, P., S. Kitchener, M. Edstein, and K. Rieckmann. 2002. Comparison of tafenoquine (WR238605) and primaquine in the post-exposure (terminal) prophylaxis of *vivax* malaria in Australian Defence Force personnel. *Trans R Soc Trop Med Hyg* 96(6):683684.

Nasveld, P. E., M. D. Edstein, M. Reid, L. Brennan, I. E. Harris, S. J. Kitchener, P. A. Leggat, P. Pickford, C. Kerr, C. Ohrt, W. Prescott, and the Tafenoquine Study Team. 2010. Randomized, double-blind study of the safety, tolerability, and efficacy of tafenoquine versus mefloquine for malaria prophylaxis in nonimmune subjects. *Antimicrob Agents Chemother* 54(2):792-798.

NIH (National Institutes of Health). 2018. Study to evaluate the efficacy and safety of tafenoquine for the treatment of *Plasmodium vivax* in adults. U.S. National Library of Medicine. NCT #01290601. Last posted February 23, 2018. https://clinicaltrials.gov/ct2/show/NCT01290601 (accessed November 14, 2019).

NIH. n.d. *Hemolytic anemia.* https://www.nhlbi.nih.gov/health-topics/hemolytic-anemia (accessed October 1, 2019).

Novitt-Moreno, A., J. Ransom, G. Dow, B. Smith, L. T. Read, and S. Toovey. 2017. Tafenoquine for malaria prophylaxis in adults: An integrated safety analysis. *Travel Med Infect Dis* 17:19-27.

Rajapakse, S., C. Rodrigo, and S. D. Fernando. 2015. Tafenoquine for preventing relapse in people with *Plasmodium vivax* malaria. *Cochrane Database Syst Rev* 2015(4):CD010458.

Rishikesh, K., and K. Saravu. 2016. Primaquine treatment and relapse in *Plasmodium vivax* malaria. *Pathog Global Health* 110(1):1-8.

Rueangweerayut, R., G. Bancone, E. J. Harrell, A. P. Beelen, S. Kongpatanakul, J. J. Möhrle, V. Rousell, K. Mohamed, A. Qureshi, S. Narayan, N. Yubon, A. Miller, F. H. Nosten, L. Luzzatto, S. Duparc, J.-P. Kleim, and J. A. Green. 2017. Hemolytic potential of tafenoquine in female volunteers heterozygous for glucose-6-phosphate dehydrogenase (G6PD) deficiency (G6PD *Mahidol* variant) versus G6PD normal volunteers. *Am J Trop Med Hyg* 97(3):702-711.

Sánchez, J. L., R. F. DeFraites, T. W. Sharp, and R. K. Hanson. Mefloquine or doxycycline prophylaxis in U.S. troops in Somalia. 1993. *Lancet* 341(8851):1021-1022.

Saunders, D. L., E. Garges, J. E. Manning, K. Bennett, S. Schaffer, A. J. Kosmowski, and A. J. Magill. 2015. Safety, tolerability, and compliance with long-term antimalarial chemoprophylaxis in American soldiers in Afghanistan. *Am J Trop Med Hyg* 93(3):584-590.

Schlagenhauf, P. 2003. Malaria in Iraq—The pitfalls of *Plasmodium vivax* prophylaxis. *Lancet Infect Dis* 3(8):460.

Shanks, G. D., and M. D. Edstein. 2005. Modern malaria chemoprophylaxis. *Drugs* 65(15):2091-2110.

Shanks, G. D., A. J. Oloo, G. M. Aleman, C. Ohrt, F. W. Klotz, D. Braitman, J. Horton, and R. Brueckner. 2001. A new primaquine analogue, tafenoquine (WR 238605) for prophylaxis against *Plasmodium falciparum* malaria. *Clin Infect Dis* 33:1968-1974.

Vandenberk, B., E. Vandael, T. Robyns, J. Vandenberghe, C. Garweg, V. Foulon, J. Ector, and R. Willems. 2016. Which QT correction formulae to use for QT monitoring? *J Am Heart Assoc* 5(6):e003264.

Walsh, D. S., C. Eamsila, T. Sasiprapha, S. Sangkharomya, P. Khaewsathien, P. Supakalin, D. B. Tang, P. Jarasrumgsichol, C. Cherdchu, M. D. Edstein, K. H. Rieckmann, and T. G. Brewer. 2004. Efficacy of monthly tafenoquine for prophylaxis of *Plasmodium vivax* and multidrug-resistant *P. falciparum* malaria. *J Infect Dis* 190(8):1456-1463.

6

Atovaquone/Proguanil

The fixed-dose combination of 250 mg atovaquone and 100 mg proguanil hydrochloride (A/P; trade name Malarone® by GlaxoSmithKline) was approved by the Food and Drug Administration (FDA) for the prophylaxis and treatment of malaria in 2000. Proguanil and an analog of atovaquone were first identified as potential antimalarial agents during the U.S. Army's drug discovery and development program during World War II (Arguin and Magill, 2017). In 1945 the first published study of proguanil reported that it was more active than quinine against avian malaria and had a better therapeutic index in animal models, prompting its use in humans (Nzila, 2006). Proguanil was approved in 1948 by FDA for use in humans as an antimalarial agent, but it was not widely used. In the 1950s the first reports of *Plasmodium* parasite resistance to proguanil when taken as monotherapy occurred; the United States stopped marketing proguanil as a single drug in the 1970s (Kitchen et al., 2006; Looareesuwan et al., 1996). Proguanil continues to be used in other countries in combination with other antimalarial agents, such as chloroquine, for malaria prophylaxis.

Once proguanil was discovered, investigated, and approved for use in the United States, other compounds, including hydroxynaphthoquinones such as atovaquone, which had been identified during the drug discovery program of World War II and had demonstrated activity against the *P. falciparum* parasite were not investigated further for several years. In the 1980s a group at Wellcome Research Laboratories reinvestigated the hydroxynaphthoquinone lapinone, an atovaquone analog, as an antimalarial agent (Nixon et al., 2013). As a result of its efforts, atovaquone was identified as an antimalarial drug candidate and in 1995 was approved for use as a monotherapy (FDA, 2019b; Nixon et al., 2013). The combination of A/P was created as a result of the emergence of resistance to proguanil and atovaquone in the

1940s and 1990s, respectively. Atovaquone is no longer used as a monotherapy to treat or prevent malaria because one-third or more of individuals with *P. falciparum* infections will recrudesce (Srivastava and Vaidya, 1999). Both drugs had been highly effective as single agents, and after laboratory testing it was discovered that they demonstrated a synergistic effect on the malaria parasite (Gorobets et al., 2017). Individuals infected with malaria that was resistant to atovaquone and proguanil as single agents could effectively take A/P as a combination for malaria prophylaxis. Although A/P was approved by FDA in 2000, it has been used in military populations since 1997, and it is considered a first-line drug for malaria prophylaxis.[1] Because of the higher cost of A/P compared with other antimalarial drugs, individuals are sometimes unable or reluctant to use it (Castelli et al., 2010).

This chapter begins with a brief description of the key changes that have been made to the FDA package insert and label for A/P since its approval in 2000, with a particular emphasis on changes to the Warnings, Precautions, and Contra-indications sections. The known mechanisms of action of A/P are then described, including its pharmacokinetic properties. Known concurrent adverse events associated with the use of A/P when used at the directed dose and interval for malaria prophylaxis are summarized, followed by detailed summaries and assessments of the post-cessation epidemiologic studies that contributed some information on persistent or latent health outcomes of A/P. As in the other chapters, the epidemiologic studies are organized by population: first, studies of military and veterans, followed by studies of members of the U.S. Peace Corps and then of travelers. A table that gives a high-level comparison of each of the four epidemiologic studies that examined the use of A/P and that met the committee's inclusion criteria is presented in Appendix C. Next, supplemental supporting evidence is presented, including other identified studies of health outcomes in populations that used A/P for prophylaxis but that did not meet the committee's inclusion criteria regarding the timing of follow-up, and information on adverse events of A/P use in specific groups, such as pregnant women and individuals with chronic health conditions. After presenting the primary and supplemental evidence in humans, the supporting literature from experimental animal and in vitro studies is then summarized. The chapter ends with a synthesis of all of the evidence presented and the inferences and conclusions that can be made from the available evidence.

FOOD AND DRUG ADMINISTRATION PACKAGE INSERT FOR ATOVAQUONE/PROGUANIL

The recommended A/P dosing regimen for malaria prophylaxis in adults begins with taking one tablet (250 mg atovaquone and 100 mg proguanil) by

---

[1] Overview of DoD antimalarial use policies. Presentation to the committee, COL Andrew Wiesen, M.D., M.P.H., Director, Preventive Medicine, Health Readiness Policy, and Oversight, Office of the Assistant Secretary of Defense (Health Affairs), January 28, 2019.

mouth 1–2 days before entering a malaria-endemic area, taking one tablet daily at the same time each day throughout the entire stay in the endemic area, and continuing for 7 days after leaving the endemic area (FDA, 2019a). It is recommended that the drug be taken with food or a milky drink to increase its absorption and efficacy and to decrease the risk of gastrointestinal adverse events. If an individual vomits within 1 hour of taking A/P, another dose should be taken.

Studies of drug adherence have found that the percentage of individuals taking A/P who were adherent to the drug regimen was higher than the percentage of individuals taking other antimalarial prophylactic drugs (Goodyer et al., 2011). This is likely due to individuals using A/P having fewer acute adverse events than individuals using other prophylactic drugs. Even greater tolerance has been reported when A/P is taken with food (Høgh et al., 2000; Kain et al., 2001). Although a Cochrane systematic review of randomized trials and observational studies that compared mefloquine to A/P found no difference in adherence between the drugs (Tickell-Painter et al., 2017), other reports indicate A/P is less likely to be discontinued due to adverse events than other antimalarial prophylactic drugs, such as mefloquine (Kain et al., 2001; Overbosch et al., 2001; Tickell-Painter et al., 2017). The regimen for A/P requires individuals to take the drug for only 7 days after leaving an endemic area; this is a much shorter period than required for other suppressive antimalarial drugs, such as doxycycline, which requires individuals to take the drug for 28 days after leaving an endemic area. Because of the shorter duration required after leaving an endemic area, the A/P regimen has also been shown to have very high post-travel adherence compared with mefloquine (Overbosch et al., 2001).

This section describes selected information that can be found in the FDA label or on the package insert for A/P. It begins with a summary of contraindications, warnings, and precautions for its use based on the most recent FDA label and package insert. This is followed by a brief synopsis of drug interactions known or presumed to occur with short-term A/P use. The final subsection provides a summary of major changes to the label or package insert from its approval in 2000 to the most recent label, updated in 2019. The presented changes are specific to A/P when used for prophylaxis (not treatment) in adults (not infants or children).

Contraindications, Warnings, and Precautions

The package insert states, "A/P is contraindicated in individuals with known hypersensitivity reactions (e.g., anaphylaxis, erythema multiforme or Stevens-Johnson syndrome, angioedema, vasculitis) to atovaquone or proguanil hydrochloride or any component of the formulation" (FDA, 2019a). A/P is also contraindicated for prophylaxis of *P. falciparum* malaria in patients with severe renal impairment (creatinine clearance <30 mL/min) because of pancytopenia in patients with severe renal impairment treated with proguanil. Users are warned that there have been reports of elevated liver laboratory tests and cases of hepatitis and one account of hepatic failure requiring liver transplantation in persons using A/P as prophylaxis.

Drug Interactions

The concomitant use of A/P and rifampin or rifabutin is not recommended because the antibiotics reduce atovaquone plasma concentrations (FDA, 2019a). Caution should be exercised when using warfarin and other coumarin-based anticoagulants when starting or stopping A/P use; proguanil can increase their anticoagulant effects, and the results of coagulation tests should be monitored closely. Concomitant use of tetracycline is associated with reduced plasma concentrations of atovaquone, so parasitemia should be monitored closely. Metoclopramide may decrease the bioavailability of atovaquone and thus should be used in A/P recipients only if other antiemetics are unavailable. Prescribing indinavir and atovaquone should be done with caution owing to the resulting reduction in trough concentrations of indinavir.

Changes to the Atovaquone/Proguanil Package Insert Over Time

A/P, marketed under the trade name Malarone®, was approved in 2000, and the most recent label was issued in 2019. It is possible that not all label updates made between 2000 and 2002 are posted on the Drugs@FDA Search site. A comparison of the original label with the posted 2002 label (a version that contained underlining and strikeouts to flag changes) showed that not all of the differences between the two labels had been flagged (FDA, 2000, 2002), so an interim label may have been issued. Only those label changes that refer to adverse reactions that occur in adults using A/P as prophylaxis are reviewed here. By 2002 a contraindication for A/P in persons with severe renal impairment (creatinine clearance <30 mL/min) appeared in the label (FDA, 2002). A/P users were also warned not to take a double dose after missing a dose. Clinical trial data were added, showing the frequency of adverse experiences in subjects receiving A/P was similar to or less than that in individuals receiving mefloquine or chloroquine plus proguanil; more specifically, fewer neuropsychiatric adverse events occurred with A/P than with mefloquine, fewer gastrointestinal adverse events occurred than with chloroquine/proguanil, and fewer adverse experiences overall than with both comparators. In 2004 the Postmarketing Adverse Reactions section added "rare cases of seizures and psychotic events (such as hallucinations)" but stated that a causal relationship had not been established (FDA, 2004). Cutaneous adverse events, including rash, photosensitivity, angioedema, urticaria, and rare cases of anaphylaxis were added to this section, as were erythema multiforme and Stevens-Johnson syndrome. The 2008 label cautioned against using atovaquone with indinavir (due to a decrease in trough levels of indinavir) and advised care when starting or stopping prophylaxis with A/P in persons taking coumarin-based anticoagulants, noting that coagulation should be monitored (FDA, 2008). The Postmarketing Adverse Reactions section added blood and lymphatic system disorders (neutropenia and rarely anemia; pancytopenia in persons with severe renal impairment treated with proguanil); immune system disorders (allergic reactions, including angioedema, urticaria, and rare cases of anaphylaxis and vasculitis); gastrointestinal disorders (stomatitis); and hepatobiliary disorders (elevated liver function tests and rare cases of hepatitis and cholestasis; a single reported case of hepatic failure requiring transplant). "Rare cases of vasculitis" was amended to "vasculitis"; angioedema and "rare cases of anaphylaxis" were deleted; and "rare cases of seizures and psychotic events" was amended to delete "rare." The 2013 label added animal studies that found no adverse fertility or pre/post-natal adverse events in animals given proguanil hydrochloride at lower than prophylactic-equivalent doses, but it noted that studies of proguanil in animals at exposures similar to or greater than those observed in humans had not been conducted (FDA, 2013). The 2019 label noted that the proguanil component of A/P acts to inhibit parasitic dihydrofolate reductase but added that pregnant women and females of reproductive potential should continue folate supplementation to prevent neural tube defects (FDA, 2019a). New data from animal studies, using doses higher than prophylaxis-equivalent doses in humans, indicated that atovaquone does not yield fetal malformations, proguanil is not associated with embryo-fetal toxicity, and the combination of atovaquone and proguanil does not yield embryo/fetal developmental effects.

PHARMACOKINETICS

The pharmacokinetics of A/P are well reviewed by Boggild et al. (2007) and Nixon et al. (2013). Atovaquone is a highly lipophilic compound with low aqueous solubility; thus taking this drug with dietary fat increases its absorption. It has an elimination half-life of 2–4 days. Atovaquone is highly bound to plasma protein (>99%) and has a high volume of distribution and low clearance (Zsila and Fitos, 2010). Elimination is primarily via the liver, with very low amounts (0.6%) of drug eliminated via the kidneys. Greater than 90% of atovaquone excreted in bile is the parent drug. Proguanil is rapidly absorbed from the gastrointestinal tract with good bioavailability. Proguanil is 75% protein bound, and it is extensively distributed in tissues. Proguanil, but not cycloguanil, is concentrated in erythrocytes, hence the five-fold difference in whole blood versus plasma concentration. Proguanil is metabolized to cycloguanil (primarily through CYP2C19) and 4-chlorophenylbiguanide, with less than 40% excreted renally (GSK, 2015). The elimination half-life of proguanil is 15 hours in both adults and children, but it may be prolonged in individuals with a genetic polymorphism in CYP2C19 (Gillotin et al., 1999; GSK, 2015; Hussein et al., 1997; Thapar et al., 2002), which may have implications for increased toxicity.

In pharmacokinetic studies conducted in healthy adults given single or multiple doses of A/P, no clinically significant interactions between atovaquone, proguanil, or its metabolite cycloguanil were observed (Gillotin et al., 1999; Hussein et al., 1997; Thapar et al., 2002). Pedersen et al. (2014) found that the pharmacokinetic properties of proguanil remained consistent even in individuals with the ultra-rapid metabolizer CYP2C19*17 single nucleotide polymorphism (SNP), indicating that the toxicity and adverse events associated with proguanil should be no different in individuals with the SNP. The pharmacokinetic parameters of A/P are similar to those of the drugs when used as single agents (Deye et al., 2012; Patel and Kain, 2005). The synergistic action of proguanil and atovaquone is thought to be due to its biguanide mode of action, not to the action of its metabolite(s), even in individuals with CYP enzyme deficiencies who are unable to metabolize proguanil to cycloguanil (Boggild et al., 2007).

ADVERSE EVENTS

The following section contains a summary of the known concurrent adverse events associated with the use of A/P. Epidemiologic studies of persistent or latent adverse events in which information was presented regarding adverse events occurring at least 28 days post-A/P-cessation are then summarized, with the emphasis on reported results of persistent or latent adverse events associated with the use of A/P, including the results of studies in which other antimalarial drugs were used as a comparison group.

Concurrent Adverse Events

The most commonly observed concurrent adverse events associated with A/P use are mild or moderate in nature and include nausea, vomiting, abdominal pain, headache, stomatitis, and diarrhea (Boggild et al., 2007; Castelli et al., 2010; Schlagenhauf et al., 2019). Many of these symptoms are avoided or relieved when A/P is taken with food (Chambers, 2003). Between 5% and 10% of individuals develop an asymptomatic elevation of hepatic transaminases (Boggild et al., 2007). There were no significant differences observed in reported adverse events in three out of six prophylaxis trials conducted in adults (Faucher et al., 2002; Shanks et al., 1998; Simons et al., 2005). Oral aphthous ulcerations are not uncommon while taking A/P, but they are rarely severe enough to warrant discontinuation (AlKadi, 2007). Discontinuation of A/P due to severe adverse events was not common (Boggild et al., 2007).

Tickell-Painter et al. (2017) performed a Cochrane systematic review in which adverse events were prespecified to include these disorders: psychiatric (abnormal dreams, insomnia, anxiety, depression, psychosis); nervous system (dizziness, headache); ear and labyrinth (vertigo); eye (visual impairment); gastrointestinal (nausea, vomiting, abdominal pain, diarrhea, dyspepsia); and skin and subcutaneous tissues (pruritus, photosensitivity, vaginal candida). The purpose of the assessment was to summarize the efficacy and safety of mefloquine for malaria prophylaxis in adult, children, and pregnant women travelers as compared with other antimalarials (including A/P), placebo, or no treatment. The dosages of mefloquine varied, as did the methods of collecting adverse event data. The authors applied categories of certainty to the results based on the five GRADE considerations (risk of bias, consistency of effect, imprecision, indirectness, and publication bias) (Higgins et al., 2019).

In the included cohort studies, no serious adverse events were reported among A/P users. Regarding neurologic adverse events, mefloquine users were more likely to report headache than A/P users, but this finding was only statistically significant across the cohort studies (RR = 3.42, 95%CI 1.71–6.82; 8 cohort studies, 4,163 participants). Similarly, dizziness was more common in mefloquine users than among A/P users in the trial (RR = 3.99, 95%CI 2.08–7.64) and in eight cohort studies (RR = 3.83, 95%CI 2.23–6.58; 3,986 participants).

In the single included trial, mefloquine users were statistically significantly more likely than A/P users to report psychiatric adverse events of abnormal dreams, insomnia, anxiety, and depressed mood. Consistent, larger effects were observed in the cohort studies. In addition, no A/P users reported abnormal thoughts or perceptions, as compared with 21 mefloquine users, but the differences between groups did not reach statistical significance.

When mefloquine users were compared with A/P users, mefloquine users were more likely to experience nausea based on one trial (RR = 2.72, 95%CI 1.52–4.86; 976 participants) and seven cohort studies (RR = 2.50, 95%CI 1.54–4.06; 3,509 participants), but there were no statistically significant differences for vomiting, abdominal pain, or diarrhea. In contrast, the risk of mouth ulcers was higher in A/P users than in mefloquine users (effect estimates recalculated to directly compare A/P with mefloquine instead of mefloquine with A/P) in two cohort studies (RR = 8.33, 95%CI 2.70–25.0; 783 participants), but not in the single trial (RR = 0.68, 95%CI 0.33–1.43; 976 participants) that included this outcome.

Other symptoms were also included when available. Based on one trial and three cohort studies, no difference between A/P and mefloquine users was found for experiencing pruritus, although the estimate was imprecise. One trial and two cohort studies found no statistically significant differences for visual impairment between mefloquine and A/P users.

Another systematic review and meta-analysis was identified that included 10 randomized trials of children and adults (but excluded studies of people with comorbidities or who were pregnant or nursing) to examine the effectiveness, safety, and tolerance of A/P as a prophylactic agent against malaria (Nakato et al., 2007). Although studies examining adverse events in individuals less than 16 years of age were excluded from the committee's consideration, because the study groups may have contained individuals 16 years of age or older the results of this review are reported. Those taking A/P did not report adverse events more frequently than those taking placebo. Only one serious adverse event was reported in an individual taking A/P, who was hospitalized after repeated vomiting. The authors reported that there were no significant differences in adverse events between individuals taking two times the approved dose of A/P used for prophylaxis and individuals taking a placebo. In several of the post-cessation epidemiologic studies, including those presented in the other antimalarial drug chapters, A/P is often used as a reference group because of its strong safety and tolerability profile.

Post-Cessation Adverse Events

A total of 960 abstracts or article titles were identified by the literature search for A/P. After screening, 418 abstracts and titles were retained, and the full text for each was retrieved and reviewed to determine whether it met the inclusion criteria, as defined in Chapter 3. The committee reviewed each article and identified four post-cessation epidemiologic studies that included some mention of adverse events that occurred ≥28 days post-A/P-cessation (Eick-Cost et al., 2017; Schneider et al., 2013, 2014; Tan et al., 2017). These are summarized below and form the basis of the body of evidence on the persistent and latent adverse events of A/P. A table that gives a high-level comparison (study design, population, exposure groups, and outcomes examined by body system) of each of these four epidemiologic studies is presented in Appendix C.

Military and Veterans

Using Department of Defense (DoD) administrative databases, Eick-Cost et al. (2017) performed a retrospective cohort study among 367,840 active-duty service members who filled at least one prescription for an antimalarial drug between 2008 and 2013: 36,538 were prescribed mefloquine, 318,421 doxycycline, and 12,881 A/P. The primary study objective was to assess and compare the risk of incident and recurrent *International Classification of Diseases, Ninth Revision, Clinical Modification* (ICD-9-CM)-coded neurologic and psychiatric outcomes (adjustment disorder, anxiety disorder, depressive disorder, posttraumatic stress disorder [PTSD], psychoses, suicide ideation, paranoia, confusion, tinnitus, vertigo, convulsions, hallucinations, insomnia, and suicide) that were reported at medical care visits during concurrent use plus 365 days after the end of the prescription for mefloquine, doxycycline, and A/P. Although the authors did not report on results for the period of ≥28 days post-cessation of antimalarial drug use, they stated that they performed several sensitivity analyses, including one in which the risk period was restricted to 30 days post-prescription. The results of that analysis were summarized in the text as, "However, none of these analyses significantly changed the results of the study and are therefore not reported" (p. 161). This statement implies (but does not show directly) that findings similar to those reported would be seen if the reporting period were restricted to the period relevant to the committee's definition of persistence (i.e., ≥28 days after cessation of exposure). The committee was unsure how to interpret the claim that different analyses did not change the results significantly (i.e., there was no information about statistical significance, the precision of effect estimates, the number of diagnoses, etc.), but given that the authors performed sensitivity analyses, the number of methodologic strengths, including a strong measurement of relevant outcomes conducted in the target population, the committee chose to include the study, despite the ambiguity in the language. If an individual had multiple prescriptions over the follow-up period, risk periods were merged. Doxycycline and A/P prescriptions were excluded if the service member previously or concurrently received mefloquine. Mefloquine risk periods were censored if an individual received a prescription for a different antimalarial. Analyses were stratified by deployment and psychiatric history. Models were adjusted for age, sex, service, grade, and the year the prescription started; analyses of deployed service members also controlled for location and combat exposure. A/P recipients had primarily served in the Army (34%), many were senior enlisted officers (23%), and a majority had prescriptions filled after 2012 (55%). Among the deployed service members, fewer individuals who had received A/P reported combat exposure (21%, compared with 29% for mefloquine and 43% for doxycycline).

With few exceptions, the adjusted incident rates were higher among the deployed than among the nondeployed for A/P as well as for the other antimalarial drugs considered. The effect estimates of neurologic and psychiatric outcomes for mefloquine and doxycycline are reported in those respective chapters. For A/P users, the highest incident rates in both deployed and nondeployed service members were for adjustment disorder (31.61 versus 13.6 per 1,000 person-years, respectively), followed by insomnia (23.21 versus 10.74 per 1,000 person-years, respectively) and anxiety disorder (14.97 versus 8.69 per 1,000 person-years, respectively). Incident depressive disorder (7.09 versus 6.86 per 1,000 person-years, respectively), convulsions (2.31 versus 0.69 per 1,000 person-years, respectively), and hallucinations (0.58 versus 0.38 per 1,000 person-years, respectively) were also higher among the deployed group. On the other hand, the incidence rates for tinnitus (10.24 versus 11.27 per 1,000 person-years, respectively), vertigo (11.24 versus 11.42 per 1,000 person-years, respectively), suicide ideation (0.71 versus 1.47 per 1,000 person-years, respectively), and psychoses (0 versus 0.17 per 1,000 person-years, respectively) were higher among the nondeployed than among the deployed. Among those prescribed A/P, the incidence rate of PTSD was 6.74 per 1,000 person-years in the deployed group and 3.81 per 1,000 person-years in the nondeployed group. Adjusted incident rate ratios (IRRs) comparing mefloquine to A/P by deployment status found that among the deployed, mefloquine users were more likely to experience tinnitus than A/P users (IRR = 1.81, 95%CI 1.18–2.79). When mefloquine and A/P users were compared among the nondeployed, mefloquine users had a significantly *higher* risk of tinnitus (IRR = 1.51, 95%CI 1.13–2.03) and PTSD (IRR = 1.83, 95%CI 1.07–3.14). No other neurologic or psychiatric outcomes were statistically significantly different between mefloquine and A/P users in either the deployed or nondeployed groups. In a second study objective, the investigators compared the risk of developing a neurologic or psychiatric outcome in mefloquine and doxycycline users with and without a neurologic or psychiatric diagnosis in the year prior to receiving antimalarial drugs; A/P was excluded from this analysis due to the small sample size.

The committee found this study to be well designed. Important factors that increased the study's quality are its large sample size; the use of an administrative data source, which provides some degree of objectivity; and a careful consideration of potential confounding variables including demographics, psychiatric history, and the military characteristics of deployment and combat exposure. Because neurologic and psychiatric diagnoses occurring during current and recent use were analyzed together without distinguishing between events that occurred within 28 days of antimalarial use and those that occurred ≥28 days post-cessation, the study provides no quantitative information regarding the persistence of most events other than the notation in text that results did not change when restricted to the post-cessation period. The use of administrative data provided a standard, consistent method to capture filled prescriptions and medical diagnoses through the use of ICD-9-CM codes. However, filled prescriptions do not equate to adherence to the drug regimens. Moreover, if the antimalarials were provided to entire units as part of force health protection measures, the use of these drugs would not be coded in individual records. Whereas medical diagnoses are likely to be more reliable than self-report for determining the outcomes, the data are dependent on the accuracy of the coding, and there was no validation of the diagnoses recorded in the administrative databases, and any symptoms or events that did not result in a medical visit or diagnosis would have been missed. For PTSD diagnoses, there was no information concerning when the index trauma occurred. Given the largely null results reported for comparisons with A/P, this implies that null results would be found for the period of interest, but the data were not presented to make it possible to examine this assumption directly.

U.S. Peace Corps

Tan et al. (2017) conducted a retrospective observational Internet-based survey of 8,931 (11% response rate) returned U.S. Peace Corps volunteers (who had served during 1995–2014) to compare the prevalence of selected health conditions after Peace Corps service between those who reported taking malaria prophylaxis (n = 5,055; 56.6%) and those who did not. The reported initial antimalarial prophylactic prescriptions were mefloquine (n = 2,981; 59.0%), A/P (n = 183; 3.6%), chloroquine (n = 674; 13.3%), doxycycline (n = 831; 16.4%), and 386 (7.6%) "other" prophylactic medications. In addition to questions on malaria prophylaxis (type, regimen, duration, and adherence), the survey included questions about the country of service, the type of assignment, and whether malaria prophylaxis was required at the assigned site. Respondents were also asked to report medical diagnoses made by a health care provider before, during, and after service in the Peace Corps and to answer questions about medications used before, during, and after Peace Corps service. In addition they were questioned about a family history of disease and psychiatric illness, any psychiatric history prior to exposure, and alcohol consumption. In total, more than 40 disease outcomes were examined for associations with each antimalarial; these included derived outcomes of major depressive disorder, bipolar disorder, anxiety disorder, insomnia, psychoses, and cancers. Outcomes were grouped by system (neuropsychologic, cardiac, ophthalmologic, dermatologic, reproductive, and gastrointestinal) or class (infectious, hematologic/oncologic) and within each group several diagnoses were listed. "Any psychiatric outcome" included all reported psychiatric diagnoses both derived and those reported as individual diagnoses, including schizophrenia, obsessive-compulsive disorder, and "other." Neuropsychologic disorders were presented as a category and that separately included dementia, migraines, seizures, tinnitus, vestibular disorder, "other" neurologic disorder, and "any" neurologic disorder. The authors reported that there were no differences in the prevalence of post-service Peace Corps disease diagnoses between those who had used A/P and those who had not. The diagnoses mentioned were those derived from reported and feared adverse events with A/P such as migraines, based on reports of headaches, fatty liver, cirrhosis, or liver failure, although the specific effect estimates were not shown. There were no statistical results presented for outcomes related to A/P exposure.

The study had many limitations, primarily stemming from its design as an Internet-based survey of people with email addresses on file. The response rate was low (11%), the authors relied on self-report for both exposure and outcome information and the timing of each, and for some participants the time between exposure and the survey was many years. Most comparisons were between specific drug exposure (i.e., mefloquine, chloroquine, doxycycline, A/P, other) and non-exposure. Thus, the comparison group for each antimalarial was a mixture of those who did not report taking any antimalarials and those who reported taking antimalarial drugs other than the one being examined. Overall, there were few details of the limited analyses presented, making it difficult to understand the groups that were being compared, how they differed with respect to important covariates, and what variables were included in the models. The reliance on self-reports that were provided years (range 2–20 years) after the exposure introduces several potential biases (selection bias, recall bias, and confounding bias) with inadequate information to determine the likely impact or direction of the potential biases acting in this study. While the use of self-reported diagnoses that were specified to be those made by a medical professional to ascertain health outcomes was arguably a better method than using a checklist of symptoms, the outcomes were not validated against any objective information. The results presented in this study do not support the presence of persistent or latent health effects—or incident neurologic or psychiatric effects specifically—after A/P cessation, but the design limitations of this study are such that any evidence provided by this study is weak.

Travelers

Schneider et al. (2013, 2014) conducted two retrospective observational studies in travelers using data from the UK-based General Practice Research Database (GPRD)—which has since changed names to the Clinical Practice Research Datalink—to assess the incidence and compare the odds of developing first-time neurologic, psychiatric, or eye disorders in individuals using A/P compared with other antimalarial drugs for malaria prophylaxis. The Clinical Practice Research Datalink, which has been active for more than 30 years, collects de-identified patient data from a network of general practitioner practices across the United Kingdom for use in public health research and clinical studies; these studies have included investigations of drug safety, the use of medications, health care delivery, and disease risk factors (CPRD, 2019). While the specific outcomes examined (neurologic, psychiatric, and eye disorders) in the two antimalarial drug studies differed, the general methodology was the same. Using the GPRD, investigators identified individuals who had at least one prescription for mefloquine, A/P, doxycycline, or chloroquine and/or proguanil in the time period of interest and who had a pre-travel consultation within 1 week of the date of the prescription that included specific codes indicating that the prescription was for malaria prophylaxis. The start of follow-up was the date of receipt of the first prescription for an individual. *Current use* was defined as between the date a prescription started and one week after the end of the time period of the drug prescription. *Current exposure time* was calculated differently for each antimalarial drug because the regimens for the antimalarial drugs differ. Investigators based the assessment on the number of tablets recorded by the general practitioner and calculated the assumed exposure time for each of the antimalarial drugs being investigated. For A/P, the current exposure time (in days) was the number of tablets plus 7 days. Investigators added 90 days to each exposure time to capture events occurring during travel that came to the attention of the general practitioner after returning to the United Kingdom. *Recent use* included periods both relevant to the committee's charge (days 28–89) and time periods that the committee considered exclusionary (days 7–27). *Past use* started at day 91 and ended at a maximum of 540 days after the end of current exposure, reflecting a time period pertinent to the committee's assessment. Non-exposed people served as controls and had no antimalarial prescription during the study period or during 540 days after their pre-travel consultation, which also served as the date of the start of their follow-up. Participants were required to have at least 12 months of information on prescribed drugs and medical diagnoses before the first prescription date for an antimalarial or their travel consultation for the non-exposed controls. An additional inclusion criterion required participants to have recorded medical activity (diagnoses or drug prescriptions) after receiving a prescription to ensure that only individuals who returned to the United Kingdom were included. A nested case–control analysis was also performed for a subset of the population in which six controls (who did not develop an outcome of interest during follow-up) were randomly selected per case; controls were matched to cases on age, sex, general practice, and calendar time (by assigning each control to the same index date as their matched case).

Overall the design of these large, retrospective studies allowed for adequate power to detect differences in outcomes and a uniform collection of exposures and outcomes that were not subject to recall bias. The nested case–control component allowed for the control of important covariates. The reliance on recorded drug prescriptions to determine exposure ensures that the assessment was applied equally to all exposure groups; however, as with any study that relies on administrative databases, the prescriptions were not a surrogate for adherence. Outcome assessment was uniform for all exposure groups and based on medical care visits coded in a database designed for both practice and research and with validated outcomes. Events that did not result in a medical care visit or that occurred outside of the national health care system would have been missed, and there may also have been some differences between the travelers who traveled to malaria-endemic areas versus areas that are not endemic for malaria, which could have led to some apparent differences in outcomes between the groups. However, it is unlikely that this would result in differential selection bias. Additional strengths and limitations that are study-specific are noted within each study summary.

Schneider et al. (2013) estimated the incidence of anxiety, stress-related disorders, or psychosis (n = 952); depression (n = 739); epilepsy (n = 86); or peripheral neuropathy (n = 56) in individuals (aged ≥1 year) with a pre-travel consultation and at least one prescription for mefloquine (n = 10,169), A/P (n = 28,502), or chloroquine and/or proguanil (n = 2,904) for malaria prophylaxis or else no antimalarial prescription (but who had a pre-travel consultation) (n = 41,573) between January 1, 2001, and October 1, 2009. Individuals were excluded if there was a record of a diagnosis of malaria prior to the start of antimalarial drug use; a history of cancer, alcoholism, or rheumatoid arthritis; or a diagnosis of an outcome of interest prior to a prescription for an antimalarial. For the unexposed group, individuals were excluded if there was a record of any of those diagnoses prior to the date of the pre-travel clinic visit. The date of the diagnosis of the first neurologic or psychiatric disorder was the index date for each case. Investigators estimated the incidence of the specified neurologic or psychiatric outcomes that occurred up to 540 days following current use of A/P compared with other antimalarials and with no use of antimalarials. Although 15.3% of the population was ≤18 years and the reported number of cases of each outcome was reported by age group, the authors presented only the associations between drugs and health outcomes for the total population (children and adults). Despite that limitation, the committee presents the results as reported because a relatively small proportion of the population was under age 18 years, and the results should approximate the associations that would have been found for adults only. The overall incidence rates for anxiety, stress-related disorders, or psychosis (presented as a group) and depression in individuals using A/P were higher than the comparable incidence rates for individuals using mefloquine but lower than incidence rates in individuals using chloroquine and/ or proguanil or who were unexposed. A nested case–control analysis was also conducted in which investigators categorized subjects into current (use of drug plus 90 days post-cessation) or past-use (91–540 days post-cessation) exposure groups and controlled for age, sex, calendar time, general practice, smoking, and body mass index (BMI). Individuals who did not develop the outcomes of interest during the follow-up period formed the control group, and six controls per case matched on sex, year of birth, general practice, and calendar time were selected. When considering current use (which includes a mixture of nonrelevant [during use to 27 days post-use] and relevant [day 28–90 post-use] time periods) compared with travelers who did not use any antimalarial prophylaxis and after adjustment for BMI and smoking, the odds of developing anxiety, stress-related disorders, or psychosis (OR = 0.92, 95%CI 0.72–1.18); epilepsy (OR = 1.42, 95%CI 0.59–3.42); and peripheral neuropathy (OR = 1.51, 95%CI 0.54–4.21) were no greater among current A/P users. However, current A/P users were found to have statistically significantly decreased odds of developing depression compared with those who did not use antimalarials (OR = 0.56, 95%CI 0.40–0.80). When considering past exposure, the odds of developing anxiety, stress-related disorders, or psychosis were statistically significantly decreased in past users of A/P compared with those who did not use an antimalarial (OR = 0.65 95%CI 0.54–0.79). There were no statistically significant differences for depression, epilepsy, or peripheral neuropathy when examining past A/P exposure with no use of antimalarials. When anxiety, psychosis, phobia, and panic attack were analyzed as separate outcomes, compared with no antimalarial users, A/P users had statistically significantly decreased odds of developing phobia (OR = 0.64, 95%CI 0.43–0.96) and anxiety (OR = 0.66, 95%CI 0.52–0.84). However, these analyses were based on any use of A/P, and it was not stratified by current or past exposure time.

This large, adequately powered study provides evidence of decreased odds of depression among current users of A/P and decreased odds of anxiety, stress-related disorders, and psychosis (combined outcome) among past users, and it found no evidence of an increase in anxiety, stress-related disorders, or psychosis (combined outcome), depression, epilepsy, or peripheral neuropathy associated with A/P use for malaria prophylaxis in travelers when assessing current use or past use and follow-up for 18 months compared with people who did not use antimalarials. The comparison group consisted of travelers as well, but they may have traveled to non-malaria-endemic areas or had unmeasured risk factors that contraindicated antimalarial prophylaxis. The 1-year medical record history used to assess psychiatric conditions is unlikely to reflect a complete psychiatric history. Overall, this was a well-designed study that found no increase in anxiety, stress-related disorders, or psychosis (combined outcome), depression, epilepsy, or peripheral neuropathy associated with A/P use for malaria prophylaxis in travelers aged ≥1 year when assessing current use and 18 months following current use.

Using the same design and administrative database as described by Schneider et al. (2013), Schneider et al. (2014) examined the incidence of clinical eye disorders (n = 652) in travelers (aged ≥1 year) with at least one prescription for mefloquine (n = 10,169), A/P (n = 28,502), or chloroquine and/or proguanil (n = 2,904) for malaria prophylaxis or no antimalarial prescription (but who had a pre-travel consultation) (n = 41,573) between January 1, 2001, and October 1, 2009. Individuals were excluded if they had a diagnosis of malaria prior to the start of antimalarial drug use; had cancer, alcoholism, or rheumatoid arthritis; or had been diagnosed with an eye disorder of interest (any eye disorder affecting the cornea, lens, uvea, iris, retina, or other parts of the eye, or glaucoma). Because only 20 of the total 652 eye disorders occurred among people ≤17 years, although the number of users of each drug was not stratified by age, the committee presents the results as reported, and it does not believe that the interpretation of findings and inferences that can be made are overly influenced by the inclusion of people ≤17 years. Among A/P users, there were a total of 244 incident eye disorders identified (54 occurred within 90 days of finishing the prescription, and 190 occurred between 91 and 540 days after the end of the prescription). The eye disorders were grouped as disorders of the cornea, cataract, glaucoma, disorders of the retina, impairment in visual acuity, vitreous detachment, disorders of the uvea, or neuro-ophthalmalogic disorders (the latter including optic neuritis, diplopia, trigeminal neuralgia, and other conditions). Incidence rates were estimated for each eye disorder category by antimalarial group, but no comparisons between groups were made. A nested case–control analysis was performed in which smoking, BMI, and a history of depression, diabetes, hypertension, sleep disorders, and use of corticosteroids and contraceptives were controlled for. Compared with travelers who did not use any antimalarial drugs, the odds of developing any of the eye disorders of interest was elevated for A/P users (OR = 1.25, 95%CI 1.03–1.52). However, when A/P use was stratified by current (defined as use of drug plus 90 days post-cessation) and past use (91–540 days post-cessation) and compared with the nonusers, for current users there were not statistically significantly increased odds (OR = 1.04, 95%CI 0.75–1.43), whereas past users had statistically significantly increased odds (OR = 1.34, 95%CI 1.08–1.66), suggesting that the overall finding was driven by the association with past exposure. When each of the individual eye disorder categories was examined, both cataracts (OR = 2.00, 95%CI 1.3–3.08) and retinal disorders (OR = 1.83, 95%CI 1.07–3.13) showed statistically significantly increased odds in relation to A/P use (these results were not stratified by current or past timing of exposure).

The strengths and limitations of this study mirror those discussed in Schneider et al. (2013). Although "current use" likely captured some events within the 28-day post-cessation window, it is unlikely to have resulted in selection bias. The finding of increased risk of cataracts and retinal disorders with A/P use was unexpected and would require confirmatory evidence. Other risk factors for retinal disorders, such as a family history of retinal disorders, were not included in the analysis and may have differed between the groups. Overall, the study suggests an increased risk of developing eye disorders in past users and an increased risk of developing cataracts and retinal disorders for users of A/P relative to nonusers of antimalarials.

OTHER IDENTIFIED STUDIES OF A/P
PROPHYLAXIS IN HUMAN POPULATIONS

The committee also reviewed several studies of A/P use in service members from the United States (Saunders et al., 2015), Colombia (Soto et al., 2006), the United Kingdom (Tuck and Williams, 2016), Sweden (Andersson et al., 2008), and Canada (Paul et al., 2003). However, these studies either did not follow military cohorts after the A/P prophylaxis was completed or did not report on adverse events that occurred post-A/P-cessation; therefore, they were not further considered.

A number of studies were designed to examine the safety or tolerability of A/P when used in nonimmune travelers, but they did not report on adverse events or other outcomes occurring at least 28 days post-cessation of A/P or distinguish the timing of those events (within or after 28 days post-cessation) (Høgh et al., 2000; Kato et al., 2013; Laverone et al., 2006; Overbosch, 2003; Overbosch et al., 2001; Schlagenhauf et al., 2003, 2009; Sharafeldin et al., 2010; van Genderen et al., 2007; van Riemsdijk et al., 2002). Similarly, several studies conducted in healthy volunteers (Deye et al., 2012; Gillotin et al., 1999; Sukwa et al., 1999; Thapar et al., 2002), endemic populations (Berman et al., 2001; Shanks et al., 1998), migrants (Ling et al., 2002; van Vugt et al., 1999), and individuals with occupation-related exposure to malaria prophylaxis (Cunningham et al., 2014; Landman et al., 2015; Nicosia et al., 2008) did not report any adverse events occurring beyond 28 days post-cessation of A/P. Simons et al. (2005) conducted a study in healthy volunteers under aircraft pressure to evaluate the impact of A/P on in-flight performance. Individuals were split into two groups in a crossover study design, resulting in different lengths of follow-up after the use of A/P; however, reported adverse events were not reported individually for each group (one group was followed for more than 28 days post-cessation of A/P), making it impossible to distinguish between adverse events that occurred <28 days post-cessation or ≥28 days post-cessation, and, as a result, this study was not further considered.

Case Reports and Case Series

A/P is relatively well tolerated, but a few moderate to severe adverse events have been reported in individuals using A/P for malaria prophylaxis. The committee reviewed three case reports, totaling three patients, which reported adverse events that persisted for at least 28 days following A/P cessation. There was one case of phototoxicity after sun exposure while taking A/P, and this condition persisted for "several months" (Amelot et al., 2014). A case of vanishing bile duct syndrome was diagnosed in a male traveler who presented with jaundice, pruritus, lethargy, dark urine, and pale stool (Abugroun et al., 2019). A liver biopsy indicated mild interface hepatitis and marked bilorubinostasis. The traveler recovered but then was re-admitted to the hospital 2 months later, and a repeat liver biopsy showed diffuse ductopenia, diagnostic of vanishing bile duct syndrome. Over 18 months of follow-up, his symptoms and laboratory values improved. Finally, Terziroli Beretta-Piccoli et al. (2017) reported a case of A/P-induced autoimmune-like hepatitis in a traveler who presented with jaundice, fatigue, and dark urine with elevated laboratory values and a liver biopsy significant for portal inflammation with plasma cell rich interface activity, severe zone 3 necrosis, but no significant fibrosis. He was treated with prednisone, and at 6-month follow-up his laboratory tests were normal, but a repeat liver biopsy was still abnormal. At 1-year follow-up, the liver biopsy was normal. These three cases suggest that though A/P is generally well tolerated, cutaneous and liver-related adverse events should be clinically monitored.

Selected Subpopulations

In the course of its review of the literature on A/P, the committee identified and reviewed available studies that reported results stratified by demographic, medical, or behavioral factors to assess whether the risk for adverse events when using A/P for prophylaxis is associated with being part of or affiliated with a specific group. This was not done exhaustively, and the evidence included in this section is generally limited to concurrent adverse events observed with A/P use. Many of these studies did not meet the inclusion criteria of following their population for at least 28 days post-A/P-cessation, but the committee considers these findings to be important indicators when considering the evidence as a whole. The following risk groups were specifically considered: pregnant women and those with comorbid diseases or disorders.

Pregnancy

Available data from the published literature and postmarketing experience with use of A/P in pregnant women are insufficient to identify a drug-associated risk for major birth defects, miscarriage, or adverse maternal or fetal outcomes. Postmarketing surveillance (Mayer et al., 2018) and registry-based cohort studies (Duffy and Fried, 2005; Kaser et al., 2015; McGready et al., 2003) have failed to find a consistent, significant association between poor birth outcomes and the use of A/P taken at any point during pregnancy or breastfeeding. For example, a large registry-based cohort study conducted in Denmark found no significant association between exposure to A/P in early pregnancy and the risk of any major birth defect (Pasternak and Hviid, 2011). A systematic review of A/P for the prevention and treatment of malaria in pregnancy showed that outcomes following A/P exposure during pregnancy are similar to the expected rates in similar populations Andrejko et al., 2019). An analysis of birth outcomes following accidental exposures to A/P during pregnancy recorded in the A/P-exposed pregnancies database (a passive reporting system) found no concerning signals of poor pregnancy outcomes, although there was a possible higher rate of congenital anomalies with no apparent pattern. There are data to suggest that adjusting the dose of A/P during pregnancy may be warranted because blood plasma levels of the drug are lower in pregnant women (Davis et al., 2010; Nosten et al., 2006) and proguanil monotherapy is considered safe during pregnancy (Mayer et al., 2018). Because of insufficient data on its safety in pregnancy, the Centers for Disease Control and Prevention does not recommend the use of A/P for the prevention or treatment of malaria during pregnancy (CDC, 2018, 2019).

Comorbid Diseases

Many travelers have comorbid medical conditions that require them to take medication. In these individuals, there is the potential for drug–drug interactions with prophylactic antimalarial drugs, which may result in harmful consequences. One study examined A/P use in individuals with renal impairment and found no issues with the use of A/P, but it noted that dosage adjustments may be needed for proguanil because of the altered pharmacokinetics (Amet et al., 2013).

BIOLOGIC PLAUSIBILITY

Whole animal studies of A/P conducted in mice, rats, and dogs found toxicity to be no greater than that observed for either drug alone (FDA, 2019a). These studies were primarily observational and examined immediate and concurrent effects; they were not designed to investigate possible mechanisms of action. The experimental animal studies administered A/P at the equivalent of treatment doses (which are about four times higher than the prophylactic dose) but did not conduct long-term post-administration follow-up (instead it was limited to hours to days), as is standard procedure for preclinical toxicology studies (NRC, 2006). The combination of A/P was not embryotoxic at clinically relevant concentrations (FDA, 2019a).

Investigators also found that there was no accumulation of atovaquone within human cells, making it less likely for adverse events to occur. However, atovaquone may reduce the elimination of proguanil in extensive metabolizer phenotypes, so that in these individuals, proguanil concentrations may be elevated (Thapar et al., 2002).

Based on the paucity of currently available scientific literature examining the biologic plausibility of persistent or latent adverse events resulting from the use of A/P for malaria prophylaxis, the committee found minimal to no evidence suggesting plausible biologic mechanisms underlying persistent or latent effects of malaria prophylaxis in humans. Further studies would be needed to ascertain whether there are persistent cellular effects associated with the use of A/P for malaria prophylaxis.

SYNTHESIS AND CONCLUSIONS

A/P as a combination drug has been approved for use as a prophylactic drug for malaria since 2000. It is generally well tolerated and has often been used as a comparator in studies of efficacy and tolerability of other antimalarial drugs because it is less likely to be discontinued due to adverse events than other prophylactic drugs for malaria, such as mefloquine (Kain et al., 2001; Overbosch et al., 2001; Tickell-Painter et al., 2017). While there have been several studies of concurrent adverse events when using A/P for malaria prophylaxis, the evidence addressing latent or persistent adverse events is quite limited in quantity and quality.

Four epidemiologic studies were identified that reported on adverse events at least 28 days post-A/P-cessation (Eick-Cost et al., 2017; Schneider et al., 2013, 2014; Tan et al., 2017). These studies considered different populations—members of the U.S. military (Eick-Cost et al., 2017); returned U.S. Peace Corps volunteers (Tan et al., 2017); and travelers (Schneider et al., 2013, 2014)—and they considered different health outcomes, with the studies' varying definitions making a synthesis of the findings challenging. For example, three of the post-cessation epidemiologic studies for A/P collected and reported information that could be categorized as psychiatric outcomes; however, these ranged from nonspecific broad categories, such as "neuropsychologic," to specific symptoms such as sleep disturbances and anxiety, and clinical diagnoses such as PTSD, depressive disorder, and psychosis, posing a challenge to the committee's ability to make an integrated assessment. Given the inherently imperfect information generated by any one study, it would be desirable to have similar studies to assess the consistency of the findings, but the diversity of the methods used within the included epidemiologic studies makes it very difficult to combine information across studies with confidence. Even when pertinent data appeared to have been collected to meet the committee's inclusion criteria of reporting on an adverse event or health outcome (or if there were none reported) 28 days post-drug-cessation, not all of the information relevant to the committee's charge was presented because it was not a main objective or a focus of the study (e.g., studies that were designed to examine long-term efficacy against clinical malaria). In some cases it was clear that the investigators collected more data than was reported, such as when the population was followed for months or even years after A/P cessation, but the only outcomes reported were on incident cases of malaria or generic statements about all adverse events having resolved. Another limitation across the included studies was that it was not always possible to identify whether concurrent adverse events persisted beyond the time of drug cessation, thus the studies did not all contribute equally to the ultimate conclusion of the association between A/P and persistent or latent adverse events of a given health outcome. In general, the reviewed epidemiologic studies were not designed to examine the persistence of adverse events in individuals, but rather they collected information on whether adverse events were detected at some time period at least 28 days after cessation of A/P. To avoid repetition for each outcome category, a short summary of the attributes of each study that was considered to be contributory to the evidence base is presented first. The evidence summaries for each outcome category refer back to these short assessment summaries.

For each health outcome category, supporting information from FDA, known concurrent adverse events, case studies, information on selected subpopulations, and experimental animal and in vitro studies are first summarized before the evidence from post-cessation epidemiologic studies is described. While the charge to the committee was to address persistent or latent adverse events, the occurrence of concurrent adverse events enhances the likelihood that problems may persist beyond the period after cessation of drug use. The synthesis of evidence is followed by a conclusion of the strength of evidence regarding an association between the use of A/P and persistent or latent adverse events and whether the available evidence would support additional research into those outcomes. The outcomes are presented in the following order: neurologic disorders, psychiatric disorders, gastrointestinal disorders, eye disorders, cardiovascular disorders, and other outcomes.

Epidemiologic Studies Presenting Contributory Evidence

Eick-Cost et al. (2017) used DoD administrative databases to perform a large retrospective cohort study of active-duty service members who filled at least one prescription for mefloquine, doxycycline, or A/P between 2008 and 2013. The primary study objective was to assess and compare the risk of incident and recurrent ICD-9-CM-coded neurologic and psychiatric outcomes that were reported at medical care visits during concurrent antimalarial use plus 365 days after the end of a prescription. This was a well-designed study and included several important factors that increased its methodologic quality: a large sample size, an administrative data source for both exposure and outcomes, and a careful consideration of potential confounders including demographics, psychiatric history, and the military characteristics of deployment and combat exposure. Because neurologic and psychiatric diagnoses occurring during current and recent use were analyzed together without distinguishing between events that occurred within 28 days of antimalarial use and those that occurred ≥28 days post-cessation, the study provides no quantitative information regarding the persistence of most events other than the notation in the text that the results did not change when restricted to the post-cessation period. Whereas medical diagnoses are likely to be more reliable for the outcomes of self-report, there was no validation of the diagnoses recorded in the administrative databases, and symptoms or events that did not result in a medical visit or diagnosis would have been missed. For PTSD diagnoses, there was no information about when the index trauma occurred.

Two large, retrospective studies of travelers (Schneider et al., 2013, 2014) were conducted using data from the UK-based GPRD to assess the incidence and compare the odds of developing first-time neurologic, psychiatric, or eye disorders in individuals aged ≥1 year using A/P compared with other antimalarial drugs for malaria prophylaxis relative to travelers who did not use an antimalarial. While the specific outcomes examined differed by study, the general design and methodology were the same. The use of data from the GPRD (a well-established platform designed for both clinical practice and research) allowed for adequate power to detect differences in outcomes and for a uniform collection of exposures (although recorded drug prescriptions do not equate to use or adherence) and outcomes (based on clinical diagnoses coded from medical care visits) that were not subject to recall bias. Events that did not result in a medical care visit or that occurred outside of the national health care system would have been missed; however, it is unlikely that this would result in differential selection bias. Diagnoses were defined a priori, which excluded other outcomes, including the potential to identify rare outcomes. The antimalarial-exposed populations were large, an appropriate comparison group of travelers not using a form of malaria prophylaxis was included, and the health outcomes were reported in defined time periods, including current use through 90 days after a prescription ended (termed *current use* or *recent use* in analyses) and 91–540 days following cessation of use (termed *past use* in analyses). Adjustments were made for several confounders, including age, sex, calendar time, practice, smoking status, and BMI using appropriate study design or analytic methods. Each study included a nested case–control component that allowed for the control of important covariates.

The primary aim of Tan et al. (2017) was to assess the prevalence of several health conditions experienced by returned Peace Corps volunteers associated with the use of prophylactic antimalarial drugs. Although the total number of participants was large, only a small proportion (n = 183; 3.6%) used A/P. A number of important covariates, such as psychiatric history and alcohol use, were collected, but the study had several methodologic limitations. These limitations included the study design itself (self-report, Internet-based survey), an exposure characterization that was based on self-report (which introduces several potential biases such as recall bias, sampling bias, and confounding), the outcome assessment (based on self-report of health provider–diagnosed conditions up to 20 years post-service), the use of mixed comparison groups, a lack of detail regarding the analysis methods, and a poor response rate (11%, which likely introduces selection bias). The evidence generated by this study was thus considered to only weakly contribute to the inferences concerning the relationship between A/P and persistent or latent adverse events or disorders.

Neurologic Disorders

The FDA package insert listed rare cases of seizures in the Postmarketing Adverse Reactions section but stated that a causal relationship had not been established; there is no other mention of neurologic disorders. A recognized concurrent adverse neurologic event associated with A/P use has been headache, but in a Cochrane systematic review, among the eight included cohort studies, A/P users were statistically significantly less likely to report headache than mefloquine users. Similarly, dizziness was statistically significantly more common in mefloquine users than in A/P users in one trial and eight cohort studies. No persistent or latent neurologic symptoms or conditions were identified in the case reports. No experimental animal or human cell culture studies were identified that examined the biologic mechanisms by which A/P might affect the central or peripheral nervous system.

Eick-Cost et al. (2017) examined neurologic outcomes of tinnitus, vertigo, convulsions, and confusion. The incidence rates of tinnitus and vertigo were higher among the nondeployed than the deployed. Adjusted IRRs comparing mefloquine with A/P by deployment status found that among both the deployed and nondeployed, mefloquine users were statistically significantly more likely to experience tinnitus than A/P users. No other statistically significant differences were found between mefloquine and A/P users for vertigo, convulsions, or confusion in either the deployed or nondeployed groups. This study provides some evidence against the presence of persistent or latent adverse events of tinnitus, vertigo, convulsions, and confusion.

Using the UK GPRD, Schneider et al. (2013) examined the association (in individuals aged ≥ 1 year) between A/P exposure (current and past) and an incident diagnosis of epilepsy and peripheral neuropathy in comparison with nonusers of antimalarials. In this large study, the authors found no statistically significant difference in the risk of an incident diagnosis of epilepsy or peripheral neuropathy for current or past use of A/P compared with individuals who did not use any antimalarial. This high-quality study provides some evidence against the presence of the persistent or latent neurologic adverse events of incident epilepsy and peripheral neuropathy. Tan et al. (2017) provide weak supportive evidence in their findings of no differences in the prevalence of any self-reported neurologic disease or symptom diagnoses for individuals who used A/P compared with those who did not.

Based on the available evidence, the committee concludes that there is insufficient or inadequate evidence of an association between the use of atovaquone/proguanil for malaria prophylaxis and persistent or latent neurologic events. Current evidence does not suggest further study of such an association is warranted, given the lack of evidence regarding biologic plausibility, adverse events associated with concurrent use, or findings from the existing epidemiologic studies.

Psychiatric Disorders

Although the FDA label states that seizures and psychotic events (such as hallucinations) have been observed, it also states that a causal relationship has not been established (FDA, 2019a). A Cochrane systematic review of concurrent adverse events in short-term travelers using mefloquine compared with other antimalarials, including A/P, found that mefloquine users were statistically significantly more likely than A/P users to report the psychologic adverse events of abnormal dreams, insomnia, anxiety, and depressed mood in one trial, and consistent, larger effects were observed in the included cohort studies. In addition, no A/P users reported abnormal thoughts or perceptions compared with 21 mefloquine users who did, but the differences between groups did not reach statistical significance (Tickell-Painter et al., 2017). No persistent or latent psychiatric symptoms or conditions were identified in the case reports. No experimental animal or human cell culture studies were identified that examined biologic mechanisms for A/P and psychiatric outcomes.

Three epidemiologic studies examining psychiatric effects met the committee's inclusion criteria. Two were well designed (Eick-Cost et al., 2017; Schneider et al., 2013), but the third was limited in that statements were made concerning "neuropsychologic outcomes" as a whole but it did not distinguish specific psychiatric outcomes (Tan et al., 2017). Eick-Cost et al. (2017) examined more psychiatric outcomes than Schneider et al. (2013), although some of the outcomes were similar. Eick-Cost et al. (2017) examined outcomes of adjustment disorder, anxiety disorder, depressive disorder, PTSD, psychoses, suicide, suicide ideation, hallucinations, paranoia, and insomnia. Schneider et al. (2013) examined anxiety, stress-related disorders, and psychosis (as a group and individually) and depression.

Eick-Cost et al. (2017) found that with the exception of suicidal ideation and psychosis, adjusted incident rates for all psychiatric outcomes were higher among the deployed than among the nondeployed for those prescribed A/P. Although incident diagnoses of PTSD were reported for both deployed and nondeployed A/P users, comparisons of mefloquine users and A/P users stratified by deployment status found that none of the psychiatric outcomes were statistically significantly different among the deployed group. Among the nondeployed, only PTSD showed a statistically significantly decreased risk for A/P users compared with mefloquine users.

Using the UK GPRD, Schneider et al. (2013) examined the relationship (in individuals aged ≥1 year) between A/P exposure (current or past) and incident anxiety, stress-related disorders, and psychosis (as a group) and depression in comparison with nonusers of antimalarials. For current use (which includes a mixture of irrelevant [during use to 27 days post use] and relevant [days 28–90 post use] time periods), the odds of developing anxiety, stress-related disorders, or psychosis were not statistically significantly different between A/P users and nonusers, but the odds were statistically significantly decreased for past A/P users compared with nonusers. For depression, current A/P users—but not past A/P users—were found to have statistically significantly decreased odds of developing depression from the comparison group that did not use antimalarials. When restricting to past exposure (91–540 days post-use), the odds of developing anxiety, stress-related disorders, or psychosis were statistically significantly decreased for past users of A/P compared with those who did not use an antimalarial, but there was no difference for depression. When anxiety, psychosis, phobia, and panic attack were analyzed as separate outcomes, compared with nonusers of antimalarials, A/P users (combined current and past use) had statistically significantly decreased odds of developing phobia and anxiety. Both Eick-Cost et al. (2017) and Schneider et al. (2013) provide some evidence against the presence of persistent or latent psychiatric conditions in the specific outcomes examined in individuals using A/P for malaria prophylaxis.

Based on the available evidence, the committee concludes that there is insufficient or inadequate evidence of an association between the use of atovaquone/ proguanil for malaria prophylaxis and persistent or latent psychiatric events. Current evidence does not suggest further study of such an association is warranted, given the lack of evidence regarding biologic plausibility, adverse events associated with concurrent use, or findings from the existing epidemiologic studies.

Gastrointestinal Disorders

The 2019 FDA package insert lists diarrhea and oral ulcers as common concurrent adverse events associated with the use of A/P. The package insert also notes that cases of hepatitis and one account of hepatic failure requiring liver transplant have been reported with the prophylactic use of A/P. In a systematic review of concurrent adverse events in short-term travelers, A/P users were statistically significantly less likely to experience concurrent nausea than mefloquine users and statistically significantly more likely to report mouth ulcers than mefloquine users. There were no statistically significant differences in vomiting, abdominal pain, or diarrhea. One case report was identified that indicated that the use of A/P may have resulted in vanishing bile duct syndrome and the subsequent development of mild interface hepatitis and marked bilorubinostasis. A second case report described auto-immune-like hepatitis in an individual using A/P for malaria prophylaxis. Experimental animal and human cell culture studies that used A/P were also examined for evidence of mechanisms that could plausibly support adverse events, and the committee was unable to identify any such mechanisms that would support persistent or latent gastrointestinal adverse events.

Tan et al. (2017) was the only epidemiologic study identified that examined gastrointestinal outcomes and the use of A/P. The included conditions were cirrhosis, esophageal ulceration, fatty liver, liver failure, peptic ulcer, and "any" liver dysfunction. The study found no association between A/P users and any of these conditions compared with people who did not use A/P, but specific frequencies or effect estimates were not reported; the limitations of this study are described above.

Based on the available evidence, the committee concludes that there is insufficient or inadequate evidence of an association between the use of atovaquone/proguanil and persistent or latent gastrointestinal events. Current evidence does not suggest further study of such an association is warranted, given the lack of evidence regarding biologic plausibility, adverse events associated with concurrent use, or findings from the existing epidemiologic studies.

Eye Disorders

The FDA label is silent on eye disorders, and no case studies of latent or persistent eye disorders were identified. A Cochrane systematic review of concurrent adverse events in short-term travelers using A/P compared with mefloquine found that, based on one trial and two cohort studies, there was no difference between A/P users and mefloquine users in experiencing visual impairment (Tickell-Painter et al., 2017). No experimental animal or human cell culture studies were identified that examined biologic mechanisms for A/P and eye disorders.

Using the UK GPRD, Schneider et al. (2014) examined the relationship (in individuals aged ≥1 year) between A/P exposure (current and past) and incident eye disorders affecting the cornea, uvea, lens, iris, retina, or other parts of the eye relative to nonusers. The primary finding was a statistically significant increase in the odds of any eye disorder among users of A/P relative to nonusers, which appeared to be driven by past use rather than current use, suggesting a latent adverse event. Further analysis of specific eye disorders revealed a statistically significant increased risk of cataracts and retinal disorders in users of A/P relative to nonusers (these results were not stratified by current or past timing of exposure). This single high-quality study provides some evidence for the presence of persistent, possibly latent, eye disorders, specifically cataract and retinal disorders; however, because there is only a single study, the evidence for eye disorders associated with use of A/P must be considered insufficient. Given its limitations, Tan et al. (2017) could only provide supportive evidence, and it reported no differences in any ophthalmologic conditions (macular degeneration, retinopathy, "any" ophthalmologic disorder) for individuals who used A/P compared with those who did not.

Based on the available evidence, the committee concludes that there is insufficient or inadequate evidence of an association between the use of atovaquone/proguanil for malaria prophylaxis and persistent or latent eye disorders. Current evidence suggests further study of such an association is warranted, given the evidence regarding biologic plausibility, adverse events associated with concurrent use, or findings from the existing epidemiologic studies.

Cardiovascular Disorders

The FDA label and package insert do not list any cardiovascular adverse events associated with the use of A/P. The label cautions that the concomitant use of A/P with warfarin and other coumarin-based anticoagulants can increase their anticoagulant effects, but no evidence for concurrent or persistent adverse blood or cardiovascular outcomes was found in any of the literature reviewed on A/P. The Cochrane review examining concurrent adverse events while using antimalarials in short-term travelers did not examine cardiovascular disorders (Tickell-Painter et al., 2017). The committee did not identify any case reports that followed an individual for ≥28 days post-A/P-cessation that reported cardiovascular adverse events.

Tan et al. (2017) was the only post-cessation epidemiologic study that examined cardiovascular events (arrhythmia, congestive heart failure, myocardial infarction, and "any" cardiac disorder), but no association was found between the use of A/P and any of the cardiovascular outcomes.

Based on the available evidence, the committee concludes that there is insufficient or inadequate evidence of an association between the use of atovaquone/ proguanil for malaria prophylaxis and persistent or latent cardiovascular events. Current evidence does not suggest further study of such an association is warranted, given the lack of evidence regarding biologic plausibility, adverse events associated with concurrent use, or findings from the existing epidemiologic studies.

Other Outcomes and Disorders

None of the three high-quality epidemiologic studies reviewed (Eick-Cost et al., 2017; Schneider et al., 2013, 2014) reported on associations between A/P use and other outcomes or disorders. In their survey of returned Peace Corps volunteers, Tan et al. (2017) reported no differences in any disease or symptom diagnoses for dermatologic, infectious, or cancer outcomes between individuals who used A/P and those who did not, but no effect estimates were reported for any of these outcomes.

REFERENCES

Abugroun, A., I. Colina Garcia, F. Ahmed, S. Potts, and M. Flicker. 2019. The first report of atovaquone/proguanil-induced vanishing bile duct syndrome: Case report and mini-review. *Travel Med Infect Dis*, June 22 [Epub ahead of print].

AlKadi, H. O. 2007. Antimalarial drug toxicity: A review. *Chemotherapy* 53(6):385-391.

Amelot, A., J. Dupouy-Camet, and M. Jeanmougin. 2014. Phototoxic reaction associated with malarone (atovaquone/proguanil) antimalarial prophylaxis. *J Dermatol* 41(4):346-348.

Amet, S., S. Zimner-Rapuch, V. Launay-Vacher, N. Janus, and G. Deray. 2013. Malaria prophylaxis in patients with renal impairment: A review. *Drug Saf* 36(2):83-91.

Andersson, H., H. H. Askling, B. Falck, and L. Rombo. 2008. Well-tolerated chemoprophylaxis uniformly prevented Swedish soldiers from *Plasmodium falciparum* malaria in Liberia, 2004-2006. *Mil Med* 173(12):1194-1198.

Andrejko, K. L., R. C. Mayer, S. Kovacs, E. Slutsker, E. Bartlett, K. R. Tan, and J. R. Gutman. 2019. The safety of atovaquone-proguanil for the prevention and treatment of malaria in pregnancy: A systematic review. *Travel Med Infect Dis* 27:20-26.

Arguin, P. M., and A. J. Magill. 2017. *For the record: A history of malaria chemoprophylaxis.* https://wwwnc.cdc.gov/travel/yellowbook/2018/infectious-diseases-related-to-travel/emfor-the-record-a-history-of-malaria-chemoprophylaxisem (accessed December 18, 2018).

Berman, J. D., R. Nielsen, J. D. Chulay, M. Dowler, K. C. Kain, K. E. Kester, J. Williams, A. C. Whelen, and M. J. Shmuklarsky. 2001. Causal prophylactic efficacy of atovaquone-proguanil (Malarone) in a human challenge model. *Trans R Soc Trop Med Hyg* 95(4):429-432.

Boggild, A. K., M. E. Parise, L. S. Lewis, and K. C. Kain. 2007. Atovaquone-proguanil: Report from the CDC expert meeting on malaria chemoprophylaxis (II). *Am J Trop Med Hyg* 76(2):208-223.

Castelli, F., S. Odolini, B. Autino, E. Foca, and R. Russo. 2010. Malaria prophylaxis: A comprehensive review. *Pharmaceuticals (Basel)* 3(10):3212-3239.

CDC (Centers for Disease Control and Prevention). 2018. *Choosing a drug to prevent malaria.* https://www.cdc.gov/malaria/travelers/drugs.html (accessed August 15, 2019).

CDC. 2019. *Guidelines for treatment of malaria in the United States.* https://www.cdc.gov/malaria/resources/pdf/treatmenttable.pdf (accessed August 15, 2019).

Chambers, J. A. 2003. Military aviators, special operations forces, and causal malaria prophylaxis. *Mil Med* 168(12):1001-1006.

CPRD (Clinical Practice Research Datalink). 2019. *Home.* https://www.cprd.com (accessed December 3, 2019).

Cunningham, J., J. Horsley, D. Patel, A. Tunbridge, and D. G. Lalloo. 2014. Compliance with long-term malaria prophylaxis in British expatriates. *Travel Med Infect Dis* 12(4):341-348.

Davis, T. M., I. Mueller, and S. J. Rogerson. 2010. Prevention and treatment of malaria in pregnancy. *Future Microbiol* 5(10):1599-1613.

Deye, G. A., R. S. Miller, L. Miller, C. J. Salas, D. Tosh, L. Macareo, B. L. Smith, S. Fracisco, E. G. Clemens, J. Murphy, J. C. Sousa, J. S. Dumler, and A. J. Magill. 2012. Prolonged protection provided by a single dose of atovaquone-proguanil for the chemoprophylaxis of *Plasmodium falciparum* malaria in a human challenge model. *Clin Infect Dis* 54(2):232-239.

Duffy, P. E., and M. Fried. 2005. Malaria in the pregnant woman. *Curr Top Microbiol Immunol* 295:169-200.

Eick-Cost, A. A., Z. Hu, P. Rohrbeck, and L. L. Clark. 2017. Neuropsychiatric outcomes after mefloquine exposure among U.S. military service members. *Am J Trop Med Hyg* 96(1):159-166.

Faucher, J. F., R. Binder, M. A. Missinou, P. B. Matsiegui, H. Gruss, R. Neubauer, B. Lell, J. U. Que, G. B. Miller, and P. G. Kremsner. 2002. Efficacy of atovaquone/proguanil for malaria prophylaxis in children and its effect on the immunogenicity of live oral typhoid and cholera vaccines. *Clin Infect Dis* 35(10):1147-1154.

FDA (U.S. Food and Drug Administration). 2000. Package insert for Malarone™ (atovaquone and proguanil hydrochloride) tablets. https://www.accessdata.fda.gov/drugsatfda_docs/nda/2000/21-078_Malarone_Prntlbl.pdf (accessed October 3, 2019).

FDA. 2002. Package insert for Malarone™ (atovaquone and proguanil hydrochloride) tablets and Malarone™ (atovaquone and proguanil hydrochloride) pediatric tablets. https://www.accessdata.fda.gov/drugsatfda_docs/label/2002/21078s3lbl.pdf (accessed October 3, 2019).

FDA. 2004. Package insert for Malarone® (atovaquone and proguanil hydrochloride) tablets and Malarone® (atovaquone and proguanil hydrochloride) pediatric tablets. https://www.accessdata.fda.gov/drugsatfda_docs/label/2004/21078s002lbl.pdf (accessed October 3, 2019).

FDA. 2008. Package insert for Malarone® (atovaquone and proguanil hydrochloride) tablets and Malarone® (atovaquone and proguanil hydrochloride) pediatric tablets. https://www.accessdata.fda.gov/drugsatfda_docs/label/2008/021078s014lbl.pdf (accessed October 3, 2019).

FDA. 2013. Package insert for Malarone® (atovaquone and proguanil hydrochloride) tablets and Malarone® (atovaquone and proguanil hydrochloride) pediatric tablets. https://www.accessdata.fda.gov/drugsatfda_docs/label/2013/021078s022lbl.pdf (accessed October 3, 2019).

FDA. 2019a. Package insert for Malarone® (atovaquone and proguanil hydrochloride) tablets and Malarone® (atovaquone and proguanil hydrochloride) pediatric tablets. https://www.accessdata.fda.gov/drugsatfda_docs/label/2019/021078s023lbl.pdf (accessed October 3, 2019).

FDA. 2019b. Drug approval letter for Atovaquone. https://www.accessdata.fda.gov/scripts/cder/daf/index.cfm?event=overview.process&ApplNo=020500 (accessed November 7, 2019).

Gillotin, C., J. P. Mamet, and L. Veronese. 1999. Lack of a pharmacokinetic interaction between atovaquone and proguanil. *Eur J Clin Pharmacol* 55(4):311-315.

Goodyer, L., L. Rice, and A. Martin. 2011. Choice of and adherence to prophylactic antimalarials. *J Travel Med* 18(4):245-249.

Gorobets, N. Y., Y. V. Sedash, B. K. Singh, Poonam, and B. Rathi. 2017. An overview of currently available antimalarials. *Curr Top Med Chem* 17(19):2143-2157.

GSK (GlaxoSmithKline). 2015. *Product monograph for Malarone*. https://ca.gsk.com/media/591413/malarone.pdf (accessed November 14, 2019).

Higgins, J. P. T., J. A. Lopez-Lopez, B. J. Becker, S. R. Davies, S. Dawson, J. M. Grimshaw, L. A. McGuinness, T. H. M. Moore, E. A. Rehfuess, J. Thomas, and D. M. Caldwell. 2019. Synthesising quantitative evidence in systematic reviews of complex health interventions. *BMJ Glob Health* 4(Suppl 1):e000858.

Høgh, B., P. D. Clarke, D. Camus, H. D. Nothdurft, D. Overbosch, M. Günther, I. Joubert, K. C. Kain, D. Shaw, N. S. Roskell, J. D. Chulay, and I. S. T. Malarone. 2000. Atovaquone-proguanil versus chloroquine-proguanil for malaria prophylaxis in non-immune travellers: A randomised, double-blind study. *Lancet* 356(9245):1888-1894.

Hussein, Z., J. Eaves, D. B. Hutchinson, and C. J. Canfield. 1997. Population pharmacokinetics of atovaquone in patients with acute malaria caused by *Plasmodium falciparum*. *Clin Pharmacol Ther* 61(5):518-530.

Kain, K. C., G. D. Shanks, and J. S. Keystone. 2001. Malaria chemoprophylaxis in the age of drug resistance. I. Currently recommended drug regimens. *Clin Infect Dis* 33(2):226-234.

Kaser, A. K., P. M. Arguin, P. L. Chiodini, V. Smith, J. Delmont, B. C. Jimenez, A. Farnert, M. Kimura, M. Ramharter, M. P. Grobusch, and P. Schlagenhauf. 2015. Imported malaria in pregnant women: A retrospective pooled analysis. *Travel Med Infect Dis* 13(4):300-310.

Kato, T., J. Okuda, D. Ide, K. Amano, Y. Takei, and Y. Yamaguchi. 2013. Questionnaire-based analysis of atovaquone-proguanil compared with mefloquine in the chemoprophylaxis of malaria in non-immune Japanese travelers. *J Infect Chemother* 19(1):20-23.

Kitchen, L. W., D. W. Vaughn, and D. R. Skillman. 2006. Role of U.S. military research programs in the development of U.S. Food and Drug Administration–approved antimalarial drugs. *Clin Infect Dis* 43(1):67-71.

Landman, K. Z., K. R. Tan, and P. M. Arguin. 2015. Adherence to malaria prophylaxis among Peace Corps volunteers in the Africa region, 2013. *Travel Med Infect Dis* 13(1):61-68.

Laverone, E., S. Boccalini, A. Bechini, S. Belli, M. G. Santini, S. Baretti, G. Circelli, F. Taras, S. Banchi, and P. Bonanni. 2006. Travelers' compliance to prophylactic measures and behavior during stay abroad: Results of a retrospective study of subjects returning to a travel medicine center in Italy. *J Travel Med* 13(6):338-344.

Ling, J., J. K. Baird, D. J. Fryauff, P. Sismadi, M. J. Bangs, M. Lacy, M. J. Barcus, R. Gramzinski, J. D. Maguire, G. Kumusumangsih, G. B. Miller, T. R. Jones, J. D. Chulay, and S. L. Hoffman. 2002. Randomized, placebo-controlled trial of atovaquone/proguanil for the prevention of *Plasmodium falciparum* or *Plasmodium vivax* malaria among migrants to Papua, Indonesia. *Clin Infect Dis* 35(7):825-833.

Looareesuwan, S., C. Viravan, H. K. Webster, D. Kyle, D. B. Hutchinson, and C. J. Canfield. 1996. Clinical studies of atovaquone, alone or in combination with other antimalarial drugs, for treatment of acute uncomplicated malaria in Thailand. *Am J Trop Med Hyg* 54:62-66.

Mayer, R. C., K. R. Tan, and J. R. Gutman. 2018. Safety of atovaquone-proguanil during pregnancy. *J Travel Med* 26(4):tay138.

McGready, R., K. Stepniewska, M. D. Edstein, T. Cho, G. Gilveray, S. Looareesuwan, N. J. White, and F. Nosten. 2003. The pharmacokinetics of atovaquone and proguanil in pregnant women with acute falciparum malaria. *Eur J Clin Pharmacol* 59:545-552.

Nakato, H., R. Vivancos, and P. R. Hunter. 2007. A systematic review and meta-analysis of the effectiveness and safety of atovaquone proguanil (Malarone) for chemoprophylaxis against malaria. *J Antimicrob Chemother* 60(5):929-936.

Nicosia, V., G. Colombo, M. Consentino, S. Di Matteo, F. Mika, S. De Sanctis, S. Ratti, and M. Vinci. 2008. Assessment of acceptability and ease of use of atovaquone/proguanil medication in subjects undergoing malaria prophylaxis. *Ther Clin Risk Manag* 4(5):1105-1110.

Nixon, G. L., D. M. Moss, A. E. Shone, D. G. Lalloo, N. Fisher, P. M. O'Neill, S. A. Ward, and G. A. Biagini. 2013. Antimalarial pharmacology and therapeutics of atovaquone. *J Antimicrob Chemother* 68(5):977-985.

Nosten, F., R. McGready, U. d'Alessandro, A. Bonell, F. Verhoeff, C. Menendez, T. Mutabingwa, and B. Brabin. 2006. Antimalarial drugs in pregnancy: A review. *Curr Drug Saf* 1(1):1-15.

NRC (National Research Council). 2006. Animal and in vitro toxicity testing. In *Toxicity testing for environmental agents*. Washington, DC: The National Academies Press. Pp. 26-70.

Nzila, A. 2006. The past, present and future of antifolates in the treatment of *Plasmodium falciparum* infection. *J Antimicrob Chemother* 57(6):1043-1054.

Overbosch, D. 2003. Post-marketing surveillance: Adverse events during long-term use of atovaquone/proguanil for travelers to malaria-endemic countries. *J Travel Med* 10(Suppl 1):S16-S20, discussion S21.

Overbosch, D., H. Schilthuis, U. Bienzle, R. H. Behrens, K. C. Kain, P. D. Clarke, S. Toovey, J. Knobloch, H. D. Nothdurft, D. Shaw, N. S. Roskell, J. D. Chulay, and the Malarone International Study Team. 2001. Atovaquone-proguanil versus mefloquine for malaria prophylaxis in nonimmune travelers: Results from a randomized, double-blind study. *Clin Infect Dis* 33(7):1015-1021.

Pasternak, B., and A. Hviid. 2011. Atovaquone-proguanil use in early pregnancy and the risk of birth defects. *Arch Intern Med* 171(3):259-260.

Patel, S. N., and K. C. Kain. 2005. Atovaquone/proguanil for the prophylaxis and treatment of malaria. *Expert Rev Anti Infect Ther* 3(6):849-861.

Paul, M. A., A. E. McCarthy, N. Gibson, G. Kenny, T. Cook, and G. Gray. 2003. The impact of Malarone and primaquine on psychomotor performance. *Aviat Space Environ Med* 74(7):738-745.

Pedersen, R. S., F. Nielsen, T. B. Stage, P. J. Vinholt, A. A. el Achwah, P. Damkier, and K. Brosen. 2014. CYP2C1917 increases clopidogrel-mediated platelet inhibition but does not alter the pharmacokinetics of the active metabolite of clopidogrel. *Clin Exp Pharmacol Physiol* 41(11):870-878.

Saunders, D. L., E. Garges, J. E. Manning, K. Bennett, S. Schaffer, A. J. Kosmowski, and A. J. Magill. 2015. Safety, tolerability, and compliance with long-term antimalarial chemoprophylaxis in American soldiers in Afghanistan. *Am J Trop Med Hyg* 93(3):584-590.

Schlagenhauf, P., A. Tschopp, R. Johnson, H. D. Nothdurft, B. Beck, E. Schwartz, M. Herold, B. Krebs, O. Veit, R. Allwinn, and R. Steffen. 2003. Tolerability of malaria chemoprophylaxis in non-immune travellers to sub-Saharan Africa: Multicentre, randomised, double blind, four arm study. *BMJ* 327(7423):1078.

Schlagenhauf, P., R. Johnson, E. Schwartz, H. D. Nothdurft, and R. Steffen. 2009. Evaluation of mood profiles during malaria chemoprophylaxis: A randomized, double-blind, four-arm study. *J Travel Med* 16(1):42-45.

Schlagenhauf, P., M. E. Wilson, E. Petersen, A. McCarthy, and L. H. Chen. 2019. Malaria chemoprophylaxis. In J. S. Keystone, P. E. Kozarsky, B. A. Connor, H. D. Nothdurft, M. Mendelson, and K. Leder (eds.), *Travel medicine, 4th ed.* New York: Elsevier. Pp. 145-167.

Schneider, C., M. Adamcova, S. S. Jick, P. Schlagenhauf, M. K. Miller, H. G. Rhein, and C. R. Meier. 2013. Antimalarial chemoprophylaxis and the risk of neuropsychiatric disorders. *Travel Med Infect Dis* 11(2):71-80.

Schneider, C., M. Adamcova, S. S. Jick, P. Schlagenhauf, M. K. Miller, H. G. Rhein, and C. R. Meier. 2014. Use of anti-malarial drugs and the risk of developing eye disorders. *Travel Med Infect Dis* 12(1):40-47.

Shanks, G. D., D. M. Gordon, F. W. Klotz, G. M. Aleman, A. J. Oloo, D. Sadie, and T. R. Scott. 1998. Efficacy and safety of atovaquone/proguanil as suppressive prophylaxis for *Plasmodium falciparum* malaria. *Clin Infect Dis* 27(3):494-499.

Sharafeldin, E., D. Soonawala, J. P. Vandenbroucke, E. Hack, and L. G. Visser. 2010. Health risks encountered by Dutch medical students during an elective in the tropics and the quality and comprehensiveness of pre-and post-travel care. *BMC Med Educ* 10:89.

Simons, R., P. J. Valk, and A. J. Krul. 2005. Malaria prophylaxis for aircrew: Safety of atovaquone/proguanil in healthy volunteers under aircraft cabin pressure conditions. *J Travel Med* 12(4):210-216.

Soto, J., J. Toledo, M. Luzz, P. Gutierrez, J. Berman, and S. Duparc. 2006. Randomized, double-blind, placebo-controlled study of Malarone for malaria prophylaxis in non-immune Colombian soldiers. *Am J Trop Med Hyg* 75(3):430-433.

Srivastava, I. K., and A. B. Vaidya. 1999. A mechanism for the synergistic antimalarial action of atovaquone and proguanil. *Antimicrob Agents Chemother* 43(6):1334-1339.

Sukwa, T. Y., M. Mulenga, N. Chisdaka, N. S. Roskell, and T. R. Scott. 1999. A randomized, double-blind, placebo-controlled field trial to determine the efficacy and safety of Malarone (atovaquone/proguanil) for the prophylaxis of malaria in Zambia. *Am J Trop Med Hyg* 60(4):521-525.

Tan, K. R., S. J. Henderson, J. Williamson, R. W. Ferguson, T. M. Wilkinson, P. Jung, and P. M. Arguin. 2017. Long term health outcomes among returned Peace Corps volunteers after malaria prophylaxis, 1995–2014. *Travel Med Infect Dis* 17:50-55.

Terziroli Beretta-Piccoli, B., G. Mieli-Vergani, R. Bertoli, L. Mazzucchelli, C. Nofziger, M. Paulmichl, and D. Vergani. 2017. Atovaquone/proguanil-induced autoimmune-like hepatitis. *Hepatol Commun* 1(4):293-298.

Thapar, M. M., M. Ashton, N. Lindegardh, Y. Bergqvist, S. Nivelius, I. Johansson, and A. Bjorkman. 2002. Time-dependent pharmacokinetics and drug metabolism of atovaquone plus proguanil (Malarone) when taken as chemoprophylaxis. *Eur J Clin Pharmacol* 58(1):19-27.

Tickell-Painter, M., N. Maayan, R. Saunders, C. Pace, and D. Sinclair. 2017. Mefloquine for preventing malaria during travel to endemic areas. *Cochrane Database Syst Rev* 10:CD006491.

Tuck, J., and J. Williams. 2016. Malaria protection in Sierra Leone during the Ebola outbreak 2014/15: The UK military experience with malaria chemoprophylaxis, Sep 14–Feb 15. *Travel Med Infect Dis* 14(5):471-474.

van Genderen, P. J., H. R. Koene, K. Spong, and D. Overbosch. 2007. The safety and tolerance of atovaquone/proguanil for the long-term prophylaxis of *Plasmodium falciparum* malaria in non-immune travelers and expatriates [corrected]. *J Travel Med* 14(2):92-95.

van Riemsdijk, M. M., M. C. Sturkenboom, J. M. Ditters, R. J. Ligthelm, D. Overbosch, and B. H. Stricker. 2002. Atovaquone plus chloroguanide versus mefloquine for malaria prophylaxis: A focus on neuropsychiatric adverse events. *Clin Pharmacol Ther* 72(3):294-301.

van Vugt, M., M. D. Edstein, S. Proux, K. Lay, M. Ooh, S. Looareesuwan, N. J. White, and F. Nosten. 1999. Absence of an interaction between artesunate and atovaquone–proguanil. *Eur J Clin Pharmacol* 55(6):469-474.

Zsila, F., and I. Fitos. 2010. Combination of chiroptical, absorption, and fluorescence spectroscopic methods reveals multiple, hydrophobicity-driven human serum albumin binding of the antimalarial atovaquone and related hydroxynaphthoquinone compounds. *Org Biomol Chem* 8:4905-4914.

7

Doxycycline

Doxycycline is a broad-spectrum bacteriostatic agent (antibiotic) synthetically derived from a naturally occurring tetracycline produced by *Streptomyces* species bacteria known as oxytetracycline; it is a member of the tetracycline class of antibiotics (Kundu et al., 2015; Thillainayagam and Ramaiah, 2016). In the early 1960s Pfizer Inc. created and clinically developed doxycycline and began marketing it under the brand name Vibramycin® (Tan et al., 2011). Doxycycline has been approved by the Food and Drug Administration (FDA) for the prevention or treatment of specific conditions within each of the following categories: rickettsial infections, sexually transmitted infections, respiratory tract infections, bacterial infections, Lyme disease, ophthalmic infections, anthrax, acute intestinal amebiasis, traveler's diarrhea, and severe acne (FDA, 2018a). It has also been investigated as a treatment for specific cancers because some studies suggest that doxycycline can inhibit cell proliferation and invasion and also induce apoptosis and block the gap phase (in which a cancerous cell grows and prepares to synthesize DNA) (Kundu et al., 2015).

While doxycycline can be used to treat a broad range of conditions, its use for malaria prophylaxis is the focus of this chapter. In 1992 Pfizer Inc. submitted a new drug application to FDA with an indication for malaria prophylaxis added to the product insert (Arguin and Magill, 2017); the indication was added in 1994 (Tan et al., 2011). The approved dosing regimen for malaria prophylaxis for adults is 100 mg per day 1–2 days before entering an endemic area, 100 mg per day while in the endemic area, and 100 mg daily for 28 days after leaving an endemic area. The FDA package insert states that this regimen is approved for up to 4 months (FDA, 2018a). Studies examining the long-term (≥4 months) use of doxycycline for malaria prophylaxis have offered mixed results on its tolerability.

Among Australian military personnel who were deployed to Cambodia (n = 600) for 12 months or Somalia (n = 900) for 4 months, doxycycline was well tolerated, and only 7 (0.6%) personnel in Cambodia and 15 (1.7%) personnel in Somalia discontinued the drug because of concurrent adverse events related to gastrointestinal symptoms or photosensitivity (Shanks et al., 1995a). However, a survey of 228 U.S. Peace Corps volunteers who had taken doxycycline on average for 19 months found that 45 (20%) of respondents reported changing medications due to severe concurrent adverse events, such as gastrointestinal symptoms, pruritic skin reactions, photosensitivity, and vaginal yeast infections (Korhonen et al., 2007).

Overall, studies suggest that adherence rates for doxycycline range from 70% to 84% when it is used for malaria prophylaxis, and adhering to the dosing regimen may be more challenging than adhering to dosing regimens for weekly prophylaxis medications (e.g., mefloquine, tafenoquine). One study found a 98% adherence for mefloquine but only an 81% adherence for doxycycline in U.S. troops in Somalia (Sánchez et al., 1993), and another study reported 70% adherence for a weekly prophylaxis regimen but only 50% adherence in people taking daily doxycycline (Watanasook et al., 1989). Furthermore, studies have shown that adherence to the doxycycline regimen decreases over time. In one study of Australian soldiers deployed to Cambodia, the adherence rate for taking doxycycline decreased from 60% at 2 months to 44% at 4 months (Shanks et al., 1995a). Studies have indicated that drugs with longer post-travel requirements tend to have worse adherence than drugs with shorter post-travel regimens (Overbosch et al., 2001); thus, doxycycline likely has poorer adherence during the post-travel period than a prophylaxis medication with a shorter post-travel regimen, such as atovaquone/proguanil (A/P).

Other studies have reported greater adherence in individuals prescribed once-daily prophylaxis than individuals prescribed once-weekly prophylaxis. Brisson and Brisson (2012) conducted an online survey in 1,200 military personnel deployed to Afghanistan between 2002 and 2012 to examine adherence rates for malaria prophylaxis in a combat zone. Of the 530 individuals who started the survey, 528 completed it (response rate of 44% to the initial survey distribution). The authors found that 3.6% of respondents were prescribed mefloquine, 90.1% received doxycycline, 0.9% received A/P, 0.2% received primaquine, and 4.4% were unsure which prophylactic drug they were prescribed. Of the individuals prescribed once-daily prophylaxis, 61% reported complete adherence; however, only 38% of individuals prescribed once-weekly prophylaxis (e.g., mefloquine) reported full adherence. Resistance of *P. falciparum* to doxycycline is not described, but breakthroughs in prophylaxis have been associated with inadequate doses, possibly inadequate serum levels, and poor adherence (Tan et al., 2011).

Beginning in the late 1980s prior to FDA's approval for doxycycline use for malaria prophylaxis, the U.S. Army conducted several field and human challenge clinical trials demonstrating the efficacy of doxycycline as malaria prophylaxis (Arguin and Magill, 2017). A 2009 Department of Defense (DoD) memorandum advised that doxycycline be used in preference to mefloquine in service members with a history of neurobehavioral disorders (DoD, 2009), and current DoD policy states that doxycycline is a first-line prophylactic agent for malaria. The U.S. military began using doxycycline as a primary agent for malaria prophylaxis after the anthrax attacks of September 2001, and it was used as a first-line agent for Operation Enduring Freedom (2001–2014) and operations Iraqi Freedom and New Dawn (2003–2011).[1] Because doxycycline provides simultaneous protection from anthrax and malaria, it is attractive for use in military operations where these are potential threats.

Doxycycline reduces the incidence and severity of traveler's diarrhea, and it has been shown to provide protection against traveler's diarrhea in 60–85% of individuals, depending on enterotoxin-producing *E. coli* resistance (Sack et al., 1984). A study comparing diarrhea rates among British and Australian medical teams deployed to Iraq in support of the 1990–1991 Gulf War found that Australians who used doxycycline for malaria prophylaxis and who had instituted an enforced plate- and hand-washing routine experienced half the rate of diarrhea as the British (36% versus 69%, respectively) and that diarrhea illness, when it occurred, was both milder and of shorter duration (p < 0.001) (Rudland et al., 1996).

This chapter begins by describing the key changes that have been made to the doxycycline package insert and label since its approval for malaria prophylaxis in 1994, with particular emphasis on changes to the Contraindications, Warnings, and Precautions sections. This is followed by an overview of the pharmacokinetic properties of doxycycline. Known concurrent adverse events associated with use of doxycycline when used at the dose and interval as directed for malaria prophylaxis are summarized, followed by a presentation of detailed summaries and assessments of the seven identified epidemiologic studies that met the committee's inclusion criteria and were able to contribute some information on persistent or latent health outcomes following the cessation of doxycycline. As in the other chapters, the epidemiologic studies are ordered by population: studies of military and veterans (U.S. followed by international forces), the U.S. Peace Corps, travelers, and endemic populations. Where available, studies of U.S. participants are presented first. A table that gives a high-level comparison of each of the seven epidemiologic studies that examined the use of doxycycline and that met the committee's inclusion criteria is presented in Appendix C. Supplemental supporting evidence is then presented, including other identified studies of health outcomes in populations that used doxycycline for malaria prophylaxis but that did not meet the committee's inclusion criteria regarding timing of follow-up. This is followed by case reports of persistent adverse events and, next, information about the adverse events of doxycycline use in specific groups, such as pregnant women and those

---

[1] Personal communication to the committee, COL Andrew Wiesen, M.D., M.P.H., Director, Preventive Medicine, Health Readiness Policy and Oversight, Office of the Assistant Secretary of Defense (Health Affairs), April 16, 2019.

with chronic health conditions. After the primary and supplemental evidence in humans is presented, supporting literature from experimental animal and in vitro studies is then summarized. The chapter ends with a synthesis of all of the evidence presented, followed by the inferences and conclusions that can be made.

FOOD AND DRUG ADMINISTRATION PACKAGE INSERT FOR DOXYCYCLINE

There have been numerous trade-name and generic formulations of doxycycline hyclate marketed in the United States. The FDA website offers a webpage for each formulation; each page lists the package insert updates, but downloadable package inserts are not available for all listed updates, and in older drugs this can mean that many years of updates are unavailable. This is also true of drugs that are currently on the market. For drugs that have been discontinued, often no downloadable package inserts are available. The oldest available package insert for doxycycline was dated 2005 (FDA, 2005a). Package inserts are listed on the webpage with an action date, but the date provided in the downloaded package insert document may occasionally differ from the action date posted on the webpage (e.g., a downloaded document listed as the 1989 mefloquine package insert was a July 2002 revision). Occasionally a downloaded document contained no date (e.g., the template's "month/year" placeholder is not filled). Because package inserts dated prior to 2005 were not available, it could not always be determined whether a formulation had ever been indicated for malaria prophylaxis or, if it was, when the indication was added. For example, the Doryx® capsule (discontinued) was approved in 1985, but the earliest package insert available for download is 2005 (FDA, 2005b), 11 years after doxycycline was approved for malaria prophylaxis.

The design and formatting of package inserts has changed for individual drugs over time, so comparisons could not always be easily made. Moreover, there continue to be differences in information sourcing and section-labeling conventions among even the most recent package inserts, although they appear to provide the same information. For example, the Adverse Reactions section for the 2018 Doryx® tablet divides its content between Clinical Trial Experience and Postmarketing Experience, while the Adverse Reactions section for 2018 Vibramycin® capsules does not cite an information source, yet matches the Postmarketing Experience of the 2018 Doryx® tablet insert. Section headings and organization may differ also; in the 2018 package inserts, Doryx® contains a single Warnings and Precautions section (FDA, 2018a); the 2018 Vibramycin® insert has two separate sections but does not indicate the differences between the two levels of guidance (FDA, 2018c). The following text contains information related to the use of doxycycline for several symptoms, illnesses, or disorders (all its approved indications) and is not limited to the use of doxycycline for malaria prophylaxis unless otherwise stated.

Contraindications, Warnings, and Precautions

Doxycycline is contraindicated in individuals who have a known hypersensitivity to tetracyclines. The Warnings and Precautions sections of package inserts for doxycycline alert users to a number of risks: permanent tooth discoloration and enamel hypoplasia during tooth development in a child if taken in the last half of the mother's pregnancy; *Clostridium difficile*–associated diarrhea and related morbidity and mortality; photosensitivity; potential overgrowth of nonsusceptible organisms, including fungi; severe skin reactions (exfoliative dermatitis, erythema multiforme, Stevens-Johnson syndrome, toxic epidermal necrolysis, and drug reaction with eosinophilia and systemic symptoms); intracranial hypertension; possible toxic effects on the developing fetus (often related to retardation of skeletal development) owing to the development of drug-resistant bacteria; the drug crossing the placenta; an increase in BUN[2] due to anti-anabolic action; incomplete suppression of the asexual blood stages of malaria *Plasmodium* parasites; and an inability to suppress *P. falciparum*'s sexual blood stage, which allows person-to-mosquito transmission of infection. Periodic laboratory evaluation of organ systems, including hematopoietic, renal, and hepatic studies, should be made when using the drug long term (FDA, 2018a).

Drug Interactions

In individuals taking oral blood thinners, tetracyclines have been shown to intensify the anticoagulant effect of these medications by interfering with the use of prothrombin and reducing vitamin K production by intestinal bacteria. In a study conducted by Penning-van Beest et al. (2008), the investigators examined the anticoagulant–doxycycline interaction by analyzing the PHARMO Record Linkage System where patients were followed through the end of coumarin treatment, and they found a 2.5-fold increased risk for increased bleeding episodes in participants who were concurrently using doxycycline and acenocoumarol or phenprocoumon; these findings have been confirmed in other studies (Hasan, 2007).

Individuals using digoxin and oral antibiotics concomitantly with doxycycline may experience increased serum digoxin concentrations. These increased concentrations are a consequence of altered gut flora and reduced conversion of digoxin to inactive metabolites. The half-life of doxycycline is believed to be reduced when barbiturates, carbamazepine, and phenytoin induce microsomal enzyme activity. Any individuals receiving the oral typhoid vaccine are advised by most experts to not use doxycycline within the 24 hours immediately following the vaccine, as the vaccine effectiveness may be reduced (Tan et al., 2011).

The FDA label also states that "concurrent use of tetracycline may render oral contraceptives less effective" (FDA, 2018a); however, some studies have shown

---

[2] BUN = blood urea nitrogen test; used to determine kidney function.

no significant association between the use of doxycycline and reduced efficacy of oral contraceptives (Dickinson et al., 2001). One study that examined the effect of doxycycline on another form of contraceptive, the subcutaneous implant, indicates that doxycycline may affect the pharmacodynamics of the levonorgestrel released from the implant; however, the results were inconclusive (Zhao et al., 2009). The use of additional contraceptive methods while taking doxycycline is advised.

Changes to the Doxycycline Package Insert Over Time

The committee established that Doryx® (tablet, capsule, and MPC formulations), Vibramycin®, Vibra-Tabs®, Acticlate® (tablet and capsule), and doxycycline hyclate are or had been indicated for malaria prophylaxis. The 2005 package inserts for the three Doryx® formulations (FDA, 2005a,b) showed no meaningful differences, nor did those for the 2007 Vibramycin® and Vibra-Tabs® formulations (FDA, 2007), nor the 2014 Acticlate® tablet (FDA, 2014) and 2016 Acticlate® capsule (FDA, 2016) formulations. Thus, the committee compared the earliest available package insert with the latest available package insert each for Doryx® tablets (FDA, 2005a, 2018a,b), Vibramycin® capsules (FDA, 2007, 2018c), and Acticlate® tablets (FDA, 2014, 2017) and summarized the major adverse-event-related updates. It is difficult to estimate how many adverse-reaction-related updates have been issued since 2005 to package inserts for doxycycline used for malaria prophylaxis. For example, during a specific period during which more than one drug formulation was being marketed for this indication, the number of label or package insert updates varied among the drugs, and it was unclear specifically which ones included changes to adverse events.

Between 2005 and 2018 several adverse reactions were added to the Warnings (or Warnings and Precautions) section for each of the formulations. One of the added adverse reactions was intracranial hypertension, in which clinical manifestations were stated to include headache, blurred vision, diplopia, vision loss, and papilledema via fundoscopy. The risk of intracranial hypertension is stated to be increased in women of childbearing age who are overweight or have a history of intracranial hypertension and in those using isotretinoin concomitantly. The warning also states that because intracranial pressure can remain elevated for weeks after drug cessation, patients should be monitored until they stabilize. Other adverse reactions added since 2005 were Stevens-Johnson syndrome, toxic epidermal necrolysis, erythema multiforme, and drug reaction with eosinophilia and systemic symptoms. The warning for *Clostridium difficile*–associated diarrhea was expanded to say that this should be considered in all patients with diarrhea after antibiotic use as it can occur more than 2 months after drug cessation and can cause increased morbidity and mortality since these infections can be refractory to antimicrobial therapy and may require colectomy. Additions to other sections of the package inserts included the alert that patients can develop watery and bloody stools (with or without stomach cramps and fever) as late as 2 or more months after antibiotic cessation, in which case patients should immediately contact a physician; reports of pancreatitis, exfoliative dermatitis, and discoloration (reversible) of adult teeth; and the advice that drugs should be taken with adequate amounts of fluid to reduce the risk of esophageal irritation and ulceration.

PHARMACOKINETICS

Compared with tetracycline, doxycycline has a longer half-life, better absorption, and a better safety profile (Shapiro et al., 1997; Thillainayagamam and Ramaiah, 2016). An oral dose of 100–200 mg of doxycycline is almost completely absorbed in the small bowel and is detectable in the blood 15–30 minutes after administration (Tan et al., 2011). Doxycycline is highly protein bound (93%), has a small volume of distribution (0.7 L/kg), and achieves relatively high blood levels (Schlagenhauf et al., 2019). Following a 200 mg oral dose of doxycycline, peak concentrations of about 2.6 µg/mL are reached at approximately 2 hours, but this may vary as gastrointestinal absorption rates differ among individuals. Doxycycline is readily transported across cell membranes, resulting in widespread distribution in body tissues and fluids. It localizes in the bone marrow, liver, and spleen; crosses the placenta; and is excreted in breast milk. Doxycycline and other tetracyclines form tetracycline-calcium orthophosphate complexes in sites of calcification such as developing teeth and bone, which may lead to permanent discoloration. The bioavailability of the monohydrate free base and of the hydrochloride salt (hyclate) forms of doxycycline has been shown to be equivalent (Tan et al., 2011).

Studies have shown that when medications composed of divalent or trivalent cations (such as antacids, laxatives, and oral iron preparations) are taken simultaneously with doxycycline, the absorption of doxycycline is decreased. Other types of medications that decrease the absorption of tetracyclines include antidiarrheal agents containing kaolin, pectin, or bismuth subsalicylate; these should be taken a few hours before ingesting doxycycline (Tan et al., 2011). Milk decreases the absorption of tetracyclines because of chelation of the calcium in the milk by the tetracyclines; however, the magnitude of this decrease varies between different tetracycline preparations, and the data for doxycycline are limited. According to FDA, the absorption of doxycycline "is not markedly influenced by simultaneous ingestion of food and milk," despite the reduced absorption observed with other tetracyclines, and taking doxycycline with food is recommended to prevent concurrent adverse gastrointestinal events.

Unlike the case with other tetracyclines, the excretion of doxycycline occurs primarily by the gastrointestinal tract and to a much lesser extent by the kidneys. The serum half-life of doxycycline (15–25 hours) is not affected by impaired renal function or hemodialysis, and in patients with renal failure all excretion of doxycycline occurs by the gastrointestinal route. There are limited to no data on sex, age, body weight, or race differences in the pharmacokinetics of doxycycline (Tan et al., 2011). One small study of healthy adult (aged 18–33 years) Vietnamese male (n = 14) and female (n = 14) volunteers found no differences in the pharmacokinetics of doxycycline by sex (Binh et al., 2009).

ADVERSE EVENTS

The following section contains a summary of the known concurrent adverse events associated with the use of doxycycline. Epidemiologic studies of persistent adverse events in which information was presented regarding the adverse events occurring at least 28 days post-doxycycline-cessation are then summarized, with the emphasis on reported results of persistent adverse events associated with the use of doxycycline, including results of studies in which other antimalarial drugs were used as a comparison group.

Concurrent Adverse Events

The FDA package insert for doxycycline uses information from trials that used doxycycline at dosages or for purposes other than for malaria prophylaxis (e.g., urogenital *Chlamydia trachomatis* infection), which are considered outside of the committee's charge. All labels provide a lengthy list of adverse reactions that appear to be based on postmarketing experience, but they are not quantified, nor is the type of use of doxycycline always specified. The committee chose to use published information on concurrent adverse events from the Cochrane Database of Systematic Reviews and other reviews in which doxycycline was used for malaria prophylaxis.

The most commonly reported adverse events associated with the use of doxycycline are gastrointestinal symptoms and photosensitivity. Gastrointestinal symptoms are typically mild to moderate and include nausea (4–33%), abdominal pain (12–33%), vomiting (4–8%), and diarrhea (6–7.5%) (Tan et al., 2011). Studies show that nausea is more likely to occur if doxycycline is taken without food (Ohrt et al., 1997; Shanks et al., 1995b). Esophageal ulcers have also been reported and are more common in individuals who take doxycycline on an empty stomach or without liquid or who lie down within an hour after ingestion (Bott et al., 1987; Carlborg et al., 1983), but this effect was not specific to its use as malaria prophylaxis. In individuals who have taken doxycycline, exposing skin to sunlight may result in an erythematous rash, which has been reported in 7.3–21.2% of individuals, depending on the population (Rieckman et al., 1993; Sánchez et al., 1993; Wallace, 1996). Individuals with lighter complexions may be more prone to photosensitivity while taking doxycycline; these individuals should remain out of the sun or use appropriate protective measures if sun exposure cannot be avoided (Smith et al., 1995). Other adverse events that have been reported in association with tetracyclines but they are less common or have not been reported during doxycycline use. These include onycholysis, benign intracranial hypertension, skin hyper-pigmentation, postinflammatory elastolysis, tooth discoloration, vertigo, ataxia, *Clostridium difficile* diarrhea, visual disturbances, and phlebitis (Klein and Cunha, 1995; Tan et al., 2011). Although *Clostridium difficile* infection is listed as an adverse event of doxycycline, current evidence suggests that doxycycline may actually provide protection against such infections (Tariq et al., 2018; Turner et al., 2014).

Tetracyclines are believed to suppress vaginal bacterial flora, resulting in an overgrowth of *Candida albicans*, and may enhance the virulence factors associated with the bacteria; the mechanism by which this occurs is unknown. Vaginitis has been reported with the use of doxycycline when taken for malaria prophylaxis, but estimates of the incidence are limited because vaginitis is often included under the category of non-specific skin reactions, and many of the early studies were conducted using populations of male military personnel. Women who are predisposed to or have a past history of candida vulvovaginitis or those taking oral contraceptives should consider carrying a self-treatment course of antifungals while taking doxycycline (Tan et al., 2011).

Cochrane Reviews

Tickell-Painter et al. (2017) performed a Cochrane systematic review in which adverse events were prespecified to include these disorders: psychiatric (abnormal dreams, insomnia, anxiety, depression, psychosis); nervous system (dizziness, headaches); ear and labyrinth (vertigo); eye (visual impairment); gastrointestinal (nausea, vomiting, abdominal pain, diarrhea, dyspepsia); and skin and subcutaneous tissue (pruritus, photosensitivity, vaginal candida). The purpose of the assessment was to summarize the efficacy and safety of mefloquine for malaria prophylaxis in adult, children, and pregnant women travelers compared with other antimalarials (including doxycycline), placebo, or no treatment. The dosages of mefloquine varied, as did the methods of collecting adverse event data. Therefore, the identified studies in this review were only those in which doxycycline was used as a comparator to mefloquine. The authors applied categories of certainty to the results based on the five GRADE considerations (risk of bias, consistency of effect, imprecision, indirectness, and publication bias) (Higgins et al., 2019). The committee recalculated the effect estimates presented below to directly compare doxycycline with mefloquine (instead of mefloquine with doxycycline).

When analyses were performed to compare doxycycline with mefloquine (4 trials totaling 1,317 participants and 20 cohort studies totaling 435,209 participants), no difference in the incidence of serious adverse events was found (RR = 0.65, 95%CI 0.10–4.35). Regarding neurologic adverse events, no differences were found for headache (RR = 0.83, 95%CI 0.34–2.90; 5 cohort studies, 3,322 participants) or dizziness (RR = 0.28, 95%CI 0.07–1.14; 5 cohort studies, 2,633 participants) when mefloquine users were compared with doxycycline users. However, for psychiatric adverse events reported in the cohort studies, doxycycline users were statistically significantly less likely than mefloquine users to report abnormal dreams, insomnia, anxiety, and depressed mood, although the pooled effect estimates were very imprecise. Whereas there were 15 episodes of abnormal thoughts and perceptions with mefloquine, no episodes were reported for doxycycline users in the cohort studies.

The 10 serious adverse events reported among doxycycline users were due to gastrointestinal disturbance (n = 6), anemia (n = 1), photosensitivity (n = 1), esophagitis (n = 1), and cough (n = 1). Among the included trials and cohort studies, there was no statistical difference in the number of discontinuations due to adverse events between mefloquine and doxycycline users. In the cohort studies reporting adverse events, doxycycline users were statistically significantly more likely to report nausea (RR = 2.70, 95%CI 2.22–3.33; 5 cohort studies, 2,683 participants), vomiting (RR = 5.55, 95%CI 3.70–8.33; 4 cohort studies, 5,071 participants), and diarrhea (RR = 3.57, 95%CI 1.37–9.09; 5 cohort studies, 5,104 participants), but in the single trial of military personnel that reported adverse events, no differences were demonstrated for these adverse gastrointestinal events.

Other symptoms were also included when available. In cohort studies reporting adverse events, photosensitivity (RR = 12.5, 95%CI 9.09–20.0; 2 cohort studies, 1,875 participants) and vaginal yeast infection in female participants (RR = 10.0, 95%CI 6.25–16.67; 1 cohort study, 1,761 participants) were more common in doxycycline users than mefloquine users. Based on two cohort studies that examined visual impairment, this adverse event was statistically significantly less commonly reported among doxycycline users than mefloquine users (RR = 0.42, 95%CI 0.25–0.71; 1,875 participants). A range of other adverse events were reported in individual cohort studies, including alopecia (hair loss), asthenia (physical weakness), balance disorder, decreased appetite, fatigue, hypoaesthesia (numbness), mouth ulcers, palpitations, and tinnitus, but for all these outcomes, there was either no difference or higher risks among mefloquine users. Risk of malaise was found to be statistically significantly higher among doxycycline users compared with mefloquine users.

Post-Cessation Adverse Events

A total of 5,672 abstracts or titles were identified by the committee's literature search for doxycycline. After an initial evaluation of the types of citations captured, the committee determined that a large portion of the literature contained information related to alternative uses of doxycycline (e.g., acne, bacterial infections). Additional search terms related to prophylaxis and malaria were added, which reduced the number of captured citations to 2,406 titles or abstracts. After screening, 568 abstracts and titles remained, and the full text for each was retrieved and reviewed to determine whether it met the committee's inclusion criteria, as defined in Chapter 3. The committee reviewed each article and identified seven epidemiologic studies that included some mention of adverse events that occurred ≥28 days post-cessation of doxycycline (Andersen et al., 1998; Eick-Cost et al., 2017; Lee et al., 2013; Meier et al., 2004; Schneiderman et al., 2018; Schwartz and Regev-Yochay, 1999; Tan et al., 2017), and these are summarized next. A table that gives a high-level comparison (study design, population, exposure groups, and outcomes examined by body system) of each of these seven epidemiologic studies is presented in Appendix C.

Military and Veterans

Using DoD administrative databases, Eick-Cost et al. (2017) performed a retrospective cohort study among 367,840 active-duty service members who filled at least one prescription for an antimalarial drug between 2008 and 2013: 36,538 were prescribed mefloquine, 318,421 doxycycline, and 12,881 A/P. The primary study objective was to assess and compare the risk of incident and recurrent *International Classification of Diseases, Ninth Revision, Clinical Modification* (ICD-9-CM)-coded neurologic and psychiatric outcomes (adjustment disorder, anxiety disorder, depressive disorder, posttraumatic stress disorder (PTSD), psychoses, suicide ideation, paranoia, confusion, tinnitus, vertigo, convulsions, hallucinations, insomnia, and death from suicide) that were reported at medical care visits during concurrent use plus 365 days after the end of the prescription for mefloquine, doxycycline, or A/P. Although the authors did not report results for the period of ≥28 days post-cessation of antimalarial drug use, they stated that they performed several sensitivity analyses, including one in which the risk period was restricted to 30 days post-prescription. The results of that analysis were summarized in the text as, "However, none of these analyses significantly changed the results of the study and are therefore not reported" (p. 161). This statement implies (but does not show directly) that similar findings to those reported would be seen if the data were restricted to the period of relevance to the committee's definition of persistence (i.e., ≥28 days after cessation of exposure). The committee was unsure how to interpret the statement that the results did not change significantly (statistical significance, precision of effect estimates, number of diagnoses, etc.), but given that the authors performed sensitivity analyses and that the study had a number of methodologic strengths, including a strong measurement of relevant outcomes conducted in the target population, the committee chose to include the study, despite the ambiguity in the language. If an individual had multiple prescriptions over the follow-up period, the risk periods were merged. Doxycycline and A/P prescriptions were excluded if the service member had previously or concurrently received mefloquine. Mefloquine risk periods were censored if an individual received a prescription for a different antimalarial. Analyses were stratified by deployment and psychiatric history. Models were adjusted for age, sex, service, grade, and year of prescription start; analyses of deployed service members also controlled for location and combat exposure. A majority of the doxycycline recipients had served in the Army (69%), many were junior enlisted (48%), and a large percentage had had their prescriptions filled after 2010 (78%). Among the deployed service members, more individuals who had received doxycycline than who had received the other antimalarial drugs reported combat exposure (43%, compared with 29% for mefloquine and 21% for A/P).

With few exceptions, the adjusted incident rates were higher among the deployed than among the nondeployed for doxycycline as well as for the other antimalarial drugs that were considered. Effect estimates of the neurologic and psychiatric outcomes for mefloquine and A/P are reported in the relevant chapters. For doxycycline users, the highest incident rates in both the deployed and nondeployed were for adjustment disorder (56.92 versus 44.35 per 1,000 person-years, respectively), insomnia (27.53 versus 22.46 per 1,000 person-years, respectively), and anxiety disorder (23.53 versus 18.47 per 1,000 person-years, respectively). Incident tinnitus (18.25 versus 15.17 per 1,000 person-years, respectively), depressive disorder (18.59 versus 18.24 per 1,000 person-years, respectively), suicide ideation (4.43 versus 4.23 per 1,000 person-years, respectively), and hallucinations (0.83 versus 0.70 per 1,000 person-years) were also higher among the deployed group. On the other hand, the incidence of vertigo (14.85 versus 15.75 per 1,000 person-years, respectively), convulsions (1.67 versus 2.16 per 1,000 person-years, respectively), paranoia (0.09 versus 0.13 per 1,000 person-years, respectively), death from suicide (0.03 versus 0.05 per 1,000 person-years, respectively), and confusion (0.03 versus 0.05 per 1,000 person-years, respectively) were higher among the nondeployed than the deployed group. Among those prescribed doxycycline, the incidence rate of PTSD was 15.55 per 1,000 person-years in the deployed group and 9.06 per 1,000 person-years in the nondeployed group. When adjusted incidence rate ratios (IRRs) were calculated comparing doxycycline to mefloquine by deployment status, the only statistically significant difference among the deployed between the two drugs was for anxiety disorder (IRR = 0.89, 95%CI 0.81–0.99). When doxycycline and mefloquine users among the nondeployed were compared, adjustment disorder (IRR = 1.44, 95%CI 1.25–1.67), insomnia (IRR = 1.49, 95%CI 1.23–1.79), anxiety disorder (IRR = 1.43, 95%CI 1.16–1.75), depressive disorder (IRR = 1.47, 95%CI 1.19–1.82), vertigo (IRR = 1.92, 95%CI 1.14–3.23), and PTSD (IRR = 1.45, 95%CI 1.10–1.92) all showed a statistically significant *higher* risk for doxycycline users. No other statistically significant differences were seen for the other outcomes examined, including psychosis, suicide ideation, and death by suicide. A subsequent analysis restricted the population to those individuals who were receiving their first mefloquine or doxycycline prescription and included individuals with a prior history of a neurologic or psychiatric diagnosis. The incidence rates and IRRs for each neurologic or psychiatric outcome were compared, stratified by those with and without a prior neurologic or psychiatric diagnosis. A diagnosis of PTSD was recorded for 2,671 (0.8%) of individuals in the doxycycline group and 131 (0.4%) of individuals in the mefloquine group in the 365 days prior to their first antimalarial prescription. For both the doxycycline and the mefloquine groups, individuals with a neuropsychiatric diagnosis in the year preceding the prescription had statistically significantly elevated risks for a subsequent diagnosis of the same condition for all conditions reported (adjustment disorder, anxiety, insomnia, depressive disorder, PTSD, tinnitus, vertigo, and convulsions) compared with individuals without a diagnosis in the prior year. However, when the IRRs were used to compare doxycycline and mefloquine users within strata of those with and without prior neuropsychiatric diagnoses, there were no statistically significant differences between doxycycline and mefloquine for any of the conditions, including PTSD (bootstrap RRR = 0.88, 95%CI 0.61–1.28).

The committee found this study to be well designed; important factors that increased the study's quality were its large size, its use of an administrative data source that provided some degree of objectivity, and its careful consideration of potential confounders including deployment and combat exposure. Because neurologic and psychiatric diagnoses occurring during current and recent use were analyzed together without distinguishing between events that occurred within 28 days of antimalarial use and those that occurred $\geq$28 days post-cessation, the study provides no quantitative information regarding the persistence of most events other than the comment in the text that the results did not change when restricted to the post-cessation period. The use of administrative data provided a standard, consistent method to capture filled prescriptions and medical diagnoses through the use of ICD-9-CM codes. However, filled prescriptions do not equate to adherence to the drug regimens. Moreover, if the antimalarials were provided to entire units as part of force health protection measures, the use of these drugs would not be coded in individual records. Whereas the use of medical diagnoses is likely to be more reliable for the identification of adverse events than self-report, the data are dependent on the accuracy of the coding, and there was no validation of the diagnoses recorded in the administrative databases, and symptoms or events that did not result in a medical visit or diagnosis would have been missed. For PTSD diagnoses, there was no information concerning when the index trauma occurred. Although the authors report higher risks for several outcomes among doxycycline users compared with mefloquine users, particularly among the nondeployed, the IRRs are not adjusted for history of neurologic or psychiatric outcomes. Given the evidence that such a history is a very strong predictor of subsequent events (as shown in table 7 of the article) and clear evidence that those with such a history were preferentially prescribed doxycycline rather than mefloquine (as shown in table 6 of the article), it is reasonable to presume that the findings of higher risk among doxycycline users in this study results from confounding by neuropsychiatric history.

Schneiderman et al. (2018) conducted a retrospective observational analysis of self-reported adverse events associated with use of antimalarial drugs in a cohort of U.S. veterans who had responded to the 2009–2011 National Health Study for a New Generation of U.S. Veterans (referred to as the "NewGen Study"). The NewGen Study is a population-based survey that sampled 30,000 veterans who had been deployed to Iraq or Afghanistan between 2001 and 2008 and 30,000 non-deployed veterans who had served during the same time period. It included a 20% oversampling of women. The survey was conducted using mail, telephone, and web-based collection, yielding a response rate of only 34.3%; while the response rate was low, the respondents nonetheless constitute a large population. For this particular analysis, 19,487 participants were included who had self-reported their history of antimalarial medication use, and this use was grouped for analysis by drug (mefloquine, chloroquine, doxycycline, primaquine, mefloquine in combination with other drugs, other antimalarials, and not specified) or no antimalarial use. Health outcomes were self-reported using standardized instruments: the Medical Outcomes Study 12-item short form (SF-12) for general health status, the PTSD Checklist-Civilian version (PCL-C), and the Patient Health Questionnaire (PHQ). These instruments yielded scores that were dichotomized for analysis on composite physical health, composite mental health (above or below the U.S. mean), PTSD (above or below screening cutoff), thoughts of death or self-harm, other anxiety disorders, and major depression. Potential confounders included in the multivariable analysis were branch of service, sex, age, education, race/ethnicity, household income, employment status, marital status, and self-reported exposure to combat. Responses were weighted to account for survey non-response. Most veterans reported no antimalarial drug exposures (61.4%, n = 11,100), and these served as the referent group. When stratified by deployment status, among the deployed (n = 12,456), of those who reported the use of an antimalarial drug (n = 6,650), 1,315 (weighted 20.5%) veterans reported using only doxycycline, and 425 (weighted 6.0%) reported using mefloquine and another antimalarial, which may have included doxycycline. Among the nondeployed (n = 7,031), 1,737 (weighted 20.8%) reported using an antimalarial drug, and of this group, 141 (weighted 8.8%) reported the use of doxycycline alone, and 52 (weighted 2.8%) used mefloquine and another antimalarial, which may have included doxycycline. Because it is not clear how many people in the mefloquine-plus-another-antimalarial group may have also used doxycycline, the results of that group are not included in the committee's assessment. The deployed doxycycline users reported increased frequencies of mental health diagnoses compared with nondeployed doxycycline users: PTSD (17.9% versus 11.1%), other anxiety disorders (11.2% versus 7.1%), major depression (9.8% versus 9.1%), and thoughts of death or self-harm (10.9% versus 10.5%), but no statistical comparisons were presented. In the adjusted logistic regression models with all covariates considered (including demographics, deployment, and combat exposure), the use of doxycycline was not associated with any of the adverse events compared with nonuse of antimalarial drugs: composite mental health score (OR = 0.96, 95%CI 0.83–1.09), composite physical health score (OR = 0.91, 95%CI 0.79–1.04), PTSD (OR = 0.96, 95%CI 0.79–1.15), thoughts of death or self-harm (OR = 0.87, 95%CI

0.69–1.09), other anxiety (OR = 0.85, 95%CI 0.67–1.07), and major depression (OR = 0.84, 95%CI 0.66–1.06). Results were similar to those of other antimalarials for analyses restricted to the deployed subset of veterans. An additional analysis was performed of the six health indicators or outcomes stratified by antimalarial exposure and a four-level measure of combat exposure intensity. The weighted prevalence estimates seem to indicate an increasing prevalence of disorders with increasing combat exposure intensity, but it is challenging to interpret the results or to compare across antimalarial exposures, given the small numbers in some cells and the lack of confidence intervals or hypothesis tests.

This analysis of the NewGen survey is highly relevant to the question of whether there are adverse events of doxycycline use that persist after the cessation of that use. The study is large enough to generate moderately precise measures of association, the specific drugs were assessed, the outcomes were based on standardized instruments (although not face-to-face diagnostic interviews), important covariates of deployment and combat exposure were considered in addition to demographics and other military characteristics, and the data were appropriately analyzed. It is noteworthy that adjusting for combat exposure consistently reduced the measures of association for adverse psychiatric events related to doxycycline use. Although the time period of drug use and the timing of adverse events were not directly addressed, given that the members of the populations were all veterans who had served between 2001 and 2008 and that the survey was not administered until 2009–2011, it is reasonable to assume that antimalarial drug use had ceased some time before the survey was conducted. Nonetheless, the study could not address explicitly the health experiences during use and in specific time intervals following the cessation of use. There are a number of methodologic concerns that limit the strength of this study's findings. The low response rate of 34% raises the concern of non-response bias, but responses were weighted to account for non-response. Selective participation by both antimalarial drug use history and health status would be required to introduce bias. The accuracy of the self-reported antimalarial drug use is unknown. Although self-reported information has some advantages over studies based on prescribed drugs in that the individual recalls using the drug, the reported drug and information on adherence are not validated. Self-reported health experience is subject to the usual disadvantages of recall bias and bias of reporting subjective experience without independent expert assessment; however, the use of standardized assessment tools may have circumvented these biases to some extent.

Lee et al. (2013) conducted a cross-sectional, web-based survey in 2009 of current and past members of the Australian Federal Police Association (AFP; a population similar to the U.S. military, but 70% male) to study the associations between deployment and exposure to doxycycline (compared with nondeployment and no exposure) and a new onset of gastrointestinal disease. Of those invited to participate, 1,300 (34%) responded, and 1,167 were eligible for analysis after the exclusion of 133 who had pre-existing gastrointestinal disease. The survey collected data on demographics, gastrointestinal health prior to joining AFP, the duration of employment, past and current overseas engagement, incident development of gastrointestinal illness, and the concurrent use of doxycycline. Adverse events were self-reported or inferred by the investigators based on reported symptoms and treatments. Respondents who reported a new gastrointestinal illness provided known diagnoses that were validated by supportive data such as appropriate investigations or appropriate treatments received for the given diagnosis; unknown diagnoses were inferred by investigators based on symptom descriptors, investigation, or treatment received. A diagnosis of inflammatory bowel disease (IBD) was supported by the description of an appropriate investigation or medication listed, and a diagnosis of irritable bowel syndrome (IBS) was either provided by the respondent, or inferred by the investigators based on the symptoms reported. Individuals were assigned to three illness groups: acute gastroenteritis, IBS, or IBD (including ulcerative colitis or Crohn's disease). All doxycycline prescriptions taken by deployed individuals were assumed to be for malaria prophylaxis; in nondeployed individuals, the timing, duration, and indication for doxycycline were not collected. Any incident illness was linked to the relevant deployment status according to its temporal relationship to the onset of symptoms. Logistic regression analyses were performed for the three adverse gastrointestinal events, stratified by deployment status and by deployment location in developing or developed countries using the classification of the United Nations Statistics Division. Of 590 deployed AFP members, 171 (30%) reported doxycycline use compared with 18 (3%) of 577 not deployed, although 21 of the 171 deployed individuals were exposed to at least one other antimalarial drug. A total of 158 incident gastrointestinal illnesses were reported during AFP employment, including acute gastroenteritis (10% deployed versus 1% not deployed; p < 0.001), IBS (5% versus 2%; p < 0.001), and IBD (2% versus 1%; p > 0.05). Compared with nondeployed AFP members with no doxycycline exposure (reference for all comparisons), nondeployed individuals who had used doxycycline reported fewer events of gastroenteritis (0 versus 4 cases, respectively), IBS (1 versus 12 cases, respectively), and IBD (0 versus 8 cases, respectively). Regression models included covariates of gender, family history of gastrointestinal illness, deployment status, deployment destination, and the use of doxycycline. For gastroenteritis, compared with nondeployed AFP members with no doxycycline exposure, those AFP members deployed to developing countries had a statistically significantly (but very imprecise) increased risk with doxycycline use (OR = 31.94, 95%CI 10.95–93.19), but the risk was not shown to be increased with doxycycline use and deployment to developed countries (OR = 7.89, 95%CI 0.83–75.05). For both deployment to developed countries (OR = 6.93, 95%CI 1.4–34.39) and to developing countries (OR = 2.47, 95%CI 0.77–7.89), the risk of IBS was statistically significantly increased for doxycycline use relative to nondeployed, non-doxycycline-exposed AFP personnel. For both deployment to developed countries (OR = 8.75, 95%CI 1.67–45.86) and to developing countries (OR = 6.99, 95%CI 3.19–15.31) the risk of IBD was statistically significantly increased for doxycycline use relative to nondeployed, non-doxycycline-exposed AFP personnel. The authors presented effect estimates for comparisons with and without the use of doxycycline between deployments to developed and developing countries relative to AFP personnel not exposed to doxycycline and not deployed, but they did not present effect estimates for comparisons between doxycycline exposed and unexposed individuals by any deployment stratum (e.g., with and without exposure to doxycycline for deployment to developed or developing countries).

This study provides a possible signal concerning persistent adverse gastrointestinal events (IBS and IBD) of doxycycline when used during deployment. It used a relatively weak study design and relied on a self-reported survey as the source of information on both exposures and outcomes, which could have occurred many years before. There was limited information on the timing of exposure, duration, and adherence, and all exposure among deployed personnel was assumed to be for malaria prophylaxis. This is potentially an important issue because, in addition to malaria prophylaxis, doxycycline may be used to prevent diarrhea and to treat a number of other infections, so the drug use may be associated with the gastrointestinal illnesses because it was prescribed to treat them. There was no information on the timing of the symptoms in relation to the exposure to doxycycline. The response rate was low (34%), raising questions about the representativeness of the respondents. There was little information on possible confounding variables other than occurrence and area of deployment and general demographic factors.

U.S. Peace Corps

Tan et al. (2017) conducted a retrospective observational Internet-based survey of 8,931 (11% response rate) returned Peace Corps volunteers (who had served during 1995–2014) to compare the prevalence of selected health conditions after Peace Corps service between those who reported taking malaria prophylaxis (n = 5,055, 56.6%) and those who did not. Reported initial antimalarial prophylactic prescriptions were mefloquine (n = 2,981; 59.0%), A/P (n = 183; 3.6%), chloroquine (n = 674; 13.3%), doxycycline (n = 831; 16.4%), and 386 (7.6%) "other" prophylactic medications. In addition to questions on malaria prophylaxis (type, regimen, duration, and adherence), the survey included questions about the country of service, the type of assignment, and whether malaria prophylaxis was required at the assigned site. Respondents were also asked to report medical diagnoses made by a health care provider before, during, and after service in the Peace Corps and to answer questions about medications used before, during, or after Peace Corps service; about family history of disease and psychiatric illness; about psychiatric history prior to exposure; and about alcohol consumption. In total, more than 40 disease outcomes were examined for associations with each antimalarial, including derived outcomes of major depressive disorder, bipolar disorder, anxiety disorder, insomnia, psychoses, and cancers. Outcomes were grouped by system (neuropsychologic, cardiac, ophthalmologic, dermatologic, reproductive, and gastrointestinal) or class (infectious, hematologic/oncologic) and within each group several diagnoses were listed. "Any psychiatric outcome" included all reported psychiatric diagnoses both derived and those reported as individual diagnoses, including schizophrenia, obsessive-compulsive disorder, and "other." Neuropsychologic disorders were presented as a category that separately included dementia, migraines, seizures, tinnitus, vestibular disorder, "other" neurologic disorder, and "any" neurologic disorder. Of the outcomes examined, the authors reported that insomnia was the only diagnosis statistically significantly more prevalent among those who used any doxycycline compared with those who did not (9.0% versus 5.4%, respectively; prevalence ratio = 1.27, 95%CI 1.02–1.59). There was no difference in the prevalence of insomnia between those with prolonged or prolonged exclusively doxycycline use and those with no doxycycline use. For exposed and unexposed groups, there were no differences in prevalence of several disease diagnoses extrapolated from adverse events derived from reported and feared adverse events with doxycycline use (i.e., recurrent yeast infections, allergic or contact dermatitis, and gastrointestinal diseases). There were no statistical results presented for adverse events related to doxycycline exposure.

The study had many limitations which stemmed primarily from its design as an Internet-based survey of people with email addresses on file. The response rate was low (11%), the authors relied on self-report for both exposure and outcome information and the timing of each, and for some participants the time between exposure and the survey was many years. Most comparisons were between those who had been exposed to a specific drug (i.e., mefloquine, chloroquine, doxycycline, A/P, other) and all of those who had not. Thus, the comparison group for each antimalarial was a mixture of those who did not report taking any antimalarials and those who reported taking antimalarial drugs other than the one being examined. Overall, there were few details of the limited analyses presented making it difficult to understand the groups that were being compared, how they differed with respect to important covariates, and what variables were included in the models. The reliance on self-report, often years (range 2–20 years) after exposure, introduces several potential biases (selection bias, recall bias, and confounding bias), with inadequate information available to determine the likely impact or direction of the potential biases acting in this study. While the use of self-reported diagnoses that were specified to be those made by a medical professional to ascertain diagnoses was arguably a better method than using a checklist of symptoms, the adverse events were not validated against any objective information.

Travelers

Meier et al. (2004) conducted a retrospective observational study in travelers using data from the UK-based General Practice Research Database (GPRD)—which has since changed names to the Clinical Practice Research Datalink—to assess the incidence of and compare the odds of developing first-time psychiatric disorders in individuals using mefloquine for malarial prophylaxis compared with individuals who used other antimalarial drugs. The Clinical Practice Research Datalink, which has now been active for more than 30 years, collects de-identified patient data from a network of general practitioner practices across the United Kingdom for use in public health research and clinical studies, which have included investigations of drug safety, the use of medications, health care delivery, and disease risk factors (CPRD, 2019). Using the GPRD, investigators identified individuals who had at least one prescription for mefloquine, A/P, doxycycline, or chloroquine and/or proguanil in the time period of interest and who had a pre-travel consultation within 1 week of the date of the prescription that included specific codes indicating that the prescription was for malaria prophylaxis. The start of the follow-up was the date of receipt of the first prescription for an individual. *Current use* was defined as between the date that a prescription was started and 1 week after the end of the time period of the drug prescription. Current exposure time was calculated differently for each antimalarial drug because the regimen for each of the antimalarial drugs differs. Investigators based their assessment on the number of tablets recorded by the general practitioner and calculated the assumed exposure time for each of the antimalarial drugs being investigated. For doxycycline the current exposure time (in days) was the number of tablets plus 7 days. Investigators added 90 days to each exposure to capture events occurring during travel that came to the attention of the general practitioner after the individual returned to the United Kingdom; this timeframe was termed *recent use*. Recent use included periods both relevant to the committee's charge (days 28–89) and time periods that the committee considered exclusionary (days 7–27). *Past use* started at day 90 and ended at a maximum of 540 days after the end of current exposure, reflecting a time period pertinent to the committee's assessment. Non-exposed people served as controls and had no antimalarial prescription during the study period or during 540 days after their pre-travel consultation, which also served as the date of the start of their follow-up. Participants were required to have at least 12 months of information on prescribed drugs and medical diagnoses before the first prescription date for an antimalarial or their travel consultation for the non-exposed controls. An additional inclusion criterion required participants to have recorded medical activity (diagnoses or drug prescriptions) after receiving a prescription to ensure that only those individuals who returned to the United Kingdom were included. A nested case–control analysis was also performed for a subset of the population in which up to six controls (who did not develop an outcome of interest during follow-up) were randomly selected per case; controls were matched to cases on age, sex, general practice, and calendar time (by assigning each control to the same index date as their matched case).

Meier et al. (2004) used the GPRD to assess the incidence of depression (n = 505), psychosis (n = 16), panic attacks (n = 57), and death by suicide (n = 2) in recent users (90 days following current use) of doxycycline compared with both current users (during active use) of mefloquine, proguanil, and/or chloroquine and past users (90–540 days) of any of these antimalarials. The study population consisted of 35,370 individuals aged 17–79 years who used antimalarials between January 1990 and December 2000: 16,491 mefloquine users, 16,129 chloroquine, and/ or proguanil users, and 4,574 doxycycline users (some individuals used multiple drugs). Investigators calculated the incidence of the four prespecified psychiatric outcomes during current, recent, and past use (people with prior diagnoses of the four psychiatric outcomes or alcoholism were excluded), and they also performed a nested case–control analysis in which both cases and controls had no history of the outcomes of interest prior to the use of any antimalarial. The incidence rates of first-time diagnoses were calculated using person-years and adjusted for age, gender, and calendar year. In total, 14 diagnoses of depression, 0 diagnoses of psychosis, 1 diagnosis of panic attack, and 0 deaths by suicide were reported for doxycycline users. The incidence rate of a first-time depression diagnosis did not differ between recent doxycycline users and all past users of antimalarials (RR = 0.8, 95%CI 0.4–1.4). In the nested case–control analysis, there was no difference in the odds of depression for recent doxycycline users compared with all other users combined after adjustment for age, gender, year, general practice, smoking status, and body mass index (BMI) (OR = 0.7, 95%CI 0.1–1.6). Regarding panic attacks, the incidence rate of a first-time diagnosis was no different for recent use of doxycycline than for past users of antimalarials (RR = 1.1, 95%CI 0.2–8.2). In the nested case–control analysis, the odds of panic attack were higher but not statistically significantly so for recent doxycycline users compared with all users (OR = 2.0, 95%CI 0.2–19.0) after adjusting for smoking status and BMI. This was a large retrospective study that found no increase in depression associated with current or recent use of doxycycline compared with the use of mefloquine, proguanil, and/or chloroquine, or all past users of antimalarials. The sample size was limited for the study of panic attacks and psychosis, leading to very imprecise estimates for those outcomes. Because current and recent use were analyzed separately, persistent outcomes were difficult to determine.

Schwartz and Regev-Yochay (1999) performed a prospective observational study, and followed 158 Israeli male and female travelers aged 22–65 years who took part in rafting trips on the Omo River, Ethiopia, and who had visited a travel clinic to obtain malaria prophylaxis. Travelers were prescribed mefloquine, primaquine, doxycycline (100 mg daily), or hydroxychloroquine by travel group. The primary aim of the study was to assess incident malaria and to compare the effectiveness of these four antimalarial drugs against both *P. falciparum* and *P. vivax*. Travelers were followed from the time of their return to Israel for an average of 16.6 months (range 8–37 months) for incident malaria. Adherence to the prophylactic regimens and the occurrence of adverse events were also collected by survey. The authors reported that "no severe side effects" were reported in any of the travelers, and one traveler withdrew from doxycycline use due to development of a rash. No other adverse events or withdrawals were noted in the doxycycline users. The strengths of this study include its design and the long duration of follow-up (an average of 16.6 months after return from a malaria-endemic country). It is limited by its small sample size, the nonrandomized design, and the lack of details on adverse events beyond reporting that no severe events occurred and only one withdrawal was reported among doxycycline users. As a result, this study provides limited information that can be used for inferences.

Endemic Populations

Andersen et al. (1998) conducted a double-blinded randomized placebo-controlled trial of azithromycin and doxycycline as prophylaxis for malaria among 232 semi-immune adults aged 18–55 years in Kenya from April through August 1995 in an area with high rates of endemic malaria. The study compared the prophylactic efficacy of three antibiotic regimens given for 10 weeks—azithromycin, 250 mg daily (n = 59); azithromycin, 1,000 mg weekly (n = 58); and doxycycline, 100 mg daily (n = 55)—versus a placebo (n = 60). Participants were determined to be in good health and were given quinine and doxycycline therapy over 7 days to clear pre-existing parasitemia. Volunteers with medical complaints, including possible cases of symptomatic malaria, were evaluated and treated at a research clinic. Pregnancy tests and enrollment blood tests were repeated after 5 and 10 weeks of drug administration. After the period of study drug administration, weekly blood smears were examined for an additional 4 weeks, and blood tests were repeated 4 weeks after the last dose of study drug. The safety and tolerability of the regimens were assessed by a daily symptom questionnaire, by review of research clinic records, and by interval hematology and serum chemistry tests. Because the timing of the adverse events was not clearly specified, the study provides little evidence as to whether adverse events were persistent following the cessation of doxycycline. There were no substantial differences between the groups in the results of the serum chemistry and hematology tests, including at the 4-week post-dosing time point, although detailed results were not presented.

OTHER IDENTIFIED STUDIES OF DOXYCYCLINE PROPHYLAXIS IN HUMAN POPULATIONS

Several studies of doxycycline use in service members from the United States (Arthur et al., 1990; Saunders et al., 2015), Australia (Kitchener et al., 2005; Rieckmann et al., 1993), France (Michel et al., 2010; Pages et al., 2002), Indonesia (Ohrt et al., 1997), Italy (Peragallo, 2001), Turkey (Sonmez et al., 2005), and the United Kingdom (Terrell et al., 2015; Tuck and Williams, 2016) were reviewed by the committee. However, because they did not follow the military cohorts after doxycycline prophylaxis was complete or did not report on adverse events that occurred post-doxycycline-cessation, these studies were not further considered.

Studies of other populations were also excluded from the final set of studies evaluated in depth because the follow-up was not at least 28 days post-doxycycline-cessation or because the authors did not distinguish between the timing of adverse events (less than or at least 28 days post-cessation). Such studies included Al-Mofarreh and Al Mofleh (2003); Bjellerup and Ljunggren (1994); Lobel et al. (2001); Meropol et al. (2008); Pang et al. (1988); Phillips and Kass (1996); Schlagenhauf et al. (2003, 2009); Shanks et al. (1995a,b); Sharafeldin et al. (2010); Story et al. (1991); Taylor et al. (2003); Vilkman et al. (2016); and Waner et al. (1999). Similarly, three studies that were designed to examine the safety or tolerability of doxycycline when used for long-term (>4 months) prophylaxis in different populations were excluded from further consideration because they did not report on adverse events or other outcomes post-cessation of doxycycline (Cunningham et al., 2014: Korhonen et al., 2007; Landman et al., 2014).

Upon full-text review and quality assessment, additional studies were excluded from further consideration. Some studies were excluded because of doxycycline's use for alternative treatment or prevention regimens (e.g., post-surgery or bacterial infection), because the reason for use of doxycycline was unclear, or because the dosage (or lack of) was determined to be irrelevant by the committee in addressing their charge (Berger, 1988; Chaabane et al., 2018).

Case Reports

The committee reviewed 14 published studies, totaling 23 cases, of adverse events related to the use of doxycycline in malaria prophylaxis. Various adverse events experienced by patients taking doxycycline resolved with discontinuation of the medication, including irritable mood and suicidality (Atigari et al., 2013), esophagitis (Geschwind, 1984), hiccups or esophageal ulceration (Morris and Davis, 2000; Tzianetas et al., 1996), diarrhea (Golledge and Riley, 1995), skin and nail issues (Cavens, 1981), and intracranial hypertension resulting in loss of vision (Lochhead and Elston, 2003), but a small number of studies reported adverse events that persisted beyond 28 days or 1 month after the discontinuation of doxycycline. The literature review produced seven published reports (nine total cases) that reported data after at least 1 month following doxycycline discontinuation (Belousova et al., 2018; Böhm et al., 2012; Gventer and Bruneti, 1985; Lim and Triscott, 2003; Lochhead and Elston, 2003; Morris and Davis, 2000; Neuberger and Schwartz, 2011). Three of these patients had skin lesions, including lymphamotoid papulosis (Belousova et al., 2018), that resolved by 5 months post-cessation of doxycycline; one patient experienced hyperpigmentation of the feet and legs (Böhm et al., 2002) that significantly improved at 1 year; and two patients had acute granuloma triggered by sun exposure (Lim and Triscott, 2003) that had resolved completely by 14 months post-cessation. Other adverse events that occurred concurrently and persisted following the cessation of doxycycline included onycholysis of the fingernails

(Gventer and Bruneti, 1985), which improved by the 3-month follow-up, and one case of diarrhea that resolved after an empirical anti-parasitic agent was prescribed (timing not provided) (Neuberger and Schwartz, 2011). One case of intracranial pressure returned to normal within 3 weeks of discontinuing doxycycline, but a consequent optic atrophy developed, resulting in a permanent loss of an estimated 70% of color vision and visual fields (Lochhead and Elston, 2003). These reports are suggestive of some persistent adverse events associated with doxycycline although the majority resolved or improved.

Selected Subpopulations

In the course of its review of the literature on doxycycline, the committee identified and reviewed available studies that reported results stratified by demographic, medical, or behavioral factors to assess whether the risk for adverse events when using doxycycline for prophylaxis is associated with being part of or affiliated with a specific group. This was not done exhaustively, and the evidence included in this section is generally limited to concurrent adverse events observed with use of doxycycline. Many of these studies did not meet the inclusion criteria of following their population for at least 28 days post-doxycycline-cessation, but the committee considers these findings to be important indicators when considering the evidence as a whole. The following risk groups were specifically considered: pregnant women and those with comorbid diseases or disorders.

Pregnancy

According to FDA, doxycycline use is classified as a pregnancy class D drug (i.e., contraindicated in pregnancy) (FDA, 2018a). Specifically, pregnancy class D indicates that there is positive evidence of human fetal risk based on adverse reaction data from investigational or postmarketing experience or studies in humans, but the potential benefits may warrant the use of the drug in pregnant women, despite the potential risks. This classification stems from a "tetracycline class effect," whereby tetracycline has been associated with teratogenicity, permanent yellowish-brown teeth discoloration after in utero exposure and in children under 8 years of age, and, more rarely, fatal hepatotoxicity reported in pregnant women (Cross et al., 2016). With respect to guidelines, according to Centers for Disease Control and Prevention malaria recommendations, doxycycline is contraindicated for use during pregnancy. Recommendations from the United Kingdom allow doxycycline for malaria prevention if other options are unsuitable, but the course of doxycycline, including the 4 weeks after travel, must be completed before 15 weeks' gestation (Public Health England, 2018). However, there is little scientific evidence of adverse pregnancy outcomes associated with doxycycline use during pregnancy. An expert review of published data on experiences with doxycycline use during pregnancy by the Teratogen Information

System concluded that therapeutic doses during pregnancy are unlikely to pose a substantial teratogenic risk (the quantity and quality of data were judged to be limited to fair), but the data are insufficient to state that there is no risk (Friedman and Polifka, 2000). Czeizel and Rockenbauer (1997) conducted a case–control study in mothers of infants with and without congenital anomalies (18,515 and 32,804, respectively) and found a weak, marginally significant association with total malformations and doxycycline use anytime during pregnancy; however, the association was not seen when the analysis was restricted to maternal treatment during the period of organogenesis (i.e., the second and third months of gestation). Other studies have reported mixed results on the impact of doxycycline use during pregnancy on congenital malformations; Cooper et al. (2008) reported no increased incidence of major congenital malformations in infants whose mothers had taken doxycycline, while Muanda et al. (2017) reported a two-fold increased risk of circulatory system malformation and cardiac malformations, and a three-fold increased risk of ventricular/atrial septal defect that may be the result of pro-inflammatory cytokines, matrix metalloprotease (MMP) inhibition, or placental anomalies related to doxycycline use.

Comorbid Conditions

While the tetracycline class of antibiotics is associated with increased blood urea levels, doxycycline specifically was shown to be safe for use in patients with renal failure or insufficiency (George and Evans, 1971). The dosage of doxycycline should be doubled in individuals taking antiepileptic drugs, such as carbamazepine, phenytoin, and phenobarbitone. These drugs cause doxycycline to be metabolized more quickly than usual and can reduce the effectiveness of this antimalarial medication; therefore, some research has suggested that twice the normal prophylactic doxycycline dose should be taken to ensure sufficient protection from malaria (Minshall, 2015).

BIOLOGIC PLAUSIBILITY

Overall, there is a lack of systematic studies of the long-term actions of doxycycline at prophylactic doses (100 mg per day in adult humans) on brain or nervous system function. There is little evidence to support or refute a role for doxycycline in promoting somatic and brain dysfunction. The committee found no evidence of persistent or latent adverse neurologic or psychiatric consequences in human or in preclinical models at doses relevant to malarial prophylaxis. In one study comparing doxycycline with other tetracyclines, evidence for vertigo was reported following minocycline, but not doxycycline, treatment (Cunha et al., 1982).

Doxycycline inhibits matrix metalloproteases (MMPs), which are enzymes that break down extracellular matrix and are associated with enhanced tissue damage and inflammation (Bench et al., 2011; Parks et al., 2004). Studies performed in multiple organisms (mice, rats, cattle, chickens) indicate beneficial effects in the prevention or treatment of connective tissue–related conditions (joint inflammation, cardiac fibrotic changes, etc.) (Bench et al., 2011; Donato et al., 2017; Haerdi-Landerer et al., 2007; Lizotte-Waniewski et al., 2016; Peters et al., 2002; Riba et al., 2017). Given their mechanism of action, interference with MMPs would not be predicted to have adverse neurologic consequences. Indeed, increased MMP activity is associated with central nervous system damage and neurodegenerative processes (Rempe et al., 2016), and MMP inhibition by doxycycline could thus be beneficial. For example, one study showed doxycycline treatment can reduce blood–brain barrier leakage following malarial infection in mice (Schmidt et al., 2018), suggesting beneficial actions on neuropathologic processes.

Long-term doxycycline is used to turn gene expression on or off in mouse models using tetracycline-responsive transgene promoters. In these types of studies, doxycycline may be either injected or administered continuously over protracted time periods (weeks) via the drinking water; the latter method is more common. The drug binds to a tetracycline-sensitive promoter in a transgene, and once bound it will promote either activation or inhibition of the expression of downstream gene products. These studies often involve a doxycycline-only control group, and doxycycline alone does not affect the reported endpoints being measured in these studies (many null effects) (Belteki et al., 2005). However, doxycycline alone has not been examined as an independent variable, and thus the neurologic and behavioral impact of doxycycline has not been tested against non-doxycycline controls.

The fact that doxycycline has antibiotic and antimicroglial activity makes it possible that the drug can alter brain inflammatory processes. Microglia are receiving a lot of attention as possible mediators of brain disorders, including depression. There is some evidence to suggest that doxycycline may be beneficial in limiting microglial-related neuroinflammatory processes, showing efficacy in reducing microglial proliferation following the intracerebral injection of toxic amyloid beta peptide and attenuating cytokine expression in a murine model of Alzheimer disease (Balducci et al., 2018). Similarly, the gut microbiome appears to modulate affective behaviors in mice and rats (Bastiaanssen et al., 2019). There are not a lot of data analyzing the impact of doxycycline on microbiota (Saarela et al., 2007). Thus, while it is possible that doxycycline could affect the brain via a rearrangement of the microbiome, there is no definitive evidence to support adverse events of long-term doxycycline exposure on brain function via this mechanism.

Doxycycline is an antibiotic that affects inflammatory processes as well as decreases gut microbiota (including beneficial probiotic bacteria) (Saarela et al., 2007). One study found that doxycycline can exacerbate colon cancer in a murine model and that it can actually enhance gut inflammation in this paradigm (Nanda et al., 2016). However, there is also evidence for gastroprotection in an ulcer model (Singh et al., 2011). The weight of the data suggest that adverse doxycycline effects on gastrointestinal function may be related to inflammatory changes in the gut, which is likely to vary substantially between individuals. These occur in a minority of users and dissipate once treatment is discontinued. Doxycycline can cause gastrointestinal symptoms in other species, including rats, mice, horses, cattle, and cats (Davis et al., 2006; German et al., 2005; Nanda et al., 2016; Riond and Riviere, 1998; Trumble, 2005). The studies often involve suprapharmacologic dosing over short time periods. Some of the consequences can be severe and usually involve the foregut (esophagus, stomach). The intensity of symptoms appears to be related to the formulation (acidity) (Malmborg, 1984).

The exact mechanism by which doxycycline produces esophagitis and esophageal ulcers is not completely understood. Its acidity has been considered a major factor with respect to its ability to damage the esophageal mucosa. Doxycycline accumulates within the basal layer of squamous epithelium in rats (Giger et al., 1978), which may inhibit protein synthesis and cause cellular degeneration. Human case reports of doxycycline-induced esophageal ulcers have supported the experimental evidence, in which diffuse degeneration of the basal layer was observed while the upper layer of esophageal mucosa was unaffected (Banisaeed et al., 2003). Other factors such as the drug dissociation rate (Bailey et al., 1990), pH (Carlborg et al., 1983), osmolarity, and intrinsic chemical toxicity (Bailey et al., 1990) are also implicated in the pathogenesis of drug-induced esophageal injury.

Doxycycline is known to produce photosensitivity in response to ultraviolet (UV)-A radiation, mediated by oxidative stress and mitochondrial toxicity. Accordingly, individuals undergoing doxycycline treatment (including for malarial prophylaxis) are warned to avoid sun exposure, and encouraged to wear protective clothing and apply broad-spectrum sunscreen (protecting against both UV-A and UV-B radiation) (Tan et al., 2011).

SYNTHESIS AND CONCLUSIONS

Although some people who take doxycycline do develop concurrent adverse events, such as photosensitivity, and there have been a few case reports of severe concurrent adverse events, the available post-cessation epidemiologic evidence does not find an association between the use of doxycycline for malaria prophylaxis and persistent or latent adverse events. The committee identified seven epidemiologic studies that included some mention of adverse events that occurred ≥28 days post-cessation of doxycycline that provided the most directly relevant information for assessing persistent health effects (Andersen et al., 1998; Eick-Cost et al., 2017; Lee et al., 2013; Meier et al., 2004; Schneiderman et al., 2018; Schwartz and Regev-Yochay, 1999; Tan et al., 2017). The studies are heterogeneous in the populations that were included (active military, veterans, U.S. Peace Corps volunteers, travelers, and endemic populations), in the modes of data collection on drug exposure, adverse events, and covariates (administrative records, researcher collected, self-report), and particularly in the nature of the health outcomes that were considered.

In most cases the focus of the studies was on neurologic or psychiatric conditions or a general assessment of adverse events of all types. Within a particular adverse event category, such as psychiatric conditions, the information elicited ranged from more minor symptoms (such as anxiety) to severe clinical disorders (e.g., psychosis, depression, PTSD), posing a challenge to the committee's ability to make an integrated assessment. Furthermore, the relevant studies were notably inconsistent in the reporting of results, and they covered different time periods in relation to the cessation of drug exposure. Given the inherently imperfect information generated by any one study, it would be desirable to have similar studies to assess the consistency of findings, but the diversity of methods used makes it very difficult to combine information across studies with confidence. Each of the included epidemiologic studies possessed strengths and limitations related to the specific methodology used, and the findings from those studies with the highest methodologic quality were given more weight when drawing conclusions. To avoid repetition for each outcome category, a short summary of the attributes of each study that was considered to be most contributory to the evidence base or that presented evidence germane to multiple outcome categories is presented first. The evidence summaries for each outcome category refer back to these short assessment summaries.

In addition to the post-cessation epidemiologic studies, the committee also considered supplemental evidence when making its conclusions, including recognized concurrent adverse events, case reports of persistent or latent adverse events, studies of adverse events in pregnant women and people with comorbid conditions, and information from experimental animal models or cell cultures. Consistent with the chapter syntheses of other antimalarial drugs, this synthesis is organized by body system category: neurologic disorders, psychiatric disorders, gastrointestinal disorders, eye disorders, cardiovascular disorders, and other outcomes and disorders, including dermatologic and biochemical parameters. Each conclusion consists of two parts: the first sentence assigns the level of association, and the second sentence offers additional detail regarding whether further research in a particular area is merited based on consideration of all the available evidence.

Epidemiologic Studies Presenting Contributory Evidence

Eick-Cost et al. (2017) used DoD administrative databases to perform a large retrospective cohort study among active-duty service members who filled at least one prescription for mefloquine, doxycycline, or A/P between 2008 and 2013. The primary study objective was to assess and compare the risk of incident and recurrent ICD-9-CM-coded neurologic and psychiatric outcomes that were reported at medical care visits during concurrent antimalarial use plus 365 days after the end of a prescription. This was a well-designed study and included several important features that increased its methodologic quality: a large sample size, the use of an administrative data source for both exposure and outcomes, and careful consideration of potential confounders including demographics, psychiatric history, and the military characteristics of deployment and combat exposure. Because neurologic and psychiatric diagnoses occurring during current and recent use were analyzed together without distinguishing between events that occurred within 28 days of antimalarial use and those that occurred ≥28 days post-cessation, the study provides no quantitative information regarding the persistence of most events other than the notation in the text that the results did not change when restricted to the post-cessation period. The use of medical diagnoses is likely to be more reliable for the outcomes than self-report, but there was no validation of the diagnoses recorded in the administrative databases, and symptoms or events that did not result in a medical visit or diagnosis would have been missed. For PTSD diagnoses there was no information on when the index trauma occurred.

Schneiderman et al. (2018) conducted an analysis of self-reported health outcomes associated with the use of antimalarials in a population-based cohort of deployed and nondeployed U.S. veterans, using information collected as part of the NewGen Study. Exposure and outcomes were systematically obtained, and psychiatric outcomes were measured by standardized assessment instruments. Antimalarial medication use was grouped by mefloquine, chloroquine, doxycycline, primaquine, mefloquine in combination with other drugs, other antimalarials, and not specified or no antimalarial drug exposures. Health outcomes were self-reported using standardized instruments: the SF-12 for general health status, PCL-C for PTSD, and the PHQ. The overall sample was large, and the researchers used a reasonably thorough set of covariates in models estimating drug–outcome associations, including deployment and combat exposure. Although the time period of drug use and the timing of health outcomes were not directly addressed, given that the population was all veterans who had served between 2001 and 2008 and that the survey was not administered until 2009–2011, it is reasonable to assume that antimalarial drug use had ceased some time before. The methodology and response rate (34% total; weighted 20.5% of deployed and weighted 8.8% of nondeployed individuals used doxycycline) for this study may have led to the introduction of non-response, recall, or selection biases; however, the committee believed that the investigators used appropriate data analysis techniques to mitigate the effects of any biases that were present.

Meier et al. (2004) conducted a study using data from the UK-based GPRD to assess the incidence and to compare the odds of first-time neurologic or psychiatric diagnoses in individuals aged 17–79 years using mefloquine compared with individuals using other antimalarial drugs, including doxycycline, for malaria prophylaxis. The use of data from GPRD (a well-established platform designed for both clinical practice and research) allowed for adequate power to detect differences in outcomes and for the uniform collection of exposures (although recorded drug prescriptions do not equate to use or adherence) and outcomes (based on clinical diagnoses coded from medical care visits) that were not subject to recall bias. Events that did not result in a medical care visit or that occurred outside of the national health care system would have been missed, and there may also be some differences between the travelers who traveled to malaria-endemic areas versus areas that are not endemic for malaria, which could lead to some apparent differences in outcomes between the groups. However, it is unlikely that this would result in differential selection bias. Diagnoses were defined a priori, which excluded other outcomes, including the potential to identify rare outcomes. The antimalarial-exposed populations were large, an appropriate comparison group of travelers not using any form of malaria prophylaxis was included, and health outcomes were reported in defined time periods, including current use through 90 days after a prescription ended (termed *recent use* in analyses) and 91–540 days following the cessation of use (termed *past use* in analyses). Adjustments were made for several confounders, including age, sex, calendar time, practice, smoking status, and BMI using appropriate study design or analytic methods. Each study included a nested case–control component that allowed for the control of important covariates.

The primary aim of Tan et al. (2017) was to assess the prevalence of several health conditions experienced by returned Peace Corps volunteers associated with the use of prophylactic antimalarial drugs. The number of participants was large (8,931 participants), and 16% of those who used an antimalarial had used doxycycline. A number of important covariates, such as psychiatric history and alcohol use, were collected, but the study had several methodologic limitations. These limitations included its study design (self-report, Internet-based survey), exposure characterization based on self-report (which introduces several potential biases such as recall bias, sampling bias, and confounding), outcome assessment (based on the self-report of health-provider-diagnosed conditions up to 20 years post-service), the use of mixed comparison groups, a lack of detail regarding the analysis methods, and poor response rate (11%, which likely introduces selection bias). The evidence generated by this study was thus considered to only weakly contribute to the inferences of doxycycline use and persistent or latent adverse events or disorders.

Neurologic Disorders

Although some studies grouped adverse events under a more general category of "neuropsychiatric effects" for discussion, the committee separated neurologic and psychiatric symptoms and conditions to the extent possible. The FDA label and package insert state that intracranial hypertension may be associated with use of doxycycline at the dose and frequency recommended for malaria prophylaxis, with clinical manifestations that include headache, blurred vision, diplopia, vision loss, and papilledema via fundoscopy. The risk of intracranial hypertension is increased in women of childbearing age who are overweight or have a history of intracranial hypertension and in those using isotretinoin concomitantly. Among the case reports that followed individuals for 28 days or more post-doxycycline-cessation, one case of intracranial pressure was reported that returned to normal within 3 weeks of discontinuing doxycycline and starting treatment, but consecutive optic atrophy developed resulting in a permanent loss of an estimated 70% of color vision and visual fields (Lochhead and Elston, 2003). Based on a systematic review of short-term travelers, there were no statistically significant differences for headache or dizziness associated with concurrent drug use when doxycycline users were compared with mefloquine users. Other concurrent neurologic adverse events were reported by individual cohort studies, including balance disorder, fatigue, hypoaesthesia (numbness), and palpitations and tinnitus, but for all of these outcomes there was either no difference in risk or a higher risk for mefloquine users than for doxycycline users (Tickell-Painter et al., 2017). Individuals with epilepsy who are taking antiepileptic drugs may need to double the dosage of doxycycline because these drugs cause doxycycline to be metabolized more quickly than usual and may reduce its effectiveness against malaria (Minshall, 2015).

Experimental animal and human cell culture studies that used doxycycline were also examined for evidence of mechanisms that could plausibly support adverse events. The committee found no evidence of persistent or latent adverse neurologic events in preclinical models at doses relevant to malaria prophylaxis. The committee found little evidence to support or refute a role for doxycycline in promoting somatic and brain dysfunction. Doxycycline may inhibit matrix metalloproteases, but this is not predicted to have adverse neurologic consequences (indeed, MMP activation is associated with central nervous system damage and neurodegenerative processes, suggesting doxycycline may be of benefit in this context).

Two epidemiologic studies included neurologic outcomes that occurred at least 28 days following the cessation of doxycycline (Eick-Cost et al., 2017; Tan et al., 2017). Both studies examined different neurologic outcomes with little overlap and used different methods to identify neurologic events. Eick-Cost et al. (2017) used ICD-9-CM-coded outcomes of confusion, tinnitus, vertigo, and convulsions, whereas Tan et al. (2017) examined "neuropsychologic" as a category that separately included dementia, migraines, seizures, tinnitus, vestibular disorder, and "other neuropsychologic" disorders. While both studies have limitations, Eick-Cost et al. (2017) provided the most evidence for potential persistent or latent neurologic outcomes.

In their analysis of data from DoD administrative databases, Eick-Cost et al. (2017) examined neurologic outcomes, and analyses were stratified by deployment and, separately, by psychiatric history. The results of a sensitivity analysis in which the risk period was restricted to 30 days post-prescription were not reported, although the authors stated that the results were similar to those of the primary analyses. Adjusted incident rates for confusion, vertigo, and convulsions—but not for tinnitus—were higher among the nondeployed than among the deployed groups who used doxycycline. When stratified by deployment, no statistically significant difference for any of the neurologic outcomes was found between deployed doxycycline users and mefloquine users. Among the nondeployed, doxycycline users had a statistically significantly increased risk of vertigo compared with mefloquine users, but no difference was found for the other three neurologic outcomes. When the population was restricted to the first mefloquine or doxycycline prescription per individual and included individuals with a prior history of a neurologic or psychiatric diagnosis, individuals with a neurologic diagnosis in the year preceding the prescription had statistically significantly elevated risks for a subsequent diagnosis of the same condition for all neurologic conditions reported (tinnitus, vertigo, and convulsions) compared with individuals without a diagnosis in the prior year. There were no statistically significant differences between mefloquine and doxycycline users for tinnitus, vertigo, or convulsions for people who had a prior neurologic diagnosis or for when users of these drugs were compared in people without a prior neurologic diagnosis. Overall, the largely null results that were reported suggest that null results would also be found if the analysis were restricted to outcomes occurring 28 days post-cessation. Tan et al. (2017) also reported no association between the use of doxycycline and any of the "neuropsychologic" adverse events examined; however, effect estimates were not presented.

Based on the available evidence, the committee concludes that there is insufficient or inadequate evidence of an association between the use of doxycycline for malaria prophylaxis and persistent or latent neurologic events. Current evidence does not suggest further study of such an association is warranted, given the lack of evidence regarding biologic plausibility, adverse events associated with concurrent use, or findings from the existing epidemiologic studies.

Psychiatric Disorders

No psychiatric adverse events are listed in the FDA label or package insert for doxycycline. In a systematic review of concurrent symptoms among short-term travelers, doxycycline users were statistically significantly less likely than mefloquine users to report psychiatric events, including abnormal dreams, insomnia, anxiety, and depressed mood, but the pooled effect estimates were very imprecise. Whereas there were 15 episodes of abnormal thoughts and perceptions among mefloquine users, no episodes were reported for doxycycline users in the cohort studies examined (Tickell-Painter et al., 2017). The committee identified 14 published case reports and case series, totaling 23 individuals, of adverse events related to the use of doxycycline for malaria prophylaxis. One case of irritable mood and suicidality was reported that resolved once doxycycline was discontinued, and no other concurrent or persistent psychiatric symptoms associated with the use of doxycycline were reported. Considering experimental animal and other biologic plausibility studies overall, systematic studies of the long-term actions of doxycycline at prophylactic doses on brain or central nervous system function are generally lacking. There is little evidence to support or refute a role for doxycycline in promoting somatic and brain dysfunction, and the committee found no evidence of persistent or latent adverse psychiatric or behavioral events in human or in preclinical models at doses relevant to malaria prophylaxis. The gut microbiome appears to modulate affective behaviors in mice and rats, but there is no definitive evidence to support an effect of doxycycline exposure on brain function via this mechanism.

Four of the epidemiologic studies with post-cessation follow-up included information on at least one adverse psychiatric outcome (Eick-Cost et al., 2017; Meier et al., 2004; Schneiderman et al., 2018; Tan et al., 2017). While all of these studies have methodologic limitations, Eick-Cost et al. (2017), Meier et al. (2004), and Schneiderman et al. (2018) provided the strongest evidence regarding the use of doxycycline and persistent or latent psychiatric outcomes. All four studies used different methods for measuring outcomes, and the psychiatric outcomes of interest varied across studies. Eick-Cost et al. (2017) examined adjustment disorder, anxiety disorder, depressive disorder, PTSD, psychoses, suicide ideation, paranoia, hallucinations, insomnia, and death by suicide using clinical diagnoses coded in DoD administrative databases. Meier et al. (2004) also used clinical diagnoses coded in a health care administrative database to examine incident depression, psychoses, panic attacks, and death by suicide. Schneiderman et al. (2018) used standardized self-report instruments to examine the outcomes of PTSD, thoughts of death or self-harm, other anxiety disorders, and major depression. Tan et al. (2017) used unverified self-reported symptoms to derive clinical diagnoses of major depressive disorder, bipolar disorder, anxiety disorder, schizophrenia, and "other."

In their analysis of active-duty service members, Eick-Cost et al. (2017) found that with the exception of paranoia and death by suicide, the adjusted incident rates for psychiatric outcomes were higher among the deployed than among the nondeployed groups who used doxycycline. When comparisons between mefloquine and doxycycline use were stratified by deployment, the only statistically significant difference for any of the psychiatric outcomes for the deployed was a slightly decreased risk for anxiety disorders among doxycycline users. Among the nondeployed, doxycycline users had statistically significantly increased risks of adjustment disorder, insomnia, anxiety disorder, depressive disorder, and PTSD compared with mefloquine users, but no difference was found for the other five psychiatric outcomes. When the population was restricted to the first mefloquine or doxycycline prescription per individual and included individuals with a prior history of a neurologic or psychiatric diagnosis, individuals with a psychiatric diagnosis in the year preceding the prescription had statistically significantly elevated risks for a subsequent diagnosis of the same condition for all of the psychiatric conditions that were reported (adjustment disorder, anxiety, insomnia, depressive disorder, and PTSD) compared with individuals without a diagnosis in the prior year. There were no statistically significant differences between mefloquine and doxycycline users for any of the psychiatric outcomes when comparisons were limited to people who had a prior psychiatric diagnosis or for when users of these drugs were compared in people without a prior psychiatric diagnosis. Schneiderman et al. (2018) also found deployed doxycycline users to have increased frequencies of mental health diagnoses compared with non-deployed doxycycline users for the four psychiatric outcomes examined. However, in the adjusted logistic regression models with all covariates considered (including demographics, deployment, and combat exposure), the use of doxycycline was not associated with any of the adverse psychiatric events in comparison with nonusers of antimalarial drugs: lower composite mental health score, PTSD, thoughts of death or self-harm, other anxiety, and major depression. When combat exposure intensity was specifically considered, the weighted prevalence estimates indicated that the prevalence of disorders increased with increasing combat exposure intensity. The results of Meier et al. (2004), which analyzed travelers, corroborated the findings of Schneiderman et al. (2018) and the deployed group of Eick-Cost et al. (2017) in finding that the use of doxycycline was not associated with a difference in depression diagnoses. Both Eick-Cost et al. (2017) and Meier et al. (2004) examined psychosis and death by suicide, and neither study found a statistically significant difference between doxycycline users and nondoxycycline users. Tan et al. (2017) also reported that in the set of psychiatric outcomes examined, none, except insomnia, was elevated among doxycycline users compared with those not using doxycycline. Regarding insomnia, Eick-Cost et al. (2017) found its risk to be statistically significantly increased among nondeployed doxycycline users compared with mefloquine users. However, Tan et al. (2017) also found no difference in the prevalence of insomnia between those with prolonged or prolonged exclusively doxycycline use and those with no doxycycline use.

Eick-Cost et al. (2017) and Schneiderman et al. (2018) examined PTSD diagnoses in active-duty U.S. military and veteran populations, respectively, and included estimates that adjusted for deployment and combat. Both studies found that deployed doxycycline users reported increased frequencies of PTSD compared with nondeployed doxycycline users. In fully adjusted models, Schneiderman et al. (2018) did not find any difference in PTSD for doxycycline users compared with those who used no antimalarials. Similarly, Eick-Cost et al. (2017) found no difference in risk for PTSD among the deployed that used doxycycline compared with those who used mefloquine. However, among the nondeployed, Eick-Cost et al. (2017) found that the risk of PTSD was statistically significantly increased for doxycycline users relative to mefloquine users. When the population was restricted to the first mefloquine or doxycycline prescription per individual and included individuals with a prior history of a neurologic or psychiatric diagnosis, individuals with a PTSD diagnosis in the year preceding the prescription had statistically significantly elevated risks for a subsequent diagnosis of PTSD compared with individuals without a diagnosis in the prior year. When comparing doxycycline and mefloquine users to those with and without prior psychiatric diagnoses, there were no statistically significant differences between mefloquine and doxycycline users for PTSD.

In sum, although there are a few findings of increased risk among specific outcomes relative to certain groups and in comparison with mefloquine, in general the results of the post-cessation epidemiologic studies provide modest evidence of no increase in risk of persistent adverse psychiatric events among individuals using doxycycline for malaria prophylaxis.

Based on the available evidence, the committee concludes that there is insufficient or inadequate evidence of an association between the use of doxycycline for malaria prophylaxis and persistent or latent psychiatric events. Current evidence does not suggest further study of such an association is warranted, given the lack of evidence regarding biologic plausibility, adverse events associated with concurrent use, or findings from the existing epidemiologic studies.

Gastrointestinal Disorders

The well-established concurrent adverse events of doxycycline on gastrointestinal symptoms, including nausea, vomiting, and diarrhea, justify a closer look at potentially persistent or latent gastrointestinal disorders following the cessation of use. The FDA label and package insert warn users of *Clostridium difficile–*associated diarrhea that can occur more than 2 months after drug cessation and further warn that this can cause increased morbidity and mortality because these infections can be refractory to antimicrobial therapy and may require colectomy. Although *Clostridium difficile* infection is listed as an adverse event of doxycycline, the current evidence suggests that doxycycline may provide protection against such infections (Tariq et al., 2018; Turner et al., 2014). The package insert also includes language warning that patients can develop watery and bloody stools (with or without stomach cramps and fever) as late as 2 or more months after antibiotic cessation, as well as pancreatitis. A systematic review in short-term travelers found that doxycycline users were statistically significantly more likely than mefloquine users to report nausea, vomiting, and diarrhea (Tickell-Painter et al., 2017).

Post-diarrheal syndromes can be associated with persistent adverse gastrointestinal events, but neither the post-cessation epidemiologic studies nor the evidence presented in the systematic reviews examining concurrent adverse gastrointestinal adverse events support such an association. There is some evidence from the biologic plausibility literature indicating that doxycycline may exert effects on the gastrointestinal tract, especially the esophagus and stomach, but the findings are inconsistent, and the studies often involve suprapharmacologic dosing over short time periods. The intensity of symptoms appears to be related to the acidity of the formulation. Human case reports of doxycycline-induced esophageal ulcers have supported the experimental evidence, in which diffuse degeneration of the basal layer was observed while the upper layer of esophageal mucosa was unaffected (Banisaeed et al., 2003). Other factors such as the drug dissociation rate, pH, osmolarity, and intrinsic chemical toxicity are also implicated in the pathogenesis of drug-induced esophageal injury (Bailey et al., 1990; Carlborg et al., 1983). Doxycycline is an antibiotic and consequently affects inflammatory processes and also decreases gut microbiota (including beneficial probiotic bacteria), suggesting that adverse doxycycline outcomes on gastrointestinal function may be related to inflammatory changes in the gut, which are likely to vary substantially among individuals. Although there is the potential for a concurrent irritant to become a chronic problem, there is no biologic-plausibility support for acute diarrhea that could be indicative of more chronic symptoms.

Two of the post-cessation epidemiologic studies provided information on gastrointestinal disorders (Lee et al., 2013; Tan et al., 2017). Lee et al. (2013) did not provide results for associations of the gastrointestinal outcomes with doxycycline use stratified by deployed versus nondeployed status and location of deployment to a developing or developed country. The only way to draw any inferences about the impact of doxycycline is by comparing the odds ratios for "doxycycline use and deployment to developing country" and "no doxycycline use and deployment to developing country" with both those estimates relative to "no doxycycline use and no deployment to a developing country." Using that indirect, approximate estimate, doxycycline appears to be associated with an increased risk for all three gastrointestinal illnesses examined (although the authors infer an association only for IBS and IBD, not gastroenteritis). Given the peculiar approach to the analysis, the inability to directly examine the impact of doxycycline, the small number of cases, exposures to doxycycline being based on self-report, and the other design limitations and likely biases, these results are quite limited in value. In a similarly methodologically limited study, Tan et al. (2017) found no association between doxycycline use and gastrointestinal diseases.

Based on the available evidence, the committee concludes that there is insufficient or inadequate evidence of an association between the use of doxycycline for malaria prophylaxis and persistent or latent gastrointestinal events. Current evidence suggests further study of such an association is warranted, given the evidence regarding biologic plausibility, adverse events associated with concurrent use, or findings from the existing epidemiologic studies.

Eye Disorders

The FDA package insert does not contain any information on eye disorders associated with the use of doxycycline, although secondary effects of blurred vision, diplopia, and vision loss may occur as a result of intracranial hypertension. A systematic review conducted in short-term travelers examining concurrent adverse events of malaria prophylaxis found that, based on two cohort studies, visual impairment was statistically significantly less commonly reported among doxycycline users than mefloquine users (Tickell-Painter et al., 2017). One case report of intracranial hypertension that resulted in a loss of vision was identified, but no other case reports that presented information on eye disorders persisting beyond 28 days post-doxycycline cessation were found. No studies of experimental animal studies were identified that examined the biologic plausibility of eye disorders.

One methodologically limited post-cessation epidemiologic study (Tan et al., 2017) was identified that presented data on eye disorders, which included macular degeneration, retinopathy, and "other." No differences in associations between eye disorders and doxycycline use compared with no doxycycline use were reported.

Based on the available evidence, the committee concludes that there is insufficient or inadequate evidence of an association between the use of doxycycline for malaria prophylaxis and persistent or latent eye disorders. Current evidence does not suggest further study of such an association is warranted, given the lack of evidence regarding biologic plausibility, adverse events associated with concurrent use, or findings from the existing epidemiologic studies.

Cardiovascular Disorders

The FDA label and package insert does not present any information regarding an association between concurrent adverse cardiovascular events and doxycycline use, and the committee did not identify any case reports reporting such an association. A systematic review conducted in short-term travelers examining concurrent adverse events found no associations between the use of doxycycline compared with mefloquine and cardiovascular disorders (Tickell-Painter et al., 2017). The committee did not identify any case reports that presented information on cardiovascular disorders persisting beyond 28 days post-doxycycline-cessation. In studies of experimental animals, doxycycline was found to inhibit matrix metalloproteases, and, as such, it may have beneficial effects in the prevention or treatment of connective-tissue-related conditions, including cardiac fibrotic changes.

One methodologically limited post-cessation epidemiologic study (Tan et al., 2017) found no association between doxycycline use and cardiovascular outcomes (arrhythmia, congestive heart failure, myocardial infarction, or "any" cardiac disorder).

Based on the available evidence, the committee concludes that there is insufficient or inadequate evidence of an association between the use of doxycycline for malaria prophylaxis and persistent or latent cardiovascular events. Current evidence does not suggest further study of such an association is warranted, given the lack of evidence regarding biologic plausibility, adverse events associated with concurrent use, or findings from the existing epidemiologic studies.

Other Outcomes and Disorders

A well-recognized concurrent adverse event of doxycycline is increased photosensitivity and skin rashes, which is thought to be mediated by oxidative stress and mitochondrial toxicity. Individuals with lighter complexions may be more prone to photosensitivity while taking doxycycline. Other adverse dermatologic events—some of which may be severe—are also presented on the FDA label and package insert and include exfoliative dermatitis, erythema multiforme, Stevens-Johnson syndrome, toxic epidermal necrolysis, and drug reaction with eosinophilia and systemic symptoms. The committee found case reports of acute skin and nail issues and persistent adverse events of onycholysis of the fingernails which improved by 3 months; skin lesions, including lymphamotoid papulosis, which resolved by 5 months post-cessation of doxycycline; hyperpigmentation of the feet and legs, which significantly improved at 1 year; and two patients with acute granuloma triggered by sun exposure, which resolved completely by a 14-month post-discontinuation follow-up. Vaginitis and yeast infections have been associated with doxycycline use, but these conditions are often included under the category of non-specific skin reactions.

Another specific and well-documented persistent adverse event of doxycycline use that results from exposure during the second half of pregnancy is permanent tooth discoloration and enamel hypoplasia in the fetus, which the potential for can persist well beyond the period of doxycycline use in the mother. There is not an obvious extrapolation of this adverse event to other types of health problems in adults. Reversible tooth discoloration in adults' teeth has also been reported, but these are cosmetic rather than clinical problems.

Tan et al. (2017) was the only epidemiologic study that met the committee's inclusion criteria that systematically examined dermatologic outcomes. Although this study had many limitations and at best can only contribute weak evidence, no differences were found in the prevalence of several disease diagnoses extrapolated from adverse events derived from reported and feared adverse events with doxycycline use (i.e., recurrent yeast infections and allergic or contact dermatitis) but no statistical results were presented for these outcomes related to doxycycline exposure. Schwartz and Regev-Yochay (1999) followed 158 Israeli travelers who took part in rafting trips on the Omo River, Ethiopia, and who had visited a travel clinic to obtain malaria prophylaxis. Of the travelers prescribed doxycycline, one traveler withdrew from doxycycline use because of the development of a rash. No other adverse events or withdrawals were noted in the doxycycline users, and the persistence of the rash was not reported. Travelers were followed for an average of 16.6 months (range 8–37 months), but no drug-associated adverse events were reported (or appeared to be collected).

In a double-blinded randomized placebo-controlled trial of azithromycin and doxycycline as prophylaxis for malaria among 232 semi-immune adults, Andersen et al. (1998) collected blood tests at baseline, at weeks 5 and 10 during drug administration, and at 4 weeks post-drug-administration for hematology and serum chemistry testing. The authors reported that there were no substantial differences between the groups regarding the results of the serum chemistry and hematology tests, including at the 4-week post-dosing time point (although detailed results were not presented). Although it met the inclusion criteria, given this limited information, this study did not provide any evidence that could be used to assess persistent or latent adverse events.

REFERENCES

Al-Mofarreh, M. A., and I. A. Al Mofleh. 2003. Esophageal ulceration complicating doxycycline therapy. *World J Gastroenterol* 9(3):609-611.

Andersen, S. L., A. J. Oloo, D. M. Gordon, O. B. Ragama, G. M. Aleman, J. D. Berman, D. B. Tang, M. W. Dunne, and G. D. Shanks. 1998. Successful double-blinded, randomized, placebo-controlled field trial of azithromycin and doxycycline as prophylaxis for malaria in western Kenya. *Clin Infect Dis* 26(1):146-150.

Arguin, P. M., and A. J. Magill. 2017. *For the record: A history of malaria chemoprophylaxis*. https://wwwnc.cdc.gov/travel/yellowbook/2018/infectious-diseases-related-to-travel/emfor-the-record-a-history-of-malaria-chemoprophylaxisem (accessed December 18, 2018).

Arthur, J. D., P. Echeverria, G. D. Shanks, J. Karwacki, L. Bodhidatta, and J. E. Brown. 1990. A comparative study of gastrointestinal infections in United States soldiers receiving doxycycline or mefloquine for malaria prophylaxis. *Am J Trop Med Hyg* 43(6):608-613.

Atigari, O. V., C. Hogan, and D. Healy. 2013. Doxycycline and suicidality. *BMJ Case Rep* 2013:bcr2013200723.

Bailey, R. T., Jr., L. Bonavina, P. E. Nwakama, T. R. DeMeester, and S. C. Cheng. 1990. Influence of dissolution rate and pH of oral medications on drug-induced esophageal injury. *DICP: The Annals of Pharmacotherapy* 24(6):571-574.

Balducci, C., G. Santamaria, P. La Vitola, E. Brandi, F. Grandi, A. R. Viscomi, M. Beeg, M. Gobbi, M. Salmona, S. Ottonello, and G. Forloni. 2018. Doxycycline counteracts neuroinflammation restoring memory in Alzheimer's disease mouse models. *Neurobiol Aging* 70:128-139.

Banisaeed, N., R. M. Truding, and C. H. Chang. 2003. Tetracycline-induced spongiotic esophagitis: A new endoscopic and histopathologic finding. *Gastrointest Endosc* 58(2):292-294.

Bastiaanssen, T. F. S., C. S. M. Cowan, M. J. Claesson, T. G. Dinan, and J. F. Cryan. 2019. Making sense of . . . the microbiome in psychiatry. *Int J Neuropsychopharmacol* 22(1):37-52.

Belousova, I. E., L. Kyrpychova, A. V. Samtsov, and D. V. Kazakov. 2018. A case of lymphomatoid papulosis type E with an unusual exacerbated clinical course. *Am J Dermatopathol* 40(2):145-147.

Belteki, G., J. Haigh, N. Kabacs, K. Haigh, K. Sison, F. Costantini, J. Whitsett, S. E. Quaggin, and A. Nagy. 2005. Conditional and inducible transgene expression in mice through the combinatorial use of Cre-mediated recombination and tetracycline induction. *Nucleic Acids Res* 33(5):e51.

Bench, T. J., A. Jeremias, and D. L. Brown. 2011. Matrix metalloproteinase inhibition with tetracyclines for the treatment of coronary artery disease. *Pharmacol Res* 64(6):561-566.

Berger, R. S. 1988. A double-blind, multiple-dose, placebo-controlled, cross-over study to compare the incidence of gastrointestinal complaints in healthy subjects given Doryx® and Vibramycin®. *J Clin Pharmacol* 28(4):367-370.

Binh, V. Q., N. T. Chinh, N. X. Thanh, B. T. Cuong, N. N. Quang, B. Dai, T. Travers, and M. D. Edstein. 2009. Sex affects the steady-state pharmacokinetics of primaquine but not doxycycline in healthy subjects. *Am J Trop Med Hyg* 81(5):747-753.

Bjellerup, M., and B. Ljunggren. 1994. Differences in phototoxic potency should be considered when tetracyclines are prescribed during summer-time. A study on doxycycline and lymecycline in human volunteers, using an objective method for recording erythema. *Br J Dermatol* 130(3):356-360.

Böhm, M., P. F. Schmidt, B. Lödding, H. Uphoff, G. Westermann, T. A. Luger, G. Bonsmann, and D. Metze. 2002. Cutaneous hyperpigmentation induced by doxycycline: Histochemical and ultrastructural examination, laser microprobe mass analysis, and cathodoluminescence. *Am J Dermatopathol* 24(4):345-350.

Bott, S., C. Prakash, and R. W. McCallum. 1987. Medication-induced esophageal injury: Survey of the literature. *Am J Gastroenterol* 82(8):758-763.

Brisson, M., and P. Brisson. 2012. Compliance with antimalaria prophylaxis in a combat zone. *Am J Trop Med Hyg* 86(4):587-590.

Carlborg, B., O. Densert, and C. Lindqvist. 1983. Tetracycline-induced esophageal ulcers: A clinical and experimental study. *Laryngoscope* 93(2):184-187.

Cavens, T. R. 1981. Onycholysis of the thumbs probably due to a phototoxic reaction from doxycycline. *Cutis* 27(1):53-54.

Chaabane, A., N. B. Fadhel, Z. Chadli, H. B. Romdhane, N. B. Fredj, N. A. Boughattas, and K. Aouam. 2018. Association of non-immediate drug hypersensitivity with drug exposure: A case control analysis of spontaneous reports from a Tunisian pharmacovigilance database. *Eur J Int Med* 53:40-44.

Cooper, W. O., S. Hernandez-Diaz, P. G. Arbogast, J. A. Dudley, S. M. Dyer, P. S. Gideon, K. S. Hall, L. A. Kaltenbach, and W. A. Ray. 2008. Antibiotics potentially used in response to bioterrorism and the risk of major congenital malformations. *Paediatr Perinat Epidemiol* 23(1):18-28.

CPRD (Clinical Practice Research Datalink). 2019. *Home.* https://www.cprd.com (accessed December 3, 2019).

Cross, R., C. Ling, N. P. Day, R. McGready, and D. H. Paris. 2016. Revisiting doxycycline in pregnancy and early childhood—Time to rebuild its reputation? *Expert Opin Drug Saf* 15(3):367-382.

Cunha, B. A., C. M. Sibley, and A. M. Ristuccia. 1982. Doxycycline. *Ther Drug Monit* 4(2):115-135.

Cunningham, J., J. Horsley, D. Patel, A. Tunbridge, and D. G. Lalloo. 2014. Compliance with long-term malaria prophylaxis in British expatriates. *Travel Med Infect Dis* 12(4):341-348.

Czeizel, A. E., and M. Rockenbauer. 1997. Teratogenic study of doxycycline. *Obstet Gynecol* 89(4):524-528.

Davis, J. L., J. H. Salmon, and M. G. Papich. 2006. Pharmacokinetics and tissue distribution of doxycycline after oral administration of single and multiple doses in horses. *Am J Vet Res* 67(2):310-316.

Dickinson, B. D., R. D. Altman, N. H. Nielsen, M. L. Sterling, and the AMA Council on Scientific Affairs. 2001. Drug interactions between oral contraceptives and antibiotics. *Obstet Gynecol* 98(5 Pt 1):853-860.

DoD (Department of Defense). 2009. *Policy memorandum on the use of mefloquine (Lariam®) in malaria prophylaxis.* September 4, #HA 09-017. Provided by COL Andrew Wiesen, M.D., M.P.H., Director, Preventive Medicine, Health Readiness Policy, and Oversight, Office of the Assistant Secretary of Defense (Health Affairs), DoD, January 25, 2019.

Donato, M., B. Buchholz, C. Morales, L. Valdez, T. Zaobornyj, S. Baratta, D. T. Paez, M. Matoso, G. Vaccarino, D. Chejtman, O. Agüero, J. Telayna, J. Navia, A. Hita, A. Boveris, and R. J. Gelpi. 2017. Loss of dystrophin is associated with increased myocardial stiffness in a model of left ventricular hypertrophy. *Mol Cell Biochem* 432(1-2):169-178.

Eick-Cost, A. A., Z. Hu, P. Rohrbeck, and L. L. Clark. 2017. Neuropsychiatric outcomes after mefloquine exposure among U.S. military service members. *Am J Trop Med Hyg* 96(1):159-166.

FDA (U.S. Food and Drug Administration). 2005a. Package insert for Doryx® (doxycycline hyclate) and Doryx® MPC delayed-release tablets. https://www.accessdata.fda.gov/drugsatfda_docs/label/2005/050795lbl.pdf (accessed July 12, 2019).

FDA. 2005b. Package insert for Doryx® (doxycycline hyclate) delayed-release capsules. https://www.accessdata.fda.gov/drugsatfda_docs/label/2005/050582s024lbl.pdf (accessed July 7, 2019).

FDA. 2007. Package insert for Vibramycyin calcium (doxycycline calcium oral suspension, USP) oral suspension syrup, Vibramycin hyclate (doxycycline hyclate, USP) capsules, Vibramycin monohydrate (doxycycline monohydrate) for oral suspension, Vibra-Tabs (doxycycline hyclate tablets, USP). https://www.accessdata.fda.gov/drugsatfda_docs/label/2008/050006s79,050007s 20,050480s42,050533s36lbl.pdf (accessed July 7, 2019).

FDA. 2014. Package insert for Acticlate™ (doxycycline hyclate USP) tablets. https://www.access-data.fda.gov/drugsatfda_docs/label/2014/205931s000lbl.pdf (accessed July 7, 2019).

FDA. 2016. Package insert for Acticlate® CAP (doxycycline hyclate) capsules. https://www.access-data.fda.gov/drugsatfda_docs/label/2014/205931s000lbl.pdf (accessed July 7, 2019).

FDA. 2017. Package insert for Acticlate® (doxycycline hyclate) tablets and Acticlate® CAP (doxy-cycline hyclate) capsules. https://www.accessdata.fda.gov/drugsatfda_docs/label/2017/205931 s003,208253s001lbl.pdf (accessed July 7, 2019).

FDA. 2018a. Package insert for Doryx® (doxycycline hyclate) and Doryx® MPC delayed-release tablets. https://www.accessdata.fda.gov/drugsatfda_docs/label/2018/050795s026lbl.pdf (ac-cessed July 12, 2019).

FDA. 2018b. Package insert for Doryx® (doxycycline hyclate) delayed-release capsules. https://www.accessdata.fda.gov/drugsatfda_docs/label/2018/050582s030lbl.pdf (accessed July 12, 2019).

FDA. 2018c. Package insert for Vibramycin® calcium (doxycycline calcium oral suspension, USP) oral suspension syrup, Vibramycin® hyclate (doxycycline hyclate capsules, USP) capsules, Vibramycin® monohydrate (doxycycline monohydrate) for oral suspension, Vibra-Tabs® (doxycycline hyclate tablets, USP) film coated tablets. https://www.accessdata.fda.gov/drug-satfda_docs/label/2018/050006s091lbl.pdf.

Friedman, J. M., and J. E. Polifka. 2000. *Teratogenic effects of drugs: A resource for clinicians (TERIS)*. Baltimore, MD: The Johns Hopkins University Press. Pp. 149-195.

George, C. R., and R. A. Evans. 1971. Tetracycline toxicity in renal failure. *Med J Aust* 1(24):1271-1273.

German, A. J., M. J. Cannon, C. Dye, M. J. Booth, G. R. Pearson, C. A. Reay, and T. J. Gruffydd-Jones. 2005. Oesophageal strictures in cats associated with doxycycline therapy. *J Fel Med Surg* 7(1):33-41.

Geschwind, A. 1984. Oesophagitis and oesophageal ulceration following ingestion of doxycycline tablets. *Med J Aust* 140(4):223.

Giger, M., A. Sormenberg, H. Brandli, M. Singeisen, R. Giiller, and A. L. Blum. 1978. Das tetra-cyclin-ulkus der speiserôhre. Klinisches Bild und in-vitro-untersuchungen [in German with English abstract]. *Dtsch Med Wschr* 103:1038-1040.

Golledge, C. L., and T. V. Riley. 1995. *Clostridium difficile*-associated diarrhoea after doxycycline malaria prophylaxis. *Lancet (London, England)* 345(8961):1377-1378.

Gventer, M., and V. A. Brunetti. 1985. Photo-onycholysis secondary to tetracycline. A case report. *J Am Podiat Med Assoc* 75(12):658-660.

Haerdi-Landerer, M. C., M. M. Suter, and A. Steiner. 2007. Intra-articular administration of doxycy-cline in calves. *Am J Vet Res* 68(12):1324-1331.

Hasan, S. A. 2007. Interaction of doxycycline and warfarin: An enhanced anticoagulant effect. *Cornea* 26(6):742-743.

Higgins, J. P. T., J. A. Lopez-Lopez, B. J. Becker, S. R. Davies, S. Dawson, J. M. Grimshaw, L. A. McGuinness, T. H. M. Moore, E. A. Rehfuess, J. Thomas, and D. M. Caldwell. 2019. Synthesising quantitative evidence in systematic reviews of complex health interventions. *BMJ Glob Health* 4(Suppl 1):e000858.

Kitchener, S. J., P. E. Nasveld, R. M. Gregory, and M. D. Edstein. 2005. Mefloquine and doxycycline malaria prophylaxis in Australian soldiers in East Timor. *Med J Aust* 182(4):168-171.

Klein, N. C., and B. A. Cunha. 1995. Tetracyclines. *Med Clin N Am* 79(4):789-801.

Korhonen, C., K. Peterson, C. Bruder, and P. Jung. 2007. Self-reported adverse events associated with antimalarial prophylaxis in Peace Corps volunteers. *Am J Prev Med* 33(3):194-199.

Kundu, C. N., S. Das, A. Nayak, S. R. Satapathy, D. Das, and S. Siddharth. 2015. Anti-malarials are anti-cancers and vice versa—One arrow two sparrows. *Acta Tropica* 149:113-127.

Landman, K. Z., K. R. Tan, P. M. Arguin, and the Centers for Disease Control and Prevention. 2014. Knowledge, attitudes, and practices regarding antimalarial chemoprophylaxis in U.S. Peace Corps volunteers—Africa, 2013. *MMWR* 63(23):516-517.

Lee, T. W., L. Russell, M. Deng, and P. R. Gibson. 2013. Association of doxycycline use with the development of gastroenteritis, irritable bowel syndrome and inflammatory bowel disease in Australians deployed abroad. *Intern Med J* 43(8):919-926.

Lim, D. S., and J. Triscott. 2003. O'Brien's actinic granuloma in association with prolonged doxycycline phototoxicity. *Australas J Dermatol* 44(1):67-70.

Lizotte-Waniewski, M., K. Brew, and C. H. Hennekens. 2016. Hypothesis: Metalloproteinase inhibitors decrease risks of cardiovascular disease. *J Cardiovasc Pharmacol Ther* 21(4):368-371.

Lobel, H. O., M. A. Baker, F. A. Gras, G. M. Stennies, P. Meerburg, E. Hiemstra, M. Parise, M. Odero, and P. Waiyaki. 2001. Use of malaria prevention measures by North American and European travelers to East Africa. *J Travel Med* 8(4):167-172.

Lochhead, J., and J. S. Elston. 2003. Doxycycline induced intracranial hypertension. *BMJ (Clin Res Ed)* 326(7390):641-642.

Malmborg, A. S. 1984. Bioavailability of doxycycline monohydrate. A comparison with equivalent doses of doxycycline hydrochloride. *Chemotherapy* 30(2):76-80.

Meier, C. R., K. Wilcock, and S. S. Jick. 2004. The risk of severe depression, psychosis or panic attacks with prophylactic antimalarials. *Drug Saf* 27(3):203-213.

Meropol, S. B., K. A. Chan, Z. Chen, J. A. Finkelstein, S. Hennessy, E. Lautenbach, R. Platt, S. D. Schech, D. Shatin, and J. P. Metlay. 2008. Adverse events associated with prolonged antibiotic use. *Pharmacoepidemiol Drug Saf* 17(5):523-532.

Michel, R., S. Bardot, B. Queyriaux, J. P. Boutin and J. E. Touze. 2010. Doxycycline–chloroquine vs. doxycycline–placebo for malaria prophylaxis in nonimmune soldiers: A double-blind randomized field trial in sub-Saharan Africa. *Trans R Soc Trop Med Hyg* 104(4):290-297.

Minshall, I. 2015. *Epilepsy and anti-malarial medication.* https://www.epilepsyresearch.org.uk/wp-content/uploads/2015/05/antimalarials4.pdf (accessed November 11, 2019).

Morris, T. J., and T. P. Davis. 2000. Doxycycline-induced esophageal ulceration in the U.S. military service. *Mil Med* 165(4):316-319.

Muanda, F. T., O. Sheehy, and A. Bérard. 2017. Use of antibiotics during pregnancy and the risk of major congenital malformations: A population based cohort study. *Br J Clin Pharmacol* 83(11):2557-2571.

Nanda, N., D. K. Dhawan, A. Bhatia, A. Mahmood, and S. Mahmood. 2016. Doxycycline promotes carcinogenesis & metastasis via chronic inflammatory pathway: An in vivo approach. *PLOS ONE* 11(3):e0151539.

Neuberger, A., and E. Schwartz. 2011. *Clostridium difficile* infection after malaria prophylaxis with doxycycline: Is there an association? *Travel Med Infect Dis* 9(5):243-245.

Ohrt, C., T. L. Richie, H. Widjaja, D. Shanks, J. Fitriadi, D. J. Fryauff, J. Handschin, D. Tang, B. Sandjaja, E. Tjitra, L. Hadiarso, G. Watt, and F. S. Wignall. 1997. Mefloquine compared with doxycycline for the prophylaxis of malaria in Indonesian soldiers: Randomized, double blind, placebo controlled trial. *Ann Intern Med* 126:963-972.

Overbosch, D., H. Schilthuis, U. Bienzle, R. H. Behrens, K. C. Kain, P. D. Clarke, S. Toovey, J. Knobloch, H. D. Nothdurft, D. Shaw, N. S. Roskell, J. D. Chulay, and the Malarone International Study Team. 2001. Atovaquone-proguanil versus mefloquine for malaria prophylaxis in nonimmune travelers: Results from a randomized, double-blind study. *Clin Infect Dis* 33(7):1015-1021.

Pages, F., J. P. Boutin, J. B. Meynard, A. Keundjian, S. Ryfer, L. Giurato, and D. Baudon. 2002. Tolerability of doxycycline monohydrate salt vs. chloroquine–proguanil in malaria prophylaxis. *Trop Med Int Health* 7(11):919-924.

Pang, L., N. Limsomwong, and P. Singharaj. 1988. Prophylactic treatment of *vivax* and *falciparum* malaria with low-dose doxycycline. *J Infect Dis* 158(5):1124-1127.

Parks, W. C., C. L. Wilson, and Y. S. Lopez-Boado. 2004. Matrix metalloproteinases as modulators of inflammation and innate immunity. *Nat Rev Immunol* 4(8):617-629.

Penning-van Beest, F. J., J. Koerselman, and R. M. Herings. 2008. Risk of major bleeding during concomitant use of antibiotic drugs and coumarin anticoagulants. *J Thromb Haemost* 6(2):284-290.

Peragallo, M. S. 2001. The Italian army standpoint on malaria chemoprophylaxis. *Med Trop (Mars)* 61(1):59-62.

Peters, T. L., R. M. Fulton, K. D. Roberson, and M. W. Orth. 2002. Effect of antibiotics on in vitro and in vivo avian cartilage degradation. *Avian Dis* 46(1):75-86.

Phillips, M. A., and R. B. Kass. 1996. User acceptability patterns for mefloquine and doxycycline malaria chemoprophylaxis. *J Travel Med* 3(1):40-45.

Public Health England. 2018. *Guidelines for malaria prevention in travelers from the UK.* https://assets.publishing.service.gov.uk/government/uploads/system/uploads/attachment_data/file/774781/ACMP_guidelines_2018.pdf (accessed December 3, 2019).

Rempe, R. G., A. M. S. Hartz, and B. Bauer. 2016. Matrix metalloproteinases in the brain and blood–brain barrier: Versatile breakers and makers. *J Cereb Blood Flow Metab* 36(9):1481-1507.

Riba, A., L. Deres, K. Eros, A. Szabo, K. Magyar, B. Sumegi, K. Toth, R. Halmosi, and E. Szabados. 2017. Doxycycline protects against ROS-induced mitochondrial fragmentation and ISO-induced heart failure. *PLOS ONE* 12(4):e0175195.

Rieckmann, K. H., A. E. Yeo, D. R. Davis, D. C. Hutton, P. F. Wheatley, and R. Simpson. 1993. Recent military experience with malaria prophylaxis. *Med J Aust* 158(7):446-449.

Riond, J. L., and J. E. Riviere. 1988. Pharmacology and toxicology of doxycycline. *Vet Hum Toxicol* 30(5):431-443.

Rudland, S., M. Little, P. Kemp, A. Miller, and J. Hodge. 1996. The enemy within: Diarrheal rates among British and Australian troops in Iraq. *Mil Med* 161(12):728-731.

Saarela, M., J. Maukonen, A. von Wright, T. Vilpponen-Salmela, A. J. Patterson, K. P. Scott, H. Hämynen, and J. Mättö. 2007. Tetracycline susceptibility of the ingested *Lactobacillus acidophilus* LaCH-5 and *Bifidobacterium animalis* subsp. lactis Bb-12 strains during antibiotic/probiotic intervention. *Int J Antimicrob Agents* 29(3):271-280.

Sack, R. B., M. Santosham, J. L. Froehlich, C. Medina, F. Orskov, and I. Orskov. 1984. Doxycycline prophylaxis of travelers' diarrhea in Honduras, an area where resistance to doxycycline is common among enterotoxigenic *Escherichia coli. Am J Trop Med Hyg* 33(3):460-466.

Sánchez, J. L., R. F. DeFraites, T. W. Sharp, and R. K. Hanson. 1993. Mefloquine or doxycycline prophylaxis in U.S. troops in Somalia. *Lancet* 341(8851):1021-1022.

Saunders, D. L., E. Garges, J. E. Manning, K. Bennett, S. Schaffer, A. J. Kosmowski, and A. J. Magill. 2015. Safety, tolerability, and compliance with long-term antimalarial prophylaxis in American soldiers in Afghanistan. *Am J Trop Med Hyg* 93(3):584-590.

Schlagenhauf, P., A. Tschopp, R. Johnson, H. D. Nothdurft, B. Beck, E. Schwartz, M. Herold, B. Krebs, O. Veit, R. Allwinn, and R. Steffen. 2003. Tolerability of malaria prophylaxis in nonimmune travellers to sub-Saharan Africa: Multicentre, randomised, double blind, four arm study. *BMJ* 327(7423):1078.

Schlagenhauf, P., R. Johnson, E. Schwartz, H. D. Nothdurft, and R. Steffen. 2009. Evaluation of mood profiles during malaria prophylaxis: A randomized, double-blind, four-arm study. *J Travel Med* 16(1):42-45.

Schlagenhauf, P., M. E. Wilson, E. Petersen, A. McCarthy, L. H. Chen, J. S. Keystone, P. E. Kozarsky, B. A. Connor, H. D. Nothdurft, M. Mendelson, and K. Leder. 2019. Malaria chemoprophylaxis. *J Travel Med* 4(15):145-167.

Schmidt, K. E., J. M. Kuepper, B. Schumak, J. Alferink, A. Hofmann, S. W. Howland, L. Renia, A. Limmer, S. Specht, and A. Hoerauf. 2018. Doxycycline inhibits experimental cerebral malaria by reducing inflammatory immune reactions and tissue-degrading mediators. *PLOS ONE* 13(2):e0192717.

Schneiderman, A. I., Y. S. Cypel, E. K. Dursa, and R. M. Bossarte. 2018. Associations between use of antimalarial medications and health among U.S. veterans of the wars in Iraq and Afghanistan. *Am J Trop Med Hyg* 99(3):638-648.

Schwartz, E., and G. Regev-Yochay. 1999. Primaquine as prophylaxis for malaria for nonimmune travelers: A comparison with mefloquine and doxycycline. *Clin Infect Dis* 29(6):1502-1506.

Shanks, G. D., P. Roessler, M. D. Edstein, and K. H. Rieckmann. 1995a. Doxycycline for malaria prophylaxis in Australian soldiers deployed to United Nations missions in Somalia and Cambodia. *Mil Med* 160(9):443-445.

Shanks, G. D., A. Barnett, M. D. Edstein, and K. H. Rieckmann. 1995b. Effectiveness of doxycycline combined with primaquine for malaria prophylaxis. *Med J Aust* 162(6):306-307, 309.

Shapiro, L. E., S. R. Knowles, and N. H. Shear. 1997. Comparative safety of tetracycline, minocycline, and doxycycline. *Arch Dermatol* 133(10):1224-1230.

Sharafeldin, E., D. Soonawala, J. P. Vandenbroucke, E. Hack, and L. G. Visser. 2010. Health risks encountered by Dutch medical students during an elective in the tropics and the quality and comprehensiveness of pre- and post-travel care. *BMC Med Educ* 10:89.

Singh, L. P., A. Mishra, D. Saha, and S. Swarnakar. 2011. Doxycycline blocks gastric ulcer by regulating matrix metalloproteinase-2 activity and oxidative stress. *World J Gastroenterol* 17(28):3310-3321.

Smith, E. L., A. al Raddadi, F. al Ghamdi, and S. Kutbi. 1995. Tetracycline phototoxicity. *Br J Dermatol* 132:316-317.

Sonmez, A., A. Harlak, S. Kilic, Z. Polat, L. Hayat, O. Keskin, T. Dogru, M. I. Yilmaz, C. H. Acikel, and I. H. Kocar. 2005. The efficacy and tolerability of doxycycline and mefloquine in malaria prophylaxis of the ISAF troops in Afghanistan. *J Infect* 51(3):253-258.

Story, M. J., P. I. McCloud, and G. Boehm. 1991. Doxycycline tolerance study. Incidence of nausea after doxycycline administration to healthy volunteers: A comparison of 2 formulations (Doryx® vs Vibramycin®). *Eur J Clin Pharmacol* 40(4):419-421.

Tan, K. R., A. J. Magill, M. E. Parise, P. M. Arguin, and the Centers for Disease Control and Prevention. 2011. Doxycycline for malaria prophylaxis and treatment: Report from the CDC expert meeting on malaria prophylaxis. *Am J Trop Med Hyg* 84(4):517-531.

Tan, K. R., S. J. Henderson, J. Williamson, R. W. Ferguson, T. M. Wilkinson, P. Jung, and P. M. Arguin. 2017. Long-term health outcomes among returned Peace Corps volunteers after malaria prophylaxis, 1995-2014. *Travel Med Infect Dis* 17:50-55.

Tariq, R., J. Cho, S. Kapoor, R. Orenstein, S. Singh, D. S. Pardi, and S. Khanna. 2018. Low risk of primary *Clostridium difficile* infection with tetracyclines: A systematic review and metaanalysis. *Clin Infect Dis* 66(4):514-522.

Taylor, W. R., T. L. Richie, D. J. Fryauff, C. Ohrt, H. Picarima, D. Tang, G. S. Murphy, H. Widjaja, D. Braitman, E. Tjitra, A. Ganjar, T. R. Jones, H. Basri, and J. Berman. 2003. Tolerability of azithromycin as malaria prophylaxis in adults in northeast Papua, Indonesia. *Antimicrob Agents Chemother* 47(7):2199-2203.

Terrell, A. G., M. E. Forde, R. Firth, and D. A. Ross. 2015. Malaria prophylaxis and self-reported impact on ability to work: Mefloquine versus doxycycline. *J Travel Med* 22(6):383-388.

Thillainayagam, M., and S. Ramaiah. 2016. Mosquito, malaria and medicines—A review. *Res J Pharm Technol* 9(8):1268-1276.

Tickell-Painter, M., N. Maayan, R. Saunders, C. Pace, and D. Sinclair. 2017. Mefloquine for preventing malaria during travel to endemic areas. *Cochrane Database Syst Rev* 10:CD006491.

Trumble, C. 2005. Oesophageal stricture in cats associated with use of the hyclate (hydrochloride) salt of doxycycline. *J Fel Med Surg* 7(4):241-242.

Tuck, J., and J. Williams. 2016. Malaria protection in Sierra Leone during the Ebola outbreak 2014/15: The UK military experience with malaria prophylaxis, Sep 14–Feb 15. *Travel Med Infect Dis* 14(5):471-474.

Turner, R. B., C. B. Smith, J. L. Martello, and D. Slain. 2014. Role of doxycycline in *Clostridium difficile* infection acquisition. *Ann Pharmacother* 48(6):772-776.

Tzianetas, I., F. Habal, and J. S. Keystone. 1996. Short report: Severe hiccups secondary to doxy-cycline-induced esophagitis during treatment of malaria. *Am J Trop Med Hyg* 54(2):203-204.

Vilkman, K., S. H. Pakkanen, T. Laaveri, H. Siikamaki, and A. Kantele. 2016. Travelers' health problems and behavior: Prospective study with post-travel follow-up. *BMC Infectious Diseases* 16(1):328.

Wallace, M. R. 1996. Malaria among United States troops in Somalia. *Am J Med* 100(1):49-55.

Waner, S., D. Durrhiem, L. E. Braack, and S. Gammon. 1999. Malaria protection measures used by in-flight travelers to South African game parks. *J Travel Med* 6(4):254-257.

Watanasook, C., P. Singharaj, V. Suriyamongkol, J. J. Karwacki, D. Shanks, P. Phintuyothin, S. Pilungkasa, and P. Wasuwat. 1989. Malaria prophylaxis with doxycycline in soldiers deployed to the Thai–Kampuchean border. *Southeast Asian J Trop Med Public Health* 20(1):61-64.

Zhao, S., C. Choksuchat, Y. Zhao, S. A. Ballagh, G. A. Kovalevsky, and D. F. Archer. 2009. Effects of doxycycline on serum and endometrial levels of MMP-2, MMP-9 and TIMP-1 in women using a levonorgestrel-releasing subcutaneous implant. *Contraception* 79(6):469-478.

8

Primaquine

Primaquine, or primaquine phosphate, was synthesized in 1945 at Columbia University under a U.S. government wartime contract (Baird, 2019), but the U.S. Army did not begin large-scale safety and efficacy studies until the early 1950s, when relapsing *Plasmodium vivax* malaria had emerged as a public health concern in troops returning from the Korean War (Kitchen et al., 2006). In 1951, while primaquine was still an experimental drug, the U.S. military performed a randomized placebo-controlled trial on shipboard veterans returning home from Korea (Baird, 2019; Brundage, 2003). The Food and Drug Administration (FDA) approved primaquine for the treatment of *P. vivax* and *P. ovale* for military use in January 1952 and for civilian use in August 1952 (Kitchen et al., 2006). The drug was manufactured by Winthrop-Stearns, Inc. (DoD, n.d.a). By 1953 more than 250,000 repatriating service members would receive primaquine, and the drug was credited with preventing the reintroduction of malaria to the United States (Alving et al., 1960).

Primaquine continues to be widely used because of the varied activity of the 8-aminoquinoline class. It can kill developing parasites of all *Plasmodium* species in the liver, as well as the dormant hypnozoites of *P. vivax* and *P. ovale*, the blood schizonts and gametocytes of *P. vivax*, and the gametocytes of *P. falciparum* (Ashley et al., 2014; Baird, 2019; Berman, 2004). Thus it can be used as primary prophylaxis, for radical cure and presumptive anti-relapse therapy, to block human-to-mosquito transmission, and finally, combined with sporozoite inoculation, to vaccinate against *Plasmodium* parasites (Ashley et al., 2014; Baird, 2019; Goh et al., 2019; Schlagenhauf et al., 2019). The role of primaquine in malaria prophylaxis has been singular; until recently it was the only available agent that could eliminate *Plasmodium* hypnozoites, a life stage of malaria that is unique to

P. vivax and *P. ovale*. Hypnozoites, which are undetectable by diagnostic tests, can lie dormant in the liver for months to years and then differentiate, traveling to the blood to cause clinical malaria and enable malaria transmission (Ackert et al., 2019; Rishikesh and Saravu, 2016). As an effective hypnozoiticide, primaquine has been of particular value to the U.S. military because *P. vivax* is endemic, or has been endemic during a military presence, in areas of military operation. Examples include Afghanistan, where *P. vivax* represents 95% of malaria cases, and Iraq, where the 1990–1991 Gulf War led to a years-long resurgence of *P. vivax* (CDC, 2019a; Schlagenhauf, 2003).

The FDA-approved indication for primaquine reads, "for the radical cure (prevention of relapse) of vivax malaria" (FDA, 2017a). The term "radical cure" generally refers to a regimen of a blood schizonticide (e.g., chloroquine) paired with a hypnozoiticide (e.g., primaquine) to treat a confirmed case of malaria by eliminating all erythrocytic and hepatic parasites in the body (Baird, 2019; Hill et al., 2006). There is some inconsistency in the literature, however, and the term "radical cure" has also been used more narrowly to refer to eliminating *P. vivax* and *P. ovale* hypnozoites from the body of an infected individual (CDC, 2019b). The dosage and administration information in the primaquine FDA package insert notes further that primaquine is recommended "following the termination of chloroquine phosphate suppressive therapy in an area where vivax malaria is endemic" (FDA, 2017a). The latter recommendation points to the use of primaquine for prophylaxis rather than for treatment. This use of primaquine differs from the way that standard blood-schizonticide antimalarials (e.g., chloroquine, doxycycline, atovoquone/proguanil, mefloquine) are used for primary prophylaxis. Instead, primaquine is used at or toward the end of primary prophylaxis to kill hypnozoites, which a blood schizonticide used as primary prophylaxis cannot kill (CDC, 2017b; Hill et al., 2006). Presumptive anti-relapse therapy (PART) is a regimen that uses an antimalarial drug to kill hypnozoites and is also referred to as terminal prophylaxis. As with the term "radical cure," the term "PART" has been used variably in the literature; it has been used both to refer to a component of a regimen to treat confirmed malaria and to a regimen added onto primary prophylaxis to kill hypnozoites (Hill et al., 2006; Vale et al., 2009). The FDA-recommended dosage is 15 mg per day for 14 days (FDA, 2017a). Since the focus of the committee is antimalarial prophylaxis, in this chapter, the term "PART" will refer to regimens for prophylaxis and not for treatment of confirmed malaria.

The remainder of this chapter follows the same structure as the other antimalarial drug chapters, beginning with a discussion of the FDA package insert, with a focus on the Contraindications, Warnings, Precautions, and Drug Interactions sections as well as a summary of the changes made to the primaquine package insert since 2003. This is followed by a summary of how the U.S. military has been using primaquine based on Department of Defense (DoD) issuances. A brief overview of the pharmacokinetic properties of primaquine is then provided. The majority of the chapter is focused on adverse events associated with its use for malaria prophylaxis, beginning with a summary of the known concurrent adverse events associated with primaquine when used as directed for PART. Next, the four identified epidemiologic studies that met the committee's inclusion criteria and provided information on persistent or latent health outcomes following the cessation of primaquine are summarized and assessed. These are ordered by population: studies of military and veterans (U.S. followed by international forces), travelers, and research volunteers. Where available, studies of U.S. participants are presented first. A table that gives a high-level comparison of each of the four epidemiologic studies that examined the use of primaquine and that met the committee's inclusion criteria is presented in Appendix C. Supplemental supporting evidence is then presented, including other identified studies of health outcomes in populations that used primaquine for prophylaxis but that did not meet the committee's inclusion criteria regarding timing of follow-up; case reports of persistent adverse events associated with primaquine use; and information on adverse events associated with primaquine use in specific groups, such as women and women who are pregnant. After presenting the primary and supplemental evidence in humans, supporting literature from experimental animal and in vitro studies is then summarized. The chapter ends with a synthesis of all of the evidence presented and the inferences and conclusions that the committee made from the available evidence.

FOOD AND DRUG ADMINISTRATION
PACKAGE INSERT FOR PRIMAQUINE

This section describes selected information in the FDA label or package insert for primaquine. It begins with information from the most recent label and package insert, detailing contraindications, warnings, and precautions as well as drug interactions known or presumed to occur with concurrent use. It then offers a chronologic overview of the changes made to the label or package insert between 2003 (the earliest label available from the Drugs@FDA Search site) and the most recent label update in November 2017.

Contraindications, Warnings, and Precautions

The adverse event of greatest concern with primaquine use is hemolysis and the resulting hemolytic anemia in glucose-6-phosphate dehydrogenase (G6PD)-deficient persons (Ashley et al., 2014; Schlagenhauf et al., 2019) (see Chapter 2). The discovery of the link between G6PD deficiency—the most common human genetic mutation—and hemolysis emerged in the 1950s during research with primaquine (Chu et al., 2018).The use of primaquine is contraindicated in persons with severe G6PD deficiency (FDA, 2017a). Because the danger of hemolysis in G6PD-deficient persons is well characterized and because primaquine use is contraindicated in those with severe G6PD deficiency, the committee did not examine the evidence of adverse events associated with G6PD deficiency in depth. Primaquine is also contraindicated in patients concurrently receiving other drugs that might cause hemolysis or depress the myeloid elements of the bone marrow. The drug is contraindicated in pregnant women and in acutely ill patients suffering from systemic disease manifested by a tendency to granulocytopenia (e.g., rheumatoid arthritis and lupus erythematosus). Primaquine is contraindicated in those who have recently taken or currently take quinacrine due to the possible potentiation of toxic effects by a structurally related compound.

Users are warned of the importance of being tested for G6PD deficiency and screened for a family history of favism prior to use, and they are advised that they should discontinue primaquine if signs of hemolytic anemia occur (FDA, 2017a). Standard screening tests for G6PD deficiency can be inexact; however, both qualitative and quantitative point-of-care tests are now being introduced (Baird, 2019; Chu et al., 2018; Pal et al., 2019). The label states that G6PD-deficiency tests have limitations and that even in the case of mild to moderate G6PD deficiency, users should consider the risks and benefits of primaquine use. In cases of mild to moderate G6PD deficiency and unknown G6PD status, baseline hematocrit and hemoglobin tests should be performed, hematologic monitoring should be performed at days 3 and 8 of drug use, and adequate medical support to manage hemolytic risk should be available. The label advises sexually active women with reproductive potential to take a pregnancy test before taking the drug and to use contraception during use.

A precaution is given against exceeding the dosage (15 mg daily for 14 days) because anemia, methemoglobinemia, and leukopenia have been observed following "large doses" of primaquine (FDA, 2017a). Routine blood examinations in G6PD-normal users are also advised. In addition, due to the potential for QT-interval prolongation with primaquine use, electrocardiogram (ECG) monitoring is advised in patients with cardiac disease, long QT syndrome, a history of ventricular arrhythmias, uncorrected hypokalemia or hypomagnesemia, or bradycardia (<50 bpm). Users are advised that no carcinogenicity and fertility studies have been conducted with primaquine.

Drug Interactions

Users are advised to use caution when taking primaquine concomitantly with other drugs that prolong the QT interval, and ECG monitoring is recommended for these recipients (FDA, 2017a).

Changes to the Primaquine Package Insert Over Time

Although the Drugs@FDA Search site lists documentation dating back to primaquine drug approval in 1952, downloadable documentation for primaquine labeling is unavailable for years prior to 2003. The most recent label available on the Drugs@FDA Search site is a June 2017 label (Sanofi-Aventis U.S. LLC) (FDA,

2017b). However, a more recent November 2017 label (Bayshore Pharmaceuticals) is available for download on the U.S. National Library of Medicine DAILYMED site (FDA, 2017a). This is the 2017 label referred to in other sections of the chapter. Although the Drugs@FDA Search site included a web page for documentation for the Bayshore Pharmaceuticals formulation of primaquine, the web page did not list or provide the most recent November 2017 label; the only documentation listed on the web page is dated 2014, and it is unavailable for download.

Only those label changes that refer to adverse reactions that occur in adults using primaquine as malaria prophylaxis are reviewed here. The changes to the primaquine label from 2003 to 2017 focused largely on strengthening language about safety concerns in patients with G6PD deficiencies (FDA, 2003, 2008, 2015, 2016, 2017a); as of 2016, routine blood tests are advised during use in G6PD-normal patients. Other updates include adding the potential for cardiac QT-interval prolongation (FDA, 2015) and strengthening warnings against use during pregnancy (FDA, 2017a). The 2017 updates advised caregivers to inform users that nonclinical studies had found evidence of adverse genetic and reproductive effects in pregnant animals and noted that no carcinogenicity or fertility studies had been conducted, but that animal studies suggested that primaquine might hold a human risk for genotoxicity (FDA, 2017a). Since 2003 the Adverse Reactions section has included gastrointestinal and hematologic categories (including methemoglobinemia) (FDA, 2003, 2017a), although the source (e.g., clinical trials, postmarketing surveillance) for the symptoms is not stated; a "nervous system" category (dizziness) was added in 2016 (FDA, 2016).

The 2003 primaquine label contained a boxed warning, sometimes informally referred to as a "black box" (FDA, 2003). This is FDA's most serious type of warning, and it appears on a prescription drug's label to call attention to serious or life-threatening risks (FDA, 2012). The boxed warning stated, "Physicians should completely familiarize themselves with the complete contents of this leaflet before prescribing primaquine phosphate" (FDA, 2003). The 2015 label did not include the warning box, and the box was absent in the 2016 and June 2017 labels (FDA, 2015, 2016, 2017b). The November 2017 label reintroduced the warning box (FDA, 2017a).

POLICIES AND INQUIRIES RELATED TO THE USE OF PRIMAQUINE BY MILITARY FORCES

The U.S. military uses primaquine prophylactically as PART in service members who serve in areas endemic for *P. vivax* or *P. ovale* (DoD, 2012, 2013a). Primaquine is used for PART more frequently in military service members than in civilian travelers (CDC, 2017b) because the drug is contraindicated in G6PD-deficient persons and requires G6PD-activity testing before use (Baird, 2019). If a service member wishes to use primaquine for the off-label purpose of primary prophylaxis, an individualized prescription by a licensed medical provider is required.[1] During the period 2007–2011, 982 prescriptions for primaquine for primary prophylaxis were written at military facilities (Kersgard and Hickey, 2013).

The FDA-approved regimen for radical cure is 15 mg primaquine daily for 14 days (FDA, 2017a). The original 1952 FDA indication was based on clinical trials showing that a 15 mg daily dose could be given without medical supervision to African Americans, who were known to be at higher risk of developing hemolytic anemia at a higher dose, who were returning from the Korean War (Hill et al., 2006). In 2003, based on available evidence, Centers for Disease Control and Prevention (CDC) guidelines recommended that 30 mg of primaquine daily for 14 days be used for PART for prophylaxis (CDC, 2017b). In the 2020 Yellow Book, CDC recommends that a 30 mg dose be used for 14 days by military service members since nonadherence and inadequate therapeutic dosing (15 mg daily) had led to outbreaks of relapsed *P. vivax* malaria in returning personnel (CDC, 2017b). Moreover, the efficacy of a primaquine dose can depend on the strain of malaria species, which vary by geography; certain strains of *P. vivax* (e.g., the Chesson strain), for example, can require higher doses to eliminate the parasite (Hill et al., 2006).

In response to a request to DoD for information about the use of primaquine as malaria prophylaxis in U.S. military service members, the committee received documents that provided information regarding policies for primaquine prophylactic use and G6PD-deficiency testing as well as about the policy and recommendations for primaquine dosages for PART.

Under the authority of force health protection (see Chapter 2) in deploying military service members, the U.S. military enforces only the FDA-approved labeled use of primaquine for PART (15 mg daily for 14 days).[2,3] The Armed Forces Epidemiology Board has recommended the use of a 30 mg dose for PART (DoD, 2003a), as has a 2019 Defense Health Agency issuance (DoD, 2019), but because the dosage remains off label, it is not enforced. A service member can be prescribed an off-label dose of primaquine (e.g., 30 mg per day) if a health care provider recommends it (based on patient interaction, including post-deployment interview from an endemic country where PART is indicated) and the service member provides consent.[4]

---

[1] Personal communication to the committee, COL Andrew Wiesen, M.D., M.P.H., Director, Preventive Medicine, Health Readiness Policy, and Oversight, Office of the Assistant Secretary of Defense (Health Affairs), DoD, September 27, 2019.

[2] Personal communication to the committee, COL Andrew Wiesen, M.D., M.P.H., Director, Preventive Medicine, Health Readiness Policy, and Oversight, Office of the Assistant Secretary of Defense (Health Affairs), DoD, August 22, 2019.

[3] Personal communication to the committee, COL Andrew Wiesen, M.D., M.P.H., Director, Preventive Medicine, Health Readiness Policy, and Oversight, Office of the Assistant Secretary of Defense (Health Affairs), DoD, September 27, 2019.

[4] Personal communication to the committee, COL Andrew Wiesen, M.D., M.P.H., Director, Preventive Medicine, Health Readiness Policy, and Oversight, Office of the Assistant Secretary of Defense (Health Affairs), DoD, August 22, 2019.

The earliest policy document provided to the committee by DoD that refers to prophylactic use of primaquine by U.S. military service members is a 2001 U.S. Central Command (CENTCOM) issuance stating that "terminal prophylaxis with primaquine is indicated for all countries in the CENTCOM area of responsibility where *P. vivax* and *P. ovale* malaria are transmitted and where prophylaxis is administered unless specifically stated by local component/Command Joint Task Force guidances" (DoD, 2001). CENTCOM covers 20 countries, including Afghanistan, Iran, Iraq, Pakistan, the countries of the Arabian Peninsula and northern Red Sea, and the five republics of Central Asia (DoD, n.d.b). Similarly, a 2006 DoD memorandum to the Third Army states that service members traveling "for even one day" to areas of operation (Afghanistan, Djibouti, Eritrea, Ethiopia, Kenya, Pakistan, Seychelles, Somalia, Sudan, and Uzbekistan) "must receive terminal malaria prophylaxis" (DoD, 2006). A 2013 DoD memorandum states that PART should be provided "when clinically and epidemiologically indicated" (DoD, 2013b).

DoD makes changes to malaria prophylaxis policy as circumstances change. For instance, a 2003 issuance stated that terminal malaria prophylaxis "is no longer required" in Iraq (DoD, 2003b), presumably because intelligence had determined that control over malaria had been regained. This was followed by a DoD policy memorandum stating, "U.S. personnel in Iraq will not take malaria chemoprophylactic medication" (DoD, 2003c).

The U.S. military sets policy that requires G6PD-deficiency testing to be performed in service members who use primaquine. A 2001 CENTCOM issuance states that testing for G6PD deficiency "will be performed prior to prescription of primaquine in accordance with service policy" (DoD, 2001). A 2006 DoD memorandum states that "Army policy now requires all soldiers to be tested for G6PD before deployment" (DoD, 2006). The memo notes further that "until G6PD screening of deploying CFLCC [Coalition Forces Land Component Command] personnel becomes reliable and routine," those taking primary prophylaxis will do so for 1 month after returning to a home station; during the first 2 weeks of that month, they will be tested for G6PD deficiency, and PART can be initiated. A 2012 issuance noted that PART will be prescribed only after proper screening and counseling to minimize the risk of adverse reactions (DoD, 2012).

In 2003 a DoD memorandum addressing antimalarials was issued by the Armed Forces Epidemiological Board (DoD, 2003a). The authors note first that DoD is subject to Section 1107 of Title 10, United States Code, regarding off-label use of force health protection medications. It then states that this would limit the prescription of CDC-recommended off-label prophylactic regimens (primary prophylaxis and PART) to the context of a doctor–patient relationship or an investigational new drug protocol, both of which could be problematic in a military setting. In its findings and recommendations, the board states that it finds the CDC consensus guidelines for malaria prevention "appropriate" for use by DoD and that as G6PD deficiency is a contraindication for primaquine, the documentation of a normal G6PD level should be available before the recommended 30 mg dosage is prescribed (DoD, 2003a).

DoD also provided the draft of a letter to the *Journal of the American Medical Association* (directed to authors of an article [Chen et al., 2007]) pointing out that the authors had not recommended an alternative PART regimen for those who are G6PD deficient, in whom a primaquine 30 mg daily dosage would be inappropriate (DoD, 2007). Though not explicit, this suggests that some service members may be using the 30 mg dosage. However, DoD issuances dating after 2003 refer only to the use of a 15 mg PART dosing regimen for force health protection (DoD, 2006, 2012).

The letter to the medical journal also referred to two cases of G6PD-deficient African American service members who, after being informed of the risks and benefits of taking primaquine, elected to take primaquine 15 mg daily and experienced no adverse reactions (DoD, 2007). An individual provider can make a clinical decision to prescribe primaquine to a G6PD-deficient military service member after weighing the risks and benefits (e.g., the risk of relapse may be high).[5] However, the service member must provide consent, and the appropriate safety monitoring must be in place.

PHARMACOKINETICS

Primaquine is rapidly absorbed in the gastrointestinal tract and is extensively distributed in tissues, with a mean volume of distribution of 3 L/kg (Baird and Hoffman, 2004). Absorption is linear with doses of 15 to 45 mg/kg (Hill et al., 2006). The elimination half-life of primaquine ranges from 4 to 9 hours (Baird and Hoffman, 2004; Myint et al., 2011). After a single 45 mg dose of primaquine, the peak serum concentration ranges from 0.13 to 0.18 µg/mL (Hill et al., 2006; Myint et al., 2011). After the administration of a 30 mg daily dose of primaquine (base) for 14 days, compared with men women had significantly higher peak serum concentrations (0.21 versus 0.12 µg/mL) and total drug exposure values (1.9 versus 0.92 µg h/mL) (Binh et al., 2009); thus, the authors suggest that women may be at an increased risk for toxicity compared with men. As reviewed by Hill et al. (2006), most authorities recommend that primaquine be given with food or after a meal to avoid gastrointestinal adverse events, especially abdominal cramps.

Primaquine is extensively metabolized (Baird, 2019; Thillainayagam and Ramaiah, 2016). Carboxyprimaquine is the major and inactive metabolite formed by the action of monoamine oxidase (Fasinu et al., 2014; Hill et al., 2006), and the level remains 10-fold higher than that of the parent drug (Hill et al., 2006). 5-Hydroxyprimaquine, formed by CYP450, primarily the CYP2D6 isoform

---

[5] Personal communication to the committee, COL Andrew Wiesen, M.D., M.P.H., Director, Preventive Medicine, Health Readiness Policy, and Oversight, Office of the Assistant Secretary of Defense (Health Affairs), DoD, September 27, 2019.

(Camarda et al., 2019; Pybus et al., 2013), is the redox-active metabolite associated with the antimalarial activity of primaquine.

ADVERSE EVENTS

This section begins with a summary of the known concurrent adverse events of primaquine, such as those that occur immediately or within a few hours or days of taking a dose of the drug. Epidemiologic studies of persistent or latent health effects in which information was available at least 28 days post-primaquine-cessation are then summarized by population category (military or veterans, travelers, and research volunteers), with an emphasis on reported results of persistent or latent events associated with use of primaquine (even if results on other antimalarial-drug comparison groups were presented).

Concurrent Adverse Events

A Cochrane review of mass drug administration for malaria prophylaxis examined 32 studies, but this review was not considered by the committee because only four studies included primaquine, there was no active adverse event surveillance in three of the four studies, and no meta-analysis was performed (Poirot et al., 2013). The committee identified one systematic review of primaquine used prophylactically that examined safety (Kolifarhood et al., 2017); this review is discussed below, along with findings from several non-systematic review papers.

Kolifarhood et al. (2017) assessed primaquine as compared with other malaria prophylactic drugs or placebo in healthy travelers. The primary outcome was confirmed parasitemia. The secondary outcome was adverse events, including both clinical and laboratory-measured events. Clinical events were categorized as neuropsychiatric and gastrointestinal complaints using the Uppsala Monitoring Center organ system classification of adverse drug reactions. Seven studies included a total of 1,710 participants from 7 to 65 years of age who had been pre-screened for G6PD deficiency. The review included five randomized controlled trials, one nonrandomized trial, and one uncontrolled before-and-after (used baseline measures as comparison) study. Only one study (Schwartz and Regev-Yochay, 1999) included in this review was also included in the final set of epidemiologic studies with long-term follow-up that the committee considered fully.

The authors computed incidence rate ratios for individual studies; they did not pool the study data for the safety outcomes (Kolifarhood et al., 2017). For the four trials that included a placebo arm, the authors found no statistically significant difference in relative risk between primaquine and placebo for gastrointestinal adverse events or for neuropsychiatric adverse events (reported in three of the four trials). Comparisons of primaquine with mefloquine, doxycycline, proguanil, and atovaquone/proguanil found no statistically significant difference in incidence rates for gastrointestinal or neuropsychiatric adverse events. In one assessed study (Baird et al., 1995), more gastrointestinal and neuropsychiatric adverse events were reported for chloroquine than for primaquine (RR = 4.13, 95%CI 1.83–9.31 and RR = 7.89, 95%CI 3.62–17.2, respectively). In another assessed study (Nasveld et al., 2002), more gastrointestinal adverse events were reported for tafenoquine than for primaquine (RR = 2.7, 95%CI 1.34–5.42).

Non-systematic reviews show that the most serious safety concern with the use of primaquine is the potential for hemolysis in persons with G6PD deficiency (Ashley et al., 2014; Hill et al., 2006; Schlagenhauf et al., 2019), an association that was recognized during its early use (Kitchen et al., 2006) and specifically defined soon after (Dern et al., 1954). Standard guidelines call for testing for G6PD deficiency before using primaquine (CDC, 2017a; DoD, 2012; FDA, 2017a). Because of primaquine's short half-life (4–9 hours) (Baird and Hoffman, 2004; Myint et al., 2011), halting the drug can quickly decrease the drug-induced hemolysis—a fact that highlights the benefit of monitoring primaquine recipients and having medical support available during use (Rishikesh et al., 2016). If severe hemolytic anemia is not treated or controlled, it can lead to serious complications, including arrhythmias, cardiomyopathy, heart failure, and death (Baird, 2019; NIH, n.d.). Released hemoglobin can also cause damage to the kidney (Ashley et al., 2014).

A common occurrence in both G6PD-normal and G6PD-deficient recipients is a mild, reversible methemoglobinemia, a condition that interferes with the ability of the blood to carry oxygen (Baird, 2019; Hill et al., 2006; Rishikesh and Saravu, 2016). Persons who are deficient in the enzyme nicotinamide adenine dinucleotide (NADH) methemoglobin reductase are extremely sensitive to primaquine (Hill et al., 2006), and if they use primaquine they should be monitored for tolerance (FDA, 2017a). High levels of methemoglobin (>15%) in red blood cells can lead to complications, including abnormal cardiac rhythms, altered mental status, delirium, seizures, coma, and profound acidosis; if the levels exceed 70%, death can occur (Denshaw-Burke et al., 2018). Methemoglobinemia in otherwise healthy persons is generally asymptomatic; symptoms such as cyanosis, dizziness, or dyspnea should prompt testing for methemoglobin levels (Hill et al., 2006, Schlagenhauf et al., 2019).

The most common adverse event in primaquine users is minor gastrointestinal upset if the drug is taken on an empty stomach (Baird, 2019; Hill et al., 2006; Schlagenhauf et al., 2019). The risk of adverse gastrointestinal events increases with increasing doses of primaquine (Hill et al., 2006), and epidemiologic studies show these may include abdominal cramps, nausea, epigastric pain, vomiting, and diarrhea (Baird et al., 2001; Ebringer et al., 2011; Nasveld et al., 2002; Soto et al., 1998). Other adverse events include headache, anorexia, skin rash, and itching (NIH, 2017).

There is little mention in the literature of primaquine in association with neuropsychiatric events. Three reviews stated that neuropsychiatric symptoms have been reported rarely with primaquine use (Ashley et al., 2014; Castelli et al., 2010; Hill et al., 2006). Two reviews (Castelli et al., 2010; Hill et al., 2006) alluded to a single case report of depression and psychosis with primaquine use. The case report described a man who experienced depression, confusion, and anorexia after being treated for malaria (Schlossberg, 1980). There is no mention of neuropsychiatric events in the FDA package insert (FDA, 2017a).

Post-Cessation Adverse Events

A total of 1,337 abstracts or titles were identified by the committee for inclusion for primaquine. After screening, 558 abstracts and titles remained, and the full text for each was retrieved and reviewed to determine whether it met the committee's inclusion criteria, as defined in Chapter 3. The committee reviewed each article and identified 25 primary epidemiologic studies that presented information indicating that the study population was followed for at least 28 days. Upon further examination, the committee found that 21 of the 25 articles did not include a comparator, did not provide information on adverse events that occurred ≥28 days after cessation of primaquine, or presented data that did not distinguish between adverse events that occurred during the use of primaquine, <28 days post-cessation of primaquine, or ≥28 days post-cessation of primaquine. These are briefly discussed later in the chapter under the heading Other Identified Studies of Primaquine Prophylaxis in Human Populations. There were four remaining epidemiologic studies that included some mention of adverse events that occurred ≥28 days post-cessation of primaquine (Nasveld et al., 2010; Rueangweerayut et al., 2017; Schneiderman et al., 2018; Schwartz and Regev-Yochay, 1999), and these are summarized below. A table that gives a high-level comparison (study design, population, exposure groups, and outcomes examined by body system) of each of these four epidemiologic studies is presented in Appendix C.

Primaquine is used as PART (within label) and as primary prophylaxis (off label). The committee sought to review any studies that could inform its understanding of the drug's safety when used as prophylaxis; thus, while the committee examined studies using PART, it also considered studies that investigated prophylactic regimens that are off label. Two studies in the final data set used primaquine regimens that are not within current FDA labeling. Nasveld et al. (2010) used primaquine as PART, but the dosage (30 mg daily for 2 weeks) was off label. Schwartz and Regev-Yochay (1999) used primaquine as primary prophylaxis.

Military and Veterans

Schneiderman et al. (2018) conducted a retrospective observational analysis of self-reported health outcomes associated with the use of antimalarial drugs in a cohort of U.S. veterans who had responded to the 2009–2011 National Health Study for a New Generation of U.S. Veterans (referred to as the "NewGen Study"). The NewGen Study is a population-based survey that sampled 30,000 veterans who had been deployed to Iraq or Afghanistan between 2001 and 2008 and 30,000 nondeployed veterans who had served during the same time period, and it included a 20% oversampling of women. The survey was conducted using mail, telephone, and web-based collection and yielded a response rate of only 34.3%. For this particular analysis, 19,487 participants were included who had self-reported their history of antimalarial medication use, and the use was grouped for analysis by drug (mefloquine, chloroquine, doxycycline, primaquine, mefloquine in combination with other drugs, other antimalarials, and not specified) or no antimalarial use. Health outcomes were self-reported using standardized instruments: the Medical Outcomes Study 12-item Short Form (SF-12) for general health status, PTSD Checklist–Civilian version, and the Patient Health Questionnaire. These instruments yielded scores that were dichotomized for analysis on composite physical health, composite mental health (above or below the U.S. mean), posttraumatic stress disorder (PTSD) (above or below screening cutoff), thoughts of death or self-harm, other anxiety disorders, and major depression. Potential confounders included in the multivariable analysis were branch of service, sex, age, education, race/ethnicity, household income, employment status, marital status, and self-reported exposure to combat. Responses were weighted to account for survey non-response. Most veterans reported no antimalarial drug exposures (61.4%, n = 11,100), and these served as the referent group. When stratified by deployment status, among the deployed (n = 12,456), of those who reported the use of an antimalarial drug (n = 6,650) only 98 (weighted 1.4%) veterans reported using primaquine alone, and 425 (weighted 6.0%) reported using mefloquine plus another antimalarial, which may have included primaquine. Among the nondeployed (n = 7,031), 1,737 reported using an antimalarial drug, and of this group only 35 (weighted 1.6%) used primaquine alone, and 52 (weighted 2.8%) used mefloquine plus another antimalarial, which may have included primaquine. Because it is not clear how many people in the mefloquine-plus group may have also used primaquine, the results of that group are not included in the committee's assessment.

When comparing outcomes among the deployed group, participants using primaquine alone reported the lowest prevalence of adverse mental and physical health outcomes among the antimalarial regimens: SF-12 mental health component scores below the U.S. mean (41.0%), SF-12 physical health component scores below the U.S. mean (28.7%), positive screens for PTSD (6.9%), thoughts of death or self-harm (6.3%), other anxiety disorders (1.4%), and major depression (3.3%). Descriptive statistics indicated that, compared with nondeployed primaquine-only users, the deployed primaquine users reported increased frequencies of positive PTSD screens (6.9% versus 3.0%); similar reported frequencies of SF-12 mental health scores below the U.S. mean (41.0% versus 40.7%), thoughts of death or self harm (6.3% versus 5.9%), and symptoms of major depression (3.3% versus 3.2%); and lower frequencies of SF-12 physical health scores below the U.S. mean (28.7% versus 42.8%) and other anxiety disorders (1.4% versus 11.0%). However, no statistical measures were presented. In the adjusted logistic regression models with all covariates considered (including demographics, deployment, and combat exposure), the use of primaquine alone was not associated with four of the health outcomes as compared with nonuse of antimalarial drugs: composite mental health score (OR = 0.74, 95%CI 0.46–1.18), PTSD (OR = 0.48, 95%CI 0.21–1.10), thoughts of death or self-harm (OR = 0.78, 95%CI 0.31–1.98), and major depression (OR = 0.46, 95%CI 0.17–1.21). The composite physical health score (OR = 0.56, 95% CI 0.35–0.87) was statistically significantly lower—an indication of better physical health—for primaquine users compared with non-users of antimalarial drugs after including demographics, deployment, and combat exposure in the model. The presence of other anxiety disorders (OR = 0.19, 95% CI 0.06–0.67) was statistically significantly lower for primaquine users than for nonusers of antimalarial drugs after including demographics, deployment, and combat exposure in the model. In a stratified analysis, primaquine was associated with a decreased risk of anxiety in the deployed (OR = 0.14, 95%CI 0.03–0.60), but not in the nondeployed (OR = 1.45, 95%CI 0.35–6.08).

Although the study was large, the number of primaquine-only users was small, yielding imprecise effect estimates for this exposure. The outcomes were based on standardized instruments (although not face-to-face diagnostic interviews), important covariates of deployment and combat exposure were considered in addition to demographics and other military characteristics, and the data were appropriately analyzed. The small number of primaquine-only users in this sample (weighted 1.4% of deployed and weighted 1.6% of nondeployed antimalarial users), coupled with the very low odds ratios for physical health and anxiety, raises concerns about the comparability of this group to nonusers of antimalarials and about the validity of associated estimates. As primaquine is commonly used prophylactically by the U.S. military in combination with other drugs (at the end of malaria exposure), it is unknown whether primaquine was actually used alone. It is noteworthy that adjusting for combat exposure consistently reduced the measures of association, potentially indicating that a strong confounding can exist due to combat exposure. Although the time period of drug use and the timing of health outcomes were not directly addressed, given that the populations were all veterans who had served between 2001 and 2008 and that the survey was not administered until 2009–2011, it is reasonable to assume that antimalarial drug use had ceased some time before. Nonetheless, the study could not address explicitly the health experiences during use and in specific time intervals following the cessation of use. There are a number of methodologic concerns that limit the strength of this study's findings. The very small sample size of the primaquine drug category raises questions about generalizability and validity. The low response rate of 34% raises concerns about non-response bias, but responses were weighted to account for this. Selective participation by both antimalarial drug use history and health status would be required to introduce bias. The accuracy of self-reported antimalarial drug use in this population is unknown. Although self-reported information has some advantages over studies based on prescriptions because self-report implies that the individual recalls using the drug, the reported drug and the information on adherence to that drug were not validated. Self-reported health experience is subject to the usual disadvantages of recall bias and to the bias of reporting subjective experience without independent expert assessment; however, by using standardized assessment tools, these biases may have been circumvented to some extent.

Nasveld et al. (2010) conducted a randomized double-blind controlled study to compare the safety and tolerability of mefloquine for 26 weeks (primary prophylaxis) followed by primaquine (30 mg per day) for 2 weeks (PART) (n = 162) with the safety and tolerability of tafenoquine for 26 weeks followed by placebo for 2 weeks (n = 492) in male and female Australian soldiers aged 18–55 years. Since tafenoquine is an 8-aminoquinoline with antihypnozoite action (like primaquine), the tafenoquine arm did not require PART and used placebo to preserve study blinding. The primaquine dose was off label; the FDA-approved dose is 15 mg per day (FDA, 2017a). The soldiers were deployed on United Nations peacekeeping duties to East Timor. They were predominantly young, Caucasian men and were judged to be healthy by a medical history and physical examination with normal hematological and biochemical values and also judged to be G6PD normal. Participants with a history of psychiatric disorders or seizures were excluded, as were women who were pregnant, lactating, or unwilling or unable to comply with contraception. A subset of 98 participants (21 mefloquine/primaquine group, 77 tafenoquine/placebo group) underwent extra safety assessments to investigate drug-induced phospholipidosis and methemoglobinemia as well as ophthalmic and cardiac safety. In addition to assessments done while taking the medication, the safety group had safety and tolerability assessment, including of hematologic and blood chemistry parameters, at week 2 and at week 12 during the follow-up phase after the last dose of primaquine or placebo. There was an additional telephone follow-up at weeks 18 and 24 post-drug-cessation. Adverse-event monitoring was supplemented by a review of the subjects' medical records. In the safety group, mean methemoglobin levels increased by 0.1% in the mefloquine primary-prophylaxis group and by 1.8% in the tafenoquine primary-prophylaxis group, but these increases resolved by week 12 of follow-up (after the primaquine/placebo stage of the study). A small increase in QT interval was seen in the mefloquine followed by primaquine recipients, and a small reduction in mean QT interval was seen in the tafenoquine recipients; whether the change in interval resolved with time is not stated, but none of these findings were considered to be clinically significant by the authors. Corneal deposits were not observed in any mefloquine primary-prophylaxis recipients in the safety group, so ophthalmic assessment was not performed in these participants after they took the primaquine. The authors stated that during the relapse follow-up phase, 53 (33.9%) of the mefloquine/primaquine subjects and 203 (41.3%) of the tafenoquine/placebo subjects reported adverse events, but no notable difference between the groups in the incidence or nature of events was observed. The adverse events are not named, nor is their timing specified. The authors do state that at follow-up, 6–8% of the participants in both arms had creatinine values that were 25% above the baseline, but few had values outside the normal range, and none were considered clinically significant.

Although the overall study design was rigorous, with randomization of the medications, a temporal ordering of the exposures and outcomes, systematic data collection, high adherence to assigned medications, little attrition from the study (94% of subjects in both arms completed the trial), a placebo control for the anti-hypnozoite (primaquine) stage of the study, and a study population that was highly relevant for the committee's task, still the study is limited in the information it provides with respect to persistent or latent adverse events for primaquine because of the limited information it provided about adverse events. Moreover, because the drug regimen involved the sequential use of mefloquine and primaquine, it is difficult to identify what, if any, role an individual drug played in the occurrence of an adverse event. Exposure assessment was fairly strong because of the consistent measurement across the arms and the use of medication logs to measure adherence prospectively. Most adverse events were not assessed in a systematic way, however, limiting the quality of these measures, and the timing of the adverse events was not clearly specified beyond the prophylaxis-use phase, and therefore it was not possible to ascertain how long the adverse events persisted. While the statistical power was sufficient for the primary goal of the study, which was to assess the antimalarial efficacy of the drugs, the sample size was insufficient for assessing the occurrence of most adverse events. In the small safety subgroup, there were no persistent adverse methemoglobin or cardiac outcomes in either group at 12 weeks. Given that there were no adverse ophthalmic outcomes during mefloquine use in the safety subgroup, these outcomes were not assessed during or following the 2 weeks of primaquine. There were no other evaluations of specific adverse outcomes.

Travelers

Schwartz and Regev-Yochay (1999) performed a prospective observational study, and followed 158 male and female Israeli travelers aged 22–65 years who took part in rafting trips on the Omo River, Ethiopia, and who had visited a travel clinic to obtain malaria prophylaxis. The travelers were prescribed mefloquine, primaquine (15 mg daily for those ≤70 kg; 30 mg daily for those >70 kg), doxycycline, or hydroxychloroquine by travel group. The primary aim of the study was to assess incident malaria and to compare the effectiveness of these four antimalarial drugs against both *P. falciparum* and *P. vivax*. The primaquine recipients (n = 106) received G6PD-deficiency testing beforehand. The travelers were followed from the time of their return to Israel for an average of 16.6 months (range 8–37 months) for incident malaria. A survey (completed by 50 of the 106 primaquine users) was used to gather information on the travelers' adherence to the prophylactic regimens and on the adverse events they experienced. Using primaquine for primary prophylaxis and at a dose >15 mg per day is not FDA approved. The authors reported that "no severe side effects" were reported in any of the travelers. One participant discontinued primaquine because of nausea and vomiting soon after beginning the drug. The strengths of this study include that it used standard recommended prophylactic drugs as comparators and that it had a long follow-up (an average of 16.6 months after return from a malaria-endemic country). It was limited by its small sample size, its nonrandomized design, and the lack of details it provided on adverse events. Although a long-term follow-up was completed to assess effectiveness, it is unclear whether specific persistent or latent adverse events would have been reported during this period. As a result, this study provides limited information that can be used for inference.

Research Volunteers

Rueangweerayut et al. (2017) used a prospective observational study design to examine the tolerability of primaquine (15 mg for 14 days) compared with tafenoquine (100, 200, or 300 mg, single dose) in healthy Thai females who were heterozygous for Mahidol variant G6PD deficiency (primaquine, n = 5; tafenoquine, n = 19) or G6PD normal (primaquine, n = 6; tafenoquine, n = 18). The primary outcome was a maximum absolute decrease in hemoglobin or hematocrit from pretreatment up to day 14 after treatment. Additional outpatient follow-up visits were at days 21, 28, and 56. In the primaquine group the G6PD-deficient participants completed 6 (2 recipients), 9, 10, and 14 days of treatment; all participants in the G6PD-normal group received 14 days of treatment. Safety assessments included adverse event monitoring, vital signs, 12-lead ECGs, clinical biochemistry, hematology (including methemoglobin determined by oximetry), and urinalysis. In the G6PD-deficient arms, dose-limiting adverse effects were reported to occur in 3 of 5 of the primaquine arm, and 3 of 3 of the highest-dose (300 mg) tafenoquine arm; of these, two recipients of each drug experienced both a decrease ≥2.5 g/dL in hemoglobin and a decrease ≥7.5% in hematocrit versus pretreatment. Among the primaquine recipients, 4 of 6 of the G6PD-normal group showed sustained elevations in methemoglobin (maximum values 5.5–13.1%); values did not exceed 3.9% in the G6PD-deficient group. No tafenoquine recipient experienced methemoglobin levels >5.0%. The authors reported that there were no accompanying clinical symptoms associated with hemolysis or increased methemoglobin levels, no other clinically important changes in laboratory measures, and no notable ECG changes. All values appeared to be in the normal range by day 28 (14 days post-drug-cessation). The study was limited by its small sample size and by the narrow range of measures it examined. In addition, although the final follow-up visit at day 56 met the inclusion criteria of ≥28 days following drug cessation, there was no information reported from that visit.

OTHER IDENTIFIED STUDIES OF PRIMAQUINE PROPHYLAXIS IN HUMAN POPULATIONS

Five additional studies of primaquine use in military service members were reviewed by the committee, including studies from Canada (Paul et al., 2003),

Australia (Ebringer et al., 2011; Nasveld et al., 2002), and Colombia (Soto et al., 1998, 1999). However, because they did not follow the military cohorts for at least 28 days after primaquine cessation or did not report on adverse events that occurred post-cessation, these studies were excluded. In addition, an early study in U.S. troops (Vivona et al., 1961) was excluded because the regimen used the "C-P pill," a combination of chloroquine and primaquine that has not been used for several decades and thus was not reviewed by the committee.

Three studies of mass drug administration were reviewed but were excluded because the drug combination (primaquine and an artemisinin) is not one that is used by the population of interest (military service members or veterans) (Landier et al., 2018; Song et al., 2010) or for the lack of a comparator (Tseroni et al., 2015). Eleven remaining studies in various populations were reviewed but were excluded because they did not include a comparator, did not follow the participants after primaquine cessation, did not report on adverse events that occurred post-cessation, or did not distinguish events occurring post-cessation from those occurring while taking the drug (Baird et al., 1995, 2001; Brito-Sousa et al., 2019; Chen et al., 2018; Chinn and Redmond, 1954; Fryauff et al., 1995, 1996; Grimmond and Cameron, 1984; Hanboonkunupakarn et al., 2014; Manning et al., 2018; Sharafeldin et al., 2010; Winkler, 1970).

Case Reports

The committee reviewed six published case reports involving primaquine used prophylactically. Most focused on hemolysis in persons with G6PD deficiency, and since this safety concern is well characterized and primaquine is contraindicated in people with severe G6PD deficiency, these were not reviewed in depth. Only one case report met the criterion of following the person for ≥28 days after primaquine cessation (Kotwal et al., 2009). The patient had taken doxycycline 100 mg daily for malaria prophylaxis before, during, and after a 3-month deployment to Afghanistan, and he took primaquine 15 mg daily concomitantly during the last 14 days of his doxycycline regimen. A month after completing the medications, the patient developed non-ischemic central retinal vein occlusion, and he continued to have mild disk and macular edema with mild vascular defects and hemorrhages after 2 years of treatment for the eye disorder. Subsequent to the development of ocular symptoms, the patient was found to have G6PD deficiency, and the authors suggest hemolysis may have contributed to diffuse microvascular thrombosis that included the eye. However, whether the central retinal vein occlusion was a result of the primaquine use remains uncertain.

Selected Subpopulations

There is little information in the literature on the use of primaquine used prophylactically in selected risk groups.

Sex Differences

A difference between women and men in the reported incidence of adverse events has been observed. In an open-label randomized study in Australian Defence Force members, Nasveld et al. (2002) compared primaquine (22.5 mg daily for 14 days) with tafenoquine (400 mg daily for 3 days) for post-deployment PART. The primaquine dose was not within FDA labeling nor was the tafenoquine dose. The volunteers also took routine doxycycline prophylaxis (100 mg daily) before and concomitantly with the PART regimens. In the doxycycline/primaquine group (women, n = 23; men, n = 193), 8 women (35%) reported nausea, compared with 22 men (12%), and 2 women (9%) reported lethargy, compared with 8 men (4%).

Pregnancy

Whether primaquine can be used safely during pregnancy has not been established. Primaquine is contraindicated in pregnancy (FDA, 2017a). Transplacental transfer of primaquine to a G6PD-deficient fetus potentially could result in life-threatening hemolytic anemia in utero. Even if a pregnant woman is G6PD normal, the fetus may not be. CDC guidelines state that primaquine cannot be used by pregnant women (CDC, 2017a). According to the package insert, animal data show reproduction-related toxicity. Nonclinical data from studies conducted in pregnant animals treated with primaquine show evidence of teratogenicity as well as injury to embryos and developing fetuses (FDA, 2017a).

BIOLOGIC PLAUSIBILITY

There are relatively few reports assessing primaquine effects on neuronal function. Very high (toxic) doses of primaquine can induce cell loss in brain regions controlling neuroendocrine (paraventricular and supraoptic nuclei) and cardiovascular function (dorsal motor nucleus of the vagus) in non-human primates, according to an early study (Schmidt and Schmidt, 1951). The authors of that study stated that "there is little likelihood that significant neuronal injury would result from clinical use of ... primaquine ... in doses such as are applied in malaria therapy."

Hypotension, cardiac contractility, and arrhythmias can be observed upon administration of toxic doses of primaquine in rats and dogs (Bass et al., 1972; Orta-Salazar et al., 2002). Cardiac effects can be linked to the blockade of sodium channels in cardiomyocytes, which results in decreased contractility (Orta-Salazar et al., 2002). Primaquine also blocks the delayed rectifier hERG potassium channels in HEK293 cells, resulting in effects that may be linked to the prolonged QT intervals or arrhythmias that occur in some individuals after taking antimalarials (Kim et al., 2010).

Like other members of the 8-aminoquinoline drug class, primaquine can cause hemolytic anemia in individuals with G6PD deficiency (Hill et al., 2006).

Moreover, high-dose treatment can cause methemoglobinemia in dogs, rats, and primates (Lee et al., 1981). Primaquine is rapidly degraded in vivo (Fasinu et al., 2019), and there is fairly good evidence that its metabolites (e.g., PQ-5,6-orthoquinone, 5-hydroxyprimaquine) can cause the generation of reactive oxygen species (in particular, hydrogen peroxide) in erythrocytes at physiologic concentrations (Bowman, 2005; Fasinu et al., 2019; Vázquez-Vivar and Augusto, 1992, 1994).

Toxic doses of primaquine increase the circulating markers of liver damage in rabbits (El-Denshary, 1969) and reduce CYP450 levels in rats (Murray and Farrell, 1986). Primaquine at more physiologic concentrations bind to antioxidant species (GSH, *N*-acetyl cysteine) in liver microsomes (Garg et al., 2011). Coupled with primaquine-induced increases in reactive oxygen species in erythrocytes, the latter studies are consistent with primaquine causing a potentiation of oxidative stress, which can impair cellular function and viability.

SYNTHESIS AND CONCLUSIONS

Despite the fact that primaquine was first approved by FDA in 1952 for malaria prophylaxis, only four epidemiologic studies were identified that included some mention of adverse events or data collection that occurred ≥28 days post-cessation of primaquine that provided directly relevant information for assessing persistent or latent adverse events (Nasveld et al., 2010; Rueangweerayut et al., 2017; Schneiderman et al., 2018; Schwartz and Regev-Yochay, 1999). The studies are heterogeneous in the populations that were used (active military or veterans, travelers, and research volunteers); the modes of data collection on drug exposure, health outcomes, and covariates (administrative records, researcher collected, self-report); the type of prophylactic regimen and dosages used; and, particularly, the nature of the health outcomes that were considered. Furthermore, the relevant studies were notably inconsistent in the reporting of results, covering different time periods in relation to the cessation of the drug exposure and, in some cases, failing to provide information specifically for the time period of interest. Given the inherently imperfect information generated by any one study, it would be desirable to have similar studies to assess the consistency of the findings, but the diversity of the methods makes it very difficult to combine information across studies with confidence.

The studies varied in methodologic quality and in the amount of usable information, so that their findings are not weighted equally in drawing conclusions. As described in Chapter 3, the committee considered several methodologic issues in assessing each study's contribution to the evidence base on persistent or latent health effects, including the overall study design, the quality of the exposure and health outcome assessment, the ability to address confounding and other potential biases, sample size, and the extent to which the post-cessation health experience was effectively isolated. Two studies were considered to contribute most to the evidence base (Schneiderman et al., 2018, and Nasveld et al., 2010), and to avoid repetition for multiple outcome categories, a short summary of each is presented first. The evidence summaries for outcome categories refer back to these short assessment summaries.

For each health outcome category, the supporting information from FDA, known concurrent adverse events, case studies, information on selected subpopulations, and experimental animal and in vitro studies is first summarized before the evidence from the post-cessation epidemiologic studies is described. While the charge to the committee was to address persistent and latent adverse events, the occurrence of concurrent adverse events enhances the likelihood that problems may persist beyond the period after cessation of drug use. The synthesis of evidence is followed by a conclusion about the strength of evidence regarding an association between the use of primaquine and persistent or latent adverse events and whether the available evidence would support additional research into those outcomes. The outcomes are presented in the following order: neurologic disorders, psychiatric disorders, gastrointestinal disorders, eye disorders, cardiovascular disorders, and other outcomes, including dermatologic and biochemical parameters.

Epidemiologic Studies Presenting Contributory Evidence

Schneiderman et al. (2018) conducted an analysis of self-reported health outcomes associated with the use of antimalarials in a population-based cohort of deployed and nondeployed U.S. veterans, using information collected as part of the NewGen Study. Exposure and outcomes were systematically obtained, and psychiatric outcomes were measured by standardized assessment instruments. The overall sample was large, and the researchers used a reasonably thorough set of covariates in models estimating the drug–outcome associations. Although the time period of drug use and the timing of health outcomes were not directly addressed, given that the population was all veterans who had served between 2001 and 2008 and that the survey was not administered until 2009–2011, it is reasonable to assume that the antimalarial drug use had ceased some time before the study. The methodology and the low response rate (34% overall, of whom when weighted, 1.4% of deployed and 1.6% of nondeployed individuals used primaquine) may have led to the introduction of nonresponse, recall, or selection biases; however, the committee believes that the investigators used appropriate data analysis techniques to mitigate the effects of any biases that were present. Of the four included epidemiologic studies examining the persistent health effects of the use of primaquine for malaria prophylaxis, the committee weighted this study most heavily when generating its conclusions.

Nasveld et al. (2010) conducted a randomized double-blind controlled study to compare the safety and tolerability of mefloquine followed by primaquine for

2 weeks (PART) with the safety and tolerability of tafenoquine for 26 weeks followed by placebo for 2 weeks in G6PD-normal Australian soldiers. A subset underwent extra safety assessments to investigate drug-induced phospholipidosis and methemoglobinemia as well as ophthalmic and cardiac safety. Drug compliance was observed and recorded for each subject using medication logs. In addition to the adverse-event assessments carried out while the soldiers were taking the drugs, there were additional assessments at 2 and 12 weeks following the completion of the regimen and telephone follow-ups at weeks 18 and 24. However, specific adverse events during the post-regimen phase were not detailed, except for the small safety subset that included only 21 primaquine users, all of whom had also taken mefloquine.

Neurologic Disorders

An examination of the associations of primaquine use with neurologic disorders does not indicate an increased risk for neurologic adverse events concurrent with primaquine use. Although dizziness was added to the FDA package insert in 2016 (FDA, 2016), there was no evidence from other sources of an association between primaquine and dizziness or any other concurrent, persistent, or latent neurologic outcome. A systematic review (Kolifarhood et al., 2017) found no significant differences in the incidence rate of concurrent neuropsychiatric adverse events between primaquine and placebo or between primaquine and other antimalarials (mefloquine, doxycycline, or atovaquone/proguanil); fewer neuropsychiatric adverse events were reported with primaquine than with chloroquine in one study and than with tafenoquine in another. Three nonsystematic reviews found that neuropsychiatric symptoms have been reported rarely with primaquine use (Ashley et al., 2014; Castelli et al., 2010; Hill et al., 2006); however, the authors did not define the symptoms or outcomes that this neuropsychiatric category would encompass. Nasveld et al. (2002) reported more lethargy in women than in men who were administered a combination of doxycycline and primaquine; however, the relationship of these symptoms to primaquine could not be determined because the two drugs were used together. Although animal studies indicate that very high doses of primaquine can induce cell loss in the brain, it is believed that such toxicity would not occur at the doses used for prophylaxis (Schmidt and Schmidt, 1951).

None of the four epidemiologic studies that met the inclusion criteria specifically examined neurologic outcomes following the cessation of primaquine.

Based on the available evidence, the committee concludes that there is insufficient or inadequate evidence of an association between the use of primaquine for malaria prophylaxis and persistent or latent neurologic events. Current evidence does not suggest further study of such an association is warranted, given the lack of evidence regarding biologic plausibility, adverse events associated with concurrent use, or findings from the existing epidemiologic studies.

Psychiatric Disorders

An examination of the associations of primaquine use with psychiatric disorders does not indicate an increased risk for psychiatric adverse events with concurrent primaquine use. There is no mention of adverse psychiatric events in the primaquine package insert (FDA, 2017a), and in a systematic review (Kolifarhood et al., 2017) no significant difference in the incidence rate of concurrent neuropsychiatric adverse events was observed between primaquine and placebo or between primaquine and other antimalarials (mefloquine, doxycycline, or atovaquone/proguanil); fewer neuropsychiatric adverse events were reported with primaquine than with chloroquine in one study and than with tafenoquine in another. Three nonsystematic reviews noted that neuropsychiatric symptoms have been reported rarely with primaquine use (Ashley et al., 2014; Castelli et al., 2010; Hill et al., 2006); however, the authors did not define the symptoms or outcomes that the neuropsychiatric category would encompass. Although animal studies indicate that very high doses of primaquine can induce cell loss in the brain, it is believed that such toxicity would not occur at the doses used for prophylaxis (Schmidt and Schmidt, 1951).

Schneiderman et al. (2018) examined mental health outcomes, including general mental health, PTSD, thoughts of death or self-harm, other anxiety, and major depression, among more than 19,400 veterans. However, only 133 of study participants used primaquine. After controlling for demographics, deployment status, and combat exposure, the use of primaquine alone was not associated with a composite mental health score, PTSD, thoughts of death or self-harm, or major depression when compared with nonusers of antimalarial drugs; however, other anxiety disorders were statistically significantly lower for primaquine users compared with nonusers of antimalarials drugs. In a subanalysis stratified by deployment status, primaquine was associated with a statistically significantly decreased risk of anxiety in the deployed but no difference was observed in the nondeployed.

Based on the available evidence, the committee concludes that there is insufficient or inadequate evidence of an association between the use of primaquine for malaria prophylaxis and persistent or latent psychiatric events. Current evidence does not suggest further study of such an association is warranted, given the lack of evidence regarding biologic plausibility, adverse events associated with concurrent use, or findings from the existing epidemiologic studies.

Gastrointestinal Disorders

The most common concurrent adverse event in primaquine users is minor gastrointestinal upset if the drug is taken on an empty stomach (Baird, 2019; Hill et al., 2006; Schlagenhauf et al., 2019). The risk of adverse gastrointestinal events increases with increasing doses of primaquine (Hill et al., 2006), and epidemiologic studies show that these events may include abdominal cramps, nausea, epigastric pain, vomiting, and diarrhea (Baird et al., 2001; Ebringer et al., 2011; Nasveld et al., 2002; Soto et al., 1998). The most recent package insert lists gastrointestinal disorders in the general adverse reactions section but not in the warnings or precautions sections. In a systematic review (Kolifarhood et al., 2017), no difference in the incidence rate of concurrent adverse gastrointestinal events was observed between primaquine and placebo or between primaquine and other antimalarials (mefloquine, doxycycline, or atovaquone/proguanil); in one study, fewer gastrointestinal adverse events were reported with primaquine than with chloroquine, and in another study, fewer gastrointestinal adverse events were reported with primaquine than with tafenoquine. Nasveld et al. (2002) reported more nausea in women than in men who were administered a combination of doxycycline and primaquine; however, the relationship of these symptoms to primaquine could not be determined because the two drugs were used together. Experimental studies suggest that primaquine can promote oxidative stress in cell culture, but it is unclear whether these actions are sufficient to impact gastrointestinal function in vivo. While primaquine exerts liver toxicity at high doses, it is unlikely to have adverse effects at doses used for malaria prophylaxis.

None of the four epidemiologic studies that met the inclusion criteria specifically examined gastrointestinal outcomes following the cessation of primaquine.

Based on the available evidence, the committee concludes that there is insufficient or inadequate evidence of an association between the use of primaquine for malaria prophylaxis and persistent or latent gastrointestinal events. Current evidence does not suggest further study of such an association is warranted, given the lack of evidence regarding biologic plausibility, serious adverse events associated with concurrent use, or findings from the existing epidemiologic studies.

Eye Disorders

An examination of the associations of primaquine use with eye disorders does not indicate an increased risk for concurrent adverse events with primaquine use. Eye disorders are not mentioned in the primaquine package insert (FDA, 2017a), systematic and non-systematic reviews did not report on eye disorders, and experimental studies did not provide biologic plausibility for persistent or latent eye disorders. One case study suggested a possible link between primaquine-related hemolysis and persistent sequelae from central retinal vein occlusion.

The Nasveld et al. (2010) study was designed to assess the ophthalmic safety of a regimen of mefloquine followed by primaquine in a subset of 21 soldiers. No adverse ophthalmic events were observed in that subset while taking mefloquine, so no ophthalmic follow-up was performed during or after primaquine use. The other three epidemiologic studies that met the committee's criteria for inclusion did not assess eye disorders.

Based on the available evidence, the committee concludes that there is insufficient or inadequate evidence of an association between the use of primaquine for malaria prophylaxis and persistent or latent eye disorders. Current evidence does not suggest further study of such an association is warranted, given the lack of evidence regarding biologic plausibility, adverse events associated with concurrent use, or findings from the existing epidemiologic studies.

Cardiovascular Disorders

The FDA package insert was updated in 2015 to include the potential for cardiac QT interval prolongation (FDA, 2015). ECG monitoring is advised in patients with cardiac disease, long QT syndrome, a history of ventricular arrhythmias, uncorrected hypokalemia or hypomagnesemia, or bradycardia (<50 bpm) and who are taking concomitant administration of QT-interval-prolonging agents (FDA, 2017a). The systematic and non-systematic reviews did not report on cardiovascular disorders. Experimental studies found that hypotension, cardiac contractility, and arrhythmias had been observed with toxic doses of primaquine in rat and dog models. Cardiac effects can be linked to the blockade of sodium channels in cardiomyocytes, which results in decreased contractility (Orta-Salazar et al., 2002). Primaquine also blocks the delayed rectifier hERG potassium channels in HEK293 cells, effects that may be linked to the prolonged QT intervals or arrhythmias that occur in some individuals after taking antimalarials (Kim et al., 2010).

Nasveld et al. (2010) assessed the cardiac safety of a regimen of mefloquine followed by primaquine in a subset of 21 soldiers. An increase in QT interval was reported in the mefloquine recipients, but no cardiac outcomes were observed at week 12 after cessation of primaquine. There is biologic plausibility for primaquine being associated with cardiac conduction problems. None of the other epidemiologic studies that met the inclusion criteria addressed the potential effects of prophylactic primaquine use and the outcomes of cardiovascular disorders.

Based on the available evidence, the committee concludes that there is insufficient or inadequate evidence of an association between the use of primaquine for malaria prophylaxis and persistent or latent cardiovascular events. Current evidence does not suggest further study of such an association is warranted, given the lack of evidence regarding biologic plausibility, adverse events associated with concurrent use, or findings from the existing epidemiologic studies.

Other Outcomes and Disorders

Because the danger of hemolysis in G6PD-deficient persons is well characterized and because primaquine use is contraindicated in those with severe G6PD deficiency, the committee did not examine the evidence of adverse events associated with G6PD deficiency in depth. Although the study was small and methodologically limited, Rueangweerayut et al. (2017) found three of five participants with moderate G6PD deficiency unable to tolerate 14 days of a prophylactic dose of primaquine. Although hemolysis does not persist once the drug is halted (Rishikesh and Saravu, 2016), untreated or uncontrolled hemolysis can result in arrhythmias, cardiomyopathy, heart failure, and death (Baird, 2019; NIH, n.d.), and released hemoglobin can cause damage to the kidney (Ashley et al., 2014), which may persist. Performing a G6PD-deficiency assessment before using primaquine is a standard guideline; however, routine testing may misclassify patients, and hemolysis may occur in those who test G6PD normal, so it is suggested that hemoglobin be monitored upon initial primaquine exposure.

A common occurrence in G6PD-normal and G6PD-deficient recipients is a mild, reversible methemoglobinemia (Baird, 2019; Hill et al., 2006; Rishikesh and Saravu, 2016). Persons who are deficient in the enzyme NADH methemoglobin reductase are very sensitive to primaquine (Hill et al., 2006), and their use of primaquine should be monitored for tolerance (FDA, 2017a). Methemoglobinemia can cause cyanosis, dizziness, or dyspnea (Hill et al., 2006; Schlagenhauf et al., 2019); more severe methemoglobinemia can lead to complications, including abnormal cardiac rhythms, altered mental status, delirium, seizures, coma, profound acidosis, and death (Denshaw-Burke et al., 2018). Nasveld et al. (2010) assessed methemoglobinemia levels in a subset of 21 G6PD-normal soldiers taking a regimen of mefloquine followed by primaquine. The mean methemoglobin levels increased by 0.1% in the participants taking mefloquine; the increases resolved by week 12 of follow-up after the cessation of primaquine. Although limited by its small sample size and the narrow range of measures examined, Rueangweerayut et al. (2017) also reported transient elevations of methemoglobin in both G6PD-normal and G6PD-deficient subjects, providing weak supportive evidence.

Rare serious outcomes including death have been attributed to primaquine-associated hemolysis; however, the committee found no controlled studies documenting persistent or latent events associated with hemolysis or methemoglobinemia resulting from prophylactic doses of primaquine.

REFERENCES

Ackert, J., K. Mohamed, J. S. Slakter, S. El-Harazi, A. Berni, H. Gevorkyan, E. Hardaker, A. Hussaini, S. W. Jones, G. C. K. W. Koh, J. Patel, S. Rasmussen, D. S. Kelly, D. E. Baranano, J. T. Thompson, K. A. Warren, R. C. Sergott, J. Tonkyn, A. Wolstenholme, H. Coleman, A. Yuan, S. Duparc, and J. A. Green. 2019. Randomized placebo-controlled trial evaluating the ophthalmic safety of single-dose tafenoquine in healthy volunteers. *Drug Saf* 42:1103-1114.
Alving, A. S., C. F. Johnson, A. R. Tarlov, G. J. Brewer, R. W. Kellermeyer, and P. E. Carson. 1960. Mitigation of the haemolytic effect of primaquine and enhancement of its action against exo-erythrocytic forms of the Chesson strain of *Plasmodium vivax* by intermittent regimens of drug administration: A preliminary report. *Bull WHO* 22:621-631.
Ashley, E. A., J. Recht, and N. J. White. 2014. Primaquine: The risks and the benefits. *Malar J* 13:418.

Baird, J. K. 2019. 8-aminoquinoline therapy for latent malaria. *Clin Microbiol Rev* 32(4):e00011-19.

Baird, J. K., and S. L. Hoffman. 2004. Primaquine therapy for malaria. *Clin Infect Dis* 39(9):1336-1345.

Baird, J. K., D. J. Fryauff, H. Basri, M. J. Bangs, B. Subianto, I. Wiady, Purnomo, B. Leksana, S. Masbar, T. L. Richie, T. R. Jones, E. Tjitra, F. S. Wignall, and S. L. Hoffman. 1995. Primaquine for prophylaxis against malaria among nonimmune transmigrants in Irian Jaya, Indonesia. *Am J Trop Med Hyg* 52(6):479-484.

Baird, J. K., M. D. Lacy, H. Basri, M. J. Barcus, J. D. Maguire, M. J. Bangs, R. Gramzinski, P. Sismadi, Krisin, J. Ling, I. Wiady, M. Kusumaningsih, T. R. Jones, D. J. Fryauff, S. L. Hoffman, and the United States Naval Medical Research Unit 2 Clinical Trials Team. 2001. Randomized, parallel placebo-controlled trial of primaquine for malaria prophylaxis in Papua, Indonesia. *Clin Infect Dis* 33(12):1990-1997.

Bass, S. W., M. A. Ramirez, and D. M. Aviado. 1972. Cardiopulmonary effects of antimalarial drugs. VI. Adenosine, quinacrine and primaquine. *Toxicol Appl Pharmacol* 21(4):464-481.

Berman, J. 2004. Toxicity of commonly-used antimalarial drugs. *Travel Med Infect Dis* 2(3-4):171-184.

Binh, V. Q., N. T. Chinh, N. X. Thanh, B. T. Cuong, N. N. Quang, B. Dai, T. Travers, and M. D. Edstein. 2009. Sex affects the steady-state pharmacokinetics of primaquine but not doxycycline in healthy subjects. *Am J Trop Med Hyg* 81(5):747-753.

Bowman, Z. 2005. Primaquine-induced hemolytic anemia: Role of membrane lipid peroxidation and cytoskeletal protein alterations in the hemotoxicity of 5-hydroxyprimaquine. *J Pharmacol Exp Ther* 4(2):838-845.

Brito-Sousa, J. D., T. C. Santos, S. Avalos, G. Fontecha, G. C. Melo, F. Val, A. M. Siqueira, G. C. Alecrim, Q. Bassat, M. V. G. Lacerda, and W. M. Monteiro. 2019. Clinical spectrum of primaquine-induced hemolysis in G6PD deficiency: A nine-year hospitalization-based study from the Brazilian Amazon. *Clin Infect Dis* 69(8):1440-1442.

Brundage, J. 2003. Conserving the fighting strength: Milestones of operational military preventive medicine research. In P. W. Kelley (ed.), *Military preventive medicine: Mobilization and deployment, Vol. 1.* Washington, DC: TMM Publications, Office of the Surgeon General, United States Army. Pp. 105-126.

Camarda, G., P. Jirawatcharadech, R. S. Priestley, A. Saif, S. March, M. H. L. Wong, S. Leung, A. B. Miller, D. A. Baker, P. Alano, M. J. I. Paine, S. N. Bhatia, P. M. O'Neill, S. A. Ward, and G. A. Biagini. 2019. Antimalarial activity of primaquine operates via a two-step biochemical relay. *Nat Commun* 10(1):3226.

Castelli, F., S. Odolini, B. Autino, E. Foca, and R. Russo. 2010. Malaria prophylaxis: A comprehensive review. *Pharmaceuticals* 3(10):3212-3239.

CDC (Centers for Disease Control and Prevention). 2017a. Chapter 4: Travel-related infectious diseases. Malaria section. In *CDC yellow book 2020: Health information for international travel.* New York: Oxford University Press.

CDC. 2017b. Chapter 9: Travel for work and other reasons. U.S. military deployments section. In *CDC yellow book 2020: Health information for international travel.* New York: Oxford University Press.

CDC. 2019a. *Malaria information and prophylaxis by country.* https://www.cdc.gov/malaria/travelers/country_table/a.html (accessed August 29, 2019).

CDC. 2019b. *Malaria glossary.* https://www.cdc.gov/malaria/glossary.html#r (accessed August 2, 2019).

Chen, L. H., M. E. Wilson, and P. Schlagenhauf. 2007. Controversies and misconceptions in malaria chemoprophylaxis for travelers. *JAMA* 297(20):2251-2263.

Chen, I., H. Diawara, A. Mahamar, K. Sanogo, S. Keita, D. Kone, K. Diarra, M. Djimde, M. Keita, J. Brown, M. E. Roh, J. Hwang, H. Pett, M. Murphy, M. Niemi, B. Greenhouse, T. Bousema, R. Gosling, and A. Dicko. 2018. Safety of single-dose primaquine in G6PD-deficient and G6PD-normal males in Mali without malaria: An open-label, phase 1, dose-adjustment trial. *J Infect Dis* 217(8):1298-1308.

Chinn, H. I., and R. F. Redmond. 1954. Effect of primaquine on hypoxia tolerance. *J Appl Physiol* 6(12):773-775.

Chu, C. S., G. Bancone, F. Nosten, N. J. White, and L. Luzzatto. 2018. Primaquine-induced haemolysis in females heterozygous for G6PD deficiency. *Malar J* 17(1):101.

Denshaw-Burke, M., A. L. Curran, D. C. Savior, and M. Kumar. 2018. Methemoglobinemia. Medscape. https://emedicine.medscape.com/article/204178-overview (accessed February 12, 2020).

Dern, R. J., E. Beutler, and A. S. Alving. 1954. The hemolytic effect of primaquine. II. The natural course of the hemolytic anemia and the mechanism of its self-limited character. *J Lab Clin Med* 44(2):171-176.

DoD (Department of Defense). 2001. *Individual protection and individual/unit (from USCENTCOM Surgeon [MC]), October 2001*. Provided by COL Andrew Wiesen, M.D., M.P.H., Director, Preventive Medicine, Health Readiness Policy, and Oversight, Office of the Assistant Secretary of Defense (Health Affairs), DoD, August 22, 2019.

DoD. 2003a. *Memorandum on antimalarials and current practice in the military (July 31, 2003)*. Provided by COL Andrew Wiesen, M.D., M.P.H., Director, Preventive Medicine, Health Readiness Policy, and Oversight, Office of the Assistant Secretary of Defense (Health Affairs), DoD, August 22, 2019.

DoD. 2003b. *FRAGO 947 Post deployment health assessment PDHA SOP (October 2003)*. Provided by COL Andrew Wiesen, M.D., M.P.H., Director, Preventive Medicine, Health Readiness Policy, and Oversight, Office of the Assistant Secretary of Defense (Health Affairs), DoD, August 22, 2019.

DoD. 2003c. *Memorandum on CJTF-7 policy on malaria prevention (December 29, 2003)*. Provided by COL Andrew Wiesen, M.D., M.P.H., Director, Preventive Medicine, Health Readiness Policy, and Oversight, Office of the Assistant Secretary of Defense (Health Affairs), DoD, August 22, 2019.

DoD. 2006. *Third U.S. Army/USARCENT/CFLCC policy memorandum on malaria chemoprophylaxis (February 18, 2006; #SUR-01AFRD-SURG)*. Provided by COL Andrew Wiesen, M.D., M.P.H., Director, Preventive Medicine, Health Readiness Policy, and Oversight, Office of the Assistant Secretary of Defense (Health Affairs), DoD, August 22, 2019.

DoD. 2007. *Letter to editor of Journal of American Medical Association*. Provided by COL Andrew Wiesen, M.D., M.P.H., Director, Preventive Medicine, Health Readiness Policy, and Oversight, Office of the Assistant Secretary of Defense (Health Affairs), DoD, August 22, 2019.

DoD. 2012. *Guidance memorandum on use of primaquine during primaquine shortages (August 2, 2012)*. Provided by COL Andrew Wiesen, M.D., M.P.H., Director, Preventive Medicine, Health Readiness Policy, and Oversight, Office of the Assistant Secretary of Defense (Health Affairs), DoD, August 14, 2019.

DoD. 2013a. *Ceasing use of mefloquine in U.S. army special operations command units (September 13, 2013)*. Provided by COL Andrew Wiesen, M.D., M.P.H., Director, Preventive Medicine, Health Readiness Policy, and Oversight, Office of the Assistant Secretary of Defense (Health Affairs), DoD, August 22, 2019.

DoD. 2013b. *Memorandum on guidance on medications for prophylaxis of malaria (April 15, 2013)*. Provided by COL Andrew Wiesen, M.D., M.P.H., Director, Preventive Medicine, Health Readiness Policy, and Oversight, Office of the Assistant Secretary of Defense (Health Affairs), DoD, January 25, 2019.

DoD. 2019. *Defense Health Agency procedural instruction (December 17, 2019, #6490.03)*. Deployment health procedures. Provided by COL Andrew Wiesen, M.D., M.P.H., Director, Preventive Medicine, Health Readiness Policy, and Oversight, Office of the Assistant Secretary of Defense (Health Affairs), DoD, December 19, 2019.

DoD. n.d.a. *Primaquine information paper*. https://webcache.googleusercontent.com/search?q =cache:fGB3q2GnczYJ:https://midrp.amedd.army.mil/pdf_files/INFO_PDF/Primaquine. pdf+&cd=1&hl=en&ct=clnk&gl=us (accessed December 10, 2019).

DoD. n.d.b. *U.S. Central Command area of responsibility.* https://www.centcom.mil/AREA-OF-RESPONSIBILITY (accessed November 14, 2019).

Ebringer, A., G. Heathcote, J. Baker, M. Waller, G. D. Shanks, and M. D. Edstein. 2011. Evaluation of the safety and tolerability of a short higher-dose primaquine regimen for presumptive anti-relapse therapy in healthy subjects. *Trans R Soc Trop Med Hyg* 105(10):568-573.

El-Denshary, E. S. M. 1969. Studies on the protective effectiveness of choline and methionine against the acute toxicity of primaquine diphosphate in mice. *J Pharm Sci (UAR)* 11(2):267-272.

Fasinu, P. S., B. L. Tekwani, N. P. Nanayakkara, B. Avula, H. M. Herath, Y. H. Wang, V. R. Adelli, M. A. Elsohly, S. I. Khan, I. A. Khan, B. S. Pybus, S. R. Marcsisin, G. A. Reichard, J. D. McChesney, and L. A. Walker. 2014. Enantioselective metabolism of primaquine by human CYP2D6. *Malar J* 13:507.

Fasinu, P. S., N. P. D. Nanayakkara, Y. H. Wang, N. D. Chaurasiya, H. M. B. Herath, J. D. McChesney, B. Avula, I. Khan, B. L. Tekwani, and L. A. Walker. 2019. Formation primaquine-5,6-ortho-quinone, the putative active and toxic metabolite of primaquine via direct oxidation in human erythrocytes. *Malar J* 18(1):30.

FDA (Food and Drug Administration). 2003. Package insert for primaquine phosphate tablets, USP. https://www.accessdata.fda.gov/scripts/cder/daf/index.cfm?event=overview.process&ApplNo=008316 (accessed August 8, 2019).

FDA. 2008. Package insert for primaquine phosphate tablets, USP. https://www.accessdata.fda.gov/scripts/cder/daf/index.cfm?event=overview.process&ApplNo=008316 (accessed August 8, 2019).

FDA. 2012. *A guide to drug safety terms at FDA.* https://www.fda.gov/media/74382/download (accessed July 8, 2019).

FDA. 2015. Package insert for primaquine phosphate tablets, USP. https://www.accessdata.fda.gov/scripts/cder/daf/index.cfm?event=overview.process&ApplNo=008316 (accessed August 8, 2019).

FDA. 2016. Package insert for primaquine phosphate tablets, USP. https://www.accessdata.fda.gov/scripts/cder/daf/index.cfm?event=overview.process&ApplNo=008316 (accessed August 8, 2019).

FDA. 2017a. Package insert for primaquine phosphate tablets, USP. https://dailymed.nlm.nih.gov/dailymed/drugInfo.cfm?setid=0c8c2bc6-428b-40b6-8114-6df80290878d (accessed August 29, 2019).

FDA. 2017b. Package insert for primaquine phosphate tablets, USP. https://dailymed.nlm.nih.gov/dailymed/drugInfo.cfm?setid=0c8c2bc6-428b-40b6-8114-6df80290878d (accessed August 8, 2019).

Fryauff, D. J., J. K. Baird, H. Basri, I. Sumawinata, Purnomo, T. L. Richie, C. K. Ohrt, E. Mouzin, C. J. Church, A. L. Richards, B. Subianto, B. Sandjaja, F. S. Wignall, and S. L. Hoffman. 1995. Randomised placebo-controlled trial of primaquine for prophylaxis of *falciparum* and *vivax* malaria. *Lancet* 346(8984):1190-1193.

Fryauff, D. J., A. L. Richards, J. K. Baird, T. L. Richie, E. Mouzin, E. Tjitra, M. A. Sutamihardja, S. Ratiwayanto, H. Hadiputranto, R. P. Larasati, N. Pudjoprawoto, B. Subianto, and S. L. Hoffman. 1996. Lymphocyte proliferative response and subset profiles during extended periods of chloroquine or primaquine prophylaxis. *Antimicrob Agents Chemother* 40(12):2737-2742.

Garg, A., B. Prasad, H. Takwani, M. Jain, R. Jain, and S. Singh. 2011. Evidence of the formation of direct covalent adducts of primaquine, 2-tert-butylprimaquine (NP-96) and monohydroxy metabolite of NP-96 with glutathione and N-acetylcysteine. *J Chromatogr B Analyt Technol Biomed Life Sci* 879(1):1-7.

Goh, Y. S., D. McGuire, and L. Renia. 2019. Vaccination with sporozoites: Models and correlates of protection. *Front Immunol* 10:1227.

Grimmond, T. R., and A. S. Cameron. 1984. Primaquine-chloroquine prophylaxis against malaria in Southeast-Asian refugees entering South Australia. *Med J Aust* 140(6):322-325.

Hanboonkunupakarn, B., E. A. Ashley, P. Jittamala, J. Tarning, S. Pukrittayakamee, W. Hanpithakpong, P. Chotsiri, T. Wattanakul, S. Panapipat, S. J. Lee, N. P. Day, and N. J. White. 2014. Open-label crossover study of primaquine and dihydroartemisinin-piperaquine pharmacokinetics in healthy adult Thai subjects. *Antimicrob Agents Chemother* 58(12):7340-7346.

Hill, D. R., J. K. Baird, M. E. Parise, L. S. Lewis, E. T. Ryan, and A. J. Magill. 2006. Primaquine: Report from CDC expert meeting on malaria chemoprophylaxis. *Am J Trop Med Hyg* 75(3):402-415.

Kersgard, C. M., and P. W. Hickey. 2013. Adult malaria chemoprophylaxis prescribing patterns in the military health system from 2007–2011. *Am J Trop Med Hyg* 89(2):317-325.

Kim, K. S., H. A. Lee, S. W. Cha, M. S. Kwon, and E. J. Kim. 2010. Blockade of hERG K(+) channel by antimalarial drug, primaquine. *Arch Pharm Res* 33(5):769-773.

Kitchen, L. W., D. W. Vaughn, and D. R. Skillman. 2006. Role of U.S. military research programs in the development of U.S. Food and Drug Administration-approved antimalarial drugs. *Clin Infect Dis* 43(1):67-71.

Kolifarhood, G., A. Raeisi, M. Ranjbar, A. A. Haghdoust, A. Schapira, S. Hashemi, H. Masoumi-Asl, H. Mozafar Saadati, S. Azimi, N. Khosravi, and A. Kondrashin. 2017. Prophylactic efficacy of primaquine for preventing *Plasmodium falciparum* and *Plasmodium vivax* parasitaemia in travelers: A meta-analysis and systematic review. *Travel Med Infect Dis* 17:5-18.

Kotwal, R. S., F. K. Butler, Jr., C. K. Murray, G. J. Hill, J. C. Rayfield, and E. A. Miles. 2009. Central retinal vein occlusion in an Army Ranger with glucose-6-phosphate dehydrogenase deficiency. *Mil Med* 174(5):544-547.

Landier, J., D. M. Parker, A. M. Thu, K. M. Lwin, G. Delmas, F. H. Nosten, and the Malaria Elimination Task Force Group. 2018. Effect of generalised access to early diagnosis and treatment and targeted mass drug administration on *Plasmodium falciparum* malaria in eastern Myanmar: An observational study of a regional elimination programme. *Lancet* 391(10133):1916-1926.

Lee, C. C., L. D. Kinter, and M. H. Heiffer. 1981. Subacute toxicity of primaquine in dogs, monkeys, and rats. *Bull WHO* 59(3):439-448.

Manning, J., C. Lon, M. Spring, M. Wojnarski, S. Somethy, S. Chann, P. Gosi, K. Soveasna, S. Sriwichai, W. Kuntawunginn, M. M. Fukuda, P. L. Smith, H. Rekol, M. Sinoun, M. So, J. Lin, P. Satharath, and D. Saunders. 2018. Cluster-randomized trial of monthly malaria prophylaxis versus focused screening and treatment: A study protocol to define malaria elimination strategies in Cambodia. *Trials* 19(1):558.

Murray, M., and G. C. Farrell. 1986. Effects of primaquine on hepatic microsomal haemoproteins and drug oxidation. *Toxicology* 42(2-3):205-217.

Myint, H. Y., J. Berman, L. Walker, B. Pybus, V. Melendez, J. K. Baird, and C. Ohrt. 2011. Review: Improving the therapeutic index of 8-aminoquinolines by the use of drug combinations: Review of the literature and proposal for future investigations. *Am J Trop Med Hyg* 85(6):1010-1014.

Nasveld, P., S. Kitchener, M. Edstein, and K. Rieckmann. 2002. Comparison of tafenoquine (WR238605) and primaquine in the post-exposure (terminal) prophylaxis of *vivax* malaria in Australian Defence Force personnel. *Trans R Soc Trop Med Hyg* 96(6):683-684.

Nasveld, P. E., M. D. Edstein, M. Reid, L. Brennan, I. E. Harris, S. J. Kitchener, P. A. Leggat, P. Pickford, C. Kerr, C. Ohrt, W. Prescott, and the Tafenoquine Study Team. 2010. Randomized, double-blind study of the safety, tolerability, and efficacy of tafenoquine versus mefloquine for malaria prophylaxis in nonimmune subjects. *Antimicrob Agents Chemother* 54(2):792-798.

NIH (National Institutes of Health). 2017. *LiverTox: Clinical and research information on drug-induced liver injury.* https://livertox.nih.gov/Primaquine.htm (accessed October 3, 2019).

NIH. n.d. *Hemolytic anemia.* https://www.nhlbi.nih.gov/health-topics/hemolytic-anemia (accessed October 1, 2019).

Orta-Salazar, G., R. A. Bouchard, F. Morales-Salgado, and E. M. Salinas-Stefanon. 2002. Inhibition of cardiac Na+ current by primaquine. *Br J Pharmacol* 135(3):751-763.

Pal, S., P. Bansil, G. Bancone, S. Hrutkay, M. Kahn, G. Gornsawun, P. Penpitchaporn, C. S. Chu, F. Nosten, and G. J. Domingo. 2019. Evaluation of a novel quantitative test for glucose-6-phosphate dehydrogenase deficiency: Bringing quantitative testing for glucose-6-phosphate dehydrogenase deficiency closer to the patient. *Am J Trop Med Hyg* 100(1):213-221.

Paul, M. A., A. E. McCarthy, N. Gibson, G. Kenny, T. Cook, and G. Gray. 2003. The impact of malarone and primaquine on psychomotor performance. *Aviat Space Environ Med* 74(7):738-745.

Poirot, E., J. Skarbinski, D.Sinclair, S. P. Kachur, L. Slutsker, and J. Hwang. 2013. Mass drug administration for malaria. *Cochrane Database Syst Rev* 2013(12):CD008846.

Pybus, B. S., S. R. Marcsisin, X. Jin, G. Deye, J. C. Sousa, Q. Li, D. Caridha, Q. Zeng, G. A. Reichard, C. Ockenhouse, J. Bennett, L. A. Walker, C. Ohrt, and V. Melendez. 2013. The metabolism of primaquine to its active metabolite is dependent on CYP 2D6. *Malar J* 12:212.

Rishikesh, K., and K. Saravu. 2016. Primaquine treatment and relapse in *Plasmodium vivax* malaria. *Pathog Glob Health* 110(1):1-8.

Rueangweerayut, R., G. Bancone, E. J. Harrell, A. P. Beelen, S. Kongpatanakul, J. J. Mohrle, V. Rousell, K. Mohamed, A. Qureshi, S. Narayan, N. Yubon, A. Miller, F. H. Nosten, L. Luzzatto, S. Duparc, J. P. Kleim, and J. A. Green. 2017. Hemolytic potential of tafenoquine in female volunteers heterozygous for glucose-6-phosphate dehydrogenase (G6PD) deficiency (G6PD *Mahidol* variant) versus G6PD-normal volunteers. *Am J Trop Med Hyg* 97(3):702-711.

Schlagenhauf, P. 2003. Malaria in Iraq—The pitfalls of *Plasmodium vivax* prophylaxis. *Lancet Infect Dis* 3(8):460.

Schlagenhauf, P., M. E. Wilson, E. Petersen, A. McCarthy, L. H. Chen, J. S. Keystone, P. E. Kozarsky, B. A. Connor, H. D. Nothdurft, M. Mendelson, and K. Leder. 2019. Malaria chemoprophylaxis. In *Travel Medicine*, 4th ed., edited by J. S. Keystone, P. E. Kozarsky, B. A. Connor, H. D. Nothdurft, M. Mendelson, and K. Leder. Edinburgh: Elsevier. Pp. 145-167.

Schlossberg, D. 1980. Reaction to primaquine. *Ann Intern Med* 92(3):435.

Schmidt, I. G., and L. H. Schmidt. 1951. Neurotoxicity of the 8-aminoquinolines. III. The effects of pentaquine, isopentaquine, primaquine, and pamaquine on the central nervous system of the rhesus monkey. *J Neuropathol Exp Neurol* 10(3):231-256.

Schneiderman, A. I., Y. S. Cypel, E. K. Dursa, and R. Bossarte. 2018. Associations between use of antimalarial medications and health among U.S. veterans of the wars in Iraq and Afghanistan. *Am J Trop Med Hyg* 99(3):638-648.

Schwartz, E., and G. Regev-Yochay. 1999. Primaquine as prophylaxis for malaria for nonimmune travelers: A comparison with mefloquine and doxycycline. *Clin Infect Dis* 29(6):1502-1506.

Sharafeldin, E., D. Soonawala, J. P. Vandenbroucke, E. Hack, and L. G. Visser. 2010. Health risks encountered by Dutch medical students during an elective in the tropics and the quality and comprehensiveness of pre-and post-travel care. *BMC Med Educ* 10:89. http://www.biomedcentral.com/1472-6920/10/89 (accessed November 14, 2019).

Song, J., D. Socheat, B. Tan, P. Dara, C. Deng, S. Sokunthea, S. Seila, F. Ou, H. Jian, and G. Li. 2010. Rapid and effective malaria control in Cambodia through mass administration of artemisinin-piperaquine. *Malar J* 9(1):57.

Soto, J., J. Toledo, M. Rodriquez, J. Sanchez, R. Herrera, J. Padilla, and J. Berman. 1998. Primaquine prophylaxis against malaria in nonimmune Colombian soldiers: Efficacy and toxicity. A randomized, double-blind, placebo-controlled trial. *Ann Intern Med* 129(3):241-244.

Soto, J., J. Toledo, M. Rodriquez, J. Sanchez, R. Herrera, J. Padilla, and J. Berman. 1999. Double-blind, randomized, placebo-controlled assessment of chloroquine/primaquine prophylaxis for malaria in nonimmune Colombian soldiers. *Clin Infect Dis* 29(1):199-201.

Thillainayagam, M., and S. Ramaiah. 2016. Mosquito, malaria and medicines—A review. *Res J Pharm Technol* 9(8):1268-1276.

Tseroni, M., A. Baka, C. Kapizioni, G. Snounou, S. Tsiodras, M. Charvalakou, M. Georgitsou, M. Panoutsakou, I. Psinaki, M. Tsoromokou, G. Karakitsos, D. Pervanidou, A. Vakali, V. Mouchtouri, T. Georgakopoulou, Z. Mamuris, N. Papadopoulos, G. Koliopoulos, E. Badieritakis, V. Diamantopoulos, A. Tsakris, J. Kremastinou, C. Hadjichristodoulou, and the MALWEST Project. 2015. Prevention of malaria resurgence in Greece through the association of mass drug administration (MDA) to immigrants from malaria-endemic regions and standard control measures. *PLOS Neglected Trop Dis* 9(11):e0004215.

Vale, N., R. Moreira, and P. Gomes. 2009. Primaquine revisited six decades after its discovery. *Eur J Med Chem* 44(3):937-953.

Vásquez-Vivar, J., and O. Augusto. 1992. Hydroxylated metabolites of the antimalarial drug primaquine. Oxidation and redox cycling. *J Biol Chem* 267(10):6848-6854.

Vásquez-Vivar, J., and O. Augusto. 1994. Oxidative activity of primaquine metabolites on rat erythrocytes in vitro and in vivo. *Biochem Pharmacol* 47(2):309-316.

Vivona, S., G. J. Brewer, M. Conrad, and A. S. Alving. 1961. The concurrent weekly administration of chloroquine and primaquine for the prevention of Korean vivax malaria. *Bull WHO* 25:267-269.

Winkler, W. P. 1970. The successful control of malaria in the 173d airborne brigade. *Mil Med* 135(2):107-111.

9

Chloroquine

Chloroquine is a 4-aminoquinoline synthetic derivative of quinine, and it displays increased tolerability and lower toxicity in trials comparing it with quinine (Berberian, 1947). Chloroquine was patented in the United States in 1941 by the Winthrop Company, a cartel partner of the IG Farbenindustrie, but its drug development was not immediately pursued (Kitchen et al., 2006). Chloroquine was synthesized in the United States during World War II by the National Research Council's malaria chemotherapy research program in cooperation with multiple pharmaceutical companies, and it was tested among Army engineers on the Bataan Peninsula shortly before the war ended (Maier, 1948). In 1949 chloroquine phosphate was approved by the Food and Drug Administration (FDA) under the trade name Aralen®. Its broad use among U.S. service members began in Korea in 1950 (Brundage, 2003; Kitchen et al., 2006), and chloroquine was commonly given in combination with primaquine for presumptive anti-relapse therapy (PART) during service members' return trip to the United States following deployment (Kitchen et al., 2006). The once-weekly dosing regimen of chloroquine for malaria prophylaxis consists of one 500 mg salt (300 mg base) tablet, which made it ideal for use in resource-limited settings such as those encountered in the military. Chloroquine was used extensively around the world until chloroquine-resistant *P. falciparum* was first reported in the late 1950s. The declining efficacy of chloroquine for the prevention of clinical malaria resulted in a decrease in its use for malaria prophylaxis for several decades. Presently, chloroquine-resistant parasites can be found in almost all areas where *P. falciparum* is transmitted (Schlagenhauf et al., 2019).

Researchers began investigating the use of chloroquine in combination with other drugs following the emergence of chloroquine-resistant parasites and identified two combinations that have been widely used for malaria prophylaxis and

PART. The combination of chloroquine and primaquine (known as the "C-P pill") was given to troops returning home from Korea as well as given for standard prophylaxis for deployed service members during the Vietnam War (Brundage, 2003; Kitchen et al., 2006). Chloroquine and proguanil (chlorproguanil) has been used by foreign militaries and is approved for use in other countries (Henderson et al., 1986; Peragallo et al., 1999; Public Health England, 2018); however, the combination is not approved for use in the United States, and the committee found no indication that chlorproguanil was ever used by American service members for malaria prophylaxis. Because it is not possible to distinguish between adverse events that might result from the use of individual drugs when administered as part of a combination and adverse events that result from interactions between drugs when ingested simultaneously, the committee eliminated from further consideration any studies examining adverse events associated with the concurrent use of chloroquine and any other antimalarial drug (e.g., proguanil, primaquine) in its assessment of persistent and latent adverse events associated with the use of chloroquine for malaria prophylaxis.

Chloroquine (and hydroxychloroquine) is used to treat diseases other than malaria, specifically rheumatoid arthritis and systemic lupus erythematosus. Serious adverse events (e.g., retinopathy, macular degeneration) have been reported in people using chloroquine for the treatment of rheumatoid arthritis and systemic lupus erythematosus; however, the chloroquine regimen for treating these diseases is 250 mg per day, a much higher dose than the once-weekly 500 mg dosing regimen used for malaria prophylaxis (Cabral et al., 2019). The result of the dosing regimen for rheumatoid arthritis and systemic lupus erythematosus is a higher cumulative dose than experienced by individuals using chloroquine for malaria prophylaxis, and the higher cumulative dose is associated with a greater severity of adverse events. The literature indicates that if an individual uses chloroquine on a long-term basis (i.e., for 5–6 years) and takes in a cumulative dose >100 g, it is possible that more severe adverse events may occur. However, the use of chloroquine for malaria prophylaxis over several years is atypical in military and veteran populations; thus, the literature examining adverse events associated with the use of chloroquine over the course of several years or as treatment of other disorders was excluded.

The remainder of this chapter follows the same structure of the other antimalarial drug chapters, beginning with a discussion of the changes that have been made to the chloroquine package insert since 1990, with a particular emphasis on the Contraindications, Warnings, and Precautions sections. This is followed by a brief overview of the pharmacokinetic properties of chloroquine. The majority of the chapter is focused on the adverse events associated with chloroquine's use for malaria prophylaxis, beginning with a summary of the known concurrent adverse events associated with its use when used at the dose and interval indicated for malaria prophylaxis in the package insert. Next, the three post-cessation epidemiologic studies that met the committee's inclusion criteria and provided information on persistent health outcomes are summarized and assessed. These are ordered by population: military and veterans, U.S. Peace Corps, and research volunteers. A table that gives a high-level comparison of the three epidemiologic studies that examined the use of chloroquine and that met the committee's inclusion criteria is presented in Appendix C. Supplemental, supporting evidence is then presented, including other identified studies of health outcomes in populations that used chloroquine for malaria prophylaxis but that did not meet the committee's inclusion criteria; case reports of persistent or latent adverse events; and information on adverse events of chloroquine use in specific groups, such as during pregnancy and in people with comorbid conditions. After the primary and supplemental evidence in humans is presented, supporting literature from experimental animal and in vitro studies is then summarized. The chapter ends with a synthesis of all evidence presented by body system and the inferences and conclusions that can be made from the available evidence.

FOOD AND DRUG ADMINISTRATION PACKAGE INSERT FOR CHLOROQUINE

This section describes selected information in the FDA label or package insert for chloroquine. It begins with information from the most recent label and package insert, detailing contraindications, warnings, and precautions as well as drug interactions known or presumed to occur with concurrent use. It then offers a chronologic overview of changes made to the label. The earliest chloroquine label available on the Drugs@FDA Search site was dated 2003. The overview of label changes is based on information from the 1990 edition of the *Physicians Desk Reference* and package inserts and letters posted on the Drugs@FDA search site dating from 2003 up to the most recent label, updated in 2018. The adverse events listed in chloroquine's FDA package insert do not distinguish between adverse events experienced by those using chloroquine for malaria prophylaxis and those using it for malaria treatment, and the list of adverse events appears to be based on non-quantified postmarketing experience (FDA, 2018).

Contraindications, Warnings, and Precautions

Chloroquine used for malaria prophylaxis is contraindicated in the presence of retinal or visual field changes of any cause (FDA, 2018). It is also contraindicated in persons with known hypersensitivity to 4-aminoquinoline compounds.

Users are warned that acute extrapyramidal disorders may occur with chloroquine; adverse reactions usually resolve after drug cessation or symptomatic treatment, or both (FDA, 2018).

The label warns that cardiomyopathy resulting in cardiac failure, sometimes fatal, has been reported with the long-term, high-dose use of chloroquine (FDA, 2018). Users should be monitored for signs and symptoms of cardiomyopathy and should stop the drug if cardiomyopathy develops. If conduction disorders (bundle branch block/atrio-ventricular heart block) are diagnosed, users should stop the drug and be assessed for toxicity. The label states that QT interval prolongation, torsades de pointes, and ventricular arrhythmias, sometimes fatal, have been reported, and that high doses increase risk. Chloroquine should be used cautiously in people with cardiac disease, a history of ventricular arrhythmias, uncorrected hypokalemia or hypomagnesemia, or bradycardia (<50 bpm) as well as in those taking QT-interval-prolonging agents owing to the potential for QT-interval prolongation.

Irreversible retinal damage has occurred with chloroquine use, and the label states that significant risk factors include daily doses of chloroquine phosphate in amounts >2.3 mg/kg of body weight, administration longer than 5 years, subnormal glomerular filtration, the use of certain concomitant drug products (e.g., tamoxifen citrate), and concurrent macular disease (FDA, 2018). Chloroquine users should receive a baseline ophthalmologic examination during year 1. Those with significant risk factors should be monitored for retinal damage, including an annual examination; those with no significant risk factors can defer the annual exam to year 5. In individuals of Asian descent, visual field testing should be performed in the central 24 degrees. If ocular toxicity is suspected in a chloroquine user, the drug should be stopped and the person observed closely since retinal changes and visual disturbances can progress after drug cessation.

The label warns that chloroquine can cause severe hypoglycemia, including a loss of consciousness that could be life threatening in people treated with or without antidiabetic medications (FDA, 2018). Chloroquine users who show clinical symptoms of hypoglycemia should be monitored. The label states that those receiving the drug over the long term should be assessed periodically for evidence of muscular weakness and that if weakness occurs, the drug should be stopped.

Individuals with psoriasis are warned that chloroquine can trigger a severe attack, and users with porphyria are warned that the drug can exacerbate the condition (FDA, 2018). A drug risk–benefit assessment should precede chloroquine use in people with these disorders. People who use the drug over the long term are advised to receive complete blood cell counts periodically. Blood monitoring may be required because chloroquine can cause hemolysis in those with glucose-6-phosphate dehydrogenase (G6PD) deficiency, particularly when the drug is taken concomitantly with drugs that cause hemolysis.

Individuals with preexisting auditory damage should take chloroquine with caution, and if hearing defects occur during use, chloroquine should be stopped and the person observed (FDA, 2018). The drug should be used with caution in those with hepatic disease or alcoholism as well as in those taking hepatotoxic drugs, as chloroquine is known to accumulate in the liver.

The label warns that experimental data showed a potential risk of chloroquine inducing gene mutations and states that there is insufficient evidence regarding the drug's carcinogenicity. In addition, there are insufficient human data to rule out an increased risk of cancer with long-term use (FDA, 2018).

Animal studies showed embryo–fetal developmental toxicity at supra-therapeutic doses of chloroquine and a potential risk of genotoxicity (FDA, 2018). Human studies, including prospective studies with chloroquine exposure during pregnancy, have found no increase in the rate of birth defects or spontaneous abortions, but an individualized risk–benefit assessment should precede the use of chloroquine by pregnant women. Users are warned that serious adverse reactions in nursing infants can occur when mothers use chloroquine. The label also advises careful dose selection and possible monitoring in those aged ≥65 years; because the drug is substantially excreted by the kidney, the risk of toxic reactions may be greater in patients with impaired renal function, and the elderly are more likely to have decreased renal function.

Drug Interactions

Drugs that interact with chloroquine include mefloquine (concomitant use increases the risk of convulsions), antacids and kaolin, cimetidine, insulin and other antidiabetic drugs, arrhythmogenic drugs (e.g., amiodarone, moxifloxacin), ampicillin, cyclosporine, praziquantel, and tamoxifen as well as primary immunization with intradermal human diploid-cell rabies vaccine (FDA, 2018).

Changes to the Chloroquine Package Insert Over Time

Although the Drugs@FDA Search site lists documentation for chloroquine phosphate dating back to the drug's initial approval in 1949, downloadable documentation for package inserts or labeling is unavailable on the site for the years prior to 2003. The most recent label available on the Drugs@FDA Search site is a 2018 label (Sanofi-Aventis US). Generic formulations of chloroquine phosphate have been manufactured, but only one label (dated 2009) is downloadable from the site. The 2009 label for Aralen® was unavailable for download, so the label from the generic formulation (Hikma Pharms) is used for that year. Aralen® (chloroquine phosphate) has been discontinued. An effort has been made to limit the discussion below to label changes that refer to adverse events that occur in adults who use chloroquine as malaria prophylaxis (not for acute attacks of malaria or treatment for other conditions).

In 2003 a boxed warning, sometimes informally referred to as a "black box" (FDA, 2003a), was removed from the label. This is FDA's most serious type of warning, and it appears on a prescription drug's label to call attention to serious or life-threatening risks (FDA, 2012). The boxed warning had stated, "Physicians should completely familiarize themselves with the complete contents of this leaflet before prescribing Aralen®" (FDA, 2003a). Based on committee review of the Aralen® label in the 1990 *Physicians Desk Reference*, it appears that updates between 1990 and 2003 included cautioning persons with epilepsy that chloroquine use could cause seizures and warning that the risk of toxic reactions was higher in persons with impaired renal function (FDA, 2003b; *Physicians Desk Reference*, 1990). Delirium, personality changes, and depression were added as adverse reactions. Other additions were cardiomyopathy, myopathy, photosensitivity, and hair loss and bleaching. No source for the adverse reactions (e.g., clinical studies) was provided (FDA, 2003b). Antacids and kaolin, cimetidine, ampicillin, and cyclosporin were added as drug interactions. Language stating that persons who take chloroquine long term be questioned and tested periodically for evidence of muscle weakness was removed from the Warnings section.

In the 2009 updates, users were warned that coadministration of chloroquine with mefloquine could increase the risk of convulsions (FDA, 2009). The label also stated that chloroquine could decrease the strength of rabies vaccine. The label added polyneuritis, anxiety, agitation, insomnia, confusion, and hallucinations as adverse reactions. Other additions were rare reports of erythema multiforme, Stevens-Johnson syndrome, toxic epidermal necrolysis, exfoliative dermatitis and similar desquamationtype events; urticaria; anaphylactic/anaphylactoid reaction including angioedema; and pancytopenia. It was noted that hepatitis can increase the gastrointestinal symptoms experienced with chloroquine use.

In the 2013 additions, users were warned that acute extrapyramidal disorders could occur with chloroquine but would usually resolve after stopping the drug or treating the symptoms (FDA, 2013). Users were also warned that retinopathy/maculopathy and macular degeneration had been reported and that irreversible retina damage in patients taking the drug for long periods or at high doses had been reported. The adverse reactions maculopathy and macular degeneration were noted to be potentially irreversible.

In 2017 chloroquine became contraindicated for malaria prophylaxis in patients with retinal or visual field changes (FDA, 2017). Users were warned that cardiac myopathy, sometimes fatal, had been reported in those taking high doses for long periods. Similarly, QT interval prolongation, torsades de pointes, and ventricular arrhythmias, including fatal cases, had been reported and that the risk increased with high doses. The label advised persons with current cardiac problems or a history of cardiac problems to use the drug with caution. Users were also warned of the risk of severe hypoglycemia, which is potentially life threatening, "in patients treated with or without antidiabetic medications." Retinopathy warnings were strengthened. Precautions regarding the use of insulin, other antidiabetic drugs, arrythmogenic drugs, praziquantel, and tamoxifen were added. Sensorimotor disorders were added as an adverse reaction, as was suicidal behavior. Hemolytic anemia in G6PD-deficient patients was noted to be an adverse reaction.

In 2018 a warning was added that preclinical data with chloroquine showed a potential risk of gene mutations, and it was noted that there were insufficient data in animals and humans to rule out an increase in cancer risk with the long-term use of chloroquine (FDA, 2018). Users were warned that embryo–fetal developmental toxicity had been observed with supratherapeutic doses; in addition, data showed a potential risk of genotoxicity (doses not provided). The label noted that prophylactic doses did not show an increased rate of birth defects or spontaneous abortions in human studies. Information was added about research on chloroquine and mutagenesis stating that there is some evidence of genotoxic potential but that discrepancies exist in the literature. The label noted that chloroquine (5 mg per day for 30 days) in male rats led to a decrease in testosterone levels and in the weight of the testes, epididymis, seminal vesicles, and prostate; in addition, untreated female rats produced fewer fetuses after mating with males that received injections (10 mg/kg chloroquine for 14 days). The label states that "based on non-Good Laboratory Practice literature reports," chloroquine at supratherapeutic doses in rats have been found to cause malformations that cause fetal mortality; to cause ocular malformations; and to accumulate in the eyes and ears when administered at the beginning or end of gestation.

PHARMACOKINETICS

Chloroquine is rapidly absorbed in the gastrointestinal tract and extensively distributed in tissues with a very large volume of distribution that ranges from 200 to 800 L/kg (Ducharme and Farinotti, 1996). As a consequence, distribution rather than elimination processes determines the blood concentration profile of chloroquine. The oral bioavailability of chloroquine ranges 75–89% (Ducharme and Farinotti, 1996; Krishna and White, 1996; White, 1985). Chloroquine is 50–65% bound to plasma proteins and is cleared equally by the kidney and the liver. Chloroquine undergoes phase I metabolism to form the pharmacologically active desethyl- and bisdesethylchloroquine metabolites. Concentrations of chloroquine and its two major metabolites decline slowly, with elimination half-lives of 20 to 60 days. Chloroquine and desethylchloroquine competitively inhibit CYP2D1/6-mediated metabolic reactions. Existing data suggest that CYP3A and CYP2D6 are the two major CYP450 isoforms affected by, or involved in, chloroquine metabolism, which may have implications for potential drug interactions (Ducharme and Farinotti, 1996). Weekly 300 mg oral doses of chloroquine used for prophylaxis result in plasma concentrations up to 0.20 µg/mL (0.62 µM) (Brohult et al., 1979).

ADVERSE EVENTS

The following section contains a summary of the known concurrent adverse events associated with the use of chloroquine for malaria prophylaxis. Epidemiologic studies in which information was presented regarding adverse events occurring at least 28 days post-chloroquine-cessation are then summarized, with the emphasis on reported results of persistent or latent adverse events associated with the use of chloroquine, including the results of studies in which other antimalarial drugs were used as a comparison group.

Concurrent Adverse Events

The dosing regimens for prophylaxis and treatment vary significantly, and, as with other drugs of interest, individuals using chloroquine for malaria treatment are exposed to a larger dose in a shorter period of time than those using it for malaria prophylaxis. As a result, some adverse events are more prevalent among those using chloroquine for treatment than among those using it for prophylaxis. The committee was unable to identify any systematic reviews examining adverse events that occurred in chloroquine users compared with placebo or nonusers of antimalarial prophylactic drugs. One Cochrane systematic review was identified (Tickell-Painter et al., 2017) that compared the adverse events associated with the use of mefloquine for prophylaxis in nonimmune travelers with adverse events from other antimalarials, including chloroquine, and it is summarized below.

Cochrane Reviews

Tickell-Painter et al. (2017) prespecified adverse events to include these disorders: psychiatric (abnormal dreams, insomnia, anxiety, depression, psychosis); nervous system (dizziness, headaches); ear and labyrinth (vertigo); eye (visual impairment); gastrointestinal (nausea, vomiting, abdominal pain, diarrhea, dyspepsia); and skin and subcutaneous tissue (pruritus, photosensitivity, vaginal candida). The purpose of the assessment was to summarize the efficacy and safety of mefloquine for malaria prophylaxis in adult, children, and pregnant women travelers compared with other antimalarials, placebo, or no treatment. The dosages of mefloquine varied, as did the dosages of chloroquine, and the methods of collecting adverse event data also varied. The authors applied categories of certainty to the results based on the five GRADE considerations (risk of bias, consistency of effect, imprecision, indirectness, and publication bias) (Higgins et al., 2019). The committee recalculated the effect estimates presented below to directly compare chloroquine with mefloquine (instead of mefloquine with chloroquine).

In the four cohort studies in the review, 13 serious adverse events were reported in 22,583 chloroquine users, and 29 serious adverse events were reported in 56,674 mefloquine users; the differences between them were not statistically significant (RR = 0.88, 95%CI 0.48–1.61; 79,257 participants). Regarding neurologic adverse events, there was no statistically significant difference between groups in the trials or cohort studies in the proportion of participants reporting headache (RR = 1.19, 95%CI 0.75–1.89; 56,998 participants). Chloroquine users reported statistically significantly less dizziness than mefloquine users in the cohort studies (RR = 0.66, 95%CI 0.59–0.75; 56,710 participants), but this was not observed in the trials (RR = 0.72, 95%CI 0.65–1.46; 569 participants). In single cohort studies, chloroquine users were less likely to report altered spatial perception (RR = 0.32, 95%CI 0.16–0.65; 2,032 participants) and unsteadiness (RR = 0.28, 95%CI 0.17–0.47; 2,137 participants) than mefloquine users. Tingling was reported in two cohort studies and was statistically significantly less common in chloroquine users than in mefloquine users (RR = 0.45, 95%CI 0.25–0.79; 2,778 participants).

Four trials were included, and no serious adverse events were reported among 471 chloroquine users, while two serious adverse events were reported among 529 mefloquine users; the difference between the groups was not statistically significant (RR = 0.36, 95%CI 0.04–2.77), but the estimate was imprecise. Chloroquine users were statistically significantly less likely than mefloquine users to report the psychologic adverse events of abnormal dreams (RR = 0.83, 95%CI 0.75–0.91), anxiety (RR = 0.16, 95%CI 0.11–0.23), depressed mood (RR = 0.32, 95%CI 0.12–0.87), and abnormal thoughts or behavior (RR = 0.18, 95%CI 0.09–0.38) across the included cohort studies. Abnormal dreams was the only psychiatric outcome reported by the trials and the risk of it was also statistically significantly decreased with chloroquine use compared with mefloquine use in the trials. Insomnia was reported by five cohort studies (RR = 0.55, 95%CI 0.22–1.37; 56,952 participants) and two trials (RR = 0.84, 95%CI 0.54–1.32; 359 participants), and there were no statistically significant differences observed between chloroquine and mefloquine users. No statistically significant differences were found between chloroquine and mefloquine users for experiencing anger, disturbance in attention, irritability, loss of appetite, malaise, or altered mood.

When mefloquine users were compared with chloroquine users, there was no statistically significant difference for nausea, vomiting, or abdominal pain. Overall, mefloquine users were less likely to report diarrhea, but that finding was based primarily on the results from a single cohort study that contributed more than 90% of the weight in the meta-analysis (RR = 0.84, 95%CI 0.74–0.95; 5 cohort studies, 5,577 participants).

Other symptoms were also included when available. No statistically significant differences were found between chloroquine and mefloquine users for experiencing pruritus or abdominal distension. Several outcomes were reported in only one or two cohort studies. For example, in single cohort studies chloroquine users were less likely than mefloquine users to report alopecia (RR = 0.59, 95%CI 0.44–0.79) and visual impairment (RR = 1.10, 95%CI 0.01–2.44; 5 cohort studies, 58,847 participants).

Post-Cessation Adverse Events

A total of 17,337 abstracts or titles were identified by the committee for inclusion for chloroquine. After an initial evaluation of the types of citations captured, the committee determined that a large portion of the literature contained information related to alternative uses of chloroquine (e.g., rheumatoid arthritis, cancer, systemic lupus erythematosus). Additional search terms related to prophylaxis and malaria were added, which reduced the number of captured citations to 4,106. After screening, 791 abstracts and titles remained, and the full text for each was retrieved and reviewed to determine whether it met the committee's inclusion criteria, as defined in Chapter 3. The committee reviewed each article and identified three primary epidemiologic studies that met its inclusion criteria, including a mention of adverse events (or that no adverse events were observed) that occurred ≥28 days post-cessation of chloroquine (Lege-Oguntoye et al., 1990; Schneiderman et al., 2018; Tan et al., 2017). A table that gives a high-level comparison (study design, population, exposure groups, and outcomes examined by body system) of each of these three epidemiologic studies is presented in Appendix C.

Military and Veterans

Schneiderman et al. (2018) conducted a retrospective observational analysis of self-reported health outcomes associated with the use of antimalarial drugs in a cohort of U.S. veterans who had responded to the 2009–2011 National Health Study for a New Generation of U.S. Veterans (referred to as the "NewGen Study"). The NewGen Study is a population-based survey that sampled 30,000 veterans who had been deployed to Iraq or Afghanistan between 2001 and 2008 and 30,000 nondeployed veterans who had served during the same time period, and it included a 20% oversampling of women. The survey was conducted using mail, telephone, and web-based collection, and it yielded a response rate of only 34.3%. For this particular analysis, 19,487 participants were included who had self-reported their history of antimalarial medication use, and the use was grouped for analysis by drug (mefloquine, chloroquine, doxycycline, primaquine, mefloquine in combination with other drugs, other antimalarials, and not specified) or no antimalarial use. Health outcomes were self-reported using standardized instruments: the Medical Outcomes Study 12-item Short Form (SF-12) for general health status, PTSD checklist–Civilian version (PCL-C), and the Patient Health Questionnaire (PHQ). These instruments yielded scores that were dichotomized for analysis on composite physical health, composite mental health (above or below the U.S. mean), posttraumatic stress disorder (PTSD) (above or below the screening cutoff), thoughts of death or self-harm, other anxiety disorders, and major depression. Potential confounders included in multivariate analysis were the branch of service, sex, age, education, race/ethnicity, household income, employment status, marital status, and self-reported exposure to combat. Responses were weighted to account for survey non-response. Most veterans reported no antimalarial drug exposures (61.4%, n = 11,100), and these served as the referent group.

When stratified by deployment status, among the deployed (n = 12,456), of those who reported using an antimalarial drug (n = 6,650), 274 (weighted 3.5%) veterans reported using only chloroquine and 425 (weighted 6.0%) reported using mefloquine and another antimalarial, which may have included chloroquine. Among the nondeployed (n = 7,031), 110 (weighted 5.8%) used chloroquine alone and 52 (weighted 2.8%) reported using mefloquine and another antimalarial, which may have included chloroquine. Because it is not clear how many people in the mefloquine-plus group may have also used chloroquine, the results of that group are not included in the committee's assessment. The deployed chloroquine users reported increased frequencies of mental health diagnoses compared with nondeployed chloroquine users: PTSD (18.9% versus 7.4%), other anxiety disorders (10.4% versus 2.5%), major depression (11.4% versus 4.5%), and thoughts of death or self-harm (12.8% versus 9.2%), but no statistical comparisons were presented. In the adjusted logistic regression models with all the covariates considered (including demographics, deployment, and combat exposure), chloroquine use was not associated with any of the health outcomes when compared with no antimalarial use: composite mental health score (OR = 1.15, 95%CI 0.88–1.50), composite physical health score (OR = 1.15, 95%CI 0.88–1.50), PTSD (OR = 0.89, 95%CI 0.6–1.33), thoughts of death or self-harm (OR = 0.94, 95%CI 0.62–1.42), other anxiety (OR = 0.66, 95%CI 0.40–1.06), and major depression (not adjusted for combat exposure) (OR = 0.96, 95%CI 0.63–1.47).

The analysis of the NewGen survey is highly relevant to the question of whether there are adverse events of chloroquine use that persist following drug cessation. The study was large enough to generate moderately precise measures of association, specific drugs were assessed, the outcomes were based on standardized instruments (although not face-to-face diagnostic interviews), important covariates of deployment and combat exposure were considered in addition to demographics and other military characteristics, and the data were appropriately analyzed. The number of chloroquine users in this sample was small. It is noteworthy that adjusting for combat exposure consistently reduced the measures of association, potentially indicating a strong confounding effect of combat exposure. Although the time period of drug use and the timing of health outcomes were not directly addressed, given that the populations were all veterans who had served between 2001 and 2008 and the survey was not administered until 2009–2011, it is reasonable to assume that antimalarial drug use had ceased some time before the survey. Nonetheless, the study could not address explicitly the health experiences during use and in specific time intervals following the cessation of use. There are a number of methodologic concerns that limit the strength of this study's findings. The low response rate of 34% raises concerns of non-response bias, but the responses were weighted to account for non-response. Selective participation by both antimalarial drug use history and health status would be required to introduce bias. The accuracy of self-reported antimalarial drug use in this population is unknown. Although self-reported information has some advantages over studies based on prescriptions in that the individual specifically recalls using the drug, the details about the reported drug and adherence are not validated. Self-reported health experience is subject to the usual disadvantages of recall bias and the bias of reporting subjective experience without an independent expert assessment; however, by using standardized assessment tools, these biases may have been circumvented to some extent.

U.S. Peace Corps

Tan et al. (2017) conducted a retrospective observational Internet-based survey of 8,931 (11% response rate) returned U.S. Peace Corps volunteers (who had served during 1995–2014) to compare the prevalence of selected health conditions after Peace Corps service between those who reported taking malaria prophylaxis (n = 5,055, 56.6%) and those who did not. The reported initial antimalarial prophylactic prescriptions were mefloquine (n = 2,981; 59.0%), atovaquone/proguanil (A/P) (n = 183, 3.6%), chloroquine (n = 674, 13.3%), doxycycline (831, 16.4%), and "other" prophylactic medications (n = 386, 7.6%). In addition to questions on malaria prophylaxis (type, regimen, duration, and adherence), the survey included questions about the country of service, the type of assignment, and whether malaria prophylaxis was required at the assigned site. Respondents were also asked to report medical diagnoses made by a health care provider before, during, and after serving in the Peace Corps; to answer questions about medications used before, during, or after Peace Corps service; to provide a family history of disease and psychiatric illness; to describe their psychiatric history prior to exposure; and to give details about alcohol consumption. In total, more than 40 disease outcomes were examined for associations with each antimalarial, including derived outcomes of major depressive disorder, bipolar disorder, anxiety disorder, insomnia, psychoses, and cancers. Outcomes were grouped by system (neuropsychologic, cardiac, ophthalmologic, dermatologic, reproductive, and gastrointestinal) or class (infectious, hematologic/oncologic) and within each group several diagnoses were listed. "Any psychiatric outcome" included all reported psychiatric diagnoses both derived and those reported as individual diagnoses, including schizophrenia, obsessive-compulsive disorder, and "other." Neuropsychologic disorders were presented as a category and separately included dementia, migraines, seizures, tinnitus, vestibular disorder, "other" neurologic disorder, and "any" neurologic disorder. Gastrointestinal diseases were the only diagnosis statistically significantly more prevalent among Peace Corps volunteers who had used any chloroquine than among those who had not (9.1% versus 6.7%, respectively; prevalence ratio = 1.40, 95%CI 1.10–1.79). There was no difference in the prevalence of gastrointestinal diseases between those with prolonged or prolonged exclusively chloroquine use and those with no chloroquine use. The study reported that the prevalences of other disease diagnoses extrapolated from adverse events derived from reported and feared adverse events were similar between the groups, including those diagnoses that previous studies had indicated might be associated with chloroquine use, such as ocular toxicity.

The study had many limitations, primarily stemming from its design as an Internet-based survey of people with an email address on file. The response rate was low (11%), the authors relied on self-report for both exposure and outcome information and the timing of each, and for some participants the time between drug exposure and the survey was many years. Most comparisons were between those who had been exposed to a specific drug (i.e., mefloquine, chloroquine, doxycycline, A/P, other) and those who had not. Thus, the comparison group for each antimalarial was a mixture of those who did not report taking any antimalarials and those who reported taking antimalarial drugs other than the one being examined. Overall, there were few details of the limited analyses presented, which made it difficult to understand the groups that were being compared, how they differed with respect to important covariates, and what variables were included in the models. The reliance on self-report, often years (range 2–20 years) after the exposure, introduced several potential biases (selection bias, recall bias, and confounding bias), with inadequate information to determine the likely impact or direction of the potential biases acting in this study. While the use of self-reported diagnoses that were specified to be those made by a medical professional to ascertain health outcomes was arguably a better method than using a checklist of symptoms, the outcomes were not validated against any objective information. While the results presented in this study do not support the presence of persistent adverse events, or neuropsychiatric events, specifically post-cessation of chloroquine, the design limitations of this study are such that any evidence provided by this study is weak.

Research Volunteers

Lege-Oguntoye et al. (1990) conducted a nonblinded randomized controlled trial to study the effect of chloroquine on the humoral and cell-mediated immunity of semi-immune adult volunteers in Zaria, Nigeria. Thirty subjects were block randomized to chloroquine (n = 20) or control (n = 10) and given weekly dosing for a period of 6 months; three individuals in the chloroquine group were excluded from analysis due to poor adherence. Drugs were orally administered under supervision from March 1986 through December 1986. Blood measures were obtained at baseline, 3 months, and 6 months after starting the prophylaxis and 2 months after drug cessation. None of the 27 enrolled individuals had detectable drug plasma concentrations at enrollment. After 3 months of chloroquine dosing, indirect immunofluorescence assay titers to *P. falciparum* declined and further decreased throughout the study; the effect lasted up to 2 months post-chloroquine-cessation. Furthermore, after 3 months of chloroquine dosing, serum concentrations of IgG and IgM were significantly reduced. Two months after drug cessation, the serum concentrations of IgG and factor B were significantly reduced. The investigators hypothesized that the secretory processes of the macrophage–monocyte system are generally inhibited by the use of chloroquine; the implication of significant short-term or long-term use of chloroquine prophylaxis may be the predisposition of the subjects to bacterial infections by organisms with capsular polysaccharide that depend on the alternative pathway for effective clearance. No changes were found for serum C_{3C} or C_4 for either group. Lymphocyte counts were unchanged throughout the study period. The details of the statistical differences between study groups in outcomes were not presented. In summary, the study found some changes in immune response that persisted for 2 months after drug cessation. However, the study had a very small sample size and presented data related to only a limited number of outcomes. The measures of immunity are intermediate, and the relationship to clinical outcomes is unknown.

OTHER IDENTIFIED STUDIES OF CHLOROQUINE PROPHYLAXIS IN HUMAN POPULATIONS

When reviewing full-text articles, the committee identified several epidemiologic articles on chloroquine use for malaria prophylaxis that could not be included because they either did not provide information on adverse events that occurred ≥28 days post-cessation of chloroquine or presented data that did not distinguish among adverse events that occurred during concurrent use of chloroquine or ≥28 days post-cessation of chloroquine. These studies include Baird et al. (1995), Barrett et al. (1996), Boudreau et al. (1991, 1993), Bustos et al. (1994), Cunningham et al. (2014), Fryauff et al. (1996), Handschin et al. (1997), Harries et al. (1988), Hill (2000), Hilton et al. (1989), Huzly et al. (1996), Korhonen et al. (2007), Laverone et al. (2006), Lobel et al. (1991, 1993), Petersen et al. (2000), Roestenberg et al. (2009, 2011), Sharafeldin et al. (2010), Sossouhounto et al. (1995), Steffen et al. (1990, 1993), Stemberger et al. (1984), Sturchler et al. (1987), Waner et al. (1999), and Winkler (1970). Additionally, three articles included for consideration within other drug chapters only reported exposure as "chloroquine and/or proguanil" in the study results. These articles did not distinguish between adverse events associated with chloroquine alone, chloroquine and proguanil, or proguanil alone; therefore, they were not considered by the committee for this chapter. The studies were Meier et al. (2004) and Schneider et al. (2013, 2014).

Upon full-text review and quality assessment, additional studies were excluded from further consideration. Bijker et al. (2014) conducted a double-blind randomized controlled trial of experimental infection 16 weeks following the administration of prophylactic doses of mefloquine (n = 10) or chloroquine (n = 5) in healthy volunteers in the Netherlands. Adverse events and their severity were recorded over the duration of the study; all adverse events were reported to have resolved by the end of the study, but because the exact timing of the resolution was not provided, this study was not included in the primary epidemiologic studies. Bunnag et al. (1992) conducted a randomized double-blind study comparing the efficacy and tolerability of Fansimef®, mefloquine, Fansidar®, and chloroquine to placebo for malaria prophylaxis in 602 healthy adult males in Thailand who were followed for 4 weeks after the final dose. The timing of the adverse events was not specified, although blood measures were reported to remain stable throughout the study period, but because the details were not presented, the study did not meet the inclusion criteria. Salako et al. (1992) conducted a randomized double-blind trial to assess the efficacy of Fansimef®, mefloquine, Fansidar®, and chloroquine compared with placebo. Follow-up was continued for 4 weeks after the cessation of prophylaxis, but neither the details of which data were collected during those 4 weeks nor the timing of adverse events were provided, and thus this study did not meet inclusion as a primary epidemiologic study. Finally, Shanks et al. (1993) compared the efficacy of post-exposure malaria prophylaxis of two dosages of halofantrine and chloroquine among copper mine workers returning from Papua New Guinea; 400 were successfully followed for 28 days post-drug-administration. Adverse events were not collected in a systematic way, and their timing was not specified.

Case Reports and Case Series

Chloroquine exposure has been associated with "chloroquine retinopathy," an eye condition that can lead to persistent visual dysfunction and even blindness. Numerous case studies of retinopathy have appeared in the literature, typically in the context of chloroquine taken in larger doses than prescribed for malaria prophylaxis; however, only adverse events in people who used chloroquine to prevent malaria are considered here. The committee reviewed three case studies and five published reports of other adverse events associated with chloroquine use (n = 80).

Neurologic disorders were found in three patients: two cases of neuromyopathy, both of which occurred in people who were taking doses of chloroquine that were much higher than the recommended dose for malaria prophylaxis (Karstorp et al., 1973; Tegner et al., 1988), and one case where an electroencephalogram was suggestive of a diagnosis of nonconvulsive complex partial status epilepticus, which resolved by 2 months post-chloroquine-cessation (Mulhauser et al., 1995). In the case reported by Karstorp et al. (1973), muscle strength and reflexes returned to normal by 3 months post-cessation, but the case reported in Tegner et al. was found to have morphologic changes in Schwann cells upon autopsy.

Other cases of adverse events were reported. Spira (1997) reported a patient with desquamation and symmetrical hypopigmentaion of the hands, which improved at 4 weeks post-chloroquine-cessation and resolved completely by 3-month follow-up. Sensory disorders were associated with chloroquine exposure in a few patients as reported in several studies. Kokong et al. (2014) found ototoxicity resulting in hearing loss in individuals taking chloroquine. Bertagnolio et al. (2001) reported persistent retinopathy in one patient, and Ferrucci et al. (1998) reported an exacerbation of retinitis pigmentosa. Lange et al. (1994) studied 588 missionaries who had previously used chloroquine for malaria prophylaxis and conducted physical examinations on a subset of 53 individuals. A detailed medical history was conducted that included medication exposures and completion of a visual examination. One participant was diagnosed with chloroquine retinopathy, including blurred vision, blind spots, photophobia, eye pain, and clinical findings of ring scotoma, retinal pigment changes endothelial dystrophy, and macular degeneration; however, this patient used chloroquine for a connective tissue disorder, and not solely for malaria prophylaxis. No other diagnoses of retinopathy were discovered. And Munera et al. (1997) wrote of a case of elevated thyroid stimulating hormone that was presumed to stem from chloroquine exposure.

Selected Subpopulations

In the course of its review of the literature on chloroquine, the committee identified and reviewed available studies that reported results stratified by demographic, medical, or behavioral factors to assess whether the risk for adverse events when using chloroquine for prophylaxis is associated with being part of or affiliated with a specific group. This was not done exhaustively, and the evidence included in this section is generally limited to adverse events observed with concurrent use of chloroquine. Many of these studies did not meet the inclusion criteria of following their population for at least 28 days post-chloroquine-cessation, but the committee considers these findings to be important indicators when considering the evidence as a whole. The following risk groups were specifically considered: pregnant women and individuals with comorbid diseases.

Pregnancy

Chloroquine is considered to be safe for malaria prophylaxis in all trimesters of pregnancy (Moore and Davis, 2018). Chloroquine has not been found to have harmful effects on the fetus when it is used in the recommended doses for malaria prophylaxis (McGready et al., 2002; Villegas et al., 2007). For example, in a cohort of U.S. government employees taking chloroquine (300 mg weekly) as prophylaxis throughout pregnancy in 1969–1978, the prevalence of newborns with congenital abnormality (1.2%, 2/169) was not different from that among those who were not exposed to chloroquine (0.9%, 4/454) (Wolfe and Cordero, 1985). The Centers for Disease Control and Prevention states that chloroquine can be used for malaria prophylaxis during all trimesters of pregnancy, but only in destinations where chloroquine resistance is not present (CDC, 2019). A pharmacokinetic study of chloroquine during pregnancy found increased drug metabolism and clearance rates and decreased blood levels as compared with a nonpregnant group, thus allowing the authors to recommend a 33% increase in chloroquine doses in pregnant women based on a detailed computational analysis (Salman et al., 2017).

Comorbid Diseases

Amet et al. (2013) suggests that reductions be made to chloroquine prophylactic dosing regimens in individuals with decreased creatinine clearance (a measure of renal compromise). Chloroquine can produce retinal effects, albeit at a very low rate (Labriola et al., 2012), a fact that reinforces the need for long-term monitoring of retinal and visual changes. In critically ill individuals, chloroquine may increase the risk of developing drug-induced acute liver failure (Lat et al., 2010). Caution should be used when prescribing chloroquine to elderly adults, particularly those suffering from blood dyscrasias, psoriasis, porphyria, or liver disease or who engage in heavy alcohol consumption (Yax et al., 2007).

BIOLOGIC PLAUSIBILITY

Some in vitro and in vivo studies suggest that chloroquine may benefit neurologic outcomes following stroke or neurotoxic challenge, perhaps via PLA2 inhibition (Farooqui et al., 2006); however, other studies in neuronal and astrocyte cell lines suggest that high doses of chloroquine result in neurotoxicity, thought to be mediated by mitochondrial oxidative stress (Woerhling et al., 2010). In addition, chloroquine promotes the generation of reactive oxygen species in human astrocyte cultures, increasing chemokine production, which is suggestive of local inflammation (Park et al., 2004). Binding studies indicate that chloroquine can bind (and act as a competitive inhibitor of) the mu (μ), delta (δ), and kappa (κ) opioid receptors with low micromolar affinity. Drug levels of chloroquine can approach 1 μM during prophylactic dosing, so it is possible that this drug perturbs opioid signaling (Liu et al., 1991). However, chloroquine does not bind GABA, serotonin, or dopamine receptors to any significant extent (Janowsky et al., 2014; Liu et al., 1991). While these data were based on generally very high doses of chloroquine, the experimental evidence suggests a means for chloroquine to affect neuronal health and viability (beneficially for some outcomes, deleteriously for others), although the specific actions on neurologic and psychiatric endpoints have not been definitively examined in vivo.

There is evidence that chloroquine can prolong QT interval at curative doses in patients, but it does not provoke overt cardiac symptoms and remits with discontinuation of therapy (Bustos et al., 1994). Chloroquine also affects action potential velocity, duration, and refractory period in sheep Purkinje fibers of the heart, a phenomenon that may be related to anti-arrhythmic actions of chloroquine in cardiac patients (thought to be linked to PLA2 inhibition) (Harris et al., 1988; Tobón et al., 2019).

There is evidence for deleterious actions of chloroquine on the retinal pigment epithelium, which can cause visual disturbances and macular degeneration in patients receiving anti-inflammatory dosing for the treatment of autoimmune diseases (e.g., systemic lupus erythematosus) for which the recommended doses are much higher than the dose used for malaria prophylaxis. It is postulated that retinal pigment changes may also be seen following short-term prophylactic dosing regimens (Rimpela et al., 2018); however, the committee did not find any evidence to support this hypothesis during the review of the available research. These changes may be the result of an elevation in the lysosomal pH in the retinal pigment epithelium (Audo and Warchol, 2012) and possibly by the binding of chloroquine to melanin (Rimpela et al., 2018).

In addition to being an efficacious antimalarial drug, chloroquine has also gained usage as an anti-inflammatory agent and is used at high doses in the treatment of autoimmune diseases, including systemic lupus erythematosus, rheumatoid arthritis, and Sjögren's syndrome (Dai et al., 2018). Its anti-inflammatory actions are thought to be mediated largely via its actions as a lysosomotrophic agent, increasing intra-lysosomal pH by acting as a diprotic weak base (Accapezzato et al., 2005; Fox and Kang, 1993). As reviewed by Galluzzi et al. (2017) and He et al. (2018), chloroquine inhibits autophagy by deacidifying the lysosome. Autophagy is a lysosome-dependent survival pathway of intracellular degradation that maintains cellular homeostasis. Chloroquine can also decrease cytokine production (e.g., TNFα, IL-6) by altering iron metabolism (Picot et al., 1993) or via the inhibition of toll-like receptor 3 signaling cascades in immune cells, indicative of anti-inflammatory actions (Aizawa et al., 2019; Cui et al., 2013; Imaizumi et al., 2017). Chloroquine also inhibits PLA2, a membrane protein important in cellular signaling cascades (Bondeson and Sundler, 1998). Some data suggests that chloroquine prophylaxis can decrease the levels of immunoglobins and T- and B-cells (Lege-Oguntoye et al., 1990); it is possible that immunosuppression actions could impair resistance to infection. Osorio et al. (1992) examined the effects of chloroquine at prophylactic doses on the phagocytic function of human monocytes and suggested that immune consequences may be associated with the use of chloroquine for malaria prophylaxis, but these results are limited and only weakly supportive of the findings of Lege-Oguntoye et al. (1990).

SYNTHESIS AND CONCLUSIONS

Even though chloroquine has been approved by FDA for malaria prophylaxis for more than 70 years, only three epidemiologic studies were identified that included some mention of adverse events or data collection that occurred ≥28 days post-cessation of chloroquine and that provided directly relevant information for assessing persistent or latent adverse events (Lege-Oguntoye et al., 1990; Schneiderman et al., 2018; Tan et al., 2017). The studies are heterogeneous in the populations that were used (endemic populations, U.S. military veterans, and returned U.S. Peace Corps volunteers, respectively); in the modes of data collection on drug exposure, health outcomes, and covariates (administrative records, researcher collected, self-report, respectively); and particularly in the nature of the health outcomes that were considered. Within a particular outcome category, such as psychiatric conditions, the information elicited ranged from more minor symptoms (such as anxiety) to severe clinical disorders (e.g., psychosis, depression, PTSD), posing a challenge to the committee's ability to make an integrated assessment. Furthermore, the relevant studies were notably inconsistent in their reporting of results, covering different time periods relative to the cessation of the drug exposure. Given the inherently imperfect information generated by any one study, it would be desirable to have similar studies to assess the consistency of the findings, but the diversity of the methods in these three studies made it very difficult to combine information across studies with confidence. Each of the post-cessation epidemiologic studies possessed strengths and weaknesses related to the specific methodology used by the investigators during the study process. The studies are notably different in methodologic quality, so their findings are not weighted equally in drawing conclusions. Based on the methodologic considerations described in Chapter 3, a brief summary of the committee's evaluation of each post-cessation epidemiologic study is described here, and findings specific to each body system are presented below, as appropriate. Each conclusion consists of two parts: the first sentence assigns the level of association, and the second sentence offers additional detail regarding whether further research in a particular area is merited based on a consideration of all the available evidence.

Epidemiologic Studies Presenting Contributory Evidence

Schneiderman et al. (2018) conducted an analysis of self-reported health outcomes associated with use of antimalarials in a population-based cohort study of deployed and nondeployed U.S. veterans, using information collected as a part of the NewGen Study. Exposures and outcomes were systematically obtained, and psychiatric outcomes were measured by standardized assessment instruments. Antimalarial medication use was grouped into mefloquine, chloroquine, doxycycline, primaquine, mefloquine in combination with other drugs, other antimalarials, and not specified or no antimalarial drug exposures. Health outcomes were self-reported using standardized instruments: the SF-12 for general health status, PCL-C for PTSD, and the PHQ. The overall sample was large, and the researchers used a reasonably thorough set of covariates in models estimating drug–outcome associations, including deployment and combat exposure. Although the time period of drug use and the timing of health outcomes were not directly addressed, given that the population comprised veterans who had served between 2001 and 2008 and that the survey was not administered until 2009–2011, it is reasonable to assume that antimalarial drug use had ceased some time before the survey. The methodology and response rate (34% total; weighted 3.5% of deployed and weighted 5.8% of nondeployed individuals used chloroquine) for this study may have led to the introduction of non-response, recall, or selection biases; however, the committee believes that the investigators used appropriate data analysis techniques to mitigate the effects of any biases that were present.

The primary aim of Tan et al. (2017) was to assess the prevalence of several conditions experienced by returned U.S. Peace Corps volunteers and their association with the use of prophylactic antimalarial medications. Although the number of participants was large (8,931 participants) and a number of important covariates, such as psychiatric history and alcohol use, were collected, the study had several methodologic issues. These limitations included the study design (self-report,

Internet-based survey), exposure characterization (reliance on self-reported exposure introduces several potential biases, such as recall bias, sampling bias, and confounding), the outcome assessment (based on self-report of health provider–diagnosed conditions up to 20 years post-service), the use of mixed comparison groups, the lack of detail regarding the analysis methods, and a poor response rate (11%, which likely introduced selection bias). Additionally, only 674 (13.3%) of the respondents reported using chloroquine for primary malaria prophylaxis. The evidence generated by this study was thus considered to only weakly contribute to the inferences of persistent adverse events or disorders associated with chloroquine use for malaria prophylaxis.

The primary objective of the study conducted by Lege-Oguntoye et al. (1990) was to examine the effects of short-term chloroquine use for malaria prophylaxis on the humoral and cell-mediated immunity of healthy semi-immune adults. Investigators analyzed changes in biochemical parameters within individuals taking chloroquine for 6 months and then followed the individuals for 2 months post-chloroquine-cessation. In the committee's view, the use of standardized laboratory testing and procedures in this study reduces the likelihood of the introduction of bias and likely indicates that the data presented are of high quality. However, the committee believed that the limitations of the endpoints tested did not allow for the conclusion that there is a significant impact of chloroquine on immune function. This study also had a very small sample size (n = 27), and investigators examined and reported only intermediate measures of immunity with unknown clinical implications, limiting the information that could be gleaned from the study findings; therefore, this study was given less weight in the committee's forming of conclusions regarding the persistent or latent adverse events of chloroquine use as malaria prophylaxis.

In addition to the epidemiologic studies, the committee also considered supplemental evidence, including recognized concurrent adverse events, case reports of persistent adverse events, studies of adverse events in pregnant women and people with comorbid conditions, and information from experimental animal models or cell cultures. Consistent with the chapter syntheses of other antimalarial drugs, the synthesis is organized by body system category: neurologic disorders, psychiatric disorders, gastrointestinal disorders, eye disorders, cardiovascular disorders, and other disorders, including immunologic and dermatologic outcomes.

Neurologic Disorders

Although some studies grouped adverse events under a more general category of "neuropsychiatric" effects for discussion, the committee separated neurologic and psychiatric symptoms and conditions to the extent possible. An examination of the associations between chloroquine use and neurologic disorders does not indicate an increased risk for current chloroquine users, with the exception of the indication in the FDA label and package insert that muscle weakness may be associated with chloroquine use and that individuals with a history of epilepsy should be warned about the risk of chloroquine provoking seizures. According to a systematic review examining concurrent adverse events experienced by short-term travelers, risk of altered spatial perception, unsteadiness, and tingling were statistically significantly reduced in individuals using chloroquine compared with mefloquine (Tickell-Painter et al., 2017). The committee identified three case reports: one case of neuromyopathy that had fully resolved by 3 months post-chloroquine-withdrawal (Karstorp et al., 1973); one case study reporting symptoms of motor dysphagia and language problems, with an electroencephalogram suggestive of a diagnosis of nonconvulsive complex partial status epilepticus (Mulhauser et al., 1995); and one case that reported autopsy findings of morphologic changes to Schwann cells (Tegner et al., 1988). Preclinical studies do not indicate that chloroquine has marked neurotoxic effects, although alterations in astrocyte function have been noted, suggesting possible neuromodulary actions.

Of the three post-cessation epidemiologic studies that examined chloroquine use, Tan et al. (2017) was the only one that examined neurologic health outcomes, including migraines, seizures, tinnitus, vestibular disorder, "other neuropsychologic" disorders, and "any neuropsychologic" disorder. The investigators reported no difference in the rates of "neuropsychological" outcomes between users of chloroquine and nonusers of chloroquine; however, the limitations of the study design, as previously described, provide weak inferences.

Based on the available evidence, the committee concludes that there is insufficient or inadequate evidence of an association between the use of chloroquine for malaria prophylaxis and persistent or latent neurologic events. Current evidence does not suggest further study of such an association is warranted, given the lack of evidence regarding biologic plausibility, adverse events associated with concurrent use, or findings from the existing epidemiologic studies.

Psychiatric Disorders

The FDA label or package insert for chloroquine lists psychosis, delirium, anxiety, agitation, insomnia, confusion, hallucinations, personality changes, and depression as potential psychiatric adverse events that may occur in individuals taking chloroquine. However, in a systematic review examining concurrent adverse events experienced by short-term travelers, chloroquine users were statistically significantly less likely than mefloquine users to report such psychologic adverse events as abnormal dreams, anxiety, depressed mood, and abnormal thoughts or behavior (Tickell-Painter et al., 2017). No statistically significant differences were found between chloroquine and mefloquine users for experiencing anger, disturbance in attention, irritability, malaise, or altered mood. No published case studies were identified that presented information on psychiatric adverse events associated with chloroquine use when used at the dosing regimen for malaria prophylaxis that developed or persisted for ≥28 days post-cessation of chloroquine. Experimental animal studies and other biologic plausibility studies identified by the committee provided no evidence of persistent or latent adverse psychiatric events associated with chloroquine use for malaria prophylaxis.

Two of the epidemiologic studies assessed included information on at least one psychiatric outcome: one in military populations (Schneiderman et al., 2018) and one in returned U.S. Peace Corps volunteers (Tan et al., 2017). The two studies used different methods for measuring outcomes—unverified self-reported clinical diagnoses (Tan et al., 2017) and standardized self-report instruments (Schneiderman et al., 2018)—with little overlap in the specific outcomes examined across the two studies. For example, PTSD was included in Schneiderman et al. (2018) but not in Tan et al. (2017). Similarly, insomnia was included in Tan et al. (2017), but not in Schneiderman et al. (2018). Notably, both studies collected data on depression and anxiety, but in different ways. Schneiderman et al. (2018) used a validated, standardized, mental health questionnaire and recorded a diagnosis based on the total score, whereas Tan et al. (2017) used unverified self-reported symptoms to derive diagnoses of major depressive disorder, bipolar disorder, anxiety disorder, schizophrenia, and a category of "other" mental health disorders from these symptoms. The diagnosis classification methods used by Tan et al. (2017) may have introduced nondifferential misclassification of the outcomes; however, the committee believed this was unlikely to affect study findings.

In terms of results, Tan et al. (2017) reported no associations between chloroquine exposure and the psychiatric outcomes examined (depressive disorder, bipolar disorder, anxiety disorder, psychosis, and insomnia). In Schneiderman et al. (2018), the deployed chloroquine users reported increased frequencies of mental health diagnoses compared with nondeployed chloroquine users: PTSD (18.9% versus 7.4%), other anxiety disorders (10.4% versus 2.5%), major depression (11.4% versus 4.5%), and thoughts of death or self-harm (12.8% versus 9.2%), but no formal statistical inferences were made. In the adjusted logistic regression models that adjusted for demographics, deployment, and combat exposure, the use of chloroquine was not statistically significantly associated with any of the psychiatric health outcomes—composite mental health score, PTSD, thoughts of death or self-harm, other anxiety, and major depression (not adjusted for combat exposure)—when compared with nonusers of antimalarial drugs. Notably, adjustment for combat exposure consistently reduced the measures of association for psychiatric outcomes related to chloroquine use. This study provides modest evidence of no increase in risk of persistent or latent psychiatric adverse events of chloroquine in terms of PTSD, anxiety disorders, major depression, or thoughts of death or self-harm.

Based on the available evidence, the committee concludes that there is insufficient or inadequate evidence of an association between the use of chloroquine for malaria prophylaxis and persistent or latent psychiatric events. Current evidence does not suggest further study of such an association is warranted, given the lack of evidence regarding biologic plausibility, adverse events associated with concurrent use, or findings from the existing epidemiologic studies.

Gastrointestinal Disorders

Chloroquine is known to accumulate in the liver, and the package insert warns that caution should be used in individuals with hepatic disease or alcoholism or who are using known hepatotoxic drugs. Likewise, chloroquine-induced hepatitis has been reported in studies examining concurrent adverse events of chloroquine use. This effect may be more likely in critically ill individuals. Experimental animal and human cell culture studies that used chloroquine were also examined for evidence of mechanisms that could plausibly support persistent or latent adverse events, and the committee found no information indicating that chloroquine use is associated with persistent or latent gastrointestinal adverse events. In a systematic review examining concurrent adverse events experienced by short-term travelers, no statistically significant differences were found between chloroquine and mefloquine users for experiencing nausea, vomiting, or abdominal pain. Chloroquine users were more likely to report diarrhea, but that finding was based primarily on the results from a single cohort study that contributed to more than 90% of the weight in the meta-analysis.

The committee identified one post-cessation epidemiologic study that examined persistent gastrointestinal adverse events associated with chloroquine use (Tan et al., 2017). Tan et al. (2017) reported that gastrointestinal disorders were 1.4 times more prevalent among those who had used any chloroquine (n = 63; 9.1%) than among those who had not used any chloroquine (n = 486; 6.7%). When stratified by prolonged exposure to chloroquine, no statistically significant difference in gastrointestinal disorders was found. The limitations of this study, as previously discussed, restricted the committee's ability to make inferences about any persistent gastrointestinal adverse events of chloroquine use.

Based on the available evidence, the committee concludes that there is insufficient or inadequate evidence of an association between the use of chloroquine for malaria prophylaxis and persistent or latent gastrointestinal events. Current evidence does not suggest further study of such an association is warranted, given the lack of evidence regarding biologic plausibility, adverse events associated with concurrent use, or findings from the existing epidemiologic studies.

Eye Disorders

There are known associations between eye disorders and concurrent use of chloroquine when used at higher doses than the recommended regimen for malaria prophylaxis or when a large cumulative dose is taken over an extended period of time. The FDA label and package insert lists maculopathy, macular degeneration, and retinal damage as potentially irreversible adverse events that may occur as a result of chloroquine use. However, the label also states that this damage usually occurs in individuals who are receiving long-term or high-dosage 4-aminoquinoline therapy, neither of which would typically be the case for individuals, including military and veteran populations, using chloroquine for malaria prophylaxis. A systematic review examining the concurrent adverse events associated with malaria prophylaxis in short-term travelers found no statistically significant differences in visual impairment between chloroquine and mefloquine users (Tickell-Painter et al., 2017). The committee identified one published case study in which an individual was diagnosed with chloroquine retinopathy and experienced adverse vision-related symptoms. The individual was using chloroquine for malaria prophylaxis; however, the study states that chloroquine was being used simultaneously to treat a connective tissue disorder, indicating that it is likely the individual was receiving a greater dose of chloroquine than recommended for malaria prophylaxis. Experiments conducted in vitro and in animal models indicate that chloroquine's effects on lysosomal function or its binding to melanin can impair the health and viability of the retinal pigment epithelium. Both actions may underlie the risks to the visual system that are associated with chloroquine treatment, although these are not necessarily observed at prophylactic doses.

Tan et al. (2017) was the only post-cessation epidemiologic study that presented data on eye disorders; these included macular degeneration, retinopathy, and "any" ophthalmologic disorder. No association between chloroquine use and ocular toxicity was found, although specific data were not reported.

Based on the available evidence, the committee concludes that there is insufficient or inadequate evidence of an association between the use of chloroquine for malaria prophylaxis and persistent or latent eye disorders. Current evidence does not suggest further study of such an association is warranted, given the lack of evidence regarding biologic plausibility, adverse events associated with concurrent use, or data from the existing epidemiologic studies.

Cardiovascular Disorders

Some studies of concurrent adverse events associated with chloroquine use (e.g., Bustos et al., 1994) as well as the FDA labels and package insert, indicate that chloroquine may result in concurrent cardiac adverse events (e.g., hypotension, prolongation of the QTc interval). There is not a substantial body of evidence that addresses the cardiac actions of chloroquine, and indeed it has been suggested that chloroquine's inhibitory effects on PLA2 may be of benefit in the treatment of arrhythmias (Tobón et al., 2019).

In terms of post-cessation epidemiologic studies examining persistent or latent adverse events, only Tan et al. (2017) examined cardiovascular outcomes. The included conditions were arrhythmia, congestive heart failure, myocardial infarction, and "any" cardiac disorder. No association was reported between chloroquine use and any of these conditions when compared with people who did not use chloroquine, but the authors did not report specific frequencies or effect estimates.

Based on the available evidence, the committee concludes that there is insufficient or inadequate evidence of an association between the use of chloroquine for malaria prophylaxis and persistent or latent cardiovascular events. Current evidence does not suggest further study of such an association is warranted, given the lack of evidence regarding biologic plausibility, adverse events associated with concurrent use, or findings from the existing epidemiologic studies.

Other Outcomes and Disorders

Lege-Oguntoye et al. (1990) examined the immune response among 27 individuals randomly assigned to chloroquine or placebo groups. Three months after these individuals had begun their chloroquine use, investigators found that immunofluorescence assay titers to *P. falciparum* had declined, and they decreased further throughout the study. The decreased titers persisted for up to 2 months post-chloroquine-cessation. Furthermore, the serum concentrations of IgG and IgM were significantly reduced 2 months after chloroquine withdrawal. These outcomes are considered to be intermediate, and the relevance to clinical outcomes is not clear. Concurrent adverse effects on immune endpoints are evident at one post-cessation time point but not thereafter, and they are in general alignment with a wealth of data demonstrating chloroquine to have anti-inflammatory actions. While these data suggest vulnerability to immune challenges, the results of the study are only weakly supported by other findings (Osorio et al., 1992). Based on this evidence, the committee believed that immune dysfunction is likely not associated with the use of chloroquine for malaria prophylaxis.

Tan et al. (2017) also examined dermatologic health outcomes and found no association between persistent adverse dermatologic events and chloroquine use; nevertheless, the committee did identify some weak signals for dermatologic disorders within the scientific literature. One case study reported a patient with desquamation and symmetrical hypopigmentation of the hands, which fully resolved by 3 months post-chloroquine-cessation. The FDA label and systematic reviews previously discussed in this chapter also list concurrent adverse events of pruritus and the exacerbating effects of chloroquine use on attacks in people with psoriasis; however, these findings were not reported in the included epidemiologic studies. Tan et al. (2017) also examined the associations between chloroquine and a number of additional persistent outcomes, including reproductive, hematologic, and cancer, and found no association.

REFERENCES

Accapezzato, D., V. Visco, V. Francavilla, C. Molette, T. Donato, M. Paroli, M. U. Mondelli, M. Doria, M. R. Torrisi, and V. Barnaba. 2005. Chloroquine enhances human CD8+ T cell responses against soluble antigens in vivo. *J Exp Med* 202(6):817-828.

Aizawa, T., T. Imaizumi, K. Hirono, S. Watanabe, K. Tsugawa, and H. Tanaka. 2019. Chloroquine attenuates TLR3-mediated plasminogen activator inhibitor-1 expression in cultured human glomerular endothelial cells. *Clin Exp Nephrol* 23(4):448-454.

Amet, S., S. Zimner-Rapuch, V. Launay-Vacher, N. Janus, and G. Deray. 2013. Malaria prophylaxis in patients with renal impairment: A review. *Drug Saf* 36(2):83-91.

Audo, I., and M. E. Warchol. 2012. Retinal and cochlear toxicity of drugs: New insights into mechanisms and detection. *Curr Opin Neurol* 25(1):76-85.

Baird, J. K., D. J. Fryauff, H. Basri, M. J. Bangs, B. Subianto, I. Wiady, Purnomo, B. Leksana, S. Masbar, T. L. Richie, T. R. Jones, E. Tjitra, F. S. Wignall, and S. L. Hoffman. 1995. Primaquine for prophylaxis against malaria among nonimmune transmigrants in Irian Jaya, Indonesia. *Am J Trop Med Hyg* 52(6):479-484.

Barrett, P. J., P. D. Emmins, P. D. Clarke, and D. J. Bradley. 1996. Comparison of adverse events associated with use of mefloquine and combination of chloroquine and proguanil as antimalarial prophylaxis: Postal and telephone survey of travellers. *Br Med J* 313(7056):525-528.

Berberian, D. A. 1947. Treatment and prophylaxis of malaria with aralen. *J Palest Arab Med Assoc* 2(6):143-151.

Bertagnolio, S., E. Tacconelli, G. Camilli, and M. Tumbarello. 2001. Case report: Retinopathy after malaria prophylaxis with chloroquine. *Am J Trop Med Hyg* 65(5):637-638.

Bijker, E. M., R. Schats, J. M. Obiero, M. C. Behet, G. J. Van Gemert, M. Van De Vegte-Bolmer, W. Graumans, L. Van Lieshout, G. J. H. Bastiaens, K. Teelen, C. C. Hermsen, A. Scholzen, L. G. Visser, and R. W. Sauerwein. 2014. Sporozoite immunization of human volunteers under mefloquine prophylaxis is safe, immunogenic and protective: A double-blind randomized controlled clinical trial. *PLOS ONE* 9(11):e112910.

Bondeson, J., and R. Sundler. 1998. Antimalarial drugs inhibit phospholipase A2 activation and induction of interleukin 1beta and tumor necrosis factor alpha in macrophages: Implications for their mode of action in rheumatoid arthritis. *Gen Pharmacol* 30(3):357-366.

Boudreau, E. F., L. W. Pang, S. Chaikummao, and C. Witayarut. 1991. Comparison of mefloquine, chloroquine plus pyrimethamine-sulfadoxine (fansidar), and chloroquine as malarial prophylaxis in eastern Thailand. *SE Asian J Trop Med* 22(2):183-189.

Boudreau, E., B. Schuster, J. Sanchez, W. Novakowski, R. Johnson, D. Redmond, R. Hanson, and L. Dausel. 1993. Tolerability of prophylactic lariam regimens. *Trop Med Parasitol* 44(3):257-265.

Brohult, J., L. Rombo, V. Sirleaf, and E. Bengtsson. 1979. The concentration of chloroquine in serum during short and long term malaria prophylaxis with standard and "double" dosage in nonimmunes: Clinical implications. *Ann Trop Med Parasitol* 73(5):401-405.

Brundage, J. 2003. Conserving the fighting strength: Milestones of operational military preventive medicine research. In P. W. Kelley (ed.), *Military preventive medicine: Mobilization and deployment, Vol. 1.* Washington, DC: TMM Publications, Office of the Surgeon General, United States Army. Pp. 105-126.

Bunnag, D., S. Malikul, S. Chittamas, D. Chindanond, T. Harinasuta, M. Fernex, M. L. Mittelholzer, S. Kristiansen, and D. Sturchler. 1992. Fansimef for prophylaxis of malaria: A double-blind randomized placebo controlled trial. *SE Asian J Trop Med* 23(4):777-782.

Bustos, M. D., F. Gay, B. Diquet, P. Thomare, and D. Warot. 1994. The pharmacokinetics and electrocardiographic effects of chloroquine in healthy subjects. *Trop Med Parasitol* 45(2):83-86.

Cabral, R. T. S., E. M. Klumb, M. I. N. N. Couto, and S. Carneiro. 2019. Evaluation of toxic retinopathy caused by antimalarial medications with spectral domain optical coherence tomography. *Arq Bras Oftalmol* 82(1):12-17.

CDC (Centers for Disease Control and Prevention). 2019. *Yellow book.* https://wwwnc.cdc.gov/travel/yellowbook/2020/travel-related-infectious-diseases/malaria (accessed September 26, 2019).

Cui, G., X. Ye, T. Zuo, H. Zhao, Q. Zhao, W. Chen, and F. Hua. 2013. Chloroquine pretreatment inhibits toll-like receptor 3 signaling after stroke. *Neurosci Lett* 548:101-104.

Cunningham, J., J. Horsley, D. Patel, A. Tunbridge, and D. G. Lalloo. 2014. Compliance with long-term malaria prophylaxis in British expatriates. *Travel Med Infect Dis* 12(4):341-348.

Dai, C., X. Xiao, D. Li, S. Tun, Y. Wang, T. Velkov, and S. Tang. 2018. Chloroquine ameliorates carbon tetrachloride-induced acute liver injury in mice via the concomitant inhibition of inflammation and induction of apoptosis. *Cell Death Dis* 9(12):1164.

Ducharme, J., and R. Farinotti. 1996. Clinical pharmacokinetics and metabolism of chloroquine. Focus on recent advancements. *Clin Pharmacokinet* 31(4):257-274.

Farooqui, A. A., W. Y. Ong, and L. A. Horrocks. 2006. Inhibitors of brain phospholipase A2 activity: Their neuropharmacological effects and therapeutic importance for the treatment of neurologic disorders. *Pharmacol Rev* 58(3):591-620.

FDA (Food and Drug Administration). 2003a. FDA letter, Aralen® chloroquine phosphate, USP package insert. https://www.accessdata.fda.gov/scripts/cder/daf/index.cfm?event=overview. process&ApplNo=006002 (accessed October 21, 2019).

FDA. 2003b. Package insert for Aralen® chloroquine phosphate, USP. https://www.accessdata.fda. gov/scripts/cder/daf/index.cfm?event=overview.process&ApplNo=006002 (accessed October 21, 2019).

FDA. 2009. Package insert for chloroquine phosphate tablets, USP. https://www.accessdata.fda.gov/ scripts/cder/daf/index.cfm?event=overview.process&ApplNo=083082 (accessed October 21, 2019).

FDA. 2012. *A guide to drug safety terms at FDA.* https://www.fda.gov/media/74382/download (accessed July 8, 2019).

FDA. 2013. Package insert for Aralen® chloroquine phosphate, USP. https://www.accessdata.fda. gov/scripts/cder/daf/index.cfm?event=overview.process&ApplNo=006002 (accessed October 21, 2019).

FDA. 2017. Package insert for Aralen® chloroquine phosphate, USP. https://www.accessdata.fda. gov/scripts/cder/daf/index.cfm?event=overview.process&ApplNo=006002 (accessed October 21, 2019).

FDA. 2018. Package insert for Aralen® chloroquine phosphate, USP. https://www.accessdata.fda. gov/scripts/cder/daf/index.cfm?event=overview.process&ApplNo=006002 (accessed October 21, 2019).

Ferrucci, S., S. F. Anderson, and J. C. Townsend. 1998. Retinitis pigmentosa inversa. *Optom Vis Sci* 75(8):560-570.

Fox, R. I., and H. I. Kang. 1993. Mechanism of action of antimalarial drugs: Inhibition of antigen processing and presentation. *Lupus* 2(Suppl 1):S9-S12.

Fryauff, D. J., A. L. Richards, J. K. Baird, T. L. Richie, E. Mouzin, E. Tjitra, M. A. Sutamihardja, S. Ratiwayanto, H. Hadiputranto, R. P. Larasati, N. Pudjoprawoto, B. Subianto, and S. L. Hoffman. 1996. Lymphocyte proliferative response and subset profiles during extended periods of chloroquine or primaquine prophylaxis. *Antimicrob Agents Chemother* 40(12):2737-2742.

Galluzzi, L., J. M. Bravo-San Pedro, B. Levine, D. R. Green, and G. Kroemer. 2017. Pharmacological modulation of autophagy: Therapeutic potential and persisting obstacles. *Nat Rev Drug Discov* 16(7):487-511.

Handschin, J. C., M. Wall, R. Steffen, and D. Sturchler. 1997. Tolerability and effectiveness of malaria chemoprophylaxis with mefloquine or chloroquine with or without co-medication. *J Travel Med* 4(3):121-127.

Harries, A. D., C. J. Forshaw, and H. M. Friend. 1988. Malaria prophylaxis amongst British residents of Lilongwe and Kasungu districts, Malawi. *Trans R Soc Trop Med Hyg* 82(5):690-692.

Harris, L., E. Downar, N. A. Shaikh, and T. Chen. 1988. Antiarrhythmic potential of chloroquine: New use for an old drug. *Can J Cardiol* 4(6):295-300.

He, S., Q. Li, X. Jiang, X. Lu, F. Feng, W. Qu, Y. Chen, and H. Sun. 2018. Design of small molecule autophagy modulators: A promising druggable strategy. *J Med Chem* 61(11):4656-4687.

Henderson, A., J. W. Simon, and W. Melia. 1986. Failure of malaria chemoprophylaxis with a proguanil-chloroquine combination in Papua New Guinea. *Trans R Soc Trop Med Hyg* 80(5):838-840.

Higgins, J. P. T., J. A. Lopez-Lopez, B. J. Becker, S. R. Davies, S. Dawson, J. M. Grimshaw, L. A. McGuinness, T. H. M. Moore, E. A. Rehfuess, J. Thomas, and D. M. Caldwell. 2019. Synthesising quantitative evidence in systematic reviews of complex health interventions. *BMJ Glob Health* 4(Suppl 1):e000858.

Hill, D. R. 2000. Health problems in a large cohort of Americans traveling to developing countries. *J Travel Med* 7(5):259-266.

Hilton, E., B. Edwards, and C. Singer. 1989. Reported illness and compliance in U.S. travelers attending an immunization facility. *Arch Intern Med* 149(1):178-179.

Huzly, D., C. Schonfeld, W. Beuerle, and U. Bienzle. 1996. Malaria chemoprophylaxis in German tourists: A prospective study on compliance and adverse reactions. *J Travel Med* 3(3):148-155.

Imaizumi, T., R. Hayakari, T. Matsumiya, H. Yoshida, K. Tsuruga, S. Watanabe, S. Kawaguchi, and H. Tanaka. 2017. Chloroquine attenuates TLR3/IFN-beta signaling in cultured normal human mesangial cells: A possible protective effect against renal damage in lupus nephritis. *Mod Rheumatol* 27(6):1004-1009.

Janowsky, A., A. J. Eshleman, R. A. Johnson, K. M. Wolfrum, D. J. Hinrichs, J. Yang, T. M. Zabriskie, M. J. Smilkstein, and M. K. Riscoe. 2014. Mefloquine and psychotomimetics share neurotransmitter receptor and transporter interactions in vitro. *Psychopharmacology* 231(14):2771-2783.

Karstorp, A., H. Ferngren, P. Lundbergh, and U. Lying-Tunell. 1973. Letter: Neuromyopathy during malaria suppression with chloroquine. *Br Med J* 4(5894):736.

Kitchen, L. W., D. W. Vaughn, and D. R. Skillman. 2006. Role of U.S. military research programs in the development of US Food and Drug Administration—Approved antimalarial drugs. *Clin Infect Dis* 43(1):67-71.

Kokong, D. D., A. Bakari, and B. M. Ahmad. 2014. Ototoxicity in Nigeria: Why it persists. *Ear Nose Throat J* 93(7):256-264.

Korhonen, C., K. Peterson, C. Bruder, and P. Jung. 2007. Self-reported adverse events associated with antimalarial chemoprophylaxis in Peace Corps volunteers. *Am J Prev Med* 33(3):194-199.

Krishna, S., and N. J. White. 1996. Pharmacokinetics of quinine, chloroquine, and amodiaquine: Clinical implications. *Clin Pharmacokinet* 30(4):263-299.

Labriola, L. T., D. Jeng, and A. A. Fawzi. 2012. Retinal toxicity of systemic medications. *Int Ophthalmol Clin* 52(1):149-166.

Lange, W. R., D. L. Frankenfield, M. Moriarty-Sheehan, C. S. Contoreggi, and J. D. Frame. 1994. No evidence for chloroquine-associated retinopathy among missionaries on long-term malaria chemoprophylaxis. *Am J Trop Med Hyg* 51(4):389-392.

Lat, I., D. R. Foster, and B. Erstad. 2010. Drug-induced acute liver failure and gastrointestinal complications. *Crit Care Med* 38(6 Suppl.):S175-S187.

Laverone, E., S. Boccalini, A. Bechini, S. Belli, M. G. Santini, S. Baretti, G. Circelli, F. Taras, S. Banchi, and P. Bonanni. 2006. Travelers' compliance to prophylactic measures and behavior during stay abroad: Results of a retrospective study of subjects returning to a travel medicine center in Italy. *J Trav Med* 13(6):338-344.

Lege-Oguntoye, L., G. C. Onyemelukwe, B. B. Maiha, E. O. Udezue, and S. Eckerbom. 1990. The effect of short-term malaria chemoprophylaxis on the immune response of semi-immune adult volunteers. *East Afr Med J* 67(11):770-778.

Liu, L., Y. Katz, R. Weizman, B. Rosenberg, G. W. Pasternak, and M. Gavish. 1991. Interactions of chloroquine with benzodiazepine, gamma-aminobutyric acid and opiate receptors. *Biochem Pharmacol* 41(10):1534-1536.

Lobel, H. O., K. W. Bernard, S. L. Williams, A. W. Hightower, L. C. Patchen, and C. C. Campbell. 1991. Effectiveness and tolerance of long-term malaria prophylaxis with mefloquine. Need for a better dosing regimen. *JAMA* 265(3):361-364.

Lobel, H. O., M. Miani, T. Eng, K. W. Bernard, A. W. Hightower, and C. C. Campbell. 1993. Long-term malaria prophylaxis with weekly mefloquine. *Lancet* 341(8849):848-851.

Maier, J. 1948. A field trial of chloroquine (SN 7618) as a suppressive against malaria in the Philippines. *Am J Trop Med Hyg* 28(3):407-412.

McGready, R., K. L. Thwai, T. Cho, L. S. Samuel, N. J. White, and F. Nosten. 2002. The effects of quinine and chloroquine antimalarial treatments in the first trimester of pregnancy. *Trans R Soc Trop Med Hyg* 96(2):180-184.

Meier, C. R., K. Wilcock, and S. S. Jick. 2004. The risk of severe depression, psychosis or panic attacks with prophylactic antimalarials. *Drug Saf* 27(3):203-213.

Moore, B. R., and T. M. E. Davis. 2018. Pharmacotherapy for the prevention of malaria in pregnant women: Currently available drugs and challenges. *Expert Opin Pharmacother* 19(16):1779-1796.

Mulhauser, P., Y. Allemann, and C. Regamey. 1995. Chloroquine and nonconvulsive status epilepticus. *Ann Intern Med* 123(1):76-77.

Munera, Y., F. C. Hugues, C. Le Jeunne, and J. F. Pays. 1997. Interaction of thyroxine sodium with antimalarial drugs. *BMJ* 314(7094):1593.

Osorio, L. M., L. Fonte, and C. M. Finlay. 1992. Inhibition of human monocyte function by prophylactic doses of chloroquine. *Am J Trop Med Hyg* 46(2):165-168.

Park, J. S., K. S. Choi, E. J. Jeong, D. H. Kwon, E. N. Benveniste, and C. H. Choi. 2004. Reactive oxygen species mediate chloroquine-induced expression of chemokines by human astroglial cells. *Glia* 47:9-20.

Peragallo, M. S., G. Sabatinelli, and G. Sarnicola. 1999. Compliance and tolerability of mefloquine and chloroquine plus proguanil for long-term malaria chemoprophylaxis in groups at particular risk (the military). *Trans R Soc Trop Med Hyg* 93(1):73-77.

Petersen, E., T. Ronne, A. Ronn, I. Bygbjerg, and S. O. Larsen. 2000. Reported side effects to chloroquine, chloroquine plus proguanil, and mefloquine as chemoprophylaxis against malaria in Danish travelers. *J Travel Med* 7(2):79-84.

Physicians Desk Reference, 44th ed. 1990. Medical Economics Company. Pp. 2305-2306.

Picot, S., F. Peyron, A. Donadille, J. P. Vuillez, G. Barbe, and P. Ambroise-Thomas. 1993. Chloroquine-induced inhibition of the production of TNF, but not of IL-6, is affected by disruption of iron metabolism. *Immunology* 80(1):127-133.

Public Health England. 2018. *Guidelines for malaria prevention in travelers from the UK.* https://assets.publishing.service.gov.uk/government/uploads/system/uploads/attachment_data/file/774781/ACMP_guidelines_2018.pdf (accessed December 7, 2019).

Rimpela, A. K., M. Reinisalo, L. Hellinen, E. Grazhdankin, H. Kidron, A. Urtti, and E. M. del Amo. 2018. Implications of melanin binding in ocular drug delivery. *Adv Drug Deliv Rev* 126:23-43.

Roestenberg, M., M. McCall, J. Hopman, J. Wiersma, A. J. F. Luty, G. J. Van Gemert, M. Van De Vegte-Bolmer, B. Van Schaijk, K. Teelen, T. Arens, L. Spaarman, Q. De Mast, W. Roeffen, G. Snounou, L. Renia, A. Van Der Ven, C. C. Hermsen, and R. Sauerwein. 2009. Protection against a malaria challenge by sporozoite inoculation. *N Engl J Med* 361(5):468-477.

Roestenberg, M., A. C. Teirlinck, M. B. B. McCall, K. Teelen, K. N. Makamdop, J. Wiersma, T. Arens, P. Beckers, G. Van Gemert, M. Van De Vegte-Bolmer, A. J. A. M. Van Der Ven, A. J. F. Luty, C. C. Hermsen, and R. W. Sauerwein. 2011. Long-term protection against malaria after experimental sporozoite inoculation: An open-label follow-up study. *Lancet* 377(9779):1770-1776.

Salako, L. A., R. A. Adio, O. Walker, A. Sowunmi, D. Sturchler, M. L. Mittelholzer, R. Reber-Liske, and U. Dickschat. 1992. Mefloquine-sulphadoxine-pyrimethamine (fansimef, Roche) in the prophylaxis of *Plasmodium falciparum* malaria: A double-blind, comparative, placebo-controlled study. *Ann Trop Med Parasitol* 86(6):575-581.

Salman, S., F. Baiwog, M. Page-Sharp, K. Kose, H. A. Karunajeewa, I. Mueller, S. J. Rogerson, P. M. Siba, K. F. Ilett, and T. M. E. Davis. 2017. Optimal antimalarial dose regimens for chloroquine in pregnancy based on population pharmacokinetic modelling. *Int J Antimicrob Agents* 50(4):542-551.

Schlagenhauf, P., M. E. Wilson, E. Petersen, A. McCarthy, L. H. Chen, J. S. Keystone, P. E. Kozarsky, B. A. Connor, H. D. Nothdurft, M. Mendelson, and K. Leder. 2019. Malaria chemoprophylaxis. *J Travel Med* 4(15):145-167.

Schneider, C., M. Adamcova, S. S. Jick, P. Schlagenhauf, M. K. Miller, H. G. Rhein, and C. R. Meier. 2013. Antimalarial chemoprophylaxis and the risk of neuropsychiatric disorders. *Travel Med Infect Dis* 11(2):71-80.

Schneider, C., M. Adamcova, S. S. Jick, P. Schlagenhauf, M. K. Miller, H. G. Rhein and C. R. Meier. 2014. Use of anti-malarial drugs and the risk of developing eye disorders. *Travel Med Infect Dis* 12(1):40-47.

Schneiderman, A. I., Y. S. Cypel, E. K. Dursa, and R. M. Bossarte. 2018. Associations between use of antimalarial medications and health among U.S. veterans of the wars in Iraq and Afghanistan. *Am J Trop Med Hyg* 99(3):638-648.

Shanks, G. D., M. D. Edstein, R. K. Kereu, P. E. Spicer, and K. H. Rieckmann. 1993. Postexposure administration of halofantrine for the prevention of malaria. *Clin Infect Dis* 17(4):628-631.

Sharafeldin, E., D. Soonawala, J. P. Vandenbroucke, E. Hack, and L. G. Visser. 2010. Health risks encountered by Dutch medical students during an elective in the tropics and the quality and comprehensiveness of pre- and post-travel care. *BMC Med Educ* 10:89.

Sossouhounto, R. T., B. N. Soro, A. Coulibaly, M. L. Mittelholzer, D. Stuerchler, and L. Haller. 1995. Mefloquine in the prophylaxis of *P. falciparum* malaria. *J Travel Med* 2(4):221-224.

Spira, A. M. 1997. Hypopigmentation and desquamation as dermatologic reactions to aralen. *J Travel Med* 4(3):189-191.

Steffen, R., R. Heusser, R. Machler, R. Bruppacher, U. Naef, D. Chen, A. M. Hofmann, and B. Somaini. 1990. Malaria chemoprophylaxis among European tourists in tropical Africa: Use, adverse reactions, and efficacy. *Bull WHO* 68(3):313-322.

Steffen, R., E. Fuchs, J. Schildknecht, U. Naef, M. Funk, P. Schlagenhauf, P. Phillips-Howard, C. Nevill, and D. Sturchler. 1993. Mefloquine compared with other malaria chemoprophylactic regimens in tourists visiting east Africa. *Lancet* 341(8856):1299-1303.

Stemberger, H., R. Leimer, and G. Wiedermann. 1984. Tolerability of long-term prophylaxis with Fansidar: A randomized double-blind study in Nigeria. *Acta Tropica* 41(4):391-399.

Sturchler, D., M. Schar, and N. Gyr. 1987. Leucopenia and abnormal liver function in travelers on malaria chemoprophylaxis. *J Trop Med Hyg* 90(5):239-243.

Tan, K. R., S. J. Henderson, J. Williamson, R. W. Ferguson, T. M. Wilkinson, P. Jung, and P. M. Arguin. 2017. Long term health outcomes among returned Peace Corps volunteers after malaria prophylaxis, 1995–2014. *Travel Med Infect Dis* 17:50-55.

Tegner, R., F. M. Tome, P. Godeau, F. Lhermitte, and M. Fardeau. 1988. Morphological study of peripheral nerve changes induced by chloroquine treatment. *Acta Neuropathol* 75(3):253-260.

Tickell-Painter, M., N. Maayan, R. Saunders, C. Pace, and D. Sinclair. 2017. Mefloquine for preventing malaria during travel to endemic areas. *Cochrane Database Syst Rev* 10:CD006491.

Tobón, C., L. Palacio, B. Chidipi, D. P. Slough, T. Tran, N. Tran, M. Reiser, Y. Lin, B. Herweg, D. Sayad, J. Saiz, and S. Noujaim. 2019. The antimalarial chloroquine reduces the burden of persistent atrial fibrillation. *Front Pharmacol* doi:10.3389/fphar.2019.01392.

Villegas, L., R. McGready, M. Htway, M. K. Paw, M. Pimanpanarak, R. Arunjerdja, S. J. Viladpai-Nguen, B. Greenwood, N. J. White, and F. Nosten. 2007. Chloroquine prophylaxis against *vivax* malaria in pregnancy: A randomized, double-blind, placebo-controlled trial. *Trop Med Int Health* 12(2):209-218.

Waner, S., D. Durrhiem, L. E. Braack, and S. Gammon. 1999. Malaria protection measures used by in-flight travelers to South African game parks. *J Trav Med* 6(4):254-257.

White, N. J. 1985. Clinical pharmacokinetics of antimalarial drugs. *Clin Pharmacokin* 10(3):187-215.

Winkler, W. P. 1970. The successful control of malaria in the 173d Airborne Brigade. *Mil Med* 135(2):107-111.

Woehrling, E. K., E. J. Hill, and M. D. Coleman. 2010. Evaluation of the importance of astrocytes when screening for acute toxicity in neuronal cell systems. *Neurotox Res* 17(2):103-113.

Wolfe, M. S., and J. F. Cordero. 1985. Safety of chloroquine in chemosuppression of malaria during pregnancy. *Br Med J Clin Res* 290(6480):1466-1467.

Yax, J. A., C. D. Collins, and P. N. Malani. 2007. Prevention and prophylaxis of malaria in older travelers. *Clin Geriatr* 15(8):36-45.

10

Improving the Quality of Research on the Long-Term Health Effects of Antimalarial Drugs

The committee was charged with reviewing the available scientific evidence regarding the prophylactic use of Food and Drug Administration (FDA)-approved antimalarial drugs, particularly those that were used by U.S. service members or were of interest to the Department of Veterans Affairs (VA), and their persistent or latent adverse health effects, with a focus on neurologic and psychiatric conditions. This report is an assessment of the evidence with a focus on the published research, supplemented with other evidence as available (such as national and foreign government reports, responses to committee-generated information requests, and information submitted by the public through invited presentations, comments, and data submissions) relating the use of antimalarial drugs to adverse health effects, with specific consideration of the quality and quantity of studies and their findings.

The previous six chapters provide comprehensive assessments of the literature pertaining to each of the individual antimalarial drugs of interest (mefloquine, tafenoquine, atovaquone/proguanil [A/P], doxycycline, primaquine, and chloroquine) and their association with adverse events that might occur in any organ system. Those chapters offer integrated summaries and assessments of the evidence for each drug and each type of adverse event, organized by body system (neurologic, psychiatric, gastrointestinal, eye, cardiovascular, and other outcomes and disorders), and those specific assessments will not be repeated here. In this chapter the committee reflects more broadly on the current overall state of scientific knowledge regarding persistent and latent adverse events of the antimalarial drugs of interest when used for malaria prophylaxis and how to best advance the understanding of possible persistent events of antimalarial drugs. The committee was not asked to design the "gold standard" epidemiologic study for future research on this topic. However, following its review of the studies, the committee was able to identify areas where the methodologic rigor could be strengthened in order to guide future research efforts that would then allow researchers to make stronger inferences and conclusions. This is in response to the penultimate sentence of its Statement of Task, "Additionally, the committee will consider approaches for identifying short-term, long-term, and persistent adverse health effects of antimalarials."

As noted in the drug-specific chapters, there is a sharp contrast between the abundant amount of literature pertaining to concurrent adverse events that are experienced while a drug is being used or shortly following its cessation and the dearth of information, especially high-quality information, pertaining to adverse experiences after the use of that drug has ended. To assess the persistent effects of exposure to antimalarial drugs the committee opted to use a conservative cutoff time of ≥28 days (which was considered equivalent to expressions of 4 weeks or 1 month) post-cessation of drug intake to differentiate between events that are concurrent (outside the committee's scope) and those that are persistent or latent (within the committee's scope). Because some terms are used interchangeably in the literature and may have very different connotations depending on their context, the committee endeavored to use language that allowed it to be as precise as possible. As such, instead of "long term," which may refer to the duration of drug use for prophylaxis or to the duration or timing of symptoms, the committee uses "persistent" and "latent" to describe associations with adverse events after the use of a drug has ended. The committee defined *persistent* adverse events as those adverse events that began during the period in which the drug was used and continued after its cessation beyond the period that the drug would still be present, which is defined as ≥28 days post-cessation. *Latent* adverse events are those adverse events that were not apparent during the period the drug was in use but that were present at any time (i.e., ≥28 days, after the cessation of antimalarial prophylaxis). The focus of the committee's assessment was research that examined persistent or latent adverse effects, both of which indicate adverse health outcomes that extend beyond user experience while taking the drug.

ATTRIBUTES OF AVAILABLE RESEARCH

The currently available body of high-quality research addressing the use of antimalarial drugs for malaria prophylaxis (some of which have been in use for more than 70 years) and persistent or latent adverse effects is quite limited, even when combined across all the drugs of interest and all organ systems and types of possible adverse events. There appears to be a disconnect between the level of concern raised—millions of people have used the drugs, and there are many known concurrent events and case reports of adverse events—and the systematic research that has been conducted, particularly in areas such as the use of mefloquine and persistent neurologic or psychiatric outcomes. As reflected in the chapter syntheses, only a small subset of studies, mostly conducted in military populations or travelers, provide the most relevant and informative evidence regarding persistent adverse events. A few of those studies compared the occurrence of adverse events across several antimalarial drugs of interest. From all of the studies considered and assessed by the committee, only about half (Ackert et al., 2019; Eick-Cost et al., 2017; Green et al., 2014; Leary et al., 2009; Meier et al., 2004; Nasveld et al., 2010; Schneider et al., 2013, 2014; Schneiderman et al., 2018; Wells et al., 2006) of the 21 epidemiologic studies that met the committee's inclusion criteria were considered to be the most informative due to their methodologic attributes of having sufficient quality of exposure and outcome information, being of sufficient size to potentially provide adequate statistical power (especially for rare outcomes), and presenting data on adverse events that occurred or persisted 28 days or more post-drug-cessation. Each of these studies has its own limitations, but they were determined to be the most informative for addressing the question of whether there is evidence of persistent or latent adverse health outcomes associated with the prophylactic use of antimalarial drugs.

A number of randomized controlled trials were identified that provide rigor in their control of confounding, but most did not extend the follow-up period to at least 28 days beyond the duration of the antimalarial drug use. For those that did, they were generally were too small to yield information on any but the most common adverse events, or the published study had poor documentation of adverse events. In addition, the committee notes that the randomized trials were primarily designed to study tolerability or efficacy, and, as a result, they were generally non-informative about persistent or latent adverse events. Although many of the randomized controlled trials and a much larger body of observational studies did not meet the committee's inclusion criteria because they did not report on or distinguish between outcomes at least 28 days post-drug-cessation, these studies do contribute to the evidence base regarding concurrent adverse events. The research base for concurrent adverse events is substantial and shows a consistent pattern of outcomes that are associated with the tolerability and safety of these drugs, as detailed in each chapter. While concurrent adverse events are only indirectly relevant to the charge of examining persistent adverse events, they do provide an indication of particular body systems, symptoms, and diagnoses to focus on, assuming that the problems most likely to be persistent are those that initially manifest during drug use. That scenario is more commonly observed and plausible in the committee's view than true latent effects which arise de novo at some time after exposure to the drug of interest has ceased. Although it would be ideal to have the entire time course available, beginning from exposure to an antimalarial drug to years post-cessation, and symptom manifestations that occurred at multiple time points, the literature is so limited that the committee was not able to be more specific about adverse events that were likely to persist in different time intervals (e.g., 1–6 months, 6–12 months, >12 months). As a result, all adverse events that persisted for at least 28 days were presented. Several published case reports and case series were identified that provided supportive information on adverse events, some of these being rare outcomes, that arose in conjunction with taking an antimalarial drug and persisted for some period after the cessation of drug use. The case reports varied in quality and detail. While these reports cannot contribute to causal inference in part because of a lack of comparison groups, they can direct attention to and inform areas or health outcomes that merit more methodologically rigorous evaluation for specific drugs.

The biologic effects of the various antimalarial drugs are relatively well understood with regard to their effectiveness in preventing clinical malaria and aspects of acute toxicity, but there is a very limited body of research that directly addresses the pathways by which these drugs might result in persistent changes that produce adverse events that may or may not be reversible. In general, while the animal and in vitro studies support different biologic actions of the antimalarials, the published experimental research has not rigorously tested biologic plausibility in its fullest sense with regard to the impact of prolonged treatment (as would occur in prophylaxis) of relevant doses on well-defined behavioral and neurologic endpoints. Most studies reviewed involve acute drug treatment, which may or may not be relevant to long-term administration in the setting of prophylaxis; involve supratherapeutic dosing in laboratory-based animal in vivo studies; or involve the use of in vitro systems that do not duplicate the full context of prophylaxis regimens. While the data provide hints of processes that may be relevant to the central question at hand (the plausibility of pathology following prolonged treatment), relatively few address it directly (which is highlighted in the drug-specific chapters where relevant). The pathways by which drug use for a defined period leads to irreversible biological changes that manifest as clinically recognizable symptoms or diagnoses have simply not been pursued. Many of the available basic science experimental studies have examined outcomes that do not directly link to recognizable clinical symptoms or manifestations in humans. As a result, there is very little information that can be gleaned from these types of basic science studies to provide information about the mechanisms of the adverse events observed in the epidemiologic studies.

Cumulatively, while the available research to date points toward possible avenues to pursue based on acute adverse events and case reports, the small number of directly pertinent studies precludes drawing firm conclusions. The committee has attempted to glean the most information that the scientific literature offers but, at most, only tentative inferences are possible.

QUALITY OF METHODS OF REVIEWED STUDIES

Several methodologic considerations were introduced in Chapter 3 that the committee used to assess the quality of individual studies. Providing a detailed appraisal of the methodologic quality of each of the identified epidemiologic studies allowed the committee to offer tentative inferences from very limited evidence with a clear appreciation of how fragile those inferences were. For the epidemiologic studies, those principles included study design (population, sample size, comparison groups), exposure assessment, outcome assessment, and confounding.

Study Design

As this work is at the request of the Department of Veterans Affairs (VA), the specific population of greatest interest is U.S. military service members and veterans. However, antimalarial prophylaxis is not limited to these two groups, and it is reasonable to assume that research conducted in other populations may provide relevant information regarding the persistence of adverse events following the prophylactic use of antimalarial drugs, and thus, studies of non-military populations were included in the committee's assessment. An important consideration in incorporating any evidence from non-military populations is the evaluation of differences between these groups and the military population of interest and assessing whether these differences may influence the interpretation of study results. In earlier chapters, results are reported of studies conducted using Peace Corps volunteers, pre-screened research volunteers (particularly those recruited for randomized clinical trials), travelers, and endemic populations. Recruitment into military service includes thorough health screenings and assessments that are likely very different from those experienced by, for instance, Peace Corps volunteers, and this pre-military screening may result in the exclusion of individuals with specific physical or psychological characteristics. If these health characteristics are contraindications to the use of specific prophylactic antimalarials, for example, then one may expect a lower incidence of the adverse outcomes in military and veteran populations as a result of screening out individuals at higher risk of adverse outcomes from the antimalarials of interest. Moreover, over the duration of their military careers, which may include multiple deployments or temporary duty assignments, service members may use a drug multiple times. People who experienced adverse outcomes while using a specific drug may elect (if given a choice) to use a different drug. This would result in a "depletion of susceptibles," which means that people who may have adverse events are no longer in the risk pool, which could result in an observed lower incidence of adverse outcomes for a certain drug. In the studies of populations of military and veterans evaluated by the committee, prior users were either excluded or the use of multiple drugs was censored.

A further consideration of the populations studied is the location and intent of the travel. For military populations, travel is usually occupation related (i.e., deployment), and it likely results in stress prior to travel and, depending on the circumstances, additional stress and possibly trauma and combat while in the deployment location. Other characteristics of the deployment location may also confound the association between antimalarial prophylaxis and adverse outcomes, including environmental or other exposures (see Concurrent Exposures of Military Service in Chapter 2) that may adversely affect health. In studies of travelers, most often the purpose of the travel is for leisure, the location of the travel is chosen (rather than mandated), the time is typically short term (weeks to few months), and the location is very unlikely to be an area of civil unrest or active conflict. There are limits to how informative studies based on leisure travelers or other populations, such as people living in malaria-endemic areas who may have naturally acquired immunity to malaria, can be to persistent adverse health effects in military or veteran populations.

Comparison Groups

The committee was asked to focus its assessment on the potential association between the use of any of the six FDA-approved antimalarial drugs for prophylaxis and persistent or latent adverse events. It was not asked to assess the efficacy of the antimalarials of interest, nor was it asked to compare the antimalarial drugs on the basis of toxicity. Ideally, research should be conducted to enable the comparison of each antimalarial separately against a meaningful comparison group. In the context of antimalarial prophylaxis, this is a difficult task, given that the indication for antimalarial use is travel to a malaria-endemic area. Antimalarials are highly recommended for such travel, so that it is difficult to identify, for comparison purposes, population subgroups who travel to malaria-endemic areas but do not take antimalarials. Furthermore, in the case of travelers to malaria-endemic areas who do not take antimalarials, the reasons for that choice could confound the associations reported from such studies unless the authors have collected information on the reasons for nonuse. For the most part, the epidemiologic studies have examined the adverse outcomes in groups that differ on which antimalarial they have used for malaria prophylaxis. Thus, the comparisons are necessarily relative (e.g., how does mefloquine compare to chloroquine?) rather than absolute (e.g., how does mefloquine compare to no antimalarial use?). The answers to both questions are relevant, but the conclusions that can be drawn about a specific antimalarial are limited by these designs: when comparing two antimalarial drugs, the inferences will be limited to statements that the two drugs are equivalent in their adverse event profile or that one drug is "more harmful" than the other drug. The latter conclusion implies that the other drug will appear as "less harmful," but the absolute impact of the drug is unknown. Within studies of military personnel there are also comparisons of deployed versus nondeployed personnel (Eick-Cost et al., 2017; Schneiderman et al., 2018; Wells et al., 2006), but study designs could also conceivably compare deployment location (endemic area versus not, as in Wells et al., 2006). The committee did not find any studies that made comparisons across different types of antimalarial drug users (e.g., leisure travelers versus military personnel).

Exposure Assessment

Assessing exposure outside of a clinical trial (i.e., where the drug is assigned to an individual by a process of randomization and is often monitored for adherence) is also challenging. Medications are prescribed by a health professional, and it is often up to the individual to fill the prescription and then to take the medication as prescribed. In research conducted using pharmacy or prescription databases, often the only available information is about the prescription dispensed (dose, regimen, number of tablets, date of prescription or dispensing), not about how well the individual adhered to the medication regimen. Details concerning medication adherence are often obtained through self-report, and individuals may be asked to recall medication details from the recent or even distant past (e.g., Schneiderman et al., 2018; Tan et al., 2017). In studies of people who are employed by or participate in organizations in which the use of antimalarial drugs for prophylaxis is required (e.g., military, Peace Corps, Department of State), reported adherence rates may be inflated. All these limitations add to the difficulty in being able to evaluate the role of the duration of medication use and the specifics of the doses taken. An additional challenge when studying adverse events of drugs is that the occurrence of adverse events may cause an individual to decide to modify the dose, or even stop the drug completely, without consulting a health professional. Individuals may decide to change their regimen when the adverse effect is minor and not serious enough to report but still is bothersome to the individual. Such changes are rarely recorded, and people may be reluctant to admit that they did not take the medication as prescribed. These individuals would still be counted in the exposed categories, but there would be no drug-associated adverse events. Another concern related to exposure assessment is the phenomenon known as the "depletion of susceptibles" (introduced under Study Design). This phenomenon can occur when the initiation of a drug is associated with acute effects early on, followed by a decrease in the frequency of the effects as time goes on. If individuals who stop taking the drug because of these early events are no longer followed, they do not contribute to the follow-up time. This is a form of selection bias in studies that do not use a new-user design and count all person-time in follow-up equally.

Along the same lines, most of the epidemiologic studies that met the committee's inclusion criteria did not collect information on any previous use of antimalarials prior to the time of the study. For example, Eick-Cost et al. (2017) identified service members filling a prescription for mefloquine, doxycycline, or A/P between January 1, 2008, and June 30, 2013, but service members could have used one of these (or other) antimalarials prior to 2008. Those individuals who previously took an antimalarial and experienced no adverse effects would be more likely to take an antimalarial again and to adhere with the regimen and also less likely to experience adverse events. Without specific information on adherence to the antimalarials, the committee has to assume good adherence when assessing the studies unless the authors specifically noted otherwise. Thus there could have been unmeasured misclassification of drug use, with nonusers or suboptimal users being classified as users, potentially attenuating the associations between antimalarial use and adverse health outcomes. Studies that used drug dispensing records as their sole way of ascertaining drug exposures have certain limitations, including uncertainty as to whether the dispensed medications were actually ingested (Eick-Cost et al., 2017; Schneider et al., 2013, 2014; Wells et al., 2006). Furthermore, as noted in Chapter 3, relying solely on dispensing records for determining exposure to medicines used to prevent a disease may lead to an overestimation of peoples' exposure to a given medicine, particularly if there is reason to believe that the drug is associated with concurrent adverse events.

Outcome Assessment

The gold standard for outcome assessment is the clinical assessment of individuals at multiple time points. This is rarely feasible in epidemiologic research, but there are a variety of both active and passive sources of information that can be used when conducting research to identify persistent or latent adverse events. The first step, however, is to specify and define the outcomes of interest, preferably using standardized diagnoses or definitions of outcomes. Given the dearth of available and informative literature on the persistent or latent adverse events associated with the use of antimalarial drugs, this area of research is in its infancy, and often the specific outcome is not defined, but instead broad classes of outcomes are included, such as "gastrointestinal effects" or "neuropsychiatric disorders." In the research that forms the basis of this report, even with broad classes of outcomes, definitions vary considerably. It is difficult to make comparisons across studies when not only the definitions or methods of adverse-event collection vary but also the sources of data are often different (i.e., self-report, medical records, administrative databases, etc.). A variety of methods were used by the different studies to elicit the occurrence of adverse events, including nonspecific questions (such as overall satisfaction of using a drug [Andersson et al., 2008]), checklists of symptoms or symptom diaries (e.g., Davis et al., 1996; Jaspers et al., 1996; Korhonen et al., 2007; Petersen et al., 2000; Rendi-Wagner et al., 2002; Tan et al., 2017), standardized instruments and tests (Boudreau et al.,1993; Schlagenhauf et al., 1996; Schneiderman et al., 2018), and *International Classification of Diseases* or other administrative coded diagnoses (e.g., Eick-Cost et al., 2017; Schneider et al., 2013, 2014; Wells et al., 2006).

A particular challenge in outcome assessment is that there needs to be clarity regarding the temporal sequence of the outcomes of interest (e.g., incident during prophylaxis, incident after cessation of prophylaxis, incident during prophylaxis and continuing after cessation, etc.). Without a known temporal sequence, the associations generated are difficult to interpret with regard to the timing of the drug use and the adverse events. In particular, measuring antimalarial exposure and outcomes at the same time (as in a cross-sectional survey) may lead to bias if respondents misremember which happened first (exposure or outcome), and, in fact, previous psychiatric conditions may actually lead to different antimalarial exposures as they are contraindicated for certain drugs.

Approaches to Assessing Neurologic and Psychiatric Outcomes

The assessment of neurologic and psychiatric outcomes, especially posttraumatic stress disorder (PTSD), which is included in the Statement of Task, may be challenging for a number of reasons. First, for a diagnosis of PTSD, the person should have been exposed to an identified traumatic event by directly experiencing it, witnessing it in person, learning that the traumatic event occurred to a close family member or close friend (with the actual or threatened death being either violent or accidental), or experiencing firsthand repeated or extreme exposure to aversive details of the traumatic event (not through media, pictures, television, or movies unless work related). The *Diagnostic and Statistical Manual of Mental Disorders, Fifth Edition* (DSM-5) criteria explicitly exclude medication from being the potentially traumatic event. Therefore, while some patients may experience symptoms of PTSD following exposure to a drug, PTSD symptoms must be related to experiencing trauma (e.g., combat). This may make a clear relationship between taking a medication and a resultant diagnosis of PTSD difficult to ascertain because the symptoms involved the exposure to trauma and their onset relative to taking a medication is hypothetical at best. It may be that exposure to a specific medication or several medications taken together confers an elevated risk for PTSD in the context of a different traumatic experience. It may be that concurrent adverse events associated with a medication may themselves be traumatic, but the current empirical literature and classification systems do not allow for such an assertion as the basis for a PTSD diagnosis. Second, for PTSD the reported symptoms should be directly related to the specific traumatic event reported by the person. Third, because there are currently no diagnostically valid and reliable biomarkers of PTSD, the diagnosis of any psychiatric outcomes is based on the patient's self-reported experiences, which may be biased or distorted by memory processes known to be influenced by stress and fear. For certain groups (e.g., service members), there may be also incentives to minimize or deny the experience of stigmatized neuropsychiatric symptoms, such as when acknowledging such symptoms may result in the individual's removal from duties, or there may be an incentive to over-report these symptoms, such as in the case of financial compensation related to disability. Symptoms or experiences such as nightmares, hallucinations, or paranoia may be particularly stigmatized and, as a result, possibly under-reported.

When PTSD was assessed in the reviewed studies (e.g., Eick-Cost et al., 2017; Schneiderman et al., 2018; Wells et al., 2006), the potentially traumatic events experienced previous to drug exposure and concurrently with drug exposure were not systematically assessed. Therefore, any associations between use of an antimalarial drug and PTSD symptoms were generally insufficiently ascertained. Confounders, for example, may influence such associations (e.g., PTSD could be wrongly diagnosed because the drug's symptoms mimic PTSD).

A systematic assessment of DSM-5 or *International Classification of Diseases, Tenth Revision* criteria by a trained clinician can improve diagnostic accuracy, as can the use of psychometrically sound self-report assessment tools. The use of standardized methods of assessment can reduce, although not completely eliminate, potential reporting biases. Assessing the timing of a potentially traumatic event, medication exposure, and symptom onset and content is critical to answering the scientific question of whether there are persistent psychiatric outcomes associated with antimalarial use. Additionally, it is important to recognize that it may be normal to experience some symptoms of depression, PTSD, anxiety, etc., but meeting the full diagnostic criteria is rarer, further making the measurement of these outcomes challenging.

Drug-Associated Neurologic and Psychiatric Adverse Effects

The committee was charged with assessing the evidence for persistent adverse events, with an emphasis on neurologic or psychiatric events, that are associated with the use of antimalarial drugs when used for prophylaxis. The concurrent use of many prescription drugs has been associated with neuropsychiatric adverse events, and therefore the manifestations associated with antimalarials are not unique. Such outcomes include depression, agitation, confusion, psychosis, seizures, a change in the level of consciousness, and nightmares (Ruha and Levine, 2014). Although the mechanisms of some drug-associated neuropsychiatric effects have been elucidated, for many drugs the mechanisms remain unknown. In addition, there is little information about persistent effects for these types of events.

There is a body of evidence concerning persistent effects following the cessation of drugs associated with addiction (Korpi et al., 2015) as well as on tardive dykinesia, a movement disorder, following the cessation of antipsychotic drugs (Macaluso et al., 2016). However, these types of studies appear to be the exception. For other drugs with well-recognized and common acute neuropsychiatric effects, there is no information about persistence. For example, glucocorticoids, which are used for a wide variety of inflammatory conditions, and efavirenz, a very effective HIV-1 antiviral, are associated with a high frequency of such effects. Judd et al. (2014) reviewed neuropsychiatric effects associated with glucocorticoids. In one large study, patients taking glucocorticoids were four to seven times more likely to develop suicide/suicide attempt, delirium/confusion, and mania than age-, gender-, practitioner-, and disease-matched controls. The incidence of such outcomes approached 20% for those on high doses. Dalwadi et al. (2018) reviewed neuropsychiatric events associated with efavirenz, including abnormal dreams, sleep disturbance, anxiety, depression, and dizziness. The incidence of such adverse outcomes exceeds 50% in most studies. Symptoms improve over time for many, but not all, and the trajectory of symptoms after withdrawal is unknown.

Thus, neuropsychiatric symptoms are associated with many prescription drugs, and for some, like mefloquine, there is good evidence that the acute events are causally related to drugs used as prescribed. It is plausible that a prolonged continuation of drugs that continue to produce disturbing neuropsychiatric signs and symptoms might lead to persistent effects after drug cessation. It is equally, if not more, plausible that drug-related signs and symptoms go away with drug withdrawal and that the persistence or recurrence of neuropsychiatric events after drug cessation would have occurred regardless of drug exposure.

Confounders

As noted above, there are medical contraindications for some of the antimalarials. While these contraindications (e.g., a previous psychiatric history) are not always followed either because this information is not available or because, when asked, the individual does not provide this information to the medical care provider, any tendency to preferentially give one drug versus another because of a history of health problems has the potential to introduce substantial confounding if not addressed explicitly in the analysis. Depending on the analysis methods used, such contraindications could possibly lead to a depletion of susceptibles, as discussed under the heading of Study Design, and result in findings of decreased risk of certain adverse events, such as specific psychiatric diagnoses, among mefloquine users compared with doxycycline or A/P users. Without the information on prior psychiatric history from the groups being studied, for example, the observed results may be confounded by the contraindication for use, and it is not possible to stratify by psychiatric history or restrict the analysis to those without a history of psychiatric disorders. Depending on the frequency of the contraindication and the difference in frequency across the comparison groups, the magnitude of this potential confounding bias will vary and thus be unknown in any given situation. Furthermore, as contraindications for selected antimalarials are introduced over time, studies will differ in their susceptibility to this bias in relation to the altered prescribing practices applicable at the time that drugs are being prescribed.

In addition, as described in earlier chapters, there are other exposures (e.g., concomitant drug exposures, combat, etc.) that may place individuals at a higher risk of experiencing adverse events. In military populations, there is a particular concern with the many other challenges associated with deployment in addition to any impact of antimalarial drug use. These would include the exposure to and threat of combat and trauma, social isolation resulting from separation from family and friends, and cultural dislocation from living in an environment notably different from home. If this information is not available for the drug groups being compared, then, again, confounding bias may result if the prevalence of these conditions differs by the type of drug used. At a minimum, it is important that the groups being compared are equally likely to have been deployed to a location potentially involved in combat in order to avoid substantial confounding. For example, in their analyses, Schneiderman et al. (2018) assessed exposure to combat as both a dichotomous variable (yes/no) and as a multiple-level variable to assess combat intensity.

COMPARISONS OF FINDINGS ACROSS ALL
ANTIMALARIAL DRUGS OF INTEREST

A total of 21 primary epidemiologic studies (Ackert et al., 2019; Andersen et al., 1998; DeSouza, 1983; Eick-Cost et al., 2017; Green et al., 2014; Laothavorn et al., 1992; Leary et al., 2009; Lee et al., 2013; Lege-Oguntoye et al., 1990; Meier et al., 2004; Miller et al., 2013; Nasveld et al., 2010; Rueangweerayut et al., 2017; Schlagenhauf et al., 1996; Schneider et al., 2013, 2014; Schneiderman et al., 2018; Schwartz and Regev-Yochay, 1999; Tan et al., 2017; Walsh et al., 2004; Wells et al., 2006) were identified that met the committee's inclusion criteria and were assessed in detail for the information they provided regarding persistent or latent adverse effects. Nine of these studies included multiple drugs of interest, and they contribute to the evidence in multiple chapters. A table that gives a high-level comparison (study design, population, exposure groups, and outcomes examined by body system) of each of these epidemiologic studies is presented in Appendix C. Just over half of the identified studies (11 primary studies) examined exposure to mefloquine. Fewer primary epidemiologic studies met inclusion for the other drugs of interest: tafenoquine, 7; A/P, 4; doxycycline, 7; primaquine, 4; and chloroquine, 3. From the perspective of biologic plausibility, the mechanistic links between antimalarial drugs and persistent or latent adverse outcomes have yet to be systematically and definitively explored through experimental studies, and the current literature in that area is not strong.

In general, five outcome categories emerged as the areas of greatest interest in the literature: neurologic, psychiatric, gastrointestinal, eye, and cardiovascular. Although for the majority of outcomes in this entire body of literature, no firm conclusions were warranted, in some cases suggestive patterns were apparent and useful to note. In its examination and assessment of the available evidence, the committee was looking for signals of associations and it endeavored to be sensitive rather than specific, so that even isolated findings that may well reflect random error from making multiple comparisons or those that have not been corroborated are reported. Ultimately, replications of results were considered indications of stronger evidence for an association that the committee considered in its weighting but in assessing the rather limited literature, some of the indications may not be confirmed with further research. The concern about neurologic and psychiatric effects was most apparent for mefloquine compared with the other antimalarials. For tafenoquine and chloroquine there was emphasis placed on adverse events associated with eye disorders. Doxycycline's known concurrent gastrointestinal adverse events, which are commonly experienced, have led to some concern about the development of chronic gastrointestinal diseases, but the only study focused on this issue had significant methodologic limitations. The major issue with primaquine and tafenoquine is the risk of hemolysis associated with glucose-6-phosphate dehydrogenase (G6PD) deficiency. A/P has the fewest concurrent adverse events reported, and there is insufficient evidence for any persistent event associated with

A/P; for that reason it is often used as a comparator in studies of other antimalarial drugs. Several of the studies (Eick-Cost et al., 2017; Nasveld et al., 2010; Schneider et al., 2013, 2014; Tan et al., 2017) used comparisons with different antimalarials rather than a placebo or nonuse. As described earlier in the report, the difficulty with conducting such comparisons is that results from analyses that compare one drug with another may result in an observed lack of difference in effect because both drugs cause the adverse events. This is concerning because the use of antimalarial drugs in malaria-endemic areas is recommended, and a user's choice of drug may be informed by the frequency and type of adverse events reported.

Of the 31 conclusions that the committee considered across all drugs and outcome categories, in all but one case the evidence of an association between the drug of interest and persistent or latent adverse events was deemed inadequate or insufficient. The committee concluded that there was sufficient evidence of an association between the use of tafenoquine and vortex keratopathy, which although it was found to persist beyond 28 days, was also found to resolve within 3 to 12 months and did not have a clinical implication, such as loss of vision. There was no convincing evidence of latent effects that did not manifest in individuals while they were taking the antimalarial and only emerged later, after drug cessation, with the exception of some eye disorders observed for A/P users. Individuals with past exposure (i.e., more than 90 days after the last day of use) to A/P were more likely to develop eye disorders than nonusers. This association was not present for current use. Based on information from studies of short-term follow-up, case reports, and biologic plausibility, the committee considers the existence of some persistent events, such as vertigo and tinnitus, to be highly plausible for certain antimalarials. For this reason, in its conclusion for each outcome category, the committee specifies whether the existing evidence warrants additional research in a specific area. For those health outcomes for which the committee concluded there is not a clear justification for additional research, the intention was to distinguish those issues for which there is presently an empirical basis for looking more closely and those for which such a basis is not present based on the currently available evidence. The committee's intention is not to dismiss any issue or outcome but rather to highlight those in which a signal has been detected that warrants further study of a potential association. As more research accumulates, the outcomes that warrant further research may change or new ones that were not previously reported may become recognized, such as from additional case reports or mechanistic studies.

ADVANCING RESEARCH ON ANTIMALARIAL DRUGS

Given the seriousness of malaria and the billions of people at risk for it, and given that the parasite continues to develop resistance to currently available prophylactic drugs, there will be a continuing need for the currently available antimalarial drugs as well as new ones. Studying the persistent and latent effects of exposures is challenging, and therefore it is important to recognize that seeking perfect or complete understanding is likely unrealistic. That said, in order to establish causal links between antimalarial exposure and persistent adverse events, it would be important to have a series of randomized trials designed to answer the specific safety questions ethically, with a long-term follow-up of participants and multiple well-designed observational studies of varying design with well-documented drug exposures and adverse event outcomes that control for confounding in rigorous ways. These studies would ideally have explicit documentation of the timing of antimalarial drug use and symptom occurrence (with clear temporal ordering), an extended follow-up that includes assessments at multiple time points, and a validated collection of information regarding potential confounders, antimalarial exposure (dose and timing), and the outcomes of potential interest, including a careful collection of neurologic and psychiatric outcomes using validated instruments. Given that some of the outcomes of concern are or may be rare, it will also be important to have sample sizes that are sufficient to detect associations if they do exist. While carrying out a large set of studies that has all of those components may not be realistic, there are strong designs that take advantage of existing data sets that would be possible. In addition, a series of well-designed studies that each has a number of (but perhaps not all) these components could be quite informative, and it could be used to triangulate the evidence to develop an understanding of the potential mechanisms and persistent adverse events. For example, studies that use large-scale electronic health records (including drug dispensing or prescribing records) with long-term follow-up of individuals could be used with strong non-experimental study designs and be complemented with studies of the biologic pathways that evaluate the link between the pharmacologic effects of drugs and the clinical conditions of interest. Additionally, if a sufficient number of studies are available, meta-analyses may be possible and very informative.

A key limitation of the existing literature is that very few studies were designed specifically to examine latent or persistent adverse events. However, more recently there has been more interest in assessing potential persistent or latent adverse events of antimalarial drugs, as compared with when the first of these drugs were approved in the 1940s and 1950s. The market authorization holder of tafenoquine is pursuing two required Phase IV trials to evaluate long-term tafenoquine safety. The first, NCT03320174, which is currently recruiting participants, is a randomized double-blind placebo-controlled study that will enroll 600 healthy G6PD-normal volunteers. Participants who meet the eligibility criteria will be randomized to receive a loading dose of either tafenoquine 200 mg (2 × 100 mg tablets) or placebo daily for 3 consecutive days, followed by study treatment (tafenoquine 200 mg or placebo) once per week for 51 weeks, with safety follow-up visits at weeks 4, 12, 24, and 52. All participants will return to the clinic at week 64 for an end-of-study visit. A participant who has an ongoing adverse event at the week 64 visit will be assessed up to three more times at approximately 12-week intervals, or until the resolution or stabilization of the adverse event, whichever comes first. In addition, a large observational study to compare the rates of rare adverse events of tafenoquine relative to A/P in travelers (>10,000 participants) is in the planning stages.[1] These studies, and others like them, offer an excellent opportunity to study a broader set of persistent or latent outcomes.

With regard to mefloquine specifically, several factors may influence whether additional studies of its use for malaria prophylaxis are conducted and how informative those results will be. Although mefloquine is still recommended for civilian use, the numbers of prescriptions for it have declined substantially, likely in part due to the 2013 FDA boxed warning, media reports of adverse events, and the availability of similarly efficacious drugs with comparatively fewer adverse events or different adverse event profiles. Since 2009, Department of Defense (DoD) policy has been to restrict the use of mefloquine for service members to people who cannot take the other available antimalarials and do not have a history of the contraindications; in those who cannot take the other available antimalarials and have a history of neurobehavioral disorders, it is to be used very cautiously with clinical follow-up. In 2017, the latest year for which current prescription information is available, mefloquine was prescribed to a total of 52 individuals on active duty (Wiesen, 2019). Therefore, any prospective or retrospective studies conducted using service members since the policies went into effect will lack generalizability, and the channeling of persons who are healthier or who have previously tolerated mefloquine may account for some of the findings of no difference in frequency of most outcomes compared with other antimalarials in the literature.

Administrative Databases

Some of the most informative studies thus far have used health care databases or other data sources that cover large populations. Therefore, a logical place to look for additional opportunities is in other large databases that include a sufficiently large number of individuals who used antimalarial drugs and provide documentation of their subsequent health experience, or else by obtaining data needed for both exposure and outcome assessment by linking several large databases. Before embarking on such studies, it will be essential to first ensure that there is sufficient information on exposure and outcomes for a population large enough to generate meaningful results.

Information on U.S. military populations has been valuable, as reflected in studies of veterans participating in the National Health Study for a New Generation of U.S. Veterans (referred to as the "NewGen Study") (Schneiderman et al., 2018), hospitalization data for active-duty service personnel (Wells et al., 2006), and a study with potentially greater value (limited because the timing of adverse events was not distinguished in the presented results) on medical encounters among

---

[1] Personal communication to the committee, Geoffrey Dow, M.B.A., Ph.D., Chairman and Chief Executive Officer of 60 Degrees Pharmaceuticals, LLC, January 28, 2019.

active-duty personnel (Eick-Cost et al., 2017). There may be value in revisiting other data resources generated for the study of military personnel to assess the feasibility of conducting informative research. Such sources might include general VA health care databases, registries such as the one developed for exposure to open burn pits, and cohorts assembled previously. Other countries, particularly those with national health care systems, may also have sufficient numbers of personnel deployed to areas in which malaria is endemic to learn from their experiences. For example, data could include which antimalarials were prescribed or used for different deployments and, for people who had multiple deployments, the health care experience during the deployed and nondeployed intervals as opposed to whether a condition or diagnosis was or was not present following the cessation of an antimalarial. However, as previously discussed, when using large databases for research, good adherence is assumed when in practice that has not been demonstrated to be the case.

Beyond the value of further observational research on military populations, the potential for randomized trials warrants serious consideration. Active-duty military and veterans currently participate in two distinct but overlapping health care systems administered by DoD and VA, respectively, which could facilitate examination of potential long-term health outcomes of exposures that occurred during active-duty service. Both DoD and VA collect a vast amount of health data on their personnel. VA has been a champion of the concept of a learning health care system, in which system factors are used to help incorporate established evidence into practice and reciprocally, in which new evidence is generated from a combination of rigorous analysis of quality improvement efforts and independent research investigations (Atkins et al., 2017). Although current ethical frameworks may distinguish the practice of quality improvement from research, some argue that research and practice should be viewed together in a learning health care environment. Furthermore, a case can be made that there is a moral obligation to incorporate important research questions into routine clinical practice so that such practice can be improved (Faden et al., 2013). An aspirational goal of both military and civilian health care systems might include transparently and prospectively incorporating large clinical trials (including pragmatic trials) and/or observational studies into routine practice. While there are an array of logistic and ethical considerations—especially because the people using and served by these systems may be considered populations with limited decision-making autonomy—the potential value of addressing possible health consequences of antimalarial prophylaxis in the population of interest using DoD and VA health information systems offers tremendous potential to advance knowledge and should be considered for future studies.

General population databases also have merit, as illustrated by the studies based on the UK General Practice Research Database (Meier et al., 2004; Schneider et al., 2013, 2014). Although a detailed evaluation would be required to assess the potential value of databases, large administrative data resources such as

Medicare, Sentinel, Kaiser-Permanente health system database, or commercially available claims databases, such as Optum, might be suitable for examining these issues, making up for a very low prevalence of exposure (and sometimes rare outcomes) with extremely large numbers of enrollees. These data sources—which are intended only to be illustrative of potential data sources and not exhaustive or directive—along with advanced statistical methods, are increasingly being used to study medication-related adverse events, and those methods could be applied to the question of persistent or latent health effects associated with the use of antimalarial drugs. However, an examination of psychiatric disorders, and the associated measurement difficulties, bring particular challenges that will need to be carefully considered, as discussed earlier in this chapter. For example, it may be particularly important to have longitudinal data on individuals so as to be able to account for pre-antimalarial exposure to mental health conditions and other exposures. One limitation of standard data sources such as these will be a lack of detailed information on non-medical factors, such as socioeconomic factors or military service. As such, large DoD and VA administrative databases that contain military health care records may be of particular use for studying antimalarial use and other exposures among service members over multiple time points.

FDA and Identifying and Evaluating Postmarketing Safety Concerns

FDA requirements for drug licensure have evolved over time. New requirements have often been driven by major safety events (Avorn, 2012; IOM, 2007). Thus, the amount and quality of data available about drugs prior to and post-licensure has improved over time. Many antimalarials were licensed decades ago, which may account in part for the relatively weak pre-licensure safety data for older drugs, such as chloroquine, which was licensed in the United States in 1949, and primaquine, which was licensed in the United States in 1952. Although FDA has the authority to require additional studies when safety concerns arise postmarketing, this authority was historically weak, and even now is used infrequently.

In addition, generic drug companies do not have the same requirements as the company responsible for the original labeled drug, leaving the responsibility for addressing concerns about older drugs unclear. Legislation in the 1980s encouraged the development of generic drugs, which are often less costly to consumers. Companies are required to demonstrate to FDA that their generic drugs are equivalent to the brand name drugs in terms of therapeutic effect, but they do not have to repeat the time-consuming and expensive clinical trials that have already been performed by brand companies to show safety and effectiveness. They are, however, required to establish and maintain records and make reports to FDA of all serious, unexpected adverse drug experiences associated with the use of their drug products (FDA, 2019a). Also, the original manufacturer is the "steward" of new safety issues, not the generic manufacturer, who is often not equipped to perform postmarketing safety studies. However, after generics are introduced, the brand company may stop manufacturing the product or radically reduce resources focused on that product, leaving a gap in responsibility for addressing new safety concerns and new labeling (Kesselheim et al., 2012).

The FDA adverse event reporting system (FAERS) is an important source for potential safety signals. However, adverse events are under-reported, these reports lack complete information, there is uncertainty about whether or not the reported event was caused by the product, and FAERS data cannot be used to calculate the incidence of an adverse event. Additionally, FAERS has little ability to detect relatively common events, such as heart attacks, when the background rate in the population using the drug is relatively high. For example, the drug rofecoxib, a non-steroidal anti-inflammatory drug (NSAID), was on the market for 5 years prior to its withdrawal after a large postmarketing safety study identified an association with cardiovascular events. The trial was designed to show that rofecoxib had superior gastrointestinal safety compared to an older NSAID. The cardiovascular signal was unexpected, and it is unclear when or if this association would have been detected without this study. An estimated 88,000 to 140,000 excess cases of serious coronary heart disease occurred over the time rofecoxib was marketed in the United States (Graham et al., 2005). This event helped stimulate development of the FDA Sentinel Initiative, a network of administrative data and electronic record system data from insurance organizations and health plans that have been transformed into a standardized format. After a pilot period (mini Sentinel), Sentinel was officially launched in 2014. It now maintains a database of medical information on more than 200 million people that includes prescription drug use and health outcomes (FDA, 2019b). FDA's Sentinel system has been designed to address gaps in knowledge about drug safety. Among those gaps is the lack of information on the possible persistent effects of antimalarials.

Collaborations

In its evaluation of the available evidence to address persistent adverse events, the committee identified studies that clearly had collected data that could be informative, but the analyses were either not conducted or not presented in a way that was informative for the committee's purposes. The clearest example of this was Eick-Cost et al. (2017), which referred only in passing to the pattern of health outcomes over time following the cessation of drug use. The investigators collected information that could have been quite helpful had they restricted the analysis to ≥28 days post-drug-cessation. For a substantial proportion of the other studies that qualified for consideration based on having collected health data pertaining to the time period of interest, the committee was unable to draw inferences regarding persistent adverse events because the experience during and after drug use was aggregated or not clearly distinguished. A possible contribution to advancing the literature might come from embarking on selected re-analyses of studies that collected data on adverse events for 28 days post-drug-cessation but did not analyze these data or report them. A re-analysis of individual studies with notable potential value would make the temporal course of drug use and health experience explicit and enable inferences regarding concomitant versus persistent adverse events. Re-analyses could also allow for the discovery of symptoms or diagnoses that covary. For example, if certain symptoms or diagnoses occur together in the same patients, there may be reason to consider a syndrome of "neuropsychiatric" symptoms that co-occur, rather than looking individually at separate neurologic or psychiatric experiences.

A pooled data analysis effort, where there is sufficient compatibility across studies and the ability to apply a standardized approach to classifying exposure and outcome and control for potential confounders, may also move this area of scientific inquiry forward. Many small studies have potentially informative data, but the researchers analyzed or presented the data in uninformative or simply different ways; therefore, assembling and re-analyzing data from these studies could also be beneficial. However, the committee recognizes that a meaningful summary estimate cannot be generated when study methods are fundamentally incompatible. By using standardized methods for making definitions of exposure, outcome, and covariates as compatible as possible and by conducting parallel or unified analyses, inferences may be drawn that go beyond the published results of the component studies.

Approaches to Research That Are Unlikely to Contribute to the Evidence Base

Based on the questions of concern and past experience, there are a number of approaches that are unlikely to provide much insight regarding persistent or latent adverse events of antimalarial drugs. Cross-sectional studies that attempt to correlate drug use and symptoms or diagnoses without the ability to explicitly consider the temporal course of events will not make it possible to separate acute from persistent or latent adverse events. The data need to lend themselves to analyses that can address the temporal sequence of drug use, cessation of drug use, and health experience.

Small clinical trials often contain detailed health information but rarely include sufficiently long follow-up periods to assess persistence, and they almost never have sufficient numbers of participants to provide the needed statistical precision to address clinically significant outcomes. Perhaps with some effort they could address common, relatively mild symptoms of interest longitudinally, but this generally is beyond the scope of what is conventionally done.

Adverse event registries and individual reports of suspected adverse events to medications, such as that used by FDA, provide limited information with regard to rigorous research. While the experiences reported may serve as signals to indicate reactions and events of concern that were not necessarily identified during clinical trials, they also serve to inform when changes to label warnings or precautions may be merited. Because adverse event registries do not provide comparative data on people with varying exposures and do not offer any quantitative data on the frequency with which side effects are experienced, at most they are case reports that offer hints of areas of outcomes to guide subsequent research that is more methodologically rigorous.

Different Strategies and Approaches for Advancing Research

For many complex issues there is no single research approach that can provide definitive answers since all strategies have varying strengths and limitations. The need for convergent evidence and triangulation (integrating results from several different approaches that have different and unrelated key sources of potential bias; see Lawlor et al., 2016) is clearly applicable to the assessment of persistent adverse events of antimalarial drugs. Beyond the continued exploitation of large administrative databases, some other designs warrant consideration for complementing such studies.

Conducting studies of "medium-term" adverse events that continue beyond the events that occur while taking a drug (such as those up to 3 or 6 months post-cessation) would be informative if focused and validated assessments of health status were performed over the subsequent weeks or months. This might involve extending clinical trials or systematically following returning travelers with such examinations as clinical evaluations that are sufficiently sensitive to discern even subclinical health status or even carefully constructed questionnaires. While such studies would not likely be large enough to identify rare, clinically significant events, such evidence would complement larger, less detailed studies. To the extent that there are hypotheses regarding which individuals are especially likely to be vulnerable based on genetics, pre-existing health conditions, or other factors, these smaller, more intensive evaluations could target such high-risk groups.

Large case–control studies of specific adverse events or health outcomes of interest could, provided there was sufficient prevalence of exposure, generate additional evidence on associations of antimalarial drugs. Such studies might be best conducted in populations that have more than background rates of exposure, enriched with military personnel, international travelers, or those whose work requires spending time in settings where malaria is endemic, such as Peace Corps volunteers, missionaries, and Department of State employees.

Finally, well-conceived studies of experimental systems, in vitro or in vivo, could provide meaningful information to help in interpreting the evidence from human populations. Attempts to establish correlations between the effects of an antimalarial drug on experimental systems and their effects on humans are particularly difficult because there are well-known species-, sex-, and outcome-specific differences in susceptibility to drug toxicity. Even in humans the data on the adverse effects of the drugs are not consistent across studies. Building on model systems for studying irreversible neurobehavioral effects of drugs—for example, a comparison across antimalarial drugs—would add to the constellation of data to help refine interpretation. Other examples of research that would be required for suitable rigor include (1) testing of the impact of prolonged exposure to biologically relevant antimalarial dosing (e.g., human dose adjusted to lab animal drug clearance/metabolism) across a battery of behavioral tests with face validity for persistent or latent psychiatric, neurologic, or other disorders and (2) in vivo testing of lasting antimalarial-induced cell loss and toxicity using contemporary standards of assessment, such as a stereologic assessment of cell loss, microglioisis, astrocytosis, and white matter loss in multiple brain regions and tissues of interest.

REFERENCES

Ackert, J., K. Mohamed, J. S. Slakter, S. El-Harazi, A. Berni, H. Gevorkyan, E. Hardaker, A. Hussaini, S. W. Jones, G. C. K. W. Koh, J. Patel, S. Rasmussen, D. S. Kelly, D. E. Baranano, J. T. Thompson, K. A. Warren, R. C. Sergott, J. Tonkyn, A. Wolstenholme, H. Coleman, A. Yuan, S. Duparc, and J. A. Green. 2019. Randomized placebo-controlled trial evaluating the ophthalmic safety of single-dose tafenoquine in healthy volunteers. *Drug Saf* 42(9):1103-1114.

Andersson, H., H. H. Askling, B. Falck, and L. Rombo. 2008. Well-tolerated chemoprophylaxis uniformly prevented Swedish soldiers from *Plasmodium falciparum* malaria in Liberia, 2004-2006. *Mil Med* 173(12):1194-1198.

Atkins, D., A. M. Kilbourne, and D. Shulkin. 2017. Moving from discovery to system-wide change: The role of research in a learning health care system: Experience from three decades of health systems research in the Veterans Health Administration. *Annu Rev Public Health* 38:467-487.

Avorn, J. 2012. Two centuries of assessing drug risks. *N Engl J Med* 367:193-197.

Boudreau, E., B. Schuster, J. Sanchez, W. Novakowski, R. Johnson, D. Redmond, R. Hanson, and L. Dausel. 1993. Tolerability of prophylactic Lariam regimens. *Trop Med Parasitol* 44(3):257-265.

Dalwadi, D. A., L. Ozuna, B. H. Harvey, M. Viljoen, and J. A. Schetz. 2018. Adverse neuropsychiatric events and recreational use of efavirenz and other HIV-1 antiretroviral drugs. *Pharmacol Rev* 70(3):684-711.

Davis, T. M., L. G. Dembo, S. A. Kaye-Eddie, B. J. Hewitt, R. G. Hislop, and K. T. Batty. 1996. Neurological, cardiovascular and metabolic effects of mefloquine in healthy volunteers: A double-blind, placebo-controlled trial. *Br J Clin Pharmacol* 42(4):415-421.

DeSouza, J. M. 1983. Phase I clinical trial of mefloquine in Brazilian male subjects. *Bull WHO* 61(5):809-814.

Eick-Cost, A. A., Z. Hu, P. Rohrbeck, and L. L. Clark. 2017. Neuropsychiatric outcomes after mefloquine exposure among U.S. military service members. *Am J Trop Med Hyg* 96(1):159-166.

Faden, R. R., N. E. Kass, S. N. Goodman, P. Pronovost, S. Tunis, and T. L. Beauchamp. 2013. An ethics framework for a learning health care system: A departure from traditional research ethics and clinical ethics. Ethical Oversight of Learning Health Care Systems, *Hastings Cent Rep.* Special Report 43 1:S16-S27.

FDA (Food and Drug Administration). 2019a. *21 CFR § 310.305: Prescription drugs marketed for human use without approved new drug applications.* https://www.accessdata.fda.gov/scripts/cdrh/cfdocs/cfcfr/CFRSearch.cfm?fr=310.305 (accessed November 1, 2019).

FDA. 2019b. *Sentinel initiative.* https://www.sentinelinitiative.org/sentinel/data/snapshot-database-statistics (accessed November 1, 2019).

Graham, D. J., D. Campen, R. Hui, M. Spence, C. Cheetham, G. Levy, S. Shoor, and W. A. Ray. 2005. Risk of acute myocardial infarction and sudden cardiac death in patients treated with cyclo-oxygenase 2 selective and non-selective non-steroidal anti-inflammatory drugs: Nested case-control study. *Lancet* 365(9458):475-481.

Green, J. A., A. K. Patel, B. R. Patel, A. Hussaini, E. J. Harrell, M. J. McDonald, N. Carter, K. Mohamed, S. Duparc, and A. K. Miller. 2014. Tafenoquine at therapeutic concentrations does not prolong Fridericia-corrected QT interval in healthy subjects. *J Clin Pharmacol* 54:995-1005.

IOM (Institute of Medicine). 2007. *The future of drug safety: Promoting and protecting the health of the public.* Washington, DC: The National Academies Press.

Jaspers, C. A., A. P. Hopperus Buma, P. P. van Thiel, R. A. van Hulst, and P. A. Kager. 1996. Tolerance of mefloquine chemoprophylaxis in Dutch military personnel. *Am J Trop Med Hyg* 55(2):230-234.

Judd, L. L., P. J. Schettler, E. S. Brown, O. M. Wolkowitz, E. M. Sternberg, B. G. Bender, K. Bulloch, J. A. Cidlowski, E. R. de Kloet, L. Fardet, M. Joëls, D. Y. Leung, B. S. McEwen, B. Roozendaal, E. F. Van Rossum, J. Ahn, D. W. Brown, A. Plitt, and G. Singh. 2014. Adverse consequences of glucocorticoid medication: Psychological, cognitive, and behavioral effects. *Am J Psychiatry* 171(10):1045-1051. Erratum in *Am J Psychiatry*. 2014. 171(11):1224.

Kesselheim, A. S., J. Avorn, and J. A. Greene. 2012. Risk, responsibility, and generic drugs. *N Engl J Med* 367(18):1679-1681.

Korhonen, C., K. Peterson, C. Bruder, and P. Jung. 2007. Self-reported adverse events associated with antimalarial chemoprophylaxis in Peace Corps volunteers. *Am J Prev Med* 33(3):194-199.

Korpi, E. R., B. den Hollander, U. Farooq, E. Vashchinkina, R. Rajkumar, D. J. Nutt, P. Hyytiä, and G. S. Dawe. 2015. Mechanisms of action and persistent neuroplasticity by drugs of abuse. *Pharmacol Rev* 67(4):872-1004.

Laothavorn, P., J. Karbwang, K. Na Bangchang, D. Bunnag, and T. Harinasuta. 1992. Effect of mefloquine on electrocardiographic changes in uncomplicated falciparum malaria patients. *Southeast Asian J Trop Med Public Health* 23(1):51-54.

Lawlor, D. A., K. Tilling, and G. Davey Smith. 2016. Triangulation in aetiological epidemiology. *Int J Epidemiol* 45(6):1866-1886.

Leary, K. J., M. A. Riel, M. J. Roy, L. R. Cantilena, D. Bi, D. C. Brater, C. van de Pol, K. Pruett, C. Kerr, J. M. Veazey, Jr., R. Beboso, and C. Ohrt. 2009. A randomized, double-blind, safety and tolerability study to assess the ophthalmic and renal effects of tafenoquine 200 mg weekly versus placebo for 6 months in healthy volunteers. *Am J Trop Med Hyg* 81:356-362.

Lee, T. W., L. Russell, M. Deng, and P. R. Gibson. 2013. Association of doxycycline use with the development of gastroenteritis, irritable bowel syndrome and inflammatory bowel disease in Australians deployed abroad. *Intern Med J* 43(8):919-926.

Macaluso, M., A. Flynn, and S. Preskorn. 2016. Determining whether a definitive causal relationship exists between aripiprazole and tardive dyskinesia and/or dystonia in patients with major depressive disorder, part 4: Case report data. *J Psychiatr Pract* 22(3):203-220.

Meier, C. R., K. Wilcock, and S. S. Jick. 2004. The risk of severe depression, psychosis or panic attacks with prophylactic antimalarials. *Drug Saf* 27(3):203-213.

Miller, A. K., E. Harrell, L. Ye, S. Baptiste-Brown, J. P. Kleim, C. Ohrt, S. Duparc, J. J. Möhrle, A. Webster, S. Stinnett, A. Hughes, S. Griffith, and A. P. Beelen. 2013. Pharmacokinetic interactions and safety evaluations of coadministered tafenoquine and chloroquine in healthy subjects. *Br J Clin Pharmacol* 76:858-867.

Nasveld, P. E., M. D. Edstein, M. Reid, L. Brennan, I. E. Harris, S. J. Kitchener, P. A. Leggat, P. Pickford, C. Kerr, C. Ohrt, W. Prescott, and the Tafenoquine Study Team. 2010. Randomized, double-blind study of the safety, tolerability, and efficacy of tafenoquine versus mefloquine for malaria prophylaxis in nonimmune subjects. *Antimicrob Agents Chemother* 54:792-798.

Petersen, E., T. Ronne, A. Ronn, I. Bygbjerg, and S. O. Larsen. 2000. Reported side effects to chloroquine, chloroquine plus proguanil, and mefloquine as chemoprophylaxis against malaria in Danish travelers. *J Travel Med* 7(2):79-84.

Rendi-Wagner, P., H. Noedl, W. H. Wernsdorfer, G. Wiedermann, A. Mikolasek, and H. Kollaritsch. 2002. Unexpected frequency, duration and spectrum of adverse events after therapeutic dose of mefloquine in healthy adults. *Acta Trop* 81(2):167-173.

Ruha, A. M., and M. Levine. 2014. Central nervous system toxicity. *Emerg Med Clin North Am* 32(1):205-221.

Rueangweerayut, R., G. Bancone, E. J. Harrell, A. P. Beelen, S. Kongpatanakul, J. J. Möhrle, V. Rousell, K. Mohamed, A. Qureshi, S. Narayan, N. Yubon, A. Miller, F. H. Nosten, L. Luzzatto, S. Duparc, J.-P. Kleim, and J. A. Green. 2017. Hemolytic potential of tafenoquine in female volunteers heterozygous for glucose-6-phosphate dehydrogenase (G6PD) deficiency (G6PD Mahidol variant) versus G6PD normal volunteers. *Am J Trop Med Hyg* 97(3):702-711.

Schlagenhauf, P., R. Steffen, H. Lobel, R. Johnson, R. Letz, A. Tschopp, N. Vranjes, Y. Bergqvist, O. Ericsson, U. Hellgren, L. Rombo, S. Mannino, J. Handschin, and D. Sturchler. 1996. Mefloquine tolerability during chemoprophylaxis: Focus on adverse event assessments, stereochemistry and compliance. *Trop Med Int Health* 1(4):485-494.

Schneider, C., M. Adamcova, S. S. Jick, P. Schlagenhauf, M. K. Miller, H. G. Rhein, and C. R. Meier. 2013. Antimalarial chemoprophylaxis and the risk of neuropsychiatric disorders. *Travel Med Infect Dis* 11(2):71-80.

Schneider, C., M. Adamcova, S. S. Jick, P. Schlagenhauf, M. K. Miller, H. G. Rhein, and C. R. Meier. 2014. Use of anti-malarial drugs and the risk of developing eye disorders. *Travel Med Infect Dis* 12(1):40-47.

Schneiderman, A. I., Y. S. Cypel, E. K. Dursa, and R. Bossarte. 2018. Associations between use of antimalarial medications and health among U. S. veterans of the wars in Iraq and Afghanistan. *Am J Trop Med Hyg* 99(3):638-648.

Schwartz, E., and G. Regev-Yochay. 1999. Primaquine as prophylaxis for malaria for nonimmune travelers: A comparison with mefloquine and doxycycline. *Clin Infect Dis* 29(6):1502-1506.

Tan, K. R., S. J. Henderson, J. Williamson, R. W. Ferguson, T. M. Wilkinson, P. Jung, and P. M. Arguin. 2017. Long term health outcomes among returned Peace Corps volunteers after malaria prophylaxis, 1995–2014. *Travel Med Infect Dis* 17:50-55.

Walsh, D. S., C. Eamsila, T. Sasiprapha, S. Sangkharomya, P. Khaewsathien, P. Supakalin, D. B. Tang, P. Jarasrumgsichol, C. Cherdchu, M. D. Edstein, K. H. Rieckmann, and T. G. Brewer. 2004. Efficacy of monthly tafenoquine for prophylaxis of *Plasmodium vivax* and multidrug-resistant *P. falciparum* malaria. *J Infect Dis* 190(8):1456-1463.

Wells, T. S., T. C. Smith, B. Smith, L. Z. Wang, C. J. Hansen, R. J. Reed, W. E. Goldfinger, T. E. Corbeil, C. N. Spooner, and M. A. Ryan. 2006. Mefloquine use and hospitalizations among US service members, 2002-2004. *Am J Trop Med Hyg* 74(5):744-749.

Wiesen, A. 2019. *Overview of DoD antimalarial use policies.* Presentation to the Committee to Review Long-Term Health Effects of Antimalarial Drugs, January 28, 2019.

Appendix A

Public Meeting Agendas

FIRST PUBLIC MEETING

January 28, 2019
National Academy of Sciences Building
2101 Constitution Avenue, NW
Washington, DC 20001
Board Room

1:00–1:10 p.m. ET   Welcome and introductions; Conduct of the Open
Session
David Savitz, Ph.D., Committee Chair

1:10–1:50 p.m.   Charge to the Committee
*Peter R. Rumm, M.D., M.P.H., Director, Pre-9/11 Era
Environmental Health Program, Department of Veterans
Affairs, with Dr. R. Loren Erickson, Chief Consultant,
Post Deployment Health*

1:50–2:20 p.m.   Overview of Antimalarials Use Policy and Monitoring in
Service Members
*COL Andrew Wiesen, M.D., M.P.H., Director, Preventive
Medicine, Health Readiness Policy and Oversight, Office
of the Assistant Secretary of Defense (Health Affairs)*

2:20–2:50 p.m.   Food and Drug Administration Adverse Events Report-
                          ing System
                          *Kelly Yoojung Cao, Pharm.D., Team Leader, Division of
                          Pharmacovigilance II, Food and Drug Administration*

2:50–3:30 p.m.   Centers for Disease Control and Prevention Monitoring
                          of Malaria and Research Related to Antimalarials Use
                          *Kathrine Tan, M.D., M.P.H., Chief, Domestic Response
                          Unit, Malaria Branch, Centers for Disease Control and
                          Prevention*

3:30–3:50 p.m.   Identifying and Evaluating Sources of Evidence of
                          Quinism: A Novel Disease Affecting U.S. Veterans
                          *Remington Nevin, M.D., M.P.H., Dr.P.H., Executive
                          Director, The Quinism Foundation*

3:50–4:20 p.m.[1]   Public Comments
                          Limited to 3 minutes per individual/organization

4:20 p.m.   **OPEN SESSION ENDS**

---

[1] To be extended if needed to accommodate those wishing to make a public statement.

SECOND PUBLIC MEETING AGENDA

March 27, 2019
OPEN SESSION
Keck Building
500 Fifth Street, NW, Washington, DC
Keck Room 105

9:30–9:35 a.m. ET	Welcome and Introductions; Conduct of the Open Session *David Savitz, Ph.D., Committee Chair*
9:35–10:05 a.m.	Overview of Antimalarials Use Policy and Monitoring in Peace Corps Volunteers *Kyle Petersen, D.O, F.I.D.S.A., F.A.C.P., Director of Epidemiology, Peace Corps*
10:05–10:25 a.m.	Antimalarials—Use Policy and Monitoring in Deployed Employees of Department of State *Kim Ottwell, M.D., Clinical Director of Clinical Services*
10:25–11:25 a.m.	Neurotoxic Mechanisms of Antimalarials *Thomas Brewer, M.D., University of Washington, and Principle, Global Enterics, LLC*
11:25–11:50 a.m.	Public Comments *Limited to 3 minutes per individual/organization*
11:50 a.m.	**OPEN SESSION ENDS**

Appendix B

Invited Presentations

The committee held two information-gathering sessions in the course of its work to help inform its deliberations. The first was held on January 28, 2019, in conjunction with its first meeting and included the formal charge of the committee's Statement of Task by representatives from the Department of Veterans Affairs (VA). The second information-gathering session was held March 27, 2019. The committee heard from presenters with knowledge of malaria chemoprophylaxis (hereafter referred to as prophylaxis) policies from the Department of Defense (DoD), Department of State, and the Peace Corps. In addition to presentations focused on antimalarial drug prophylaxis policies among different government agencies, representatives from the Food and Drug Administration (FDA) gave an overview of their postmarketing pharmacovigilance system of adverse events and how that information is used to monitor for signals of safety issues. A representative of the Centers for Disease Control and Prevention (CDC) explained how the agency assembles and weights data for making country-specific recommendations for malaria prophylaxis for U.S. travelers. Because those recommendations are based largely on the published literature, the second part of the CDC presentation reviewed some of the common strengths and limitations of pertinent literature. The committee heard from an advocacy organization that presented a hypothesis for the existence of a neuropsychiatric disease they believe to be associated with the use of mefloquine prophylaxis in U.S. military service members. Finally, the committee heard a detailed presentation on the neurotoxic mechanisms of some antimalarials, particularly artemisinins. Each open session also included time for attendees to make statements for the committee's consideration. The themes of those statements are summarized in Chapter 3, under the heading of public comments.

COL Andrew Wiesen, M.D., M.P.H., provided a historical overview of malaria prophylaxis in the U.S. military from World War II to the present, describing the toll of malaria that made efforts to provide effective prophylaxis a strategic imperative and the pharmacologic characteristics of the antimalarials used over the timeline of military engagements. He discussed the side effects of the antimalarials and how they have affected and continue to affect compliance. Mefloquine (Lariam®) was developed at the Walter Reed Army Institute of Research during the Vietnam War and approved for use as prophylaxis in 1989. It was used as a first-line prophylactic agent only for deployments to high-malaria-risk areas in sub-Saharan Africa, such as for the Liberian Task Force in 2003, and used as a second-line agent in Operation Iraqi Freedom (OIF) and Operation Enduring Freedom (OEF). Doxycycline was used as the first-line agent in OIF and OEF, and continues to be used in deployments to Southwest Asia. COL Wiesen explained that geographic combatant commanders set the "requirements for entry" for forces serving in their areas; the commanders decide whether and what antimalarial prophylaxis is required based on DoD Health Affairs guidelines, and they may modify requirements as intelligence comes in. The use of a medical product that is not FDA approved requires approval from DoD Health Affairs and must be accomplished via an emergency use authorization process. COL Wiesen told the committee that there are challenges to establishing the causation of drug-related adverse events. For example, poor record-keeping, especially in a combat zone, can hamper the accurate assessment of service members' exposure to a drug. He stated that an objectively definable, measurable case definition would help to determine whether there are long-term effects related to the use of any of the antimalarials used for malaria prophylaxis.

Kelley Cao, Pharm.D., provided an overview of the FDA Adverse Event Reporting System (FAERS), a computerized database used for postmarketing monitoring and pharmacovigilance of approved drugs. FDA defines pharmacovigilance as the science and activities relating to the detection, assessment, understanding, and prevention of adverse effects or any other drug-related problems. Owing to the large numbers and broad populations of people who use a drug after it goes on the market, a wider array of adverse events can be detected and over longer periods of time than were observed during clinical trials. The FAERS database stores reports of adverse events for all U.S.-marketed human drugs and therapeutic biologics, and the data include both FDA-approved and off-label uses. Patients, consumers, and health care professionals can voluntarily submit reports of adverse events either to the manufacturer or to the FAERS database via MedWatch. Manufacturers are required to send adverse event reports to FDA, and these are channeled to FAERS. Dr. Cao observed that adverse event reporting trends can be affected by multiple factors, including media reports, the length of time on the market (reports tend to decline over time and rise after approval of new indications), and modifications to reporting requirements. FAERS reporting is especially strong for detecting rare adverse events and events that occur shortly after drug exposure. FAERS data do have limitations. The incidence of adverse events cannot be estimated because of the under-reporting of events and the inability to determine the actual numbers of events and drug exposures. Case reports may lack detail, limiting their usefulness. Distinguishing a drug-related adverse event from a treated or pre-existing disease and detecting events with a long latency period are also challenges. FDA safety evaluators monitor the database for "safety signals"—information that suggests a new potentially causal association, or a new aspect of a known association—between an intervention and an event or set of related events, either adverse or beneficial. Data mining is used to identify higher-than-expected frequencies of product–adverse event combinations, to generate hypotheses, and to evaluate the strength of a potential safety signal. After a safety signal is identified, safety evaluators follow a protocol to search the database and literature for cases, formulate a case definition, and evaluate for a drug–event association. Detailed case reports, a consistency of effects within a drug class, ruling out alternative etiologies, and biologic plausibility can support causality. Depending on the severity of the safety signal, regulatory actions could include label changes, postmarketing requirements or epidemiologic studies, strategies to restrict use, and market withdrawal.

Kathrine Tan, M.D., M.P.H., reviewed the activities that CDC pursues to monitor malaria in the United States, to inform guidelines for malaria prophylaxis, and to review the strengths and limitations of current research. To develop malaria prophylaxis guidelines that are data driven and country specific, CDC monitors malaria transmission, parasite type, and the presence or emergence of drug resistance, and it performs systematic literature reviews and monitors literature and drug labeling. CDC systemic literature reviews have yielded articles on primaquine (Hill et al., 2006), atovaquone/proguanil (Boggild et al., 2007), doxycycline (Tan et al., 2011), and the safety of atovaquone/proguanil in pregnancy (Andrejko et al., 2019). Dr. Tan pointed to two CDC-run observational studies of malaria prophylaxis with safety outcomes. Lobel et al. (1993) compared taking mefloquine and chloroquine for 1 year by Peace Corps volunteers; there were no serious adverse reactions, and the frequency of mild adverse events was the same across the two drugs. Dr. Tan also presented the results of a study (Tan et al., 2017) that examined long-term outcomes in returned Peace Corps volunteers, comparing the prevalence of more than 40 disease outcomes in those who used malaria prophylaxis drugs with those who did not. Dr. Tan noted that in this study psychiatric side effects were slightly more prevalent in those who took mefloquine than in all those who did not; after excluding those with a prior psychiatric diagnosis, there was no difference in prevalence. The authors concluded that malaria prophylaxis has few latent effects, but recommended that persons with prior psychiatric disease avoid using mefloquine. Dr. Tan observed that there are several challenges to conducting studies of malaria prophylaxis and then used published articles to illustrate some of the challenges. For example, in studies based on self-report of exposure or outcome, a placebo effect or media attention to a drug may lead to an elevated baseline of reported adverse events. Also, malaria-prophylaxis studies do not typically use standardized screening tools or medical examination to verify neuropsychiatric outcomes, and thus it is difficult to compare findings among studies. Dr. Tan noted that accounting for confounding factors can be a challenge; in addition to the normal stresses of travel, for example, service members experience the stressors of deployment or combat. Dr. Tan observed that while using administrative data for public health studies is becoming more common, that approach also has limitations. For example, drug exposure cannot be validated, a drug may have been taken for a different indication, and diagnostic codes may have been used incorrectly. Finally, Dr. Tan observed that there is an evidence gap for studies of the long-term health effects of long-term malaria prophylaxis; of the available data, the Peace Corps and military data are the strongest. Literature on the safety of malaria prophylaxis in pregnant women and in children is also limited.

Remington Nevin, M.D., M.P.H., Dr.P.H., chief executive officer and founder of The Quinism Foundation, presented an overview of a syndrome termed "quinism," which the organization attributes to exposure to the quinoline class of drugs used for malaria prophylaxis. He described quinism as an "idiosyncratic chronic disabling syndrome of encephalopathy due to focal brainstem and limbic neurotoxicity injury caused by quinoline poisoning." He further hypothesized that the onset of quinism is predicted by prodromal symptoms such as insomnia, nightmares, acute anxiety, and confusion. Although he focused on the drug mefloquine, he stated that evidence of quinoline toxicity dates to the early days of the U.S. military's use of the drug class for malaria prophylaxis. He indicated that he believes that the National Academies of Sciences, Engineering, and Medicine's literature review is "premature" because insufficient research has been performed on quinoline toxicity. Dr. Nevin proposed reframing the diagnostic paradigm that deems stressors such as combat trauma as the cause of a spectrum of neuropsychiatric symptoms; he identified mefloquine as the confounding factor in this paradigm and as the potential actual cause of symptoms that have been attributed to combat trauma. He noted that mefloquine use by military service members correlates with exposure to stressors as well as with symptoms the original drug manufacturer stated should prompt drug discontinuation. Dr. Nevin views retrospective studies as an inadequate approach to investigating mefloquine and quinism. He stated that failing to include quinoline toxicity as a possible confounder in diagnoses may have long compromised the assessment of posttraumatic stress disorder (PTSD), traumatic brain injury, and other conditions in veterans. He pointed specifically to exclusion Criterion H of the diagnosis of PTSD in the fifth edition of the *Diagnostic and Statistical Manual of Mental Disorders*, which requires that symptoms not be attributable to medication, substance use, or other illness. He stated that in vitro and in vivo evidence of a pathophysiology for quinism exists, citing his publications as sources. He recommended that VA begin screening veterans for exposure to mefloquine and, if exposure has occurred, to assess specific side effects. He said that conflicts of interest—such as the role of antimalarial drugs in maintaining national security and the potential for legal liability and disability claims—constrict VA and DoD and that these have likely have impeded the pursuit and publication of research on quinism.

Kyle Petersen, D.O., FACP, FIDSA, provided an overview of Peace Corps malaria-prophylaxis policies. Volunteers serve 27-month tours in 61 countries, operating in rural villages with limited health care. The Peace Corps mandates malaria prophylaxis for volunteers in partially or highly malaria-endemic areas. Approximately 10% of malaria cases reported annually in U.S. citizens by CDC occur in Peace Corps volunteers; most cases originate in Africa and are due to *P. falciparum*. Two malaria deaths have occurred in the Peace Corps since 2000; both occurred in persons who were nonadherent with prophylaxis. Malaria prophylaxis is provided from the first day of service in country for volunteers in malaria-endemic countries; they are also issued a malaria rapid diagnostic test and malaria treatment medication. The Peace Corps does not monitor malarial chemoprophylactic adherence in volunteers other than by confirming medication receipt and tracking malaria cases. Nonadherence to prophylaxis is investigated and can be grounds for dismissal. Dr. Petersen was unable to find Peace Corps policy on malaria prophylaxis prior to 2004, but he pointed to a 1993 article (Lobel et al.) stating that volunteers "are encouraged, but not obliged, to use mefloquine" and that alternative agents were available. The 2004 Peace Corps technical guidelines identified mefloquine as the drug of choice in areas where chloroquine-resistant *P. falciparum* exists. The 2014 technical guidelines state that there is no first-line prophylactic malaria drug and that the Peace Corps medical officers who provide primary care to volunteers should individualize prophylaxis selection to the volunteer. Dr. Petersen explained that volunteers are provided with information describing available prophylactic drugs, and each meets with a medical officer to discuss the drugs' risks and benefits in order to make a choice. Peace Corps volunteers who use mefloquine are given a detailed description of side effects; in addition, they must sign that they received the information and that they will promptly report side effects to their medical officer. Dr. Petersen noted that it is common for people to underreport their psychiatric histories. A 2019 addendum to the 2014 technical guidelines included a medical officer checklist that requires a 3-week follow-up call to volunteers who take mefloquine. Therefore, in 2019 for volunteers who elect to take mefloquine, by policy they should receive information and have seven interactions with medical personnel before beginning their first dose. The Federal Employees' Compensation Act enables Peace Corps volunteers to file for compensation for illness or injury attributed to their service. The statute of limitations for a claim is 3 years from end of service or from the date of onset of symptoms believed to be associated with service. Because compensation is administered by the Department of Labor, Peace Corps medical records do not contain this claim information. The Peace Corps has not sought information on long-term disability claims related to malaria prophylaxis filed by its volunteers. While it receives an aggregated quarterly report of Federal Employees' Compensation Act claims, the diagnostic-coding methodology and limits to the searchability of the report make identifying claims related to malaria prophylaxis difficult. Dr. Petersen stated that the Peace Corps plans to discuss future research of long-term effects of antimalarials with CDC.

Kimberly K. Ottwell, M.D., reviewed the malaria prevention strategies of the Department of State Bureau of Medical Services. Less than 5,000 employees and their family members are currently posted in high-risk malaria areas, and an estimated 2,000 travel to such areas for temporary duty assignments. Dr. Ottwell said that Department of State employees are not required to take malaria prophylaxis and that in 2018 there were 21 cases of malaria in the Department of State population; the majority of these patients acknowledged nonadherence to prophylaxis. Dr. Ottwell described a 0–5 ranking system for malaria risk and recommended prophylaxis at posts. According to a 2013 survey of Department of State employees living in the high-risk posts, adherence with malaria prophylaxis was 78% for staff, 70% for children, and 66% for spouses. Mefloquine is the most commonly used drug, followed by atovaquone/proguanil and doxycycline; 50% of users reported that they never miss a dose, while 45% miss one out of four doses. The reasons given for not taking prophylaxis included fear of long-term side effects, colleagues' nonadherence, the belief that malaria is not serious and is curable, and neglecting to "follow up." Dr. Ottwell said that Department of State populations that live abroad and take prophylaxis for long periods are not monitored for health issues related to the long-term use of malaria prophylaxis. As multiple health care providers serve this population, it would be difficult to track. Dr. Ottwell stated that Department of State has no records of antimalarial-related disability claims. She said that a review of mental health medical evacuation and local hospitalization data did not turn up any diagnoses directly attributed to antimalarial prophylaxis or any anecdotal reports of related major mental health concerns. A review of general medical evacuation and local hospitalization data yielded the same results. She said that there have been anecdotal reports of minor antimalarial side effects, including mild depression, vivid dreams, sun sensitivity, pill esophagitis, and colitis but that these effects were managed effectively by health care providers. She stated that while tafenoquine has fewer psychiatric effects than mefloquine and has the ability to treat all stages of malaria infection, the drug's contraindications (age <18 years, pregnancy, and glucose-6-phosphate dehydrogenase deficiency) and limited long-term safety data mean it cannot yet be used to completely replace mefloquine in the Department of State population.

Thomas Brewer, Ph.D., described to the committee experimental work being done on the neurotoxicity of antimalarial drugs. Although the presentation focused on artemisinin, which is not one of the committee's drugs of interest because it is only approved for the treatment of malaria, the types of experiments used and the associated findings gave the committee a better foundation for its review of animal and other experimental studies related to the mechanisms of effect for the antimalarials used for prophylaxis. The artemisinin family of antimalarial drugs was long used in Chinese medicine because it was found that this compound (called Qinhaosu) was often lifesaving in malarial infections and it was reported to reverse malarial coma, show activity against resistant parasites, and not demonstrate toxicity concerns when used for the treatment of malaria. After it was "discovered" by the Western nations, it was targeted for research and development by the U.S. Army and the World Health Organization. Two analogs of artemisinin were quickly developed: artemether and arteether. Techniques of modern pharmacology were applied to the development of all analogs, including drug quantification, measures of treatment sensitivity and specificity, and preclinical neuroscience methodologies applied to understand its mechanism of action and any toxicity. In vivo, each of these drugs is metabolized to dihydro-artemisinin. Research on artemisinin established its efficacy, and initial 14- and 28-day studies in animals and humans showed no evidence of toxicity. However, the artemether and arteether analogs showed an unexpected toxicity in high-dose studies, defined by a sudden death syndrome in a small proportion of the animals (dogs) studied. Additional, focused toxicity studies using dogs, rats, mice, and monkeys using lactate dehydrogenase as the marker of cell death were conducted to explain the deaths; the deaths were traced to central nervous system actions, which were identified as a circumscribed toxicity limited to the brainstem, with lesions in the auditory vestibular nucleus and in the reticular and the visceral autonomic brainstem nuclei. The artemisinin analogs showed an increase in lactate dehydrogenase in situ in some of the dogs, indicating selective neuronal damage in these brainstem neurons. In addition, evidence of cell death in neuronal cell cultures suggested a common neuronal target. Similar neurochemical outcomes were observed between glutamate-induced cell death and the kind of toxicity observed with artemether and arteether, but no specific glutamatergic target has been found. These tests confirmed that the duration of drug administration and drug dose, as well as species specificity, were factors in the toxicity. The toxicity was specific for neurons and showed a particular structure–activity relationship between this adverse lactate dehydrogenase outcome and the structure of the drug; specifically, a ketone in the hydroxyl group site or an epoxide in the endoperoxide site both resulted in a loss of this cellular toxicity. It was clear that these small changes in structure resulted in dramatic changes in toxicity and translated into a poor therapeutic index. Mefloquine and halofantrine also showed some of this toxicity when tested in the same assay system, but whether these mechanisms are the same as those for the artemisinins was not determined. Although no clinical (human) evidence of neurotoxicity with artemisinin drugs has been reported, including any evidence of unusual damage to specific brainstem nuclei as seen in experimental animals receiving high doses of artemether and arteether, the animal data suggest relevance to mammalian systems that are potentially pertinent to human use. Therefore, the artemisinin drugs were further examined using audiometry in animals and humans because the brainstem auditory-evoked potential patterns have been clearly worked out. In an area in Vietnam with high malarial infectivity, 242 individuals who had previously received more than 21 courses of antimalarial treatment were compared with 108 never-treated controls to determine whether there was clinical or electrophysiologic evidence of brainstem neurotoxicity in humans previously exposed to artemisinin compounds. No evidence of brainstem toxicity or adverse effects of brainstem function was found with episodic use of artemisinins for treatment of malaria in humans.

In summary, the evidence thus far shows that in laboratory animals the route of administration, oil/water solubility, and concentration-duration of drug level are critical determinants of the animal toxicity and should be given appropriate consideration in the clinical decisions regarding route, choice of drug used, and drug regimens. Based on the experimental evidence, an oral, water-soluble drug with moderately rapid clearance may be the most attractive choice in the absence of significant differences in efficacy. However, the specific reports of this remarkable animal brain pathology in some animal species persists. In one study, rats treated with arteether (not artemisinin or artemether) showed a progressive and severe decline in performance on auditory discrimination. The deficit was characterized by decreases in accuracy, increases in response time, and, eventually, response suppression in the rodents. When auditory performance was suppressed, rats also showed gross behavioral signs of toxicity that included tremor, gait disturbances, and lethargy with arteether treatment. Subsequent histologic assessment of arteether-treated rats revealed marked damage in the brainstem nuclei, ruber, superior olive, trapezoideus, and inferior vestibular. The damage included chromatolysis, necrosis, and gliosis. These results demonstrate distinct differences in the ability of artemisinins to produce neurotoxicity in animals. No human toxicity has been described to date. Studies have not yet focused on testing the brainstem neurotoxicity of chronic artemisinin (and analogs and metabolites) administration for prophylactic use in animals or in humans. However, with evidence of this magnitude and consequence for mammalian brain toxicity with these drugs, human toxicity testing in all paradigms of administration is indicated. It is also important to consider testing with extended duration of action and in the relevant dose range pertinent to prophylactic usage.

REFERENCES

Andrejko, K. L., R. C. Mayer, S. Kovacs, E. Slutsker, E. Bartlett, K. R. Tan, and J. R. Gutman. 2019. The safety of atovaquone–proguanil for the prevention and treatment of malaria in pregnancy: A systematic review. *Travel Med Infect Dis* 27:20-26.

Boggild, A. K., M. E. Parise, L. S. Lewis, and K. C. Kain. 2007. Atovaquone–proguanil: Report from the CDC Expert Meeting on Malaria Chemoprophylaxis. *Am J Trop Med Hyg* 76(2):208-223.

Brewer, T. G. 2019. Overview of artemisinin neurotoxicity: Research and development findings to policy impacts. Presentation to the Committee to Review Long-Term Health Effects of AntimalarialDrugs. March 27.

Cao, K. 2019. Introduction to postmarketing drug safety surveillance: Pharmacovigilance in FDA/CDER. Presentation to the Committee to Review Long-Term Health Effects of Antimalarial Drugs. January 28.

Hill, D. R., J. K. Baird, M. E. Parise, L. S. Lewis, E. T. Ryan, and A. J. Magill. 2006. Primaquine: Report from CDC Expert Meeting on Malaria Chemoprophylaxis I. *Am J Trop Med Hyg* 75(3):402-415.

Lobel, H. O., M. Miani, T. Eng, K. W. Bernard, A. W. Hightower, and C. C. Campbell. 1993. Long-term malaria prophylaxis with weekly mefloquine. *Lancet* 341(8849):848-851.

Nevin, R. 2019. Identifying and evaluating sources of evidence of quinism: A novel disease affecting U.S. veterans. Presentation to the Committee to Review Long-Term Health Effects of Antimalarial Drugs. January 28.

Ottwell, K. K. 2019. Department of State Bureau of Medical Services malaria prevention strategies. Presentation to the Committee to Review Long-Term Health Effects of Antimalarial Drugs. March 27.

Petersen, K. 2019. Malaria in the Peace Corps. Presentation to the Committee to Review Long-Term Health Effects of Antimalarial Drugs. March 27.

Tan, K. R. 2019. CDC's activities in examining adverse events of antimalarials. Presentation to the Committee to Review Long-Term Health Effects of Antimalarial Drugs. January 28.

Tan, K. R., A. J. Magill, M. E. Parise, and P. M. Arguin. 2011. Doxycycline for malaria chemoprophylaxis and treatment: Report from the CDC Expert Meeting on Malaria Chemoprophylaxis. *Am J Trop Med Hyg* 84(4):517-531.

Tan, K. R. S. J. Henderson, J. Williamson, R. W. Ferguson, T. M. Wilkinson, P. Jung, and P. M. Arguin. 2017. Long-term health outcomes among returned Peace Corps volunteers after malaria prophylaxis, 1995-2014. *Travel Med Infect Dis* 17:50-55.

Wiesen, A. 2019. Overview of DoD antimalarial use policies. Presentation to the Committee to Review Long-Term Health Effects of Antimalarial Drugs. January 28.

Appendix C

Epidemiologic Studies That Met the Committee's Inclusion Criteria

Reference	Design	Population	Study Groups‡	Body Systems Examined
Ackert et al., 2019*	Randomized controlled trial	Healthy male and female adult volunteers (ages 18–45) in the United States	Tafenoquine (n = 306) Placebo (n = 161)	Eye
Andersen et al., 1998	Randomized controlled trial	Semi-immune male and female adult volunteers (ages 18–55) in Kenya	Doxycycline (n = 55) Azithromycin (n = 117) 250 mg daily (n = 59) 1,000 mg weekly (n = 58) Placebo (n = 60)	Other
DeSouza, 1983	Clinical trial	Healthy male adult volunteers (age range not reported) in Brazil	Mefloquine 1,000 mg (n = 10) Sulfadoxine (1,000 mg) and pyrimethamine (500 mg) (n = 10)	Gastrointestinal Cardiovascular
Eick-Cost et al., 2017*	Retrospective observational study	Male and female active-duty U.S. service members (ages ≥17)	Deployed (n = 275,097) Mefloquine (n = 25,691) A/P (n = 2,620) Doxycycline (n = 246,786) Nondeployed (n = 92,743) Mefloquine (n = 10,847) A/P (n = 10,261) Doxycycline (n = 71,635)	Neurologic Psychiatric
Green et al., 2014*	Randomized controlled trial	Healthy male and female adult volunteers (ages 18–65) in the United States	Tafenoquine (n = 156) Supratherapeutic dose of 1,200 mg (n = 52) Therapeutic dose of 300 mg (n = 52) Therapeutic dose of 600 mg (n = 52) Moxifloxacin (400 mg) (n = 52) Placebo (n = 52)	Cardiovascular

Reference	Study Design	Population	Intervention (n)	Outcomes
Laothavorn et al., 1992	Prospective observational study	Male patients with malaria and healthy male adult volunteers (ages 26–46) in Thailand	Mefloquine (750 mg) (n = 18) Patients with malaria (n = 102)	Cardiovascular
Leary et al., 2009*	Randomized controlled trial	Healthy male and female adult volunteers (ages 18–55) recruited from the United States and the United Kingdom	Tafenoquine (n = 81) Placebo (n = 39)	Eye Other
Lee et al., 2013	Cross-sectional survey	Current and former male and female adult members of the Australian Federal Police Association (ages 35–45)	Doxycycline (n = 189) Deployed (n = 171) Nondeployed (n = 18)	Gastrointestinal
Lege-Oguntoye et al., 1990	Randomized controlled trial	Semi-immune male and female adult volunteers (ages 25–34) in Nigeria	Chloroquine (n = 20) Ascorbic acid (200 mg) (n = 10)	Other
Meier et al., 2004*	Retrospective observational study	Male and female adult travelers (ages 17–79) in the United Kingdom	Mefloquine (n = 16,491) Doxycycline (n = 4,574) Proguanil and/or chloroquine (n = 16,129)	Neurologic Psychiatric Eye
Miller et al., 2013	Randomized controlled trial	Healthy male and female adult volunteers (ages 18–55) in the United States	Chloroquine (600 mg) and placebo for tafenoquine (n = 20) Placebo for chloroquine and tafenoquine (450 mg) (n = 20) Chloroquine (600 mg) and tafenoquine (450 mg) (n = 20)	Eye Other
Nasveld et al., 2010*	Randomized controlled trial	Healthy male and female Australian soldiers (ages 18–55)	Mefloquine followed by primaquine (30 mg) (n = 162) Tafenoquine followed by placebo (n = 492)	Psychiatric Gastrointestinal Eye Cardiovascular Other

continued

Reference	Design	Population	Study Groups‡	Body Systems Examined
Rueangweerayut et al., 2017	Prospective observational study	Healthy female adult volunteers (ages 18–45) in Thailand	Tafenoquine (n = 51) 100 mg (n = 12) 200 mg (n = 19) 300 mg (n = 9) Primaquine (n = 11)	Other
Schlagenhauf et al., 1996†	Prospective observational study	Healthy male and female adult Swiss travelers (ages 18–65)	Mefloquine (n = 394)	Neurologic Psychiatric
Schneider et al., 2013*	Retrospective observational study	Male and female travelers (ages ≥1) from the United Kingdom	Mefloquine (n = 10,169) A/P (n = 28,502) Chloroquine and/or proguanil (n = 2,904) Unexposed (n = 41,573)	Neurologic Psychiatric
Schneider et al., 2014*	Retrospective observational study	Male and female travelers (ages ≥1) from the United Kingdom	Mefloquine (n = 10,169) A/P (n = 28,502) Chloroquine and/or proguanil (n = 2,904) Unexposed (n = 41,573)	Eye
Schneiderman et al., 2018*	Cross-sectional survey	Post 9/11 male and female U.S. military veterans (ages ≥24)	Deployed (n = 12,456) No antimalarial use (n = 5,806) Mefloquine (n = 307) Doxycycline (n = 1,315) Primaquine (n = 98) Chloroquine (n = 274) Mefloquine + other antimalarial (n = 425) Other antimalarial (n = 525) Type not specified (n = 3,706) Nondeployed (n = 7,031) No antimalarial use (n = 5,294) Mefloquine (n = 39)	Psychiatric

Study	Study design	Population	Prophylaxis	Outcomes
			Chloroquine (n = 110) Doxycycline (n = 141) Primaquine (n = 35) Mefloquine + other antimalarial (n = 52) Other antimalarial (n = 114) Type not specified (n = 1,246)	Unknown
Schwartz and Regev-Yochay, 1999	Prospective observational study	Non-immune adult Israeli travelers (ages 22–65) (sex distribution not reported)	Mefloquine (n = 25) Doxycycline (n = 19) Primaquine (n = 106) 15 mg daily for individuals with a body weight of <70 kg 30 mg daily for individuals with a body weight of >70 kg Hydroxychloroquine (200 mg) (n = 8)	
Tan et al., 2017	Cross-sectional survey	Male and female returned U.S. Peace Corps volunteers (age range not reported)	Mefloquine (n = 2,981) A/P (n = 183) Doxycycline (n = 831) Chloroquine (n = 674) Other prophylactic medication (n = 386) No antimalarial use (n = 3,876)	Neurologic Psychiatric Gastrointestinal Eye Cardiovascular Other
Walsh et al., 2004	Randomized controlled trial	Thai soldiers (ages 18–55) (sex distribution not reported)	Tafenoquine (n = 104) 400 mg for 3 consecutive days, followed by 400 mg once monthly Placebo (n = 101)	Other

continued

Reference	Design	Population	Study Groups‡	Body Systems Examined
Wells et al., 2006*	Retrospective observational study	Male and female U.S. active-duty service members (ages ≥17)	Mefloquine (n = 8,858) U.S. active-duty service members prescribed at least seven tablets of mefloquine and deployed to operational theater or combat zone No antimalarial drug use U.S. active-duty service members assigned to Europe or Japan (n = 156,203) U.S. active-duty service members deployed for at least one month (n = 232,381)	Neurologic Psychiatric Gastrointestinal Cardiovascular Other

* Denotes epidemiologic studies considered to provide the most contributory evidence to address the committee's charge.

† Although study investigators did not make a traditional comparison between exposed and unexposed groups, they did compare individuals who experienced adverse events with those who did not experience adverse events in the data analysis; thus, the committee included this study in their evaluation of the available scientific evidence.

‡ For the six antimalarial drugs of interest the dosing regimen used follows standard FDA guidance unless otherwise noted.

Appendix D

Committee Member and Staff Biographies

COMMITTEE MEMBERS

David A. Savitz, Ph.D. (*Chair*), is a professor of epidemiology in the Brown University School of Public Health, where he serves as the interim chair of the Department of Epidemiology and holds joint appointments as a professor of obstetrics and gynecology and pediatrics in the Alpert Medical School. From 2013 to 2017, Dr. Savitz served as the vice president for research at Brown University. He came to Brown in 2010 from the Mount Sinai School of Medicine, where he had served as the Charles W. Bluhdorn Professor of Community and Preventive Medicine and the director of the Disease Prevention and Public Health Institute since 2006. Before that appointment, he taught and conducted research at the University of North Carolina School of Public Health and at the Department of Preventive Medicine and Biometrics at the University of Colorado School of Medicine. Dr. Savitz received his undergraduate training in psychology at Brandeis University, holds a master's degree in preventive medicine from The Ohio State University, and received his Ph.D. in epidemiology from the University of Pittsburgh Graduate School of Public Health. His epidemiologic research has addressed a wide range of environmental and perinatal health issues, including exposures related to military deployments, the environmental effects of energy development, pesticides and breast cancer, risks from environmental exposures during pregnancy, and drinking water safety. Dr. Savitz has directed 31 doctoral dissertations and 15 master's theses. He is the author of nearly 350 papers in professional journals and the editor or author of 3 books on environmental epidemiology. He has served as the editor at the *American Journal of Epidemiology and Epidemiology* and as a member of the Epidemiology and Disease

Control-1 study section of the National Institutes of Health. He has served as the president of the Society for Epidemiologic Research, the Society for Pediatric and Perinatal Epidemiologic Research, and the North American Regional Councilor for the International Epidemiological Association. Dr. Savitz is a member of the National Academy of Medicine and has previously served on 11 National Academies consensus committees, five of which he chaired or was the vice-chair, in addition to serving on several other National Academies convening activities.

Sara L. Dolan, Ph.D., is an associate professor of psychology and neuroscience and the graduate program director at Baylor University. She completed her Ph.D. in clinical psychology at the University of Iowa and completed her clinical internship in the Division of Substance Abuse at Yale University, and her postdoctoral fellowship at Brown University. Her early research primarily focused on substance use disorders, but more recently her work has focused on neurocognitive function in substance use disorders, posttraumatic stress disorder (PTSD), and traumatic brain injury (TBI). The goal of her research is to improve diagnosis and treatment of substance use disorders, PTSD, and TBI to improve overall functioning and well-being. Dr. Dolan has authored or co-authored more than 40 peer-reviewed journal articles.

Marie R. Griffin, M.D., M.P.H., is a professor of health policy and medicine, holds the directorship in public health research and education, and directs the master of public health program at Vanderbilt University. She received her M.D. from Georgetown University and her master's in public health from Johns Hopkins University. Dr. Griffin completed her medical residency at Emory University, served as an epidemic intelligence service officer through the Centers for Disease Control and Prevention, and was a clinical epidemiology fellow at Johns Hopkins. She is a general internist and pharmacoepidemiologist whose research focuses on the safety and effectiveness of drugs and vaccines, program evaluation, and methods in pharmacoepidemiology. She has served on Food and Drug Administration committees, including the Nonprescription Drugs Advisory Committee and the Vaccine and Related Products Advisory Committee, and she continues to serve as a member of the Drug Safety and Risk Management Advisory Committee. She also serves as a work group member of the Centers for Disease Control and Prevention's Advisory Committee on Immunization Practices for respiratory syncytial virus vaccine. She has worked extensively with administrative data from the Tennessee Medicaid program and the Department of Veterans Affairs to analyze data on the comparative effectiveness and safety of drugs and vaccines. Her work has consistently provided scientific evidence that has been used to drive policy. Dr. Griffin has authored or co-authored more than 350 peer-reviewed journal articles. She has previously served as a member of the National Academies' Committee to Review the Adverse Consequences of Pertussis and Rubella Vaccines.

James P. Herman, Ph.D., is the Flor van Maanen professor, the chair of the Department of Pharmacology and Systems Physiology, and the director of the Neurobiology Research Center and the Stress Neurobiology Laboratory at the University of Cincinnati. Dr. Herman's research examines the relationship between the physiologic actions of central nervous system stress circuits and their place in the central nervous system. His work primarily focuses on two areas. The first area is limbic system regulation of the stress response and, consequently, on the generation of stress-related disorders, ranging from major depressive illness to posttraumatic stress disorder to essential hypertension, to neurodegeneration and aging. The second focus of his research is on defining the role of central adrenocorticosteroid receptors in transducing stress-related signals in normal physiology, aging, and disease states. Dr. Herman completed his Ph.D. at the University of Rochester and his postdoctoral training at the Mental Health Research Institute at the University of Michigan. He has received several awards for his research and he has authored or co-authored more than 240 peer-reviewed journal articles.

Yuval Neria, Ph.D., is a professor of medical psychology in the Department of Psychiatry and Epidemiology at the Columbia University Medical Center and the director of the PTSD Research Program at the New York State Psychiatric Institute. Dr. Neria completed his doctoral studies at the Haifa University in Israel and has led and collaborated on numerous epidemiologic, clinical, and neuroimaging studies of trauma and PTSD. His research focuses on translational research aiming to identify behavioral and neural markers for trauma-related psychopathology. Dr. Neria uses multimodal brain imaging and a number of novel paradigms focusing on fear circuitry to probe new biomarkers of PTSD and to identify structural and functional neural markers of clinical response to PTSD treatment. He is primarily interested in clarifying the clinical, behavioral, and neural signatures of trauma and PTSD. He is the recipient of the Medal of Valor for his military service in Israel. Dr. Neria is the author of more than 180 peer-reviewed articles and book chapters and a war novel and co-edited 4 textbooks focusing on the mental health consequences of exposure to trauma.

Andy Stergachis, Ph.D., M.S., directs the Global Medicines Program in the Department of Global Health at the University of Washington (UW). He is professor of pharmacy and global health and an associate dean in the School of Pharmacy. His research focuses on pharmacoepidemiology, global drug and vaccine safety, and pharmaceutical outcomes research. He is the author of 160 peer-reviewed publications in areas such as pharmacovigilance, pharmacoepidemiology, pharmaceutical outcomes, and clinical epidemiology, and he served as the editor-in-chief of the *Journal of the American Pharmacists Association*. He presently serves as a co-investigator with the UW Institute for Health Metrics and Evaluation for a study on Mapping and Monitoring the Global Burden of Antimicrobial Resistance. He recently directed a study on the safety of antimalarial drugs used during pregnancy conducted in three sub-Saharan African countries and has developed novel approaches for malaria and HIV pharmacovigilance and strengthening pharmacy services in that region. Through his affiliation with the Northwest Center for Public Health Practice, he works on workforce development and public health systems research in emergency preparedness with the public health community. He is also affiliated with the UW Comparative Health Outcomes, Policy, and Economics (CHOICE) Institute. He is the chair of the Expert Panel to Review Surveillance and Screening Technologies for the Quality Assurance of Medicines for USP and the chair of the Low-Dose Primaquine Safety Study Group for the WorldWide Antimalarial Resistance Network, and he has served as a member of the Access and Product Management Advisory Committee for Medicines for Malaria Venture. He is a fellow of the International Society for Pharmacoepidemiology and of the American Pharmacists Association-Academy of Pharmaceutical Research and Science. Dr. Stergachis is a member of the National Academy of Medicine (elected 2012). He has served on numerous National Academies committees, including the Committee on Interactions of Drugs, Biologics, and Chemicals in U.S. Military Forces and the Committee on the Assessment of the U.S. Drug Safety System. Dr. Stergachis received his bachelor's of pharmacy from Washington State University and both his master's degree in pharmacy administration and his doctorate in social and administrative pharmacy from the University of Minnesota.

Elizabeth A. Stuart, Ph.D., is a professor in the Department of Mental Health in the Johns Hopkins Bloomberg School of Public Health (JHSPH) with joint appointments in the departments of biostatistics and of health policy and management, and she is also the associate dean for education at JHSPH. Dr. Stuart has an undergraduate degree in mathematics from Smith College and completed her Ph.D. in statistics at Harvard University. Her research focuses on the use of different design and analysis methods for estimating causal effects, especially in terms of improving the internal validity of non-experimental studies and the external validity of randomized studies. She also researches methods for addressing missing data and non-compliance. She has made important contributions to collaborative and methodologic research in the area of causal inference applied to mental health, substance use, health care policy, and education. Dr. Stuart is affiliated with several Johns Hopkins centers, including the Center for Drug Safety and Effectiveness, the Center for Mental Health and Addiction Policy Research (which she co-directs), and the Bloomberg American Health Initiative. She is an elected fellow of the American Statistical Association, for which she was a founding member of the Mental Health Statistics Section and has received the Gertrude Cox Award for applied statistics and the Myrto Lefkopoulou award from the Harvard University Department of Biostatistics, and she has been consistently recognized for her teaching and mentoring. She is an associate editor and a reviewer for several journals related to statistics, epidemiologic methods, and mental health, and she has contributed to more than 200 peer-reviewed publications. Dr. Stuart has previously served as a panel member for the National Academies on an activity related to methodologies for studying commercial motor vehicle driver fatigue.

Carol Tamminga, M.D., is a professor, chairman of psychiatry, and chief of translational neuroscience research in schizophrenia at the University of Texas (UT) Southwestern Medical School. She holds the Communities Foundation of Texas Chair in Brain Science along with the Lou and Ellen McGinley Distinguished Chair in Psychiatric Research. She directs clinical and preclinical research in schizophrenia focused on identifying disease mechanisms and on improving treatments. Dr. Tamminga graduated from Vanderbilt Medical School and completed a psychiatry residency at the University of Chicago and spent many years at the University of Maryland's Maryland Psychiatric Research Center, then moved to UT Southwestern Medical School to continue her research. Dr. Tamminga has been the recipient of numerous federal and foundation grants as well as awards in the field. She has served on the National Advisory Mental Health Council of the National Institute of Mental Health and on the Council of the National Institute of Drug Abuse. Dr. Tamminga was elected to the National Academy of Medicine in 1998 and has served on several Institute of Medicine committees in that capacity. The goal of Dr. Tamminga's research is to examine and understand the mechanisms underlying schizophrenia, especially its most prominent symptoms, psychosis and memory dysfunction, in order to build rational treatments for the illness. She evaluates the function of the living human brain in individuals with and without schizophrenia using brain imaging techniques. Then, building on this knowledge, she uses human postmortem brain tissue to translate the functional alterations from the living human patient into molecular observations of the illness. Now she is using case-specific neuronal cultures to address molecular and cellular questions. Her ultimate goal is to use the alterations in in vivo imaging, postmortem molecular changes, and cultured neuronal characteristics as biomarkers and targets for identifying animal models of disease and novel active pharmaceuticals for psychosis.

Jonathan L. Vennerstrom, Ph.D., is a professor in the Department of Pharmaceutical Sciences in the College of Pharmacy at the University of Nebraska Medical Center. He received his Ph.D. in medicinal chemistry from the University of Minnesota and completed his postdoctoral training at Walter Reed. Dr. Vennerstrom's work focuses on anti-infective drug discovery, particularly the medicinal chemistry of antiparasitic agents and the investigation of heme as a mechanistic intersection for antimalarial drugs. His work has led to the discovery of new mechanisms of action of chloroquine (and other antimalarial quinolines) and new understanding of mechanisms of how hemozoin is formed in the malaria parasite.

His research has comprehensively characterized the structural features of chloroquine associated with its antimalarial properties and shown that peroxide antimalarial activity depends on parasite hemoglobin digestion. Two antimalarial drug candidates were discovered during his work with the Medicines for Malaria Venture; one is now available in India and the other is in phase IIb trials as a potential single-dose malaria treatment. Both of these drugs are outside of the committee's Statement of Task. Dr. Vennerstrom continues to use the knowledge generated by his research to discover other antimicrobial drug candidates for several infectious diseases, including malaria. He is a member of the American Society for Microbiology, the American Society of Tropical Medicine and Hygiene, and the American Chemical Society (ACS) from which he received the ACS Award for Creative Innovation in 2019. He has received several other awards, including the Medicines for Malaria Venture Project of the Year Award twice (2001, 2006), the Alvin M. Earle Outstanding Health Science Educator Award, the University of Nebraska Medical Center Distinguished Scientist Award, the UNeMed Lifetime Achievement Award, and the University of Nebraska Innovation, Development, and Engagement (IDEA) Award. His work continues to drive innovation in the drug discovery field. Dr. Vennerstrom has authored or co-authored more than 130 peer-reviewed journal articles.

Christina M. Wolfson, Ph.D., is a professor in the Department of Medicine and the Department of Epidemiology, Biostatistics and Occupational Health at McGill University and a senior scientist in the Brain Repair and Integrative Neuroscience (BRAIN) Program at the Research Institute of the McGill University Health Centre. She is an associate member in the departments of neurology and neurosurgery and mathematics and statistics at McGill University. A neuroepidemiologist, her program of research lies in population-based research in neurodegenerative disorders, including multiple sclerosis (MS), Parkinson disease, and epilepsy. She is a co-principal investigator on the Canadian Longitudinal Study on Aging (CLSA), a 20-year study of 50,338 participants aged 45–85 in which she leads the Neurological Conditions Initiative and the Veterans' Health Initiative and is the director of the CLSA Statistical Analysis Centre. Dr. Wolfson is a co-principal investigator on a five-country MS risk factor study (Environmental Risk Factors in Multiple Sclerosis, EnvIMS) completed in Canada, Italy, Norway, Serbia, and Sweden. She is also the program director of the endMS National Training Program. Dr. Wolfson received her undergraduate degree in mathematics, her master's degree in mathematical statistics, and her Ph.D. in epidemiology and biostatistics from McGill University. She has published more than 220 peer-reviewed journal articles and has previously served as a member on four National Academies' consensus committees related to health effects in U.S. veterans who served in the 1990–1991 Gulf War and post-9/11 conflicts.

STAFF

Anne N. Styka, M.P.H., study director, is a senior program officer in the Health and Medicine Division of the National Academies. Over her tenure she has worked on more than 10 studies, 5 of which she has directed or co-directed, on a broad range of topics related to the health of military and veteran populations. The subjects of the studies have included mental health treatment offered in the Department of Defense and the Department of Veterans Affairs; designing and evaluating epidemiologic research studies of health outcomes and their association with deployment-related exposures, including burn pits, herbicides, and other chemicals; and directing a research program that fostered new research studies using data and biospecimens collected as part of the 20-year Air Force Health Study. Before coming to the National Academies, Ms. Styka spent several years working as an epidemiologist for the New Mexico Department of Health and the Albuquerque Area Southwest Tribal Epidemiology Center specializing in survey design and the analysis of behavioral risk factors and injury. She also spent several months in Zambia as the epidemiologist on a study of silicosis and other nonmalignant respiratory diseases among copper miners. She has written several peer-reviewed publications and has contributed to numerous state and national reports. She received her B.S. in cell and tissue bioengineering from the University of Illinois at Chicago and has an M.P.H. in epidemiology from the University of Michigan. Ms. Styka was the 2017 recipient of the Division of Earth and Life Sciences Mt. Everest Award, the 2015 recipient of the Institute of Medicine and National Academy of Medicine Multitasker Award, and a member of the 2011 National Academies' Distinguished Group Award.

Kristin E. White is an associate program officer in the Health and Medicine Division of the National Academies. Previously a medical writer and editor, she worked across numerous medical specialties and drug classes to create materials for, and resulting from, continuing medical education programs, international medical symposia, and drug and research advisory board meetings. She worked on programs at the annual meetings of the American Academy of Allergy, American College of Cardiology, American College of Gastroenterology, American College of Rheumatology, American Congress of Obstetricians and Gynecologists, American Heart Association, American Diabetes Association, Asthma & Immunology, European College of Cardiology, European Society for Sexual and Impotence Research, Heart Failure Society of America, and International Congress of Cardiology. She received an A.B. from Princeton University.

Stephanie J. Hanson, M.P.H., is a research associate in the Health and Medicine Division of the National Academies. Before joining the National Academies, Ms. Hanson worked at Save the Children U.S. in the Department of Humanitarian Response where she assisted on contracts related to food aid in complex emergencies. She also worked with the Peace Corps headquarters to conduct a gap analysis on training objectives and outcomes for information given to new Peace Corps volunteers before they begin their roles at post. Her work focused on training materials for malaria, mental health, substance and alcohol use, and HIV/AIDS. Ms. Hanson completed her B.S. in biology at the University of Nebraska–Omaha and has an M.P.H. in global health epidemiology and disease control from The George Washington University. Ms. Hanson has an interest in maternal mental health and has examined existing barriers in low- and middle-income countries surrounding the discussion, diagnosis, or treatment of mental illness, with a focus on postpartum depression, and the exacerbating effects of a complex emergency on these barriers. She plans to pursue her doctoral degree in epidemiology and continue her work on mental illness in low- and middle-income countries.

Rebecca F. Chevat is a senior program assistant in the Health and Medicine Division of the National Academies. Ms. Chevat is a graduate of American University where she received her B.A. in public health with concentrations in psychology and political science. During her undergraduate career, she worked in the Office of the Secretary and in the Office of Health Affairs at the Department of Homeland Security where she examined public–private partnerships and their role on point-of-dispensing models during emergencies. Ms. Chevat also has experience working on Capitol Hill and on a political campaign. She plans to pursue her M.P.H. in global health. Ms. Chevat is a recipient of a 2019 Health and Medicine Division Spot Award.

Rose Marie Martinez, Sc.D., has been senior board director of the National Academies' Board on Population Health and Public Health Practice (BPH) since 1999. BPH has a vibrant portfolio of studies that address high-profile and cutting-edge issues that affect population health. It addresses the science base for population health and public health interventions and examines the capacity of the health system, particularly the public health infrastructure, to support disease prevention and health promotion activities, including the education and supply of health professionals necessary for carrying them out. BPH has examined such topics as the safety of childhood vaccines and other drugs; systems for evaluating and ensuring drug safety postmarketing; the health effects of cannabis and cannabinoids; health effects of environmental exposures; population health improvement strategies; integration of medical care and public health; women's health services; health disparities; health literacy; tobacco control strategies; and chronic disease prevention, among others. Dr. Martinez was awarded the 2010 Institute of Medicine (IOM) Research Cecil Award for significant contributions to IOM reports of exceptional quality and influence. Prior to joining the National Academies, Dr. Martinez was a senior health researcher at Mathematica Policy Research (1995–1999) where she conducted research on the impact of health system change on public health infrastructure, access to care for vulnerable populations, managed care, and the health care workforce. Dr. Martinez is a former assistant director for health financing and policy with the U.S. General Accounting Office, where she directed evaluations and policy analysis in the area of national and public health issues (1988–1995). Her experience also includes 6 years directing research studies for the Regional Health Ministry of Madrid, Spain (1982–1988). Dr. Martinez is a member of the Council on Education for Public Health, the accreditation body for schools of public health and public health programs. She received the degree of doctor of science from the Johns Hopkins School of Hygiene and Public Health.